河南省癌症中心，河南省肿瘤医院

Henan Cancer Center，Henan Cancer Hospital

2023
河南省肿瘤登记年报

Cancer Report in Henan，2023

主编　伊文刚　张韶凯

河南科学技术出版社

· 郑州 ·

图书在版编目（CIP）数据

2023河南省肿瘤登记年报 / 伊文刚，张韶凯主编. -- 郑州：河南科学技术出版社，2024.11. -- ISBN 978-7-5725-1782-2

Ⅰ. R73-54

中国国家版本馆CIP数据核字第202480LK93号

出版发行：河南科学技术出版社

地址：郑州市郑东新区祥盛街27号　　邮编：450016

电话：（0371）65788686

网址：www.hnstp.cn

策划编辑：李振方

责任编辑：李振方

责任校对：黄亚萍

整体设计：李　娟

责任印制：徐海东

印　　刷：河南省环发印务有限公司

经　　销：全国新华书店

开　　本：889 mm × 1 194 mm　1/16　　印张：19.5　　字数：450千字

版　　次：2024年11月第1版　　2024年11月第1次印刷

定　　价：128.00元

《2023 河南省肿瘤登记年报》编委会

Editorial Board

序

肿瘤随访登记是一项收集、分析、评价民众肿瘤发病、死亡和生存状况的制度。通过肿瘤随访登记制度，研究人员可以全面、准确并及时掌握民众肿瘤的发生与死亡等相关信息，是肿瘤预防和控制的基础，能为国家制定卫生事业发展规划、进行肿瘤防治和防治效果评价提供科学依据。

1988年，河南省癌症中心在林县（现林州市）建立了第一个全人群肿瘤登记系统。2015年2月5日，国家卫计委和国家中医药管理局联合印发了《肿瘤登记管理办法》，河南省卫计委和省中医管理局结合实际情况，组织制定了《河南省肿瘤登记实施方案》（豫卫疾控【2015】10号）。根据《河南省肿瘤登记实施方案》的要求，河南省制定了具体的实施方案和规章制度，建立了河南省肿瘤随访登记网络直报系统，要求全省各地市和省直管县（市）成立肿瘤登记处，开展肿瘤随访登记工作，通过河南省肿瘤随访网络直报系统上报当地的肿瘤发病、死亡和随访数据。

随着“健康中国2030”工作的不断推进，肿瘤登记监测数据在肿瘤防控中的重要性日益凸显，河南省肿瘤登记工作也迅速发展。截至2023年12月31日，河南省已在所有县（市、区）开展了以人群为基础的肿瘤登记工作，初步形成了反映河南省城乡居民恶性肿瘤发病与死亡基本信息的肿瘤随访登记系统。自2013年起，河南省癌症中心和河南省肿瘤医院发布的河南省肿瘤登记年报成为河南省癌症预防控制的重要资料，也是河南省肿瘤登记监测工作的标志性成果之一。

《2023河南省肿瘤登记年报》报告了2020年河南省肿瘤登记地区人群肿瘤发病与死亡的流行情况，可以为肿瘤的控制与研究提供基础数据。

河南省卫生健康委员会

2024年1月

Preface

Cancer registration is a statistical system to collect, analyze and evaluate related information including cancer incidence, mortality, and survival data in the population, through which cancer occurrence and death could be obtained completely, accurately, and timely. It is the basis for cancer prevention and control, and it also provides scientific evidence for health development planning, cancer prevention and control and the effect evaluation.

Henan Cancer Center / Henan Cancer Hospital established the first population–based Cancer Registry in Lin county (now Linzhou city) in 1988. The National Health and Family Planning Commission and the National Administration of Traditional Chinese Medicine issued "Approaches for Cancer Registration Management" on February 5th, 2015. Henan Province Health and Family Planning Commission and the Administration of Traditional Chinese Medicine made the implementation plan according to the Approaches. Henan Cancer Center / Henan Cancer Hospital made the regulations and relevant specific procedures, and we established the Provincial Information System of Cancer Registration System. All the city and provincial county in Henan are required to set up cancer registries, and to carry out cancer registration project and report new cancer cases through the information system.

Now population–based cancer registration had been carried out in all counties in Henan Province, China, and the data basically reflected the cancer incidence and mortality in Henan, China.

Cancer Report in Henan, 2023 reported systematically the cancer incidence and mortality in Henan cancer registration areas in 2020, and it provided basic data for cancer control and research.

Henan Province Health Commission

January,2024

前　言

肿瘤随访登记报告是肿瘤预防控制工作的基础工程，完整、有效的肿瘤登记数据可以系统地反映肿瘤登记地区居民发病、死亡和生存状况，揭示肿瘤流行规律和变化趋势，找出病因，为政府制定肿瘤控制措施和防治效果评价提供科学依据。

随着“健康中国 2030”工作的不断推进，肿瘤登记监测数据在肿瘤防控中的重要性日益突出，河南省肿瘤登记工作也得到迅速发展。截至 2023 年 12 月 31 日，河南省已在所有县（市、区）开展了以人群为基础的肿瘤登记工作，初步形成了反映河南省城乡居民恶性肿瘤发病与死亡基本信息的肿瘤随访登记系统。自 2013 年起，河南省癌症中心 / 河南省肿瘤医院每年以年报的形式及时发布河南省肿瘤登记监测数据，河南省肿瘤登记年报成为河南省癌症预防控制的重要资料，也是河南省肿瘤登记监测工作的标志性成果之一。

《2023 河南省肿瘤登记年报》收录了 55 个肿瘤登记处提交的资料，其中 53 个登记处的资料由市县疾病预防控制中心上报，2 个由肿瘤防治专业机构上报，覆盖人口 43 145 743 人，约占河南省 2020 年人口总数的 37.43%。

《2023 河南省肿瘤登记年报》共分六章：

第一章简要介绍了河南省肿瘤登记系统及居民全死因登记系统的发展历程；第二章介绍资料的来源及资料的收集方法；第三章阐述登记数据质量控制指标、评价方法和常用统计学指标的计算方法；第四章描述河南省恶性肿瘤的发病和死亡情况；第五章对各部位恶性肿瘤的发病和死亡情况进行描述；第六章为年报表格附录，包含河南省各个登记处发病和死亡的主要统计结果数据。

为便于阅读，本书采用中英文对照的形式进行编排，但中英文并非完全对应，请广大读者理解。

《2023 河南省肿瘤登记年报》的顺利出版，凝聚着全省各登记处工作人员的辛勤劳动，在此谨向他们表示衷心的感谢！

伊文刚

2024 年 1 月

Foreword

Cancer registration is vital for cancer prevention and control. Complete and effective cancer registration data can reflect cancer incidence, mortality, and survival, and the epidemic characteristics and temporal trend were also acquired. Therefore, it could provide evidence to inform strategies for cancer prevention and control.

The importance of cancer registration in cancer prevention and control has become increasingly prominent along with the continuous development of "Healthy China 2030" policy. The Cancer Registration was also developed sharply along with the progress, and it had been carried out in all counties in Henan Province. Henan Cancer Center/ Henan Cancer Hospital reported the cancer surveillance data annually in the format of "Annual Cancer Report", and it provided import data for cancer control and prevention, and it has been one prominent achievement of cancer registration in Henan Province, China.

In 2023, the Cancer Annual Report for Henan Province included data of 2020 submitted by 55 cancer registries data in Henan province, among which 53 cancer registries belong to the Centers for Disease Control and Prevention and 2 belong to offices for cancer control and prevention, with a population coverage of 43,145,743, accounting for 37.43% of the total population in the end of 2020 in Henan, China.

Cancer Report in Henan, 2023 includes six chapters:

Chapter 1 introduced the development of cancer registration system and the vital statistics system in Henan Province; Chapter 2 introduced data source and collecting methods; Chapter 3 introduced the index system of data quality, methods for evaluating data quality and the statistical methods; Chapter 4 described the cancer incidence and mortality in Henan Province; Chapter 5 described incidence and mortality of cancers in each site, and chapter 6 is appendix, which described the incidence and mortality of each cancer registry in Henan Province.

For ease of reading, this book is aranged in Chinese and English, but the English and Chinese are not exactly corresponding, please understand.

The work presented in this report derived from data collected by all registries in Henan Province. We are grateful to all the staffs who had contributed to and supported the work of Henan cancer registry and looking forward to close cooperation in the future.

Wengang Yi

January, 2024

致　谢

Acknowledgement

河南省肿瘤登记年报编委会对河南省各肿瘤登记处的工作人员在本次年报出版过程中给予的大力协助，尤其是在数据收集、整理、补充、审核登记资料，以及建档、建库等方面所做出的贡献表示感谢！衷心感谢编写组成员在本次年报撰写工作中付出的辛苦努力！

The editorial committee of Henan cancer annual report express their gratitude to all the staff working in cancer registries of Henan province, who made great contribution to data collecting, sorting, completing, crediting and filing. Sincere thanks to all compilation group members for their hard working.

河南省各肿瘤登记处工作人员名单

地区	肿瘤登记处	登记处所在单位	成员
郑州市	郑州市	郑州市疾控中心	宋彩娟 李建彬 闫瑞平 郭向娇 黄婼璇
	中原区	中原区疾控中心	孙文娟 尚小钰 焦诣珂 杨　峻
	二七区	二七区疾控中心	杨金秀 齐梦媛 孙贝贝
	管城回族区	管城回族区疾控中心	张晓丹 叶贺丹
	金水区	金水区疾控中心	苌道亮 杨　岚 李　想 张秀美 郑丽红 董宛露 刘雅斐 冀绚珂 莫晓红
	上街区	上街区疾控中心	张旭婷 张一帆 刘慧青 张文芳
	惠济区	惠济区疾控中心	冯春明 王燕云 马子健 王晶晶
	中牟县	中牟县疾控中心	乔富可 刘　宁 陈海瑞 张　芳 王新蕾 罗巧莉
	荥阳市	荥阳市疾控中心	崔　强 江吕玮 张　瑞
	新密市	新密市疾控中心	陈姬霞 孙会娟 王慧玲 陈新娥
	新郑市	新郑市疾控中心	王　玲 乔伊娜 赵小红 黄俊勇
	登封市	登封市疾控中心	王玲鹤 郑　苗 付　研
	巩义市	巩义市疾控中心	王亚彬 王月明 张文君 李优仕 翟莉艳
开封市	开封市	开封市疾控中心	温　瑞 刘　悦 杨　雯 王久悦
	祥符区	祥符区疾控中心	马　师 田艳玲 李慎榜 朱芳敏
洛阳市	洛阳市	洛阳市疾控中心	闫云燕 马　凯 常　颖
	老城区	老城区疾控中心	齐虹飞 夏中生 赵晓丽 刘青青 张素伟
	西工区	西工区疾控中心	石晓红 刘婷婷 平　莉
	瀍河回族区	瀍河回族区疾控中心	邢建乐 张佳楠
	涧西区	涧西区疾控中心	马昊翔 魏冰燕
	洛龙区	洛龙区疾控中心	袁瑞姣 吴志豪 孙冷宁 魏宇娜 王一雯 李　博
	孟津区	孟津区疾控中心	许瑞瑞 张菲菲 赵玉红

续表

地区	肿瘤登记处	登记处所在单位	成员
	新安县	新安县疾控中心	关　勇　龚进国　李　辉　付文莉　翟亚楠　卢昊洁
	栾川县	栾川县疾控中心	刘爱坡　刘杏杏　崔妙丽　郭钊均　唐巾阁　关　珂
	嵩县	嵩县疾控中心	马振卫　杨欣欣　乔　幸　石梦瑶　杨静媛　梁秋娟　姜开霞　万晓琦
	汝阳县	汝阳县疾控中心	李白鸟　耿振强
	宜阳县	宜阳县疾控中心	楚玉梅　楚淑英　苏雅维　李若男
	洛宁县	洛宁县疾控中心	段乐永　杨荷亚　刘龙安
	伊川县	伊川县疾控中心	刘　峰
	偃师区	偃师区疾控中心	秦延锦　杨慧芳　周　鹏　陈军芳　张　丹
平顶山市	平顶山市	平顶山市疾控中心	王　轶　宋　波　张泽华　许艺苑　吴　娟　郭晏强　马西平
	新华区	新华区疾控中心	仲晓伟　张小亚　平高迪
	卫东区	卫东区疾控中心	张慧卿　李新鹏　刘　琳　高巍然
	湛河区	湛河区疾控中心	温红旭　杨建伟　李文灿　郭淑乐
	鲁山县	鲁山县疾控中心	李保瑞　杜延高　王一博
	郏县	郏县疾控中心	孙　颖　王晓艳　陈旭姣
	舞钢市	舞钢市疾控中心	刘青兰　尹馨可　李晓杰
安阳市	安阳市	安阳市肿瘤医院	刘佳欣　张媛媛　闫焕勤　张晓星　秦永超　蔺志杰
	林州市	林州市肿瘤医院	秦富强　王　强　侯　凯　于晓东　王　丽　刘　畅　郝梓汝
鹤壁市	鹤壁市	鹤壁市人民医院	钞利娜　王冰冰　王梦媛　秦爱萍　胡凤琴　任红勤　郭雪琴　裴树英
	浚县	浚县疾控中心	韩晓康　张士民　杨　莹
	淇县	淇县疾控中心	李艳辉　王颖超
焦作市	焦作市	焦作市疾控中心	任　东　孟春辉　史靖靖
	解放区	解放区疾控中心	梁　瑞　张丹华　田茂林
	中站区	中站区疾控中心	王娜娜　许利娟
	山阳区	山阳区疾控中心	李雯雯　张　晓　马继勤
新乡市	新乡市	新乡市中心医院	李碧波　张　林　曹河璐
	辉县市	辉县市疾控中心	孙花荣　赵小聪　李　颖
濮阳市	濮阳市	濮阳市疾控中心	梁　森　张玉华　张洪磊　孟庆浩
	华龙区	华龙区疾控中心	王培贤　王新杰　毛利娟
	濮阳县	濮阳县疾控中心	郭秋献　穆晓红　谷红纺　李瑞霞
	范县	范县疾控中心	田军艳　邢秀娟　薛　辉　段晓琦
	清丰县	清丰县疾控中心	高铁柱　李　宁　刘　欢
	南乐县	南乐县疾控中心	王青辉　宋黎霞　徐晓文
许昌市	许昌市	许昌市疾控中心	谭莉娜　康　宁　侯灿灿　杨彦彦　牛兵雪　刘　洋
	魏都区	魏都区疾控中心	信保祥　崔亚辉　郑云枝　廖　飞　张　方　白　雪
	禹州市	禹州市疾控中心	王全新　常红丽　郭　影　李　蔚　张亚楠　赵琳琳
漯河市	漯河市	漯河市疾控中心	黄道靖　代　莹　孙路平　孟　蕾　胡　昕　代君君
	源汇区	源汇区疾控中心	王宏博　张　祥　牛艳丽　叶　静　刘一培　王春玲
	召陵区	召陵区疾控中心	任东洋　崔一齐　樊永立　鞠晨云
	郾城区	郾城区疾控中心	李爱会　汪　真　杨莹莹　邓　捷　孟云鹤　常帅奇　张　楠
	舞阳县	舞阳县疾控中心	何　洁　马永晓　周小佳　谷来君　杨艳芳　陈丹丹

续表

地区	肿瘤登记处	登记处所在单位	成员
	临颍县	临颍县疾控中心	米富德 罗婷 吴真 马玉智 秦苏丹 张彩玲 祁亚丽
三门峡	三门峡市	三门峡市疾控中心	刘天福 刘旭 郭振平 郑爽
	湖滨区	湖滨区疾控中心	王红梅 段宏霞 李粉妮 刘润娣 罗丹
	渑池县	渑池县疾控中心	赵建国 张晓 张伟霞 王翠
	陕州区	陕州区疾控中心	贺波 郑斌 成波 孙鹏 乔金霞
南阳市	南阳市	南阳市疾控中心	杨阳 张锶赫 李志颖 何建磊 李璐璐
	卧龙区	卧龙区疾控中心	武霞 谢九汉 谷芳 王庆 陈星伊 郭博伦 刘泽政
	宛城区	宛城区疾控中心	段学敬 王昌举 王冲 马旭晓 冉欣 李天锁 李娟 邓莹 李静
	内乡县	内乡县疾控中心	李亚波 金花 黄健 代阳
	方城县	方城县疾控中心	贾浩 马璟颖 李谱 倪林静 田向阳 李业成 张娟 张禄军
	南召县	南召县疾控中心	靳万春 王珂 陈立明 朱广博 樊璞 黄靖杨
	镇平县	镇平县疾控中心	李宛均 黄勇 尹佳良 侯玲 张素音 米海奇 姚少斐
	新野县	新野县疾控中心	董帅 熊祎娜 范淘丽
	桐柏县	桐柏县疾控中心	王方方 郑向辉 石金月 王敏 李蕤
商丘市	虞城县	虞城县疾控中心	高为民 冯金洪 马宁 毕兴华 刘威 江培
	睢县	睢县疾控中心	徐强 韩敬华 袁帅 刘艳
信阳市	信阳市	信阳市疾控中心	杨岩岩 王缓 谢会敏 徐鑫鑫 张晨 张文泰 薛瑜
	浉河区	浉河区疾控中心	兰宏旺 周娣 楚尚兰 耿祎祎 李梦
	罗山县	罗山县疾控中心	江坤 徐蔚静 张世威 王明阳
周口市	周口市	周口市疾控中心	冷冰 费培筠 马培云 许炀 苏英瀚 张溪 武志强
	郸城县	郸城县疾控中心	张吉志 孙忠 郭德银 马慧 李慧珍
	沈丘县	沈丘县疾控中心	徐玲 李庆文 郭丽花 李旭东 孙梦洋
	项城市	项城市疾控中心	李波 马冠军 王玉华 袁媛 朱琳 靳冰洁
驻马店	驻马店市	驻马店市疾控中心	宋静 李渊 王若溪
	驿城区	驿城区疾控中心	简杰 佟继玲 张艺严
	西平县	西平县疾控中心	周丽萍 邵天堂 刘彩霞 毛小辉
济源市	济源市	济源市疾控中心	马璐瑶 黄艳芳 郑飞飞 张雷锋

目　录

Contents

第一章 概 述

Chapter 1 Summary

一、河南省肿瘤登记系统介绍

肿瘤登记报告是按照统一的技术与方法，在目标人群中开展经常性的收集、储存、整理、统计分析肿瘤发病、死亡及生存资料的统计制度。肿瘤登记报告是国际通用的关于人群肿瘤发病信息收集的标准方法，目的是了解人群的肿瘤发病、死亡和生存状况，为肿瘤病因研究提供依据，为制定卫生工作规划和肿瘤防治计划、评价和考核肿瘤防治效果提供基础数据。

20 世纪 50 年代末，由河南省癌症中心 / 河南省肿瘤医院的科研人员组成的河南省食管癌防治研究协作组深入林县（现林州市）山区，开展了食管癌流行病学的调查和防治研究工作，组织实施了林县食管癌和贲门癌的发病及死亡登记工作。1959~1962 年林县人群食管癌发病、死亡病例的收集主要依靠回顾性调查。随着县、乡、村三级肿瘤防治网的建立，1963~1966 年食管癌 / 贲门癌的发病、死亡登记报告工作基本稳定。1967~1969 年，由于历史的原因，登记工作受到了严重影响，发病、死亡登记资料漏报严重，经后期回顾调查补报得以完善。1977 年，根据全国的统一部署，河南省卫生厅组织实施了覆盖河南省 6 000 多万人口、为期三年（1974~1976 年）的全死因回顾性调查。

在三年全死因回顾性调查的基础上，河南省肿瘤医院 / 研究院于 1983 年在全省抽样选取了林县、济源、禹州、洛阳、偃师、罗山、鲁山、内乡等 15 个县市、约占河南省人口 1/10 的地区

1. Introduction to the Henan cancer registration system

The cancer registration is a statistical system for the consistent collection, storage, sorting and analysis to evaluate cancer incidence, mortality and survival data in a target population according to unified methods and technologies. Cancer registration is internationally recognized as a standardized method for collecting information on cancer incidence.The purpose of cancer registration is to determine cancer incidence, mortality, and survival within the population, provide a scientific basis for cancer etiology research, and supply essential data for formulating health work plans and cancer prevention and control strategies, as well as for evaluating and assessing cancer prevention and control efforts.

In the late 1950s, a cooperative esophageal cancer screening program in Northern China was organized by the Chinese Academy of Medical Sciences. The Henan research cooperative group was mainly from Henan Medical College Henan College of Traditional Chinese Medicine and Henan Provincial People's Hospital. They penetrated the mountainous areas of Lin County and carried out esophageal cancer epidemiological investigations to explore cancer prevention and control strategies. From then on, esophageal cancer incidence and mortality registrations were initiated in Lin County. From 1959 to 1962 information was mainly collected based on retrospective surveys. From 1963 to 1966 the cancer registration and reporting system spread across the three administrative levels of county, township and village. From 1967 to 1969 the cancer registration system was severely affected by the historical reasons and many cases escaped surveillance. Nevertheless the missed cases were incorporated later through a retrospective investigation. In 1977 the Henan Provincial Health Commission organized a retrospective survey on all causes of death from 1974 to 1976 covering 60,000,000 of the population according to national records. In order to record all the deaths caused by cancers, and other

开展了居民全死因登记工作，建立起了以肿瘤为主的全死因登记报告系统。

1988 年，林县在全死因登记系统的基础上，参照国际癌症中心（IARC）/ 国际癌症登记协会（IACR）推荐的肿瘤随访登记方法与原则，建立起了以人群为基础的肿瘤发病登记报告系统，对恶性肿瘤及中枢神经系统良性肿瘤进行登记报告。2004 年 4 月 1 日，河南省癌症及生命统计中心成立，并在 15 个市县建立了癌症及生命统计登记处。2004 年 10 月 7 日，河南省卫生厅印发《河南省癌症及生命统计登记工作规范》，下发到市、县卫生局及各登记处并落实执行。

2008 年，河南省癌症中心 / 河南省肿瘤医院在偃师、禹州、内乡、开封、鲁山开始实施人群肿瘤登记报告工作。2009 年，卫生部在全国范围内启动了中央财政转移支付地方的肿瘤随访登记项目工作，中央财政对肿瘤登记地区给予经费支持。河南省林州、洛阳、偃师、禹州、西平和沈丘被纳入国家肿瘤随访登记项目市县。在 2009 年的基础上，2010 年将济源市、鲁山县、漯河市、内乡县、郸城县、罗山县、三门峡市、虞城县列入河南省肿瘤登记系统。2012~2013 年又有开封县、鹤壁市区、睢县及郑州市四个市县纳入全省的肿瘤登记系统。

为进一步加强全国肿瘤登记工作规范化管理，获得及时、统一、准确的肿瘤发病、死亡和生存信息，2015 年 2 月 5 日，国家卫计委和国家中医药管理局联合印发了《肿瘤登记管理办法》，河南省卫计委和省中医管理局结合我省实际情况，组织制定了《河南省肿瘤登记实施方案》（豫卫疾控〔2015〕10 号）。河南省肿瘤防治研究办公室按照《河南省肿瘤登记实施方案》的要求对全省各级医疗机构相关人员进行了业务培训，在各市县成立肿瘤登记处，开展肿瘤随访登记工作，并通过河南省网络直报系统上报当地的肿瘤发病、死亡和随访数据。

各级肿瘤登记处履行肿瘤登记报告职责，建立健全肿瘤登记报告工作管理制度，明确肿瘤

causes, Henan Cancer Hospital/Henan Cancer Institute established a cancer centered vital statistics system in 1983. It covered one tenth of the Henan provincial population and comprised 15 selected counties/cities including LinCounty, Jiyuan City, YuCounty, Luoyang City, Yanshi County, Luoshan County, Lushan County and Neixiang County.

In 1988, the first population-based cancer registration system was established based on the vital statistics system of Lin County. Under this system, all cancer registration and follow-up recommendations were referred to the International Agency for Research on Cancer (IARC)/International Association of Cancer Registries (IACR) and all cancers (including central nervous system benign cancers) were classified and reported by the codes in accordance with the International Classification of Disease. On April 1, 2004, the Henan Provincial Cancer and Vital Statistics Center was established. Meanwhile, 15 city/county cancer and vital statistics registries were opened. On October 7, 2004, the Henan Provincial Health Bureau issued the "*Methods for Cancer and Vital Statistics Registration Henan*" which was sent to each registry as a work specification.

In 2008, the Henan Cancer Center/Henan Cancer Hospital built the population-based cancer registration and reporting system in Yanshi City, Yuzhou City, Neixiang County, Kaifeng City and Lushan County. In 2009, the registries were supported by the central government finance as the Ministry of Health launched the transfer payments on cancer follow-up registration programs to local governments. In Henan province the funded registries were Linzhou City, Luoyang City, Yanshi City, Yuzhou City, Xiping County and Shenqiu County. Funded registries were added gradually. In 2010 Jiyuan City, Lushan County, Luohe City, Neixiang County, Dancheng County, Luoshan County, Sanmenxia City and Yucheng County were added and Hebi City, Kaifeng County, Sui County and Zhengzhou City were added during 2012 ~ 2013.

To strengthen the cancer registration specification to obtain accurate, prompt and unified cancer incidence, mortality and survival data, the National Health and Family Planning Commission and National Administration of Traditional Chinese Medicine issued "*Cancer Registration Management and Methods*" on February 5,2015. The Henan province Health and Family Planning Commission and Henan Province Administrative Departments for Traditional Chinese Medicine issued "Cancer Registration Management and Specifications" applicable to Henan province. Correspondingly the Henan Cancer Center/ Henan Cancer Hospital trained all the staff who worked in cancer registries or the

登记报告管理科室及责任人，明确诊疗机构科室责任。

从早期林县食管癌/贲门癌的单癌种登记系统，发展到目前的全部位的肿瘤随访登记系统，河南省逐步建立起了人群肿瘤监测系统，为肿瘤预防控制与研究奠定了基础。肿瘤随访登记工作以政府为主导，河南省卫健委作为项目主管单位全面负责肿瘤登记报告工作，制定相关政策和规划，组织开展考核和评估工作。

河南省癌症中心/河南省肿瘤医院作为技术指导单位，负责全省肿瘤登记系统的建立和工作的实施，制定并修订肿瘤登记报告实施方案和年度工作计划，负责开展全省肿瘤登记工作业务培训、技术指导等工作。河南省各市、县（区）卫生行政部门负责辖区内肿瘤登记报告系统的建立及项目工作的实施与管理，对肿瘤登记报告工作进行督导检查和考核评估，协调相关机构和部门，为肿瘤登记报告工作的正常运行提供保障。

河南省各市、县（区）肿瘤登记处负责制定本辖区肿瘤登记报告实施方案和工作计划，指导辖区内各级医疗机构开展肿瘤登记报告工作，确定辖区内肿瘤登记报告单位、报告人、联系方式并登记建档，负责肿瘤登记的业务管理和技术指导等工作。

各级医疗机构为登记病例的上报单位，要在当地肿瘤登记处的指导下，利用河南省肿瘤随访登记网络直报系统开展肿瘤登记报告工作，按照项目内容要求，提供完整、准确、及时的肿瘤登记信息。建立健全机构内的登记报告管理组织制度和技术规范，将资料登记及死亡报告工作纳入单位考核管理内容，并制定相关的管理措施。

relevant medical institutions regarding cancer follow-up and reporting management specifications and the Henan Cancer Reporting System which was the dedicated network for the registries to report all the cancer incidences deaths and survival.

All the registries took responsibility for cancer reporting such as drawing up cancer reporting management specifications assigning the person-in-charge and specifying the work in medical institutions.

Whether it is for the early stage of a single type of esophageal cancer in Lin County or the present status for all cancer types, the cancer reporting system is designed to meet the actual needs of cancer prevention and control. The work of the cancer follow-up registry was led by the government. The Henan Provincial Health Commission is oversees the entire project and responsible for formulating relevant regulations and plans, and organizing work appraisal.

The Henan Cancer Center/Henan Cancer Hospital is in charge of technical support and guidance. It is also responsible for developing a cancer reporting and registration system and its application developing implementation schedules and annual work plans and carrying out relevant professional and technological training.The city or county administrative agencies are responsible for establishing the local cancer registration reporting system. They are also responsible for the operation management supervision inspection and appraisal of the work and coordinating agencies for the operation of the cancer registration system.

The city or county cancer registries are responsible for cancer registration management and technical guidance within their jurisdictions. They formulate the specifications and work plan supervise medical institutions in carrying out cancer registration and designate cancer reporting institutions and record-reporting personnel.

Medical institutions are responsible for reporting cancer cases. They report cancer registration data under the supervision of cancer registries through cancer registration and reporting systems in a timely and precise manner. They establish and improve the mechanism of the registration management system and technical specifications and they incorporate cancer registration and death reports into the internal examination records to formulate relevant management measures.

二、河南省居民死因登记系统简介

居民病伤死因登记是系统性、经常性收集居民病伤死亡信息的统计制度，目的是了解城乡居民各种疾病的死亡原因、分布状况和流行动态。完整、准确的人群死亡信息，对于制定人口和卫生政策、合理配置资源具有非常重要的意义。

河南省在 1975~1977 年第一次死因回顾性调查的基础上，于 1983 年在 15 个县市建立了居民病伤死亡登记报告制度。在当地政府和卫生行政部门配合下，经过多年不断的努力，现在已经形成县、乡、村三级死因登记上报体系，建立、完善了各项登记报告制度。死因统计资料基本可以反映河南省人群各种死亡原因的死亡水平。

肿瘤随访登记是在完整、有效的居民全死因登记的基础上建立的，肿瘤随访登记中肿瘤死亡数据来源于人群全死因登记系统。死因登记是肿瘤随访登记补充、完善发病、随访资料的重要途径，健全、完整的死因登记系统是肿瘤随访登记资料质量保证的基础。

死因统计按照国际疾病分类（International Classification of Diseases, ICD-10）方法进行分类编码，将死因分类为 18 大类、101 种疾病进行统计。

2. Introduction to the vital statistics system in Henan

The vital statistics system is a systematic and statistical system to collect residents'death information caused by diseases or injuries on a recurring basis and aims to monitor death causes distribution and disease epidemic dynamics in urban and rural areas. The integrity and accuracy of vital information are of great significance for population health policies and resource allocation.

Vital statistics systems in Henan province were in place in 15 cities and counties up until 1983 since the first retrospective death survey was conducted between 1975 and 1977. With 30 years of continuous effort in coordination with support from local government and the health administration, the vital statistics system has formed the county-township-village registration and reporting network under the appropriate management regulations and now records all deaths among Henan residents.

Cancer registries are based on the standard and perfect vital statistics system, as cancer registration contains cancer death cases. Additionally, the vital statistics system is an important route to supplement cancer incidences and passive follow-up. Hence, a perfect vital statistics system is vital for cancer registration when assessing its data quality.

Vital statistics were classified into 18 categories, 101 diseases according to the International Classification of Diseases ICD-10.

第二章　肿瘤登记的方法和统计学指标

Chapter 2　Methods and statistical indices of cancer registration

肿瘤登记是系统性、经常性收集有关肿瘤及肿瘤患者信息的统计制度。目的是了解城乡居民癌症发病、死亡情况和生存状态，掌握癌症的疾病负担与变化趋势，以及在不同地区和人群中的分布特征，为政府和卫生行政部门制定癌症防治策略、规划与计划、研究及评价控制措施效果提供数据支撑。

一、建立肿瘤登记处

肿瘤登记处是收集、储存、整理及报告肿瘤发病、死亡和生存信息的部门。肿瘤登记地区应具备完善的县、乡、村三级死因登记系统，同时能够获取准确的人口学资料。肿瘤登记应覆盖辖区内全部户籍人口。当地政府或卫生行政部门制定和颁布实行肿瘤登记报告制度的法律法规或规范性文件，设立肿瘤登记处，并配备相应的工作人员、经费及设备，同时制定肿瘤登记报告实施细则。

二、登记资料收集方法

河南省肿瘤登记地区资料收集采用被动收集和主动收集相结合的方法，由各医疗机构定期报送肿瘤发病登记卡片到肿瘤登记处，或由登记处工作人员主动到各医疗单位查阅肿瘤新发病例的诊疗病史，摘录肿瘤发病信息。同时，登记处定期通过医疗保险机构（新农合医疗保险、城镇居民医疗保险、职工医疗保险及商业医疗保险）和居民死因报告系统，获取相关因肿瘤疾病报销或死亡医学证书中提及肿瘤发病信息的个案记录，以补充新发病例登记，保证肿瘤登记的完整性。

Cancer registration is a statistical system for gathering information on cancer and cancer cases systematically and consistently. It aims to collect data on cancer incidence, mortality and survival in the urban and rural areas of Henan province; to analyze cancer burden, dynamic trends and distribution characteristics in different regions and populations; to provide evidence for formulating strategies for cancer prevention and control for government and health administrative departments; as well as to provide basic information for fundamental and clinical cancer research and evaluation of control measures.

1. Establishment of a cancer registry

The cancer registry is an organization that bears the responsibility of collecting, storing, sorting analyzing, appraising, elaborating and reporting dynamic cancer incidence, mortality and survival information. A cancer registry should possess a perfect three-level county-township-village death surveillance system and have the capability of obtaining demographic data accurately. A cancer registry should cover all the registered population in the whole administrative region either in urban area cancer registries or in rural area cancer registries. The local governments or health administrative departments should make and issue the specification and regulations on cancer registration and reporting systems; set up the cancer registries; allocate necessary personnel funds and equipment; and draw up the relevant implementing measures.

2. Methods of cancer registration data collection

Cancer registration data are mainly collected through a combination of passive and active collection methods. On the one hand, medical institutions report cancer incidence registration cards to the cancer registry periodically, or the staff at the cancer registry collate cancer information by abstracting newly

（一）建立信息收集渠道

肿瘤登记处从相关部门收集辖区内肿瘤新发病例、死亡病例、生存信息和相关人口资料。病例资料的收集渠道包括登记地区各级医疗机构、死因监测数据库、新型农村合作医疗及城镇居民 / 职工医疗保险数据库等。人口资料的来源包括人口普查资料、公安及统计部门有关资料等。

（二）开展病例核实工作

肿瘤登记处负责肿瘤病例的建卡和分类编码、剔除重复记录病例。应用死因监测数据库进行死亡补发病流程。

（三）开展随访工作

通过电话、书信、电子邮件，以及社区居委会、基层医疗卫生机构开展随访工作，获取病例的生存情况。肿瘤登记工作流程见图 2–1。

diagnosed cancer case files from medical institutions. On the other hand, cancer registries supplement and complete cancer incidence information through the related death certification in the death surveillance system or the related reimbursement data from medical assurance agencies, including new rural cooperative medical insurance, medical insurance for urban residents, basic medical insurance for urban workers, and commercial medical insurance.

2.1 Sources of data collection

Cancer registries collect cancer incidence, mortality, survival and related demographic data from certain departments. Cancer information collection channels include medical institutions at different levels, medical insurance databases, death surveillance databases, rural cooperative medical systems, urban residents and employee medical insurance databases. The demographic data sources include census data public security and statistics bureau.

2.2 Cancer cases ascertainment

Cancer registries establish and classify registration cards. The cases are ascertained with identified card numbers as identification codes and duplicates are deleted. The cases are verified by the death surveillance database, to which the missed cases have been added.

2.3 Cancer case follow-up

Cancer follow–up methods mainly include home visits, phone calls, letters, or email correspondence for survival information collection by the community committee or primary health care institutions. The cancer registration process is shown in Figure 2–1.

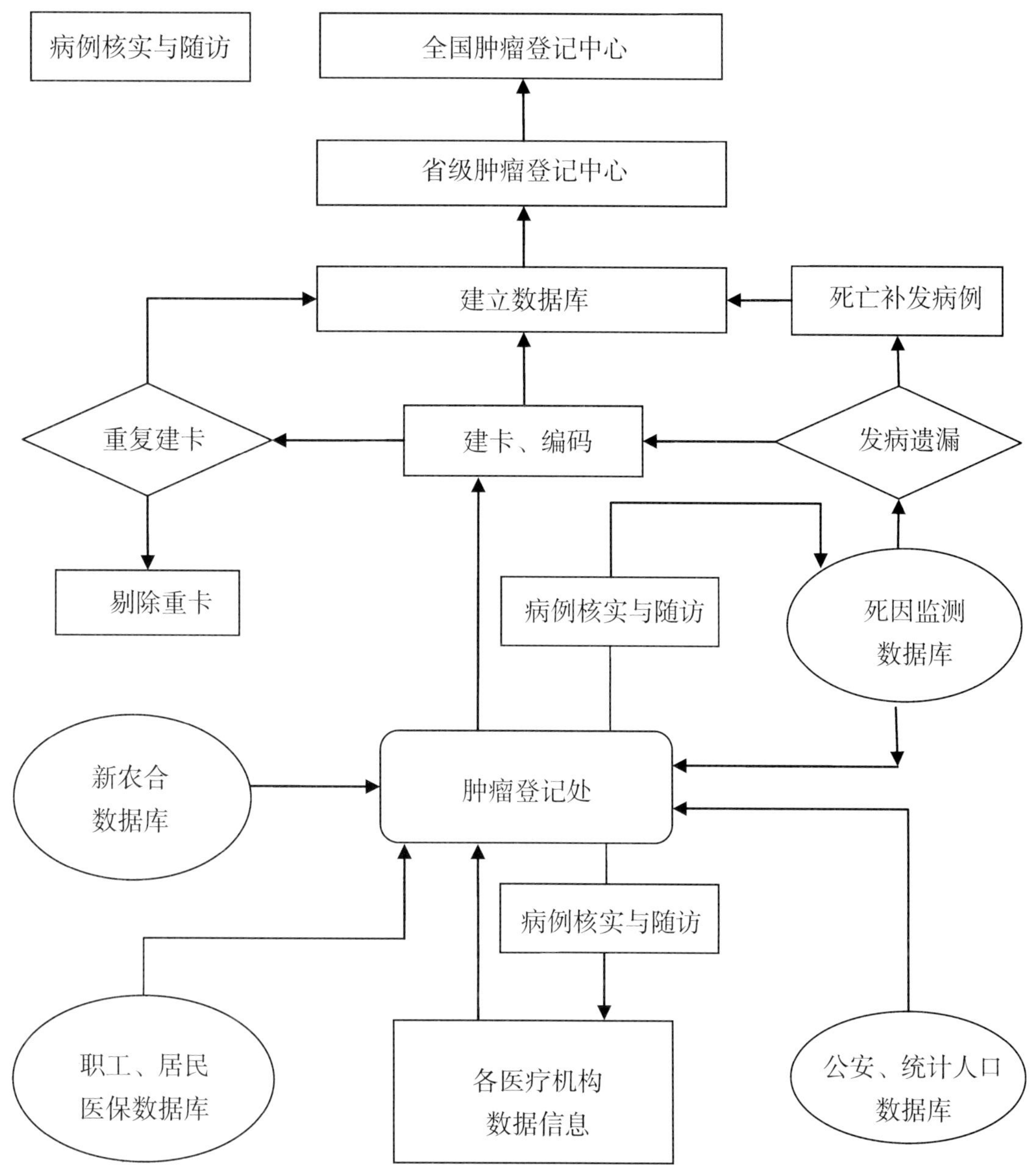

图 2–1 肿瘤登记工作流程

三、登记资料收集内容

肿瘤登记主要收集的信息是登记覆盖地区范围内全部恶性肿瘤（ICD–10：C00–C96）、原位癌、中枢神经系统良性肿瘤和中枢神经系统动态未定或者未知的肿瘤（ICD–10：D32–D33.9，D42.0–D43.9）的发病、死亡和生存信息，以及登记处覆盖人群的人口资料。

3. Information collected in cancer registration

The cancer registry mainly collects the incidence, mortality, and survival data of all cancer cases (ICD–10: C00–C96), neoplasms, and unusual conditions of the central nervous system (ICD–10: D32–D33.9, D42.0–D43.9) in the registration areas, as well as the related demographic information of the covering population.

（一）新发病例资料

个人信息包括姓名、性别、出生日期、年龄、身份证号码、住址、出生地、民族、婚姻状况、职业等；肿瘤信息包括发病日期、解剖学部位（亚部位）、组织学类型、诊断依据、临床分期等；报告单位信息包括报告日期、诊断单位、报告单位、报告医生等；随访信息包括随访病人的死亡日期及生命状态等。

（二）死亡资料

死亡资料来源于全人口死因登记报告，包括根本死因为非肿瘤原因的肿瘤病例的死亡资料。除发病信息外，还应包括死亡日期、实足年龄、死亡原因、主要诊断、诊断级别和依据、死亡地点等。

（三）人口资料

人口指辖区覆盖的户籍人口。资料来源于我国人口普查资料和公安、统计部门逐年提供的人口资料。人口资料应包括居民人口总数及其性别、年龄构成。年龄组按 0~1、1~4、5~9、10~14、……、75~79、80~84、85+ 分组。

四、登记数据的质量控制

质量控制贯穿肿瘤登记工作的全过程。肿瘤登记地区应在各个环节制定工作规范和质量控制程序，并严格执行。质量控制从登记资料的可比性、完整性、有效性和时效性等四个方面进行系统评估。

（一）登记资料的质量控制

1. 可比性

数据结果真实可比的基本先决条件是采用通用的标准或定义。通常而言，可比性是指不同地区或不同时间人群发病率的差异不是因登记数据质量、采用的编码标准及运用规则不同所产生。可比性涉及以下几个指标：对“发病”的定义，对原发、复发和转移的诊断标准，分类与编码，死亡证明等。

3.1 Incidence data

Incidence data include the following: personal information including name, gender, date of birth, age, identity card number, address, place of birth, ethnicity, marital status, professional career etc.; cancer information including date of onset, anatomical site and subsite, histological type, diagnostic evidence, clinical stages etc.; reporting unit information including reporting date, diagnosing department, institution, physician etc.; and follow-up information including survival status and date of death.

3.2 Mortality data

Mortality data are obtained from vital statistics systems including cancer cases with causes of death other than cancer. In addition to incidence information, mortality data should also include date and age at death, cause of death, place of death, major diagnoses, diagnostic level, diagnostic evidence etc.

3.3 Population information

The population refers to the household-registered people included in the registration area. The data originate from census data public security or bureaus of statistics. Population information includes overall population coverage gender and age composition. The population is divided into groups by age as follows: 0~1, 1~4, 5~9, 10~14, …, 75~79, 80~84, and 85+ years age groups.

4. Quality control in the cancer registration data

Quality control goes on throughout the cancer registration process. Each step of cancer registration adheres to the specified regulations and procedures for quality control. Quality control of registration data is systematically assessed from four aspects: comparability, validity, completeness and timeliness.

4.1 Quality control of registration data

4.1.1 Comparability

The basic prerequisite for the true comparability of data results is the use of universal standards or definitions. Comparability refers to population differences in different regions or at different times not because of the quality of registration data, the different coding standards, or the rules of use. Comparability involves the following indicators: the definition of “onset” ; diagnostic criteria for primary recurrent and metastatic; classification and coding; and death certification.

2. 完整性

完整性是指在登记地区资料库中目标人群内所有新发病例被记录的完整程度。常用的评价指标有死亡 / 发病比（M/I）、只有死亡证明比例（DCO%）、组织学诊断确认比例（MV%）、病例的来源数与报告单数、不同时间发病率的稳定性、不同人群发病率的比较、年龄别发病率曲线、儿童癌症发病率评价等。

3. 有效性

有效性是指登记病例中具有给定特征（例如肿瘤部位、年龄）真正属性的病例所占的比例。常用的评价指标有组织学诊断确认比例（MV%）、只有死亡证明比例（DCO%）、部位不明的百分比 (UK%)、年龄不明的百分比等。对各登记处的数据进行内部一致审核，检查数据库中无效编码或组合以及可疑的编码组合，如年龄 / 出生日期，性别 / 部位，部位 / 组织学，部位 / 组织学 / 年龄等。

4. 时效性

时效性一般指发病日期（诊断日期）到数据被利用时（年报、研究报告、论文）的间隔。登记地区及时获取并报告癌症信息，会提高肿瘤登记工作的效率，但是新发病例登记流程自身存在滞后性，时效性考虑就是在效率与完整性间取得平衡。目前对时效性无统一的国际标准。为平衡与完整性和准确性的关系，全国肿瘤登记中心要求各登记地区于诊断年份后的 30 个月内提交数据。

（二）登记资料的审核流程

河南省肿瘤登记中心收到各登记地区上报的资料后，首先检查资料的完整性。在确认资料完整后，使用 IARC/IACR 工具软件中的 Check 程序逐一检查所有记录的变量是否完整和有效，同时对不同变量之间是否合乎逻辑的一致性进行检查。然后使用数据分析软件及数据库软件生成统一表格，对登记数据的完整性和可靠性做出评估。各登记地区根据评估结果，对登记资料进行核实、补充与修改，将修改后的资料再次上报省级肿瘤登记中心。河南省肿

4.1.2 Completeness

Completeness refers to the extent to which all incident cancers are included and recorded within the population covered by registration areas. Common evaluation indicators include mortality/incidence ratio (M/I), the percentage of death certification only (DCO%), the percentage of morphologically verified cases (MV%), the number of sources/notifications per case, the stability of incidence rates over time a comparison of incidence rates in different populations age-specific incidence curves and incidence rate of childhood cancer evaluation.

4.1.3 Validity

Validity is defined as the proportion of cases in a dataset with a given characteristic that truly has an attribute. Common evaluation indicators include the percentage of morphologically verified cases (MV%), percentage of the death certification only (DCO%), percentage of unspecific site diagnoses (UK%), unspecific age etc. Cancer registries must evaluate the validity of data for information consistency for example age/date of birth, gender/anatomic site, anatomic site/histologic diagnosis, anatomic site/histologic diagnosis/age, and the completeness of all basic variables.

4.1.4 Timeliness

Timeliness refers to the time interval between the date of onset/diagnosis and data utilization (annual reports, research reports or papers). Timely accessing to and reporting cancer information will improve the efficiency of the cancer registry but the new case registration process has its own inherent time lag; timeliness must be balanced against efficiency and integrity. However, there are no international guidelines for the timeliness of cancer registration data. Currently the National Central Cancer Registry (NCCR) requires a reporting interval within 30 months after diagnosis considering data integrity.

4.2 Audit process of registration data

After receiving cancer registration data, the HNCCR first checks the completeness of the data. The IARC/IACR checking software can be used to determine whether all variables are complete and valid. The internal logical consistency of the dataset is also checked. The HNCCR further generates a unified form and assess the integrity and reliability of the registration data with the use of data analysis software and database software. The local registries then revise the cancer datasets following the evaluation report until they fulfill the requirements. Qualified cancer datasets were

瘤登记中心将全省各登记地区数据进行汇总分析，并撰写年度报告。肿瘤登记资料的审核流程见图 2-2。

pooled together for the Henan provincial annual cancer report analysis. (Figure 2-2)

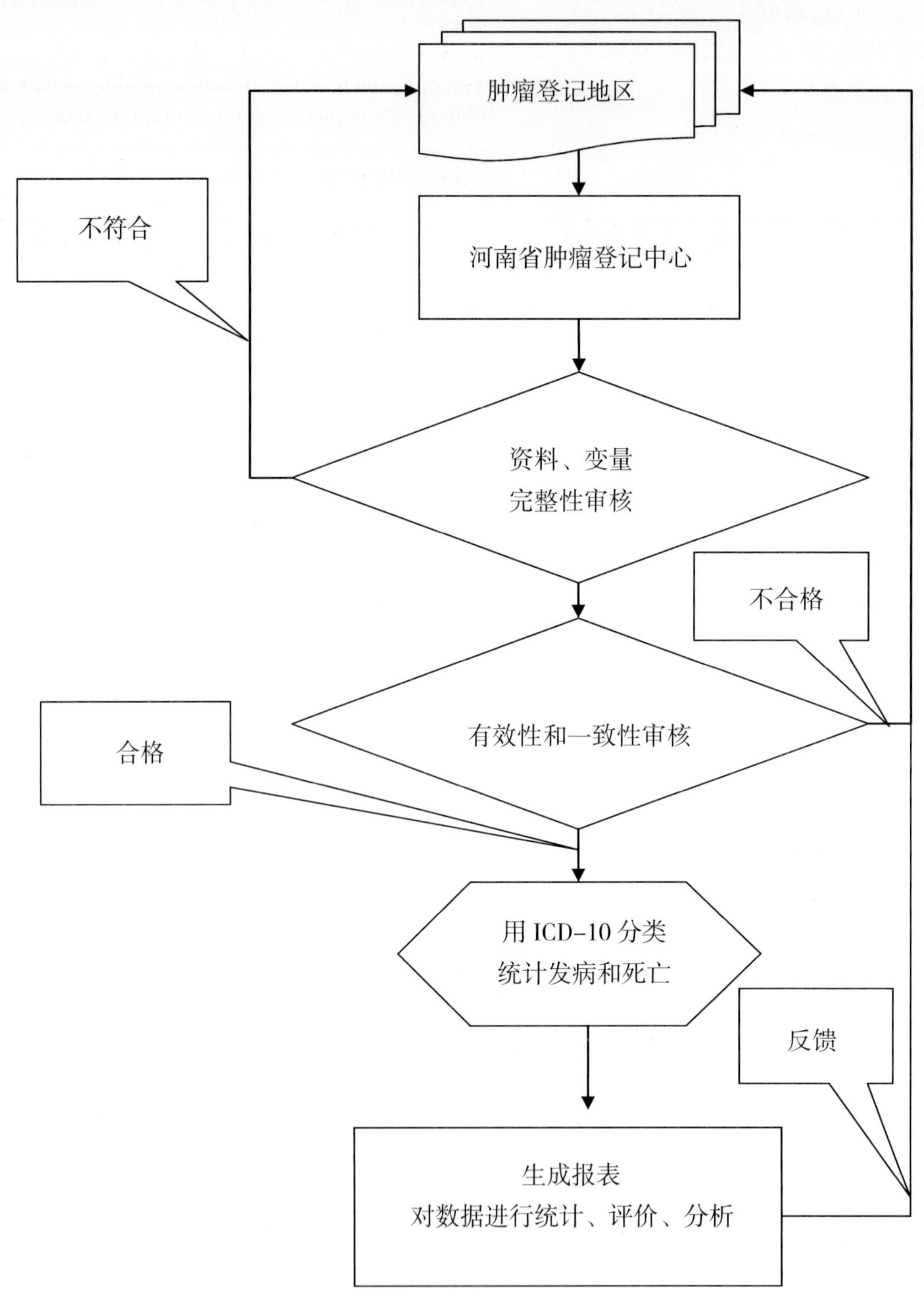

图 2-2　肿瘤登记资料的审核流程

（三）统计分类

1. 肿瘤分类

参照 ICD-10 统计分类的肿瘤学类目内容，学界将包括男、女性肿瘤细分为 59 部位，25 个大类，其中脑和神经系统包括良性及良恶性未定肿瘤。（表 2-1、表 2-2）

4.3 Data classification and coding

4.3.1 Cancer classification and coding

Based on the ICD-10 International Statistical Classification of Oncology categories, male and female cancers are subdivided into 59 types and 25 major categories, amony which the brain and central nervous system included benign tumors as well as benign and malignant undetermined tumors. (Table 2-1, Table 2-2)

表 2-1　常见肿瘤分类统计表

部位	编码范围（ICD-10）	部位	编码范围（ICD-10）
唇	C00	间皮瘤	C45
舌	C01-C02	卡波西肉瘤	C46
口	C03-C06	周围神经、其他结缔组织、软组织	C47;C49
唾液腺	C07-C08	乳房	C50
扁桃体	C09	外阴	C51
其他的口咽	C10	阴道	C52
鼻咽	C11	子宫颈	C53
喉咽	C12-C13	子宫体	C54
咽，部位不明	C14	子宫，部位不明	C55
食管	C15	卵巢	C56
胃	C16	女性其他的生殖器	C57
小肠	C17	胎盘	C58
结肠	C18	阴茎	C60
直肠	C19-C20	前列腺	C61
肛门	C21	睾丸	C62
肝脏	C22	男性其他的生殖器	C63
胆囊及其他	C23-C24	肾	C64
胰腺	C25	肾盂	C65
鼻、鼻窦及其他	C30-C31	输尿管	C66
喉	C32	膀胱	C67
气管、支气管、肺	C33-C34	其他的泌尿器官	C68
其他的胸腔器官	C37-C38	眼	C69
骨	C40-C41	脑、神经系统	C70-C72
皮肤的黑色素瘤	C43	甲状腺	C73
其他的皮肤	C44	肾上腺	C74
其他的内分泌腺	C75	髓样白血病	C92-C94
霍奇金病	C81	白血病，未特指	C95
非霍奇金淋巴瘤	C82-C85; C96	其他的或未指明部位	O&U
免疫增生性疾病	C88	骨髓增殖性疾病	MPD
多发性骨髓瘤	C90	骨髓增生异常综合征	MDS
淋巴样白血病	C91		
合计	ALL	C44 以外的部位	ALL but C44

表 2-2　常见肿瘤分类统计表（大类）

部位	编码范围（ICD-10）
口腔和咽(鼻咽和喉除外)	C00-10,C12-14（除外 C10.1）
鼻咽	C11
食管	C15
胃	C16
结直肠、肛门	C18-21
肝脏	C22
胆囊及其他	C23-C24
胰腺	C25
喉	C32，C10.1
气管、支气管、肺	C33-C34
骨	C40-C41
乳房	C50
子宫颈	C53
子宫体及子宫部位不明	C54-55
卵巢	C56
前列腺	C61
睾丸	C62
肾及泌尿系统不明	C64-66，68
膀胱	C67
脑、神经系统	C70-C72
甲状腺	C73
淋巴瘤	C81-85,88,90,96
白血病	C91-C95
其他	Other（除外以上）
所有部位合计	ALL

2. 登记地区分类

城市与农村的分类标准：国家标准《中华人民共和国行政区划代码》（GB/T 2260—2009），将地级以上城市归于城市地区，县及县级市归于农村地区。按照此项标准，我们把洛阳市、三门峡市、鹤壁市、漯河市（召陵区和源汇区）、郑州市、安阳市、濮阳市华龙区、南阳市归类为城市地区；林州市、开封市（祥符区）、内乡县等地区归类为农村地区。具体地区分类见表 3-1。

4.3.2 Cancer registration area classification

The definition standards for urban areas and rural areas are as follows: according to national standard GB/T 2260—2009, prefecture-level cities are classified as urban areas, whereas counties and county-level cities are classified as rural areas. Accordingly, the urban areas include Luoyang City, Sanmenxia City, Hebi City, and Luohe City (Shaoling District and Yuanhui District), and the rural areas include Linzhou City, Kaifeng City (Xiangfu District), and Neixiang County. (Table 3-1)

（四）常用统计指标

1. 年均人口数

年均人口数是计算发病（死亡）率指标的分母，常用年初和年末人口数的算术平均数作为年平均人口数的近似值。计算公式为：

$$\text{年均人口数} = \frac{\text{年初（上年末）人口数} + \text{年末人口数}}{2}$$

2. 性别、年龄别人口数

性别、年龄别人口数是指按男女性别和不同年龄分组的人口数。性别年龄的分组，除0岁组、1~4岁组及85岁及以上年龄组外，其余年龄组按5岁，分为19个年龄组。19个年龄分组分别为：0~1岁、1~4岁、5~9岁、10~14岁……75~79岁、80~84岁、85岁及以上组。

3. 发病（死亡）率

发病（死亡）率又称为粗发病（死亡）率，是人口发病（死亡）情况的基本指标，反映了人群的疾病发病（死亡）水平。发病（死亡）率是一定期间内，某人群发生某疾病新病例（死亡）的频率，通常以十万分率表示，整数后保留小数点后两位。计算公式为：

$$\text{恶性肿瘤发病（死亡）率} = \frac{\text{某年某地恶性肿瘤新病例（死亡）数}}{\text{某年某地平均人口数}} \times 100\,000(1/10^5)$$

4. 性别年龄别发病（死亡）率

人口的性别年龄结构是影响癌症发病（死亡）水平的重要因素，性别年龄别发病（死亡）率是统计研究的重要指标，计算公式如下：

$$\text{某年龄组发病（死亡）率} = \frac{\text{某年龄组发病（死亡）人数}}{\text{同年龄组人口数}} \times 100\,000(1/10^5)$$

5. 年龄调整率（标准化率）

年龄是癌症发病率和死亡率的重要影响因素，因此在分析比较不同地区的发病（死亡）率或同一地区人群不同时期的发病（死亡）水平时，为消除人口年龄结构对发病（死亡）水平的影响，需要计算年龄标准化发病（死亡）率，

4.4 Common statistical indicators

4.4.1 Average annual population

The average annual population is the denominator of incidence (mortality) rates. We often use the arithmetic mean of the population at the beginning of the year and the end of the year as the approximate value of the annual average population. The formula is:

$$\text{Average annual population} = \frac{\text{Population at the beginning of the year} + \text{Population at the end of the year}}{2}$$

4.4.2 Sex and age-specific population

The sex and age-specific population is the population categorized by sex and age groups, and it can be calculated by interpolation. The age-specific population is grouped by age groups of 5 years as follows: <1 years, 1~4 years, 5~9 years, 10~14 years ... 75~79 years, 80~84 years and 85+ years.

4.4.3 Incidence (mortality) rate

Incidence (mortality) rate, also known as the crude incidence (mortality) rate, is a measure of the frequency of an event such as a new case of cancer (cancer death) occurring in a population over a period of time. The incidence is usually expressed as per 100,000 of the population and two decimal digits are retained after an integer. The formula is:

$$\text{The incidence(mortality)rate per 100,000} = \frac{\text{New case(cancer deaths)occuring during a given time period}}{\text{Population at risk during the same time period}} \times 100{,}000(1/10^5)$$

4.4.4 Sex-specific and age-specific incidence (mortality) rates

Sex and age are important factors that influence cancer incidence and mortality. Sex-specific and age-specific rates are important indicators of cancer statistics. The formula is:

$$\text{Age-specific incidence(mortality)rate per 100,000} = \frac{\text{Case in a specific incidence (mortality) age group}}{\text{Population in the age group}} \times 100{,}000(1/10^5)$$

4.4.5 Age-standardized rate or age-adjusted rate (ASR)

Standardization is necessary when comparing several populations with different age structures because age has a powerful influence on cancer incidence and mortality. ASR is a summary measure of the rate that a population would have if it had a

即指按照某一标准人口的年龄结构所计算的发病（死亡）率。本年报使用的中国标准人口是2000 年全国第五次人口普查的人口年龄构成，世界标准人口采用 Segi's 标准人口构成。具体人口构成详见表 2-3。

standard age structure. In this report, the population standards we used are Segi's population and the fifth Chinese national census of 2000 for the world and China respectively (Table 2-3).

表 2-3　标准人口构成

年龄组（岁）	中国人口构成（2000 年）	世界人口构成（Segi's）
0~	13 793 799	2 400
1~4	55 184 575	9 600
5~9	90 152 587	10 000
10~	125 396 633	9 000
15~	103 031 165	9 000
20~	94 573 174	8 000
25~	117 602 265	8 000
30~	127 314 298	6 000
35~	109 147 295	6 000
40~	81 242 945	6 000
45~	85 521 045	6 000
50~	63 304 200	5 000
55~	46 370 375	4 000
60~	41 703 848	4 000
65~	34 780 460	3 000
70~	25 574 149	2 000
75~	15 928 330	1 000
80~	7 989 158	500
85+	4 001 925	500
合计	1 242 612 226	100 000

年龄标化发病（死亡）率的计算（直接法）：

（1）计算年龄组发病（死亡）率。

（2）以各年龄组发病（死亡）率乘以相应的标准人口年龄构成百分比，得到相应的理论发病（死亡）率。

（3）将各年龄组的理论发病（死亡）率相加，即是年龄标化发病（死亡）率。

Calculating ASR incidence (mortality) (direct method):

1. Calculation of the incidence (mortality) rates in each age group.

2. The multiplying incidence (mortality) rate of each age group by the corresponding age group composition of the standard population is the theoretical incidence (mortality) rate.

3. The age-standardized incidence (mortality) rate is obtained by adding the theoretical incidence (mortality) rate in each age group.

$$标化发病(死亡)率 = \frac{\sum 标准人口年龄构成 \times 年龄别发病(死亡)率}{\sum 标准人口年龄构成} \times 100\,000(1/10^5)$$

6. 分类构成

癌症发病（死亡）构成百分比可以反映各类癌症对居民健康危害的情况。癌症发病（死亡）分类构成百分比的计算公式如下：

$$某癌症构成 = \frac{某癌症发病(死亡)人数}{总发病(死亡)人数} \times 100\%$$

7. 累积发病（死亡）率

累积发病（死亡）率是指某病在某一年龄阶段内的按年龄（岁）的发病（死亡）率进行累积的总指标。累积发病（死亡）率消除了年龄构成不同的影响，故不需要标准化便可以与不同地区直接进行比较。癌症一般是计算 0~74 岁的累积发病（死亡）率。计算公式为：

$$累积发病(死亡)率 = \sum 年龄组发病(死亡)率 \times 年龄组距 \times 100\%$$

8. 截缩发病（死亡）率

通常是截取 35~64 岁癌症高发年龄段计算，其标准人口常用世界人口年龄构成。癌症在 35 岁以前发生率较低，在 65 岁以后因其他疾病发生率高，干扰较大，采用 35~64 岁这一阶段的发病（死亡）率比较稳定（截缩率是标化率），便于进行率的比较。计算公式为：

$$截缩发病(死亡)率 = \frac{\sum 截缩段各年龄组发病(死亡)率 \times 各段标准年龄构成}{\sum 各段标准年龄构成} \times 100\,000\ (1/10^5)$$

$$\text{Age-standardized rate} = \frac{\sum \text{Standard population in the correspond age group} \times \text{Age-standardized rate}}{\sum \text{Standard population}} \times 100{,}000\ (1/10^5)$$

4.4.6 Proportions

Proportional distribution indicates the site-specific percentage level of incident cases (deaths) compared with total cases (deaths) recorded reflecting the hazards of various cancer types to human health. The formula is:

$$\text{Proportion of a certain type of cancer} = \frac{\text{Cases of a particular cancer}}{\text{Cases of all cancers}} \times 100\%$$

4.4.7 cumulative incideince (mortality) rate

A cumulative incidence or death rate indicates the probability of cancer onset between birth and a specific age. The rate can be compared without age standardization because it is not affected by age structures. Cancer generally shows cumulative rates at 0~74 years of age. The formula is:

$$\text{Cumulative incideince (mortality) rate} = \sum [(\text{Age-specific incidence (Cmortality) rate} \times \text{Width of the age group})] \times 100\%$$

4.4.8 Truncated incidence (mortality) rate

The truncated rate is the calculation of rates over the truncated age of 35~64 years generally for cancer using the WHO world standard population. The data are presented as truncated rates mainly because the accuracy of age-specific rates in the elderly may be much less certain and the rates in the younger age groups may below. The formula is:

$$\text{Truncated incidence (mortality) rate} = \frac{\sum \text{Truncated in a specific age group} \times \text{Standard proportion of the age group}}{\sum \text{Standard proportion}} \times 100{,}000\ (1/10^5)$$

第三章　数据质量评价

Chapter 3　Data quality evaluation

一、数据来源

《2023 年河南省肿瘤登记年报》纳入了 2020 年 55 个市、县登记处的肿瘤登记资料，分别来自郑州市城区、中牟县、巩义市、荥阳市、登封市，开封市祥符区，洛阳市城区、洛阳市孟津区、新安县、栾川县、嵩县、汝阳县、宜阳县、洛宁县、伊川县、洛阳市偃师区，平顶山市城区、鲁山县、郏县、舞钢市，林州市，鹤壁市城区、浚县、淇县、辉县市，焦作市城区，濮阳市华龙区、范县、濮阳县，许昌市魏都区、禹州市，漯河市城区、舞阳县、临颍县，三门峡市湖滨区、渑池县、三门峡市陕州区，南阳市宛城区、南阳市卧龙区、南召县、方城县、镇平县、内乡县、新野县、桐柏县，睢县、虞城县，信阳市浉河区、罗山县，周口市沈丘县、郸城县、项城市，驻马店市驿城区、西平县以及济源市。（表 3–1）

1. Data sources

Cancer Report for Henan Province in 2023 included cancer registration data in 2020 from 55 Cancer Registries in Henan Province, China, Which were from Zhengzhou City Areas, Zhongmu County, Gongyi City, Xingyang City, Dengfeng City, Kaifeng Xiangfu District, Luoyang Mengjin District, Xin'an County, Luanchuan County, Song County, Ruyang County, Yiyang County, Luoning County, Yichuan County, Luoyang Yanshi District, Pingdingshan City Areas, Lushan County, Jia County, Wugang City, Linzhou City, Hebi City Areas, Xun County, Qi County, Huixian City, Jiaozuo City Areas, Puyang Hualong District, Fan County, Puyang County, Xuchang Weidu District, Yuzhou City, Luohe City Areas, Wuyang County, Linying County, Sanmenxia Hubin District, Mianchi County, Sanmenxia Shanzhou District, Nanyang Wancheng District, Nanyang Wolong District, Nanzhao County, Fangcheng County, Zhenping County, Neixiang County, Xinye County, Tongbai County, Sui County, Yucheng County, Xinyang Shihe District, Luoshan County, Shenqiu County, Dancheng County, Xiangcheng City, Zhumadian Yicheng District, Xiping County, and Jiyuan City .（Table 3–1）

表 3–1　《2023 河南省肿瘤登记年报》纳入的地区

编号	地区	登记地区	地区类型	登记机构名称
1	郑州市	郑州市城区	城市地区	郑州市疾控中心
2	郑州市	中牟县	农村地区	中牟县疾控中心
3	郑州市	巩义市	农村地区	巩义市疾控中心
4	郑州市	荥阳市	农村地区	荥阳市疾控中心
5	郑州市	登封市	农村地区	登封市疾控中心
6	开封市	开封市祥符区	农村地区	祥符区疾控中心
7	洛阳市	洛阳市城区	城市地区	洛阳市疾控中心
8	洛阳市	洛阳市孟津区	农村地区	孟津区疾控中心
9	洛阳市	新安县	农村地区	新安县疾控中心
10	洛阳市	栾川县	农村地区	栾川县疾控中心
11	洛阳市	嵩县	农村地区	嵩县疾控中心
12	洛阳市	汝阳县	农村地区	汝阳县疾控中心

续表

编号	地区	登记地区	地区类型	登记机构名称
13	洛阳市	宜阳县	农村地区	宜阳县疾控中心
14	洛阳市	洛宁县	农村地区	洛宁县疾控中心
15	洛阳市	伊川县	农村地区	伊川县疾控中心
16	洛阳市	洛阳市偃师区	农村地区	偃师区疾控中心
17	平顶山市	平顶山市城区	城市地区	平顶山市疾控中心
18	平顶山市	鲁山县	农村地区	鲁山县疾控中心
19	平顶山市	郏县	农村地区	郏县疾控中心
20	平顶山市	舞钢市	农村地区	舞钢市疾控中心
21	安阳市	林州市	农村地区	林州市肿瘤医院
22	鹤壁市	鹤壁市城区	城市地区	鹤壁市人民医院
23	鹤壁市	浚县	农村地区	浚县疾控中心
24	鹤壁市	淇县	农村地区	淇县疾控中心
25	新乡市	辉县市	农村地区	辉县市疾控中心
26	焦作市	焦作市城区	城市地区	焦作市疾控中心
27	濮阳市	濮阳市华龙区	城市地区	华龙区疾控中心
28	濮阳市	范县	农村地区	范县疾控中心
29	濮阳市	濮阳县	农村地区	濮阳县疾控中心
30	许昌市	许昌市魏都区	城市地区	魏都区疾控中心
31	许昌市	禹州市	农村地区	禹州市疾控中心
32	漯河市	漯河市城区	城市地区	漯河市疾控中心
33	漯河市	舞阳县	农村地区	舞阳县疾控中心
34	漯河市	临颍县	农村地区	临颍县疾控中心
35	三门峡市	三门峡市湖滨区	城市地区	湖滨区疾控中心
36	三门峡市	渑池县	农村地区	渑池县疾控中心
37	三门峡市	三门峡市陕州区	农村地区	陕州区疾控中心
38	南阳市	南阳市城区	城市地区	宛城区疾控中心
39	南阳市	南召县	农村地区	南召县疾控中心
40	南阳市	方城县	农村地区	方城县疾控中心
41	南阳市	镇平县	农村地区	镇平县疾控中心
42	南阳市	内乡县	农村地区	内乡县疾控中心
43	南阳市	新野县	农村地区	新野县疾控中心
44	南阳市	桐柏县	农村地区	桐柏县疾控中心
45	商丘市	睢县	农村地区	睢县疾控中心
46	商丘市	虞城县	农村地区	虞城县疾控中心
47	信阳市	信阳市浉河区	城市地区	浉河区疾控中心
48	信阳市	罗山县	农村地区	罗山县疾控中心
49	周口市	沈丘县	农村地区	沈丘县疾控中心
50	周口市	郸城县	农村地区	郸城县疾控中心
51	周口市	项城市	农村地区	项城市疾控中心
52	驻马店市	驻马店市城区	城市地区	驿城区疾控中心
53	驻马店市	西平县	农村地区	西平县疾控中心
54	省直辖县级行政区划	济源市	城市地区	济源市疾控中心

二、有效覆盖人口数、发病数和死亡数

2020 年，纳入年报分析的登记地区人口为 43 145 743 人（其中，男性 22 034 819 人，女性 21 110 924 人），约占河南省 2020 年人口总数的 37.43%。其中城市地区为 12 291 881 人，占登记人口的 28.49%；农村地区为 30 853 862 人，占 71.51%。

2020 年，报告癌症新发病例数合计 120 694 例，其中：城市地区 36 690 例，占 30.4%；农村地区 84 004，占 69.6%。上报癌症死亡病例合计 70 338 例，其中：城市地区 19 697 例，占 28.00%；农村地区 50 641 例，占 72.00%。（表 3–2）

2. Population coverage, new cancer cases and cancer deaths

Population coverage of Cancer Registries in Henan Province was 43,145,743 (including 22,034,819 males and 21,110,924 females), accounting approximately for 37.43% of the provincial population in 2020, with 12,291,881(28.49%) in urban areas and 30,853,862 (71.51%) in rural areas.

A total of 120,694 new cancer cases were reported in 2020, among which 36,690 (30.40%) were from urban areas, and 84,004 (69.60%) were from rural areas. There were 70,338 new cancer deaths in 2020, with 19,697 (28.00%) in urban areas and 50,641 (72.00%) in rural areas. (Table 3–2)

表 3–2 2020 年河南省肿瘤登记地区有效覆盖人口数、发病数和死亡数

编号	登记地区	人口数	发病数	死亡数
1	郑州市城区	2 181 039	7 132	3 039
2	中牟县	510 361	1 469	667
3	巩义市	850 134	1 909	1 191
4	荥阳市	709 674	1 783	875
5	登封市	742 357	1 689	958
6	开封市祥符区	670 302	1 723	989
7	洛阳市城区	1 848 001	5 699	3 348
8	洛阳市孟津区	553 454	1 634	958
9	新安县	542 158	1 574	1 057
10	栾川县	360 259	952	615
11	嵩县	645 183	1 723	1 195
12	汝阳县	532 077	1 359	819
13	宜阳县	716 873	2 027	1 303
14	洛宁县	511 878	1 405	879
15	伊川县	935 470	2 192	1 367
16	洛阳市偃师区	636 564	1 758	1 112
17	平顶山市城区	923 724	2 891	1 407
18	鲁山县	961 279	2 246	1 371
19	郏县	644 260	1 467	1 035
20	舞钢市	330 419	993	443
21	林州市	1 132 122	3 883	2 455
22	鹤壁市城区	660 842	1 853	1 154
23	浚县	678 912	1 708	999
24	淇县	272 031	915	412
25	辉县市	912 127	2 229	1 440
26	焦作市城区	662 422	1 708	962
27	濮阳市华龙区	457 781	1 355	836

续表

编号	登记地区	人口数	发病数	死亡数
28	范县	588 856	1 619	884
29	濮阳县	1 140 815	3 716	1 769
30	许昌市魏都区	326 763	1 238	495
31	禹州市	1 336 585	3 564	2 286
32	漯河市城区	1 376 880	4 093	2 397
33	舞阳县	595 600	1 760	1 075
34	临颍县	589 805	2 055	1 234
35	三门峡市湖滨区	288 010	951	527
36	渑池县	356 364	834	539
37	三门峡市陕州区	350 239	799	529
38	南阳市宛城区	596 946	1 952	1 064
39	南阳市卧龙区	943 110	2 567	1 584
40	南召县	560 770	1 544	964
41	方城县	1 132 215	3 495	2 200
42	镇平县	916 956	2 530	1 740
43	内乡县	724 078	2 068	1 273
44	新野县	696 919	2 417	1 710
45	桐柏县	393 942	1 045	590
46	睢县	865 838	2 033	1 204
47	虞城县	1 149 885	2 987	1 845
48	信阳市浉河区	661 757	1 460	920
49	罗山县	765 147	1 985	1 176
50	沈丘县	1 202 226	3 247	1 941
51	郸城县	1 399 224	3 814	2 199
52	项城市	1 349 781	3 492	1 821
53	驻马店市驿城区	633 485	1 714	716
54	西平县	890 723	2 362	1 522
55	济源市	731 121	2 077	1 248
56	全省	43 145 743	120 694	70 338
57	城市地区	12 291 881	36 690	19 697
58	农村地区	30 853 862	84 004	50 641

三、肿瘤登记地区 2016~ 2020 年癌症发病率与死亡率稳定性评价

2009 年，卫生部在全国范围内启动了中央财政转移支付地方的肿瘤随访登记项目，河南省洛阳市、偃师市、禹州市、济源市、鲁山县、内乡县等地区先后被纳入国家肿瘤随访登记项目点。除了林州市开展肿瘤登记工作较早以外，河南省其他地区的登记处于 2008 年以后开始实施

3. Incidences and mortality of cancer in cancer registries, 2016~2020

The local cancer registries were initiated at central financing by the Ministry of Health in 2009, Luoyang City, Yanshi City, Yuzhou City, Jiyuan City, Lushan County and Neixiang County have been successively including into national cancer follow-up registration project. In addition to the earlier cancer registration in Linzhou City, other cancer registries in Henan Province carried out population-based

人群肿瘤登记。

2009年肿瘤登记地区覆盖人口只有600万，占当时全省人口的6%左右，由于覆盖人口较少，各项统计指标的代表性不能全面反映我省肿瘤的发病率、死亡率和生存状态。2010年新增加10个登记点，上报点数为16个，登记地区覆盖人口达1 300多万，占当年全省人口的15%左右。

2011年没有新增登记点，肿瘤登记工作重点是加强了肿瘤登记基础工作建设，包括制度建设与落实、机构建设、人员培训、岗位职责、人员配备及增强稳定性等，目的是建立起完善、及时、系统的肿瘤登记报告系统，能准确、及时反映我省城乡居民肿瘤发病率、死亡率和生存状态，并提供满足我省肿瘤防治需求的基本信息。2012~2013年增加鹤壁市、开封县（现为开封市祥符区）、睢县及郑州市为肿瘤登记点，肿瘤登记处总数达到20个。

近年来，河南省肿瘤登记年报覆盖人口的范围不断增大，2014年覆盖人口约为21 044 835人，占河南省当年人口总数的19.73%；2015年覆盖人口为23 421 609人，约占河南省当年人口总数的21.84%；2016年覆盖人口为29 300 098人，约占河南省当年人口总数的27.16%；2020年覆盖人口为43 145 743人，约占河南省当年人口总数的37.43%。

2016~2020年河南省肿瘤发病率分别是268.31/10万、264.00/10万、272.33/10万、279.71/10万和279.74/10万；死亡率分别是162.02/10万、166.23/10万、162.16/10万、162.14/10万和163.02/10万，发病率与死亡率基本处于稳定状态。随着登记系统和登记制度的不断完善，各个登记处登记质量明显提高，漏报减少。河南省各肿瘤登记地区2016~2020年恶性肿瘤发病率和死亡率数据见表3-3和表3-4。数据显示，各个登记处发病率及死亡率没有明显的波动，都呈现小幅上升，率的水平基本稳定，显示各个地方的登记质量在不断提高、漏报逐渐减少。肿瘤登记资料的可比性、完整性与有效性得到了保证。

cancer registration in 2008. In 2009, the registered population were only 6 million, covering about 6% of the province's population (6,000,000). Due to the low population coverage lead to the representativeness of various statistical indicators cannot sufficiently reflect the incidence, mortality, and survival conditions. Subsequently, 10 new registration sites added, and the number of cancer registries increased to 16. The registered areas covered more than 13 million individuals, accounting for about 15% of the provincial population, 2010.

There were no new cancer registries site established in 2011. Cancer registration focused on construction of system implementation, institution, personnel training, job responsibility, staff stabilization, etc, aiming at constructing a complete, timely and systematic cancer registration and reporting system with the capability of reflecting cancer incidence, mortality and survival Conditions of Henan residents to provide basic information for cancer control and research. In 2012 and 2013, new cancer registries of Hebi City, Kaifeng County, Sui County and Zhengzhou City developed, and the number of cancer registries increased to 20 in Henan Province.

The coverage of the Cancer Registration in Henan Province were increasing in recent years. In 2014, the population covered by Cancer Registration was 21,044,835, and accounted for 19.73% of the total population, and the number in 2015 and 2016 were 23,421,609(21.84%) and 29,300,098(27.16%), respectively. In 2020, the population covered was 43,145,743 which accounted for 37.43% of the total population.

During 2016 to 2020, cancer incidences in Henan Province were 268.31 per 100,000 population, 264.00 per 100,000 population, 272.33 per 100,000 population, 279.71 per 100,000 population, and 279.74 per 100,000 population, respectively, and the mortality were 162.02 per 100,000 population, 166.23 per 100,000 population, 162.16 per 100,000 population, 162.14 per 100,000 population,and 163.02 per 100,000 population which were relatively stable. With the construction of registration system and regularities, data quality improved greatly, under-reporting has decreased. Table 3-3, Table 3-4 showed the changes in cancer incidence and mortality each year since cancer registration had been carried out. From the statistical data, the incidence and mortality rates kept stable relatively and the cases increased slightly, which reflected an increasing trend of data quality and a decreasing trend of case omissions. The comparability, completeness and validity of cancer registration data are basically guaranteed.

表 3-3　河南省各肿瘤登记地区 2016~ 2020 年恶性肿瘤发病率（1/10 万）

编号	登记地区	2020 年	2019 年	2018 年	2017 年	2016 年
1	全省	279.74	279.71	272.33	264.00	268.31
2	城市地区	298.49	292.70	287.83	269.43	276.82
3	农村地区	272.26	275.00	266.64	262.41	266.09
4	濮阳市华龙区	295.99	295.31	363.95	307.21	350.55
5	巩义市	224.55	—	235.73	228.48	335.54
6	林州市	342.98	349.37	334.41	307.01	305.19
7	南阳市卧龙区	272.18	268.95	269.21	267.74	303.95
8	洛阳市孟津区	295.24	294.05	296.00	289.49	292.19
9	虞城县	259.77	246.25	217.86	242.88	287.81
10	洛阳市城区	308.39	301.51	316.06	289.25	285.56
11	济源市	284.08	284.47	285.17	270.19	284.21
12	三门峡市湖滨区	330.20	330.99	339.28	308.22	280.10
13	鹤壁市城区	280.40	273.04	273.67	277.39	279.57
14	沈丘县	270.08	281.13	274.28	279.93	278.60
15	内乡县	285.60	281.77	277.37	265.26	275.65
16	嵩县	267.06	276.23	275.19	253.76	272.18
17	方城县	308.69	233.74	231.42	248.03	270.64
18	漯河市城区	297.27	278.19	256.38	267.41	270.48
19	辉县市	244.37	261.44	266.45	271.44	267.73
20	濮阳县	325.73	325.20	290.78	275.23	267.41
21	洛阳市偃师区	276.17	272.52	301.56	286.24	264.17
22	宜阳县	282.76	274.84	279.97	269.45	262.25
23	新安县	290.32	293.47	283.65	255.70	256.69
24	睢县	234.80	—	262.77	245.73	247.99
25	信阳市浉河区	220.62	249.24	242.48	223.94	246.60
26	西平县	265.18	269.30	264.18	254.56	242.40
27	洛宁县	274.48	266.38	262.62	254.96	239.59
28	罗山县	259.43	288.20	249.88	277.39	237.42
29	栾川县	264.25	270.85	273.52	247.97	236.09
30	郸城县	272.58	275.09	251.41	263.29	235.45
31	鲁山县	233.65	232.64	249.90	251.65	234.49
32	禹州市	266.65	254.45	261.46	251.17	233.37
33	平顶山市城区	312.97	297.59	296.53	232.42	231.66
34	汝阳县	255.41	256.88	234.86	242.18	229.43
35	开封市祥符区	257.05	254.35	247.34	229.00	228.28
36	伊川县	234.32	223.65	222.12	226.89	220.92
37	南召县	275.34	288.54	314.83	266.00	—
38	舞阳县	295.50	256.40	239.07	261.62	—
39	郏县	227.70	274.12	274.89	237.48	—
40	郑州市城区	327.00	321.53	284.88	—	—
41	范县	274.94	265.81	284.77	—	—

续表

编号	登记地区	2020 年	2019 年	2018 年	2017 年	2016 年
42	许昌市魏都区	378.87	344.44	—	—	—
43	项城市	258.71	313.09	—	—	—
44	舞钢市	300.53	292.13	—	—	—
45	临颍县	348.42	270.41	—	—	—
46	浚县	251.58	247.28	—	—	—
47	新野县	346.81	—	—	—	—
48	淇县	336.36	—	—	—	—
49	南阳市宛城区	327.00	—	—	—	—
50	中牟县	287.84	—	—	—	—
51	镇平县	275.91	—	—	—	—
52	驻马店市驿城区	270.57	—	—	—	—
53	桐柏县	265.27	—	—	—	—
54	焦作市城区	257.84	—	—	—	—
55	荥阳市	251.24	—	—	—	—
56	渑池县	234.03	—	—	—	—
57	三门峡市陕州区	228.13	—	—	—	—
58	登封市	227.52	—	—	—	—

表 3-4 河南省各肿瘤登记地区 2016~ 2020 年恶性肿瘤死亡率（1/10 万）

编号	登记地区	2020 年	2019 年	2018 年	2017 年	2016 年
1	全省	163.02	162.14	162.16	166.23	162.02
2	城市地区	160.24	160.57	157.48	161.82	157.44
3	农村地区	164.13	162.71	163.88	167.52	163.21
4	林州市	216.85	206.93	202.54	199.31	195.63
5	鲁山县	142.62	136.05	189.42	200.05	194.77
6	漯河市城区	174.09	168.45	172.19	170.23	192.42
7	罗山县	153.70	158.64	127.83	174.32	190.33
8	内乡县	175.81	181.09	183.23	181.79	189.00
9	沈丘县	161.45	182.17	182.21	171.26	187.06
10	禹州市	171.03	163.25	179.10	201.73	183.92
11	洛阳市城区	181.17	166.77	168.44	179.47	178.90
12	方城县	194.31	142.16	138.37	150.08	178.08
13	嵩县	185.22	178.08	184.48	174.01	176.75
14	鹤壁市城区	174.63	178.42	173.83	175.57	174.96
15	辉县市	157.87	155.14	160.87	183.76	173.83
16	济源市	170.70	167.83	175.32	168.21	173.16
17	三门峡市湖滨区	182.98	191.75	178.95	184.86	169.55
18	洛阳市孟津区	173.09	174.87	171.06	172.32	168.88
19	虞城县	160.45	136.73	152.28	142.98	165.73
20	西平县	170.87	175.82	172.89	162.74	163.83
21	郸城县	157.16	176.66	172.64	178.25	161.22

续表

编号	登记地区	2020 年	2019 年	2018 年	2017 年	2016 年
22	睢县	139.06	—	127.37	153.77	160.39
23	宜阳县	181.76	180.01	178.67	173.39	157.15
24	濮阳市华龙区	182.62	161.10	167.86	145.56	154.51
25	栾川县	170.71	165.30	174.85	159.85	153.34
26	新安县	194.96	182.06	176.75	163.02	151.60
27	开封市祥符区	147.55	126.80	125.17	136.44	151.36
28	洛阳市偃师区	174.69	164.39	167.06	164.31	149.49
29	汝阳县	153.93	146.01	131.58	147.17	148.81
30	南阳市卧龙区	167.95	162.20	159.62	162.73	147.29
31	濮阳县	155.06	158.68	149.15	162.28	143.66
32	洛宁县	171.72	164.29	165.85	153.61	142.52
33	伊川县	146.13	154.94	155.07	146.68	133.26
34	信阳市浉河区	139.02	135.67	127.64	130.22	125.70
35	巩义市	140.10	—	142.53	127.12	125.66
36	平顶山市城区	152.32	158.34	145.09	130.88	122.00
37	舞阳县	180.49	170.99	155.87	167.26	—
38	南召县	171.91	172.62	159.22	159.60	—
39	郏县	160.65	170.90	161.27	138.77	—
40	范县	150.12	167.91	140.85	—	—
41	郑州市城区	139.34	144.89	126.13	—	—
42	项城市	134.91	163.84	—	—	—
43	浚县	147.15	161.48	—	—	—
44	临颍县	209.22	158.23	—	—	—
45	舞钢市	134.07	148.52	—	—	—
46	许昌市魏都区	151.49	138.68	—	—	—
47	新野县	245.37	—	—	—	—
48	镇平县	189.76	—	—	—	—
49	南阳市宛城区	178.24	—	—	—	—
50	淇县	151.45	—	—	—	—
51	渑池县	151.25	—	—	—	—
52	三门峡市陕州区	151.04	—	—	—	—
53	桐柏县	149.77	—	—	—	—
54	焦作市城区	145.22	—	—	—	—
55	中牟县	130.69	—	—	—	—
56	登封市	129.05	—	—	—	—
57	荥阳市	123.30	—	—	—	—
58	驻马店市驿城区	113.03	—	—	—	—

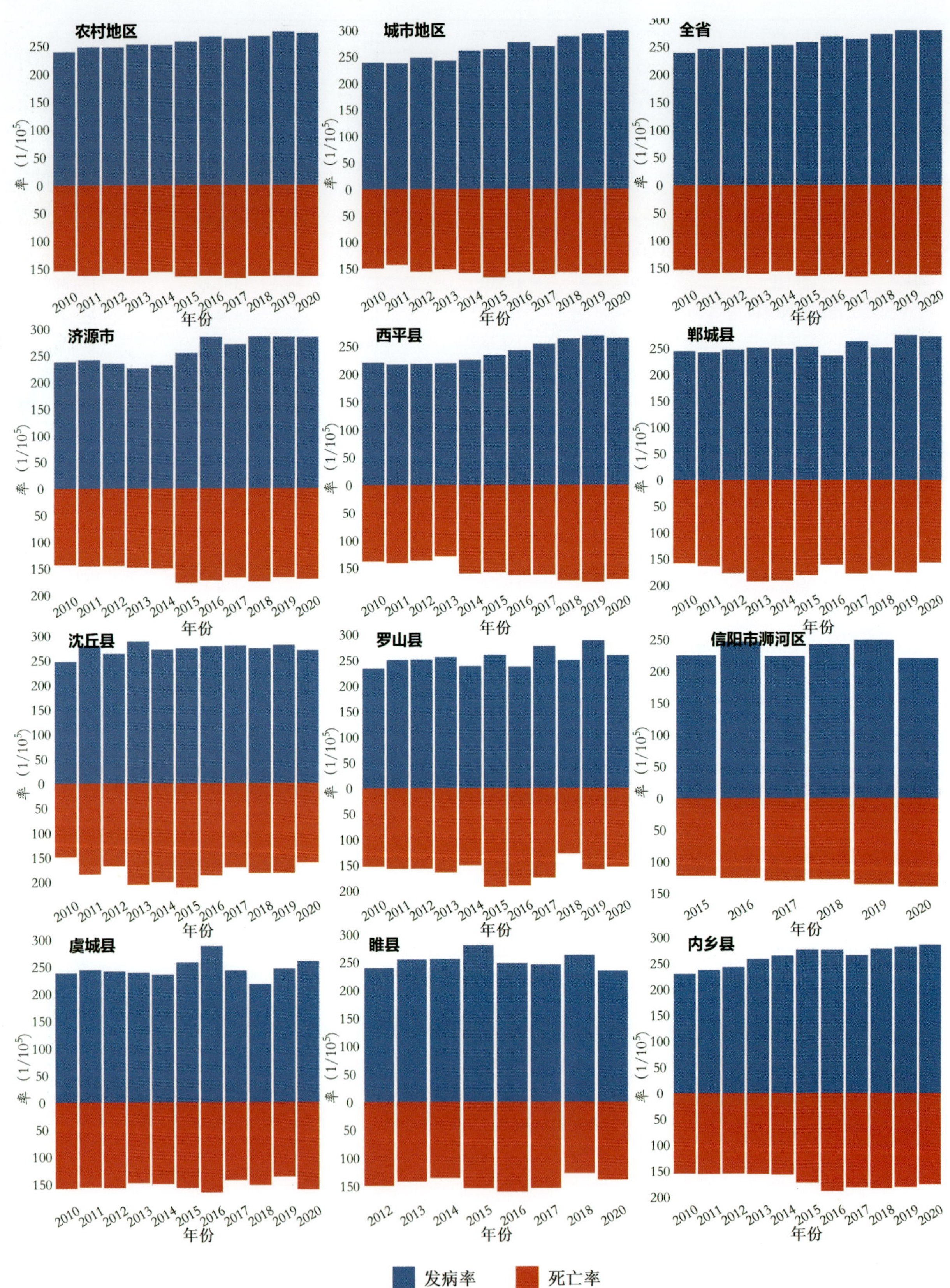

图 3-1　河南省各地近年肿瘤发病和死亡情况（1）

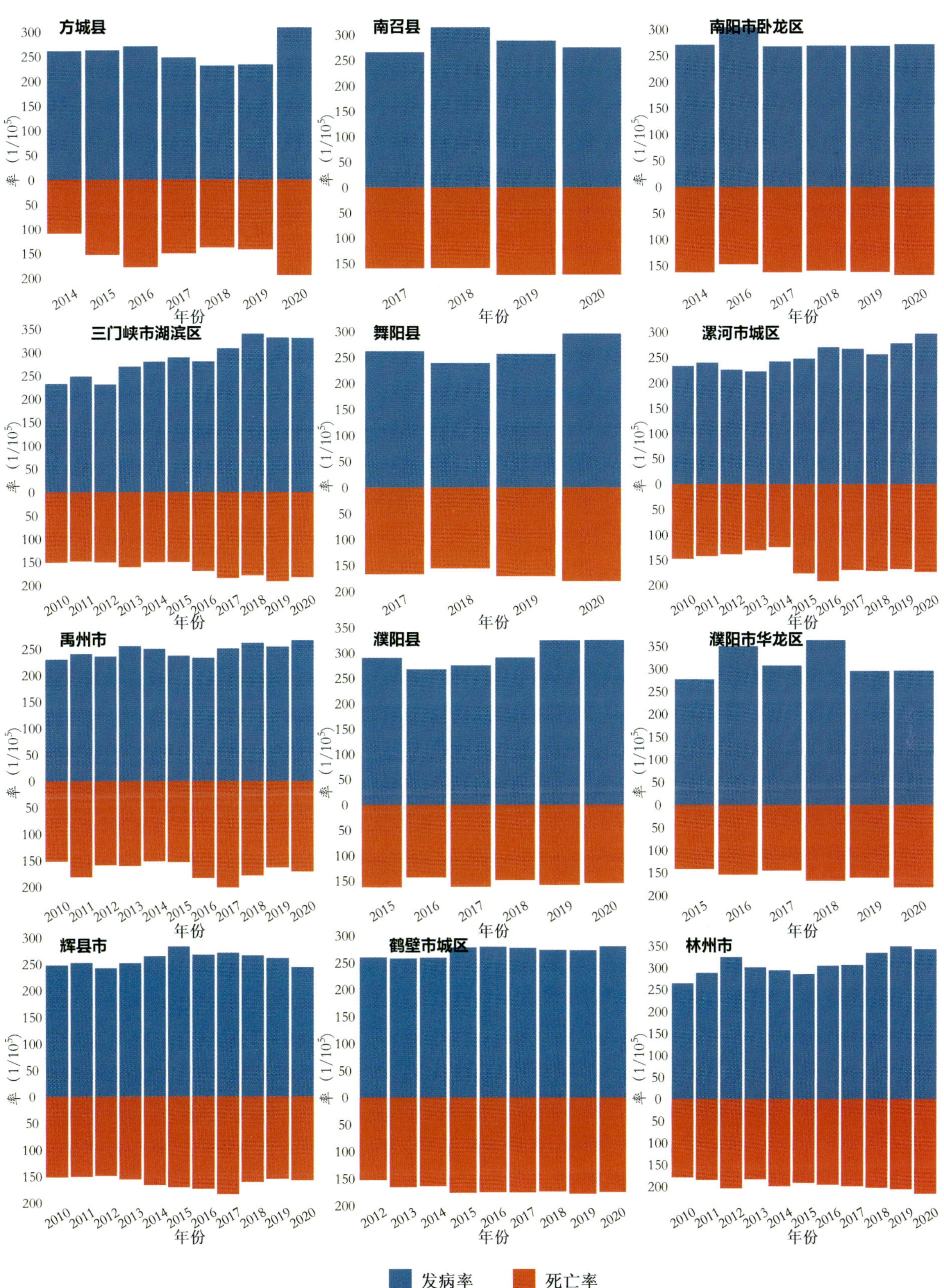

图 3-1　河南省各地近年肿瘤发病和死亡情况（2）

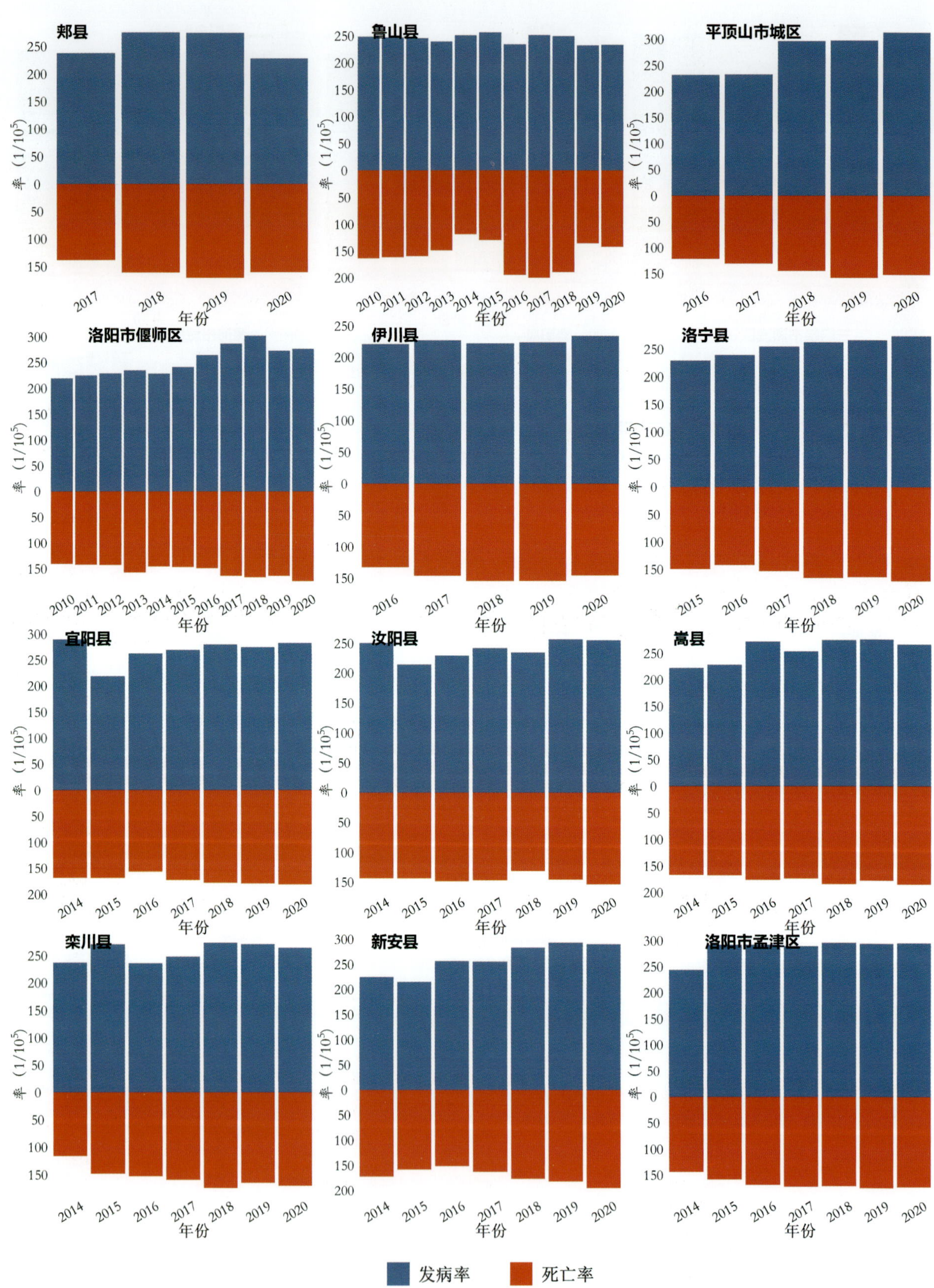

图 3-1 河南省各地近年肿瘤发病和死亡情况（3）

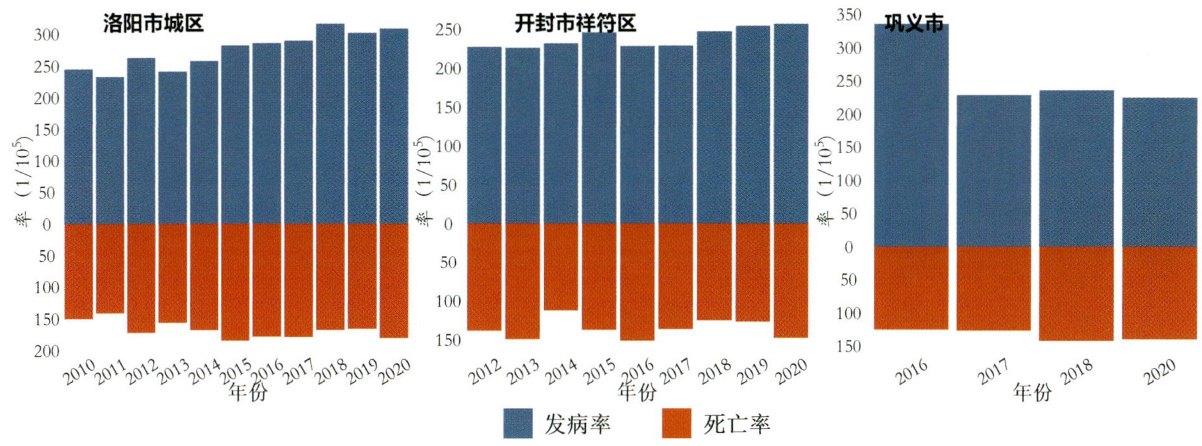

图 3-1　河南省各地近年肿瘤发病和死亡情况（4）

四、肿瘤登记地区数据质量评价

死亡发病比（M/I）、病理诊断比例（MV%）、只有死亡医学证明书比例（DCO%）是评价肿瘤登记资料完整性和有效性的重要指标。河南省肿瘤登记地区合计 M/I 为 0.58，MV% 为 74.39%，DCO% 为 1.56%。河南省城市登记地区合计 M/I 为 0.54，MV% 为 77.02%，DCO% 为 1.54%；河南省农村登记地区合计 M/I 为 0.6，MV% 为 73.24%，DCO% 为 1.57%。（表 3-5、表 3-6）

4. Data quality evaluation of cancer registries

The incidence mortality ratio (M/I), proportion of cases pathological diagnosed (MV%), and proportion of cases have only death certificate (DCO%) are important indicators that evaluating the completeness and effectiveness of cancer registration data. In Henan Cancer Registration areas, the M/I was 0.58, MV% was74.39%, and DCO% was 1.56%. In urban registration areas, they were 0.54, 77.02%, and 1.54%, respectively; In rural areas, the numbers were 0.6, 73.24%, and 1.57%, respectively. (Table 3-5, Table 3-6)

表 3-5　2020 年河南省各肿瘤登记处主要质控指标

编号	登记地区	人口数	MV%	DCO%	M/I
1	郑州市城区	2 181 039	79.51	0.86	0.43
2	中牟县	510 361	80.39	0.00	0.45
3	巩义市	850 134	55.37	3.77	0.62
4	荥阳市	709 674	80.87	0.00	0.49
5	登封市	742 357	77.68	0.06	0.57
6	开封市祥符区	670 302	80.03	0.41	0.57
7	洛阳市城区	1 848 001	76.29	1.47	0.59
8	洛阳市孟津区	553 454	71.97	1.84	0.59
9	新安县	542 158	71.92	0.44	0.67
10	栾川县	360 259	76.16	1.05	0.65
11	嵩县	645 183	71.33	0.87	0.69
12	汝阳县	532 077	72.70	0.88	0.60
13	宜阳县	716 873	69.56	0.84	0.64
14	洛宁县	511 878	74.38	0.14	0.63
15	伊川县	935 470	75.36	0.36	0.62
16	洛阳市偃师区	636 564	78.50	0.28	0.63
17	平顶山市城区	923 724	84.99	1.49	0.49
18	鲁山县	961 279	84.86	0.13	0.61
19	郏县	644 260	67.89	0.27	0.71
20	舞钢市	330 419	66.06	1.21	0.45

续表

编号	登记地区	人口数	MV%	DCO%	M/I
21	林州市	1 132 122	82.87	1.57	0.63
22	鹤壁市城区	660 842	69.78	2.43	0.62
23	浚县	678 912	80.33	0.12	0.58
24	淇县	272 031	69.95	0.11	0.45
25	辉县市	912 127	79.54	0.09	0.65
26	焦作市城区	662 422	87.76	4.33	0.56
27	濮阳市华龙区	457 781	80.52	0.66	0.62
28	范县	588 856	66.34	0.99	0.55
29	濮阳县	1 140 815	73.95	0.11	0.48
30	许昌市魏都区	326 763	80.05	2.99	0.40
31	禹州市	1 336 585	68.80	0.93	0.64
32	漯河市城区	1 376 880	72.69	3.84	0.59
33	舞阳县	595 600	75.51	3.52	0.61
34	临颍县	589 805	76.25	4.67	0.60
35	三门峡市湖滨区	288 010	74.55	0.42	0.55
36	渑池县	356 364	79.14	0.00	0.65
37	三门峡市陕州区	350 239	77.60	0.13	0.66
38	南阳市宛城区	596 946	66.14	1.79	0.55
39	南阳市卧龙区	943 110	71.06	0.08	0.62
40	南召县	560 770	75.13	1.23	0.62
41	方城县	1 132 215	78.51	3.66	0.63
42	镇平县	916 956	72.09	1.54	0.69
43	内乡县	724 078	73.55	1.74	0.62
44	新野县	696 919	89.66	0.54	0.71
45	桐柏县	393 942	62.97	13.40	0.56
46	睢县	865 838	58.14	0.00	0.59
47	虞城县	1 149 885	66.45	0.00	0.62
48	信阳市浉河区	661 757	88.56	0.00	0.63
49	罗山县	765 147	68.16	0.05	0.59
50	沈丘县	1 202 226	68.46	9.39	0.60
51	郸城县	1 399 224	65.10	2.18	0.58
52	项城市	1 349 781	69.04	0.03	0.52
53	驻马店市驿城区	633 485	78.70	0.76	0.42
54	西平县	890 723	71.72	2.84	0.64
55	济源市	731 121	70.73	0.10	0.60
56	全省	43 145 743	74.39	1.56	0.58
57	城市地区	12 291 881	77.02	1.54	0.54
58	农村地区	30 853 862	73.24	1.57	0.60

表 3–6　2020 年河南省肿瘤登记数据质量评价指标

部位	ICD–10 编码范围	全省			城市			农村		
		MV%	DCO%	M/I	MV%	DCO%	M/I	MV%	DCO%	M/I
唇	C00	74.23	1.03	0.45	71.43	0.00	0.29	75.81	1.61	0.55
舌	C01–C02	78.66	0.40	0.44	76.29	1.03	0.44	80.13	0.00	0.44
口	C03–C06	80.74	0.99	0.41	82.39	1.41	0.45	79.85	0.76	0.38
唾液腺	C07–C08	67.87	0.00	0.30	75.36	0.00	0.36	65.38	0.00	0.28
扁桃体	C09	77.55	0.00	0.47	88.24	0.00	0.53	71.88	0.00	0.44
其他的口咽	C10	60.23	1.14	0.57	63.33	0.00	0.47	58.62	1.72	0.62
鼻咽	C11	73.44	1.67	0.53	83.18	2.80	0.61	70.10	1.29	0.51
喉咽	C12–C13	79.31	0.69	0.52	84.51	0.00	0.39	74.32	1.35	0.64
咽，部位不明	C14	68.70	1.74	0.71	78.57	7.14	0.71	65.52	0.00	0.71
食管	C15	79.24	1.32	0.78	77.66	2.13	0.84	79.61	1.13	0.77

续表

部位	ICD-10编码范围	全省合计			城市			农村		
		MV%	DCO%	M/I	MV%	DCO%	M/I	MV%	DCO%	M/I
胃	C16	78.52	2.05	0.78	78.37	1.82	0.77	78.57	2.12	0.79
小肠	C17	76.31	1.99	0.56	80.46	1.72	0.59	74.41	2.11	0.55
结肠	C18	83.31	0.72	0.48	80.99	0.97	0.47	84.82	0.55	0.48
直肠	C19–C20	81.68	1.10	0.46	81.29	1.43	0.44	81.86	0.94	0.47
肛门	C21	76.97	1.82	1.03	66.67	6.67	0.53	79.26	0.74	1.14
肝脏	C22	48.83	3.39	0.87	52.04	3.23	0.90	47.71	3.45	0.87
胆囊及其他	C23–C24	63.49	0.95	0.80	63.32	0.80	0.80	63.57	1.02	0.80
胰腺	C25	54.47	2.15	0.84	56.41	2.11	0.87	53.37	2.17	0.83
鼻、鼻窦及其他	C30–C31	69.12	1.96	0.52	71.93	0.00	0.40	68.03	2.72	0.57
喉	C32	77.18	1.31	0.51	81.25	1.44	0.53	75.06	1.25	0.51
气管、支气管、肺	C33–C34	67.20	2.47	0.75	71.96	2.52	0.73	65.22	2.45	0.76
其他的胸腔器官	C37–C38	65.81	1.03	0.59	73.45	0.00	0.65	62.68	1.45	0.57
骨	C40–C41	57.56	1.79	0.61	63.46	1.92	0.59	55.77	1.75	0.61
皮肤的黑色素瘤	C43	100.00	0.00	0.45	100.00	0.00	0.31	100.00	0.00	0.56
其他的皮肤	C44	86.08	0.92	0.40	87.14	1.07	0.33	85.57	0.85	0.44
间皮瘤	C45	100.00	0.00	0.84	100.00	0.00	1.70	100.00	0.00	0.58
卡波西肉瘤	C46	100.00	0.00	0.33	0.00	0.00		100.00	0.00	0.33
周围神经、其他结缔组织、软组织	C47;C49	72.64	0.00	0.36	79.51	0.00	0.35	68.60	0.00	0.36
乳房	C50	86.40	0.38	0.21	86.84	0.56	0.20	86.16	0.28	0.21
外阴	C51	82.56	0.00	0.38	87.50	0.00	0.53	79.63	0.00	0.30
阴道	C52	81.82	0.00	0.40	86.36	0.00	0.41	80.00	0.00	0.40
子宫颈	C53	87.28	0.63	0.29	86.62	0.57	0.29	87.54	0.65	0.28
子宫体	C54	87.61	0.22	0.18	87.61	0.00	0.18	87.61	0.31	0.19
子宫，部位不明	C55	70.66	0.28	0.36	69.77	0.00	0.33	70.94	0.38	0.38
卵巢	C56	82.83	0.53	0.41	84.83	0.40	0.51	82.00	0.58	0.37
女性其他的生殖器	C57	69.03	0.88	0.24	76.47	2.94	0.24	65.82	0.00	0.24
胎盘	C58	81.82	0.00	0.00	100.00	0.00	0.00	71.43	0.00	0.00
阴茎	C60	85.81	1.35	0.28	92.31	0.00	0.28	83.49	1.83	0.28
前列腺	C61	78.40	0.95	0.44	79.39	1.19	0.45	77.66	0.78	0.44
睾丸	C62	72.37	0.00	0.29	94.12	0.00	0.24	66.10	0.00	0.31
男性其他的生殖器	C63	75.00	0.00	0.46	92.31	0.00	0.46	54.55	0.00	0.45
肾	C64	75.05	0.58	0.40	83.19	0.18	0.38	70.36	0.81	0.42
肾盂	C65	74.24	0.76	0.56	91.49	0.00	0.53	64.71	1.18	0.58
输尿管	C66	76.41	1.03	0.55	73.08	1.28	0.63	78.63	0.85	0.50
膀胱	C67	77.56	0.68	0.39	81.25	0.85	0.35	75.41	0.58	0.42
其他的泌尿器官	C68	62.50	0.00	0.53	63.64	0.00	0.64	61.90	0.00	0.48
眼	C69	67.95	1.28	0.40	72.73	4.55	0.41	66.07	0.00	0.39
脑、神经系统	C70–C72	50.14	2.45	0.65	59.42	3.19	0.67	47.00	2.20	0.64
甲状腺	C73	91.89	0.07	0.04	93.39	0.08	0.03	90.54	0.05	0.06
肾上腺	C74	50.81	4.03	0.60	62.22	2.22	0.40	44.30	5.06	0.71
其他的内分泌腺	C75	67.07	0.00	0.37	74.19	0.00	0.29	62.75	0.00	0.41
霍奇金病	C81	100.00	0.00	0.53	100.00	0.00	0.45	100.00	0.00	0.57
非霍奇金淋巴瘤	C82–C85;C96	96.97	0.00	0.52	95.71	0.00	0.48	97.75	0.00	0.54
免疫增生性疾病	C88	100.00	0.00	0.18	100.00	0.00	0.00	100.00	0.00	0.20
多发性骨髓瘤	C90	98.56	0.00	0.61	99.08	0.00	0.52	98.24	0.00	0.66
淋巴样白血病	C91	100.00	0.00	0.57	100.00	0.00	0.55	100.00	0.00	0.59
髓样白血病	C92–C94	100.00	0.00	0.51	100.00	0.00	0.55	100.00	0.00	0.49
白血病，未特指	C95	92.17	1.04	0.66	87.17	2.65	0.79	93.93	0.47	0.61
其他的或未指明部位	O&U	44.69	3.29	0.59	38.09	3.95	0.61	48.46	2.91	0.59
骨髓增殖性疾病	MPD	100.00	0.00	0.32	100.00	0.00	0.27	100.00	0.00	0.36
骨髓增生异常综合征	MDS	100.00	0.00	5.61	100.00	0.00	19.33	100.00	0.00	3.55
合计	ALL	74.39	1.56	0.58	77.02	1.54	0.54	73.24	1.57	0.60
除 C44 外的其他部位	ALL but C44	74.31	1.56	0.58	76.95	1.55	0.54	73.15	1.57	0.60

第四章　河南省肿瘤登记地区肿瘤发病与死亡情况

Chapter 4　Incidence and mortality in Henan cancer registries

2023 年，河南省肿瘤登记年报共纳入 55 个市、县肿瘤登记处提交的 2020 年的肿瘤发病和死亡数据。全省各登记处数据合并得到的河南省肿瘤发病与死亡的统计指标，基本反映了我省人群恶性肿瘤的流行情况。

In 2023, cancer registration data from a total of 55 cancer registries in 2020 were included and analyzed in Henan cancer registration annual report. The data can basically reflect cancer prevalence in Henan Province, China.

一、河南省肿瘤登记地区覆盖人口

2023 年，纳入年报分析的登记地区人口为 43 145 743 人（其中，男性 22 034 819 人，女性 21 110 924 人），约占河南省 2020 年人口总数的 37.43%。其中城市地区为 12 291 881 人，占登记人口的 28.49%；农村地区为 30 853 862 人，占 71.51%。（表 4–1，图 4–1）

1. Population coverage in Henan cancer registries

The population in Henan Province cancer registration areas in 2020 was 43,145,743 (22,034,819 males and 21,110,924 females), accounting for 37.43% of the provincial population in 2020, with 12,291,881 (28.49%) in urban areas and 30,853,862 (71.51%) in rural areas. (Table 4–1, Figure 4–1)

表 4–1　2020 年河南省肿瘤登记地区覆盖人口

年龄组	全省			城市			农村		
	合计	男性	女性	合计	男性	女性	合计	男性	女性
合计	43 145 743	22 034 819	21 110 924	12 291 881	6 132 973	6 158 908	30 853 862	15 901 846	14 952 016
	447 664	233 403	214 261	127 846	66 710	61 136	319 818	166 693	153 125
1–	2 171 757	1 150 904	1 020 853	607 290	317 837	289 453	1 564 467	833 067	731 400
5–	2 894 483	1 540 543	1 353 940	767 430	403 248	364 182	2 127 053	1 137 295	989 758
10–	3 023 439	1 613 098	1 410 341	775 749	411 639	364 110	2 247 690	1 201 459	1 046 231
15–	2 802 137	1 479 302	1 322 835	737 854	383 982	353 872	2 064 283	1 095 320	968 963
20–	2 975 282	1 543 746	1 431 536	796 631	401 797	394 834	2 178 651	1 141 949	1 036 702
25–	3 253 541	1 664 835	1 588 706	929 425	451 663	477 762	2 324 116	1 213 172	1 110 944
30–	3 476 391	1 768 811	1 707 580	973 057	471 083	501 974	2 503 334	1 297 728	1 205 606

续表

年龄组	全省			城市			农村		
	合计	男性	女性	合计	男性	女性	合计	男性	女性
35–	3 136 991	1 604 218	1 532 773	935 633	455 681	479 952	2 201 358	1 148 537	1 052 821
40–	3 150 385	1 601 490	1 548 895	969 403	479 741	489 662	2 180 982	1 121 749	1 059 233
45–	3 321 437	1 682 129	1 639 308	1 036 568	516 873	519 695	2 284 869	1 165 256	1 119 613
50–	3 085 591	1 568 310	1 517 281	892 989	449 310	443 679	2 192 602	1 119 000	1 073 602
55–	2 586 094	1 298 826	1 287 268	759 424	377 735	381 689	1 826 670	921 091	905 579
60–	2 074 419	1 043 184	1 031 235	586 539	290 407	296 132	1 487 880	752 777	735 103
65–	1 766 383	873 924	892 459	491 930	238 350	253 580	1 274 453	635 574	638 879
70–	1 243 451	596 387	647 064	363 253	170 560	192 693	880 198	425 827	454 371
75–	831 960	388 045	443 915	257 608	117 008	140 600	574 352	271 037	303 315
80–	527 466	236 739	290 727	173 618	83 390	90 228	353 848	153 349	200 499
85–	376 872	146 925	229 947	109 634	45 959	63 675	267 238	100 966	166 272

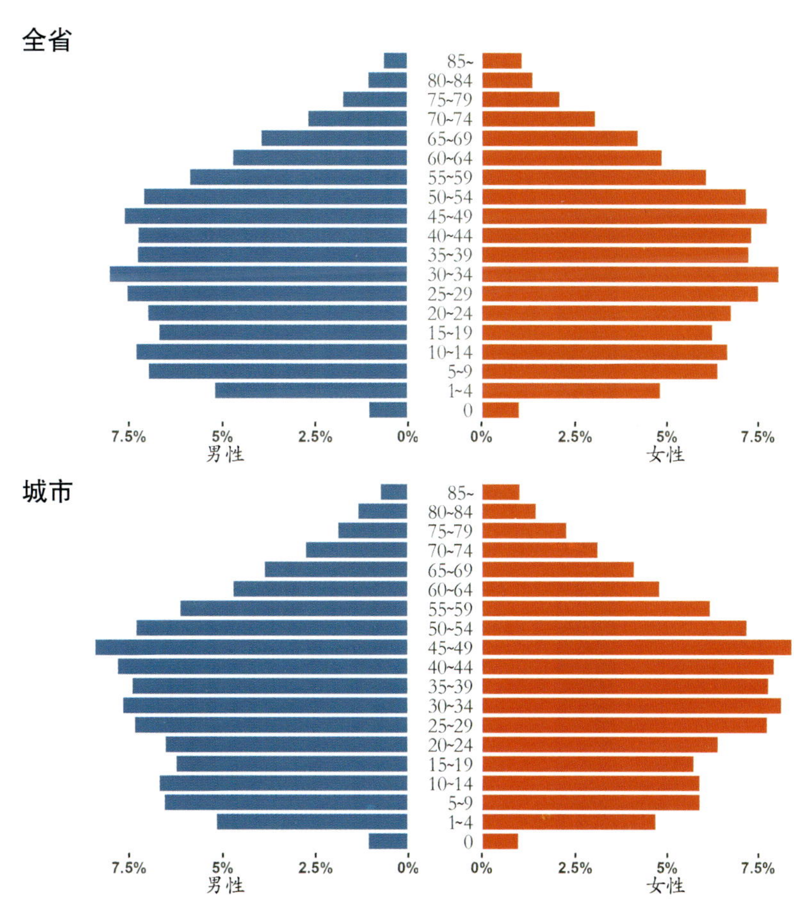

图 4–1　河南省肿瘤登记地区人口金字塔

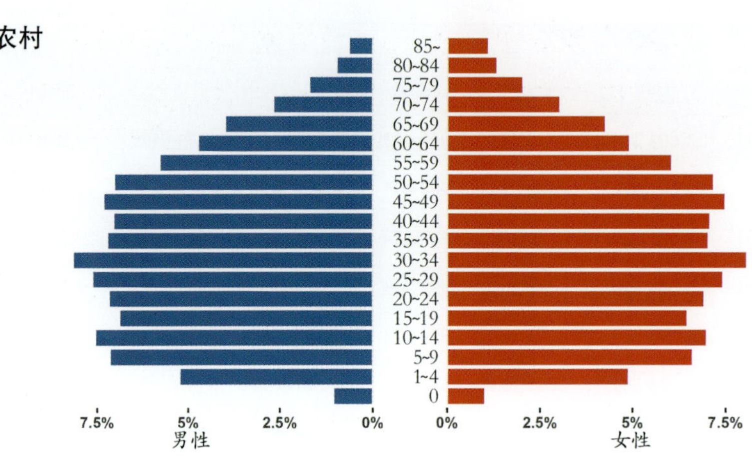

图 4-1 河南省肿瘤登记地区人口金字塔（续）

二、恶性肿瘤发病（ICD-10：C00-C96）

（一）恶性肿瘤发病情况

河南省肿瘤登记地区 2020 年报告癌症新发病例数合计为 120 694 例，其中男性 61 820 例，女性 58 874 例。城市地区上报 36 690 例，占 30.4%；农村地区上报 84 004 例，占 69.6%。

河南省肿瘤登记地区恶性肿瘤发病率为 279.74/10 万（男性 280.56/10 万，女性 278.88/10 万），中标率 200.69/10 万，世标率 196.11 /10 万，累积率（0~74 岁）22.93%。城市地区发病率为 298.49 /10 万（男性 298.14/10 万，女性 298.84/10 万），中标率 208.46/10 万，世标率 203.25/10 万，累积率（0~74 岁）为 23.46%；农村地区发病率为 272.26/10 万（男性 273.77/10 万，女性 270.66/10 万），中标率 197.40/10 万，世标率 193.08/10 万，累积率（0~74 岁）为 22.71%。城市与农村相比，城市地区男性、女性及男女合计中标发病率均高于农村地区。（表 4-2）

2. Cancer incidences （ICD-10：C00-C96）

2.1 Cancer incidences of all sites

The total number of new cancer cases reported in the Henan cancer registration areas in 2020 was 120,694 (Male: 61,820, Female: 58,874) among which 36,690 (30.4%) were from urban areas and 84,004 (69.6%) from rural areas.

The incidence rate of all cancer sites was 279.74 per 100,000 population (280.56 per 100,000 population for males and 278.88 per 100,000 population for females). The ASR China was 200.69 per 100,000 population and ASR World was 196.11 per 100,000 population. The cumulative incidence (0~74 years old) for both sexes was 22.93%.

The incidence rate of all cancers in urban areas was 298.49 per 100,000 population (298.14 per 100,000 population for males and 298.84 per 100,000 population for females). The ASR China was 208.46 per 100,000 population and ASR World was 203.25 per 100,000 population. The cumulative rate (0~74 years old) for both sexes was 23.46%.

The incidence rate of all cancer sites in rural areas was 272.26 per 100,000 population (273.77 per 100,000 population for males and 270.66 per 100,000 population for females). The ASR China was 197.40 per 100,000 population and ASR World was 193.08 per 100,000 population. The cumulative incidence (0~74 years old) for both sexes was 22.71%. In urban areas, the crude incidence rates for both genders of all cancer sites were higher than those in rural areas. (Table 4-2)

表 4-2 2020 年河南省肿瘤登记地区恶性肿瘤（C00-C96）发病主要指标

地区	性别	发病数	发病率（1/10^5）	中标率（1/10^5）	世标率（1/10^5）	累积率 0～74(%)
全省	合计	120 694	279.74	200.69	196.11	22.93
	男性	61 820	280.56	204.39	203.26	24.69
	女性	58 874	278.88	200.08	191.92	21.39
城市地区	合计	36 690	298.49	208.46	203.25	23.46
	男性	18 285	298.14	207.60	207.19	25.00
	女性	18 405	298.84	211.39	201.65	22.17
农村地区	合计	84 004	272.26	197.40	193.08	22.71
	男性	43 535	273.77	203.15	201.68	24.57
	女性	40 469	270.66	195.06	187.61	21.05

（二）恶性肿瘤年龄别发病率

河南省肿瘤登记地区 2020 年年龄别发病率在 0~29 岁年龄段发病率处于较低水平，低于 50/10 万，30 岁及以上年龄组发病率明显升高，在 85 岁年龄组时达到最高峰。男、女性年龄别发病率的年龄变化趋势基本相同，二者均在 30 岁年龄组开始快速上升，并均在 85 岁年龄组时达到峰值。

对比性别间的年龄别发病率可以看出，15~54 岁女性的发病率高于男性，55 岁以后则发生逆转，男性的发病率明显高于女性，城市和农村登记地区男、女性的年龄别发病率也呈现基本一致的变化趋势。

城乡间的年龄别发病率比较显示，70 岁以下大部分年龄组城市地区年龄别发病率略高于农村地区，70 岁及以上各年龄组城市地区的发病率明显高于农村地区；男性和女性的年龄别发病率的分布特征基本一致。（表 4-3，图 4-2）

2.2 Age-specific cancer incidence of all sites

The age-specific cancer incidence rate of all sites in Henan cancer registration areas were low at 0~29 age group. It increased dramatically after 30 years old, reaching the peak at the age group of 85+. The age-specific cancer incidence rate for males was similar to that for females, they all increase sharply since 30 years old, and reached the peak at 85 years old.

When comparing the age-specific cancer incidence rates between males and females, they were lower for males than for females at the age groups of 15 to 54, while obviously higher for males than those for females after 55 years old. This characteristic was seen in both urban areas and rural areas.

When compare the age-specific incidence rates between the urban areas and the rural areas, the age-specific rates in urban areas were slightly higher than those in rural areas before 70 years old and reversely, they were obviously higher in urban areas than in rural areas after 70 years old. There were similar trends in both males and females. (Table 4-3, Figure 4-2)

表 4-3　2020 年河南省肿瘤登记地区恶性肿瘤年龄别发病率（1/10 万）

年龄组	全省			城市			农村		
	合计	男性	女性	合计	男性	女性	合计	男性	女性
合计	279.74	280.56	278.88	298.49	298.14	298.84	272.26	273.77	270.66
0–	8.27	7.71	8.87	10.95	6.00	16.36	7.19	8.40	5.88
1–	11.88	13.29	10.29	13.17	17.62	8.29	11.38	11.64	11.07
5–	10.16	10.19	10.12	10.42	8.18	12.91	10.06	10.90	9.09
10–	9.92	10.17	9.64	9.54	9.96	9.06	10.05	10.24	9.84
15–	12.95	12.51	13.46	11.11	11.98	10.17	13.61	12.69	14.65
20–	18.96	13.41	24.94	15.94	13.94	17.98	20.06	13.22	27.59
25–	35.71	21.56	50.54	37.01	21.48	51.70	35.20	21.60	50.05
30–	72.58	43.48	102.72	89.82	54.13	123.31	65.87	39.61	94.14
35–	92.64	52.11	135.05	113.19	65.84	158.14	83.90	46.67	124.52
40–	143.19	88.42	199.82	172.68	102.35	241.60	130.08	82.46	180.51
45–	246.07	170.44	323.67	259.90	166.97	352.32	239.79	171.98	310.38
50–	389.97	314.10	468.40	396.31	308.25	485.49	387.39	316.44	461.34
55–	517.77	494.83	540.91	557.92	543.50	572.19	501.08	474.87	527.73
60–	673.10	761.71	583.48	736.52	818.16	656.46	648.10	739.93	554.07
65–	1 067.55	1 268.07	871.19	1 030.43	1 246.07	827.75	1 081.88	1 276.33	888.43
70–	1 284.65	1 664.52	934.53	1 237.43	1 612.92	905.07	1 304.14	1 685.19	947.02
75–	1 367.97	1 756.50	1 028.35	1 251.13	1 577.67	979.37	1 420.38	1 833.70	1 051.05
80–	1 539.63	1 948.14	1 206.97	1 639.23	1 946.28	1 355.46	1 490.75	1 949.15	1 140.16
85–	1 561.27	2 009.87	1 274.64	1 695.64	2 260.71	1 287.79	1 506.15	1 895.69	1 269.61

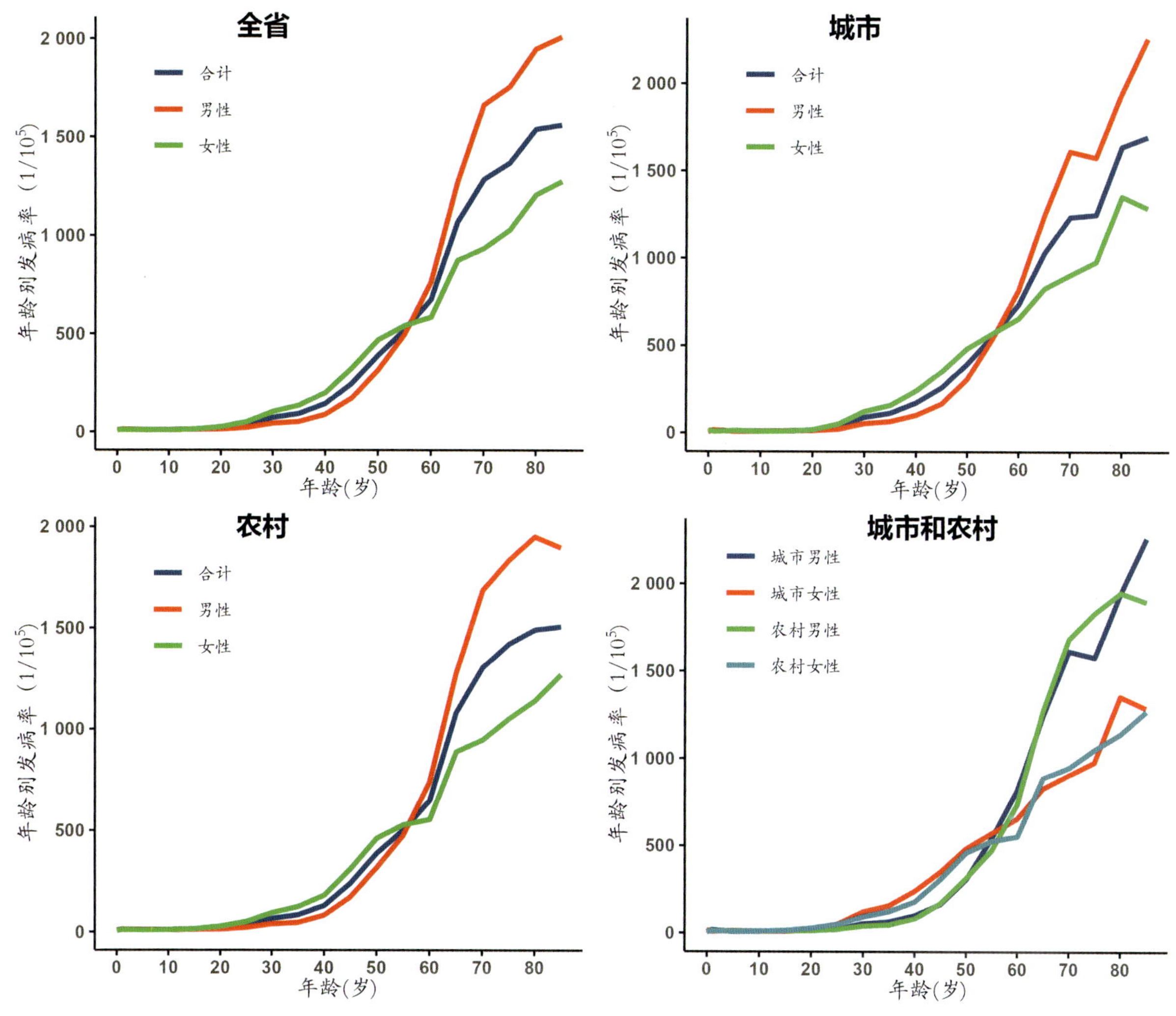

图 4-2 河南省肿瘤登记地区恶性肿瘤年龄别发病率

（三）河南省前 10 位恶性肿瘤发病情况

2020 年，河南省肿瘤登记地区恶性肿瘤发病第 1 位的是肺癌，其次为乳腺癌、胃癌、食管癌和肝癌，前 10 位恶性肿瘤占全部恶性肿瘤的 78.06%。男性恶性肿瘤发病第 1 位的是肺癌，其次为胃癌、肝癌、食管癌和结直肠癌，男性前 10 位恶性肿瘤占全部恶性肿瘤的 84.06 %；女性恶性肿瘤发病第 1 位的是乳腺癌，其次为肺癌、甲状腺癌、食管癌和子宫颈癌，女性前 10 位恶性肿瘤占全部恶性肿瘤的 81.59 %。（表 4-4，图 4-3）

2.3 Incidence of the top 10 most common cancers

In Henan cancer registration areas in 2020, Trachea, Bronchus & Lung cancer was the most common cancer, followed by cancers of Breast, Stomach, Esophagus and Liver. The 10 most common cancers accounted for 78.06% of all cancers. For males, Trachea, Bronchus & Lung cancer was the most common cancer followed by cancers of Stomach, Liver, Esophagus and Conlon,Rectum & Anus. The 10 most common cancers accounted for 84.06% of all cancers in males. For females, Breast cancer was the most common cancer followed by cancers of Trachea, Bronchus & Lung, Thyroid Gland, Esophagus and Cervix Uteri. The 10 most common cancers accounted for 81.59% of all cancers in females. (Table 4–4, Figure 4–3)

表 4-4 2020 年河南省肿瘤登记地区前 10 位恶性肿瘤发病情况

顺序	合计				男性				女性			
	癌种	发病率 (1/10^5)	构成 (%)	中标率 (1/10^5)	癌种	发病率 (1/10^5)	构成 (%)	中标率 (1/10^5)	癌种	发病率 (1/10^5)	构成 (%)	中标率 (1/10^5)
1	肺癌 (C33–C34)	54.23	19.39	36.31	肺癌 (C33–C34)	71.15	25.36	50.17	乳腺癌 (C50)	48.62	17.44	38.26
2	乳腺癌 (C50)	48.62	8.50	38.26	胃癌 (C16)	41.51	14.80	29.37	肺癌 (C33–C34)	36.56	13.11	23.39
3	胃癌 (C16)	30.35	10.85	20.34	肝癌 (C22)	32.87	11.71	24.17	甲状腺癌 (C73)	27.64	9.91	24.23
4	食管癌 (C15)	27.07	9.68	17.68	食管癌 (C15)	32.85	11.71	22.95	食管癌 (C15)	21.03	7.54	12.71
5	肝癌 (C22)	24.44	8.74	17.03	结直肠癌 (C18–C21)	22.65	8.07	16.53	子宫颈癌 (C53)	21.01	7.53	16.38
6	结直肠癌 (C18–C21)	21.07	7.53	14.56	甲状腺癌 (C73)	8.16	2.91	7.51	结直肠癌 (C18–C21)	19.43	6.97	12.69
7	子宫颈癌 (C53)	21.01	3.67	16.38	前列腺癌 (C61)	8.09	2.88	5.50	胃癌 (C16)	18.70	6.70	11.84
8	甲状腺癌 (C73)	17.69	6.32	15.76	膀胱癌 (C67)	6.76	2.41	4.74	肝癌 (C22)	15.65	5.61	9.95
9	子宫体癌 (C54)	10.86	1.90	7.96	脑癌 (C70–C72)	6.39	2.28	5.23	子宫体癌 (C54)	10.86	3.89	7.96
10	前列腺癌 (C61)	8.09	1.48	5.50	肾及泌尿系统不明癌（C64–66，C68）	5.43	1.93	4.08	卵巢癌 (C56)	8.06	2.89	6.39

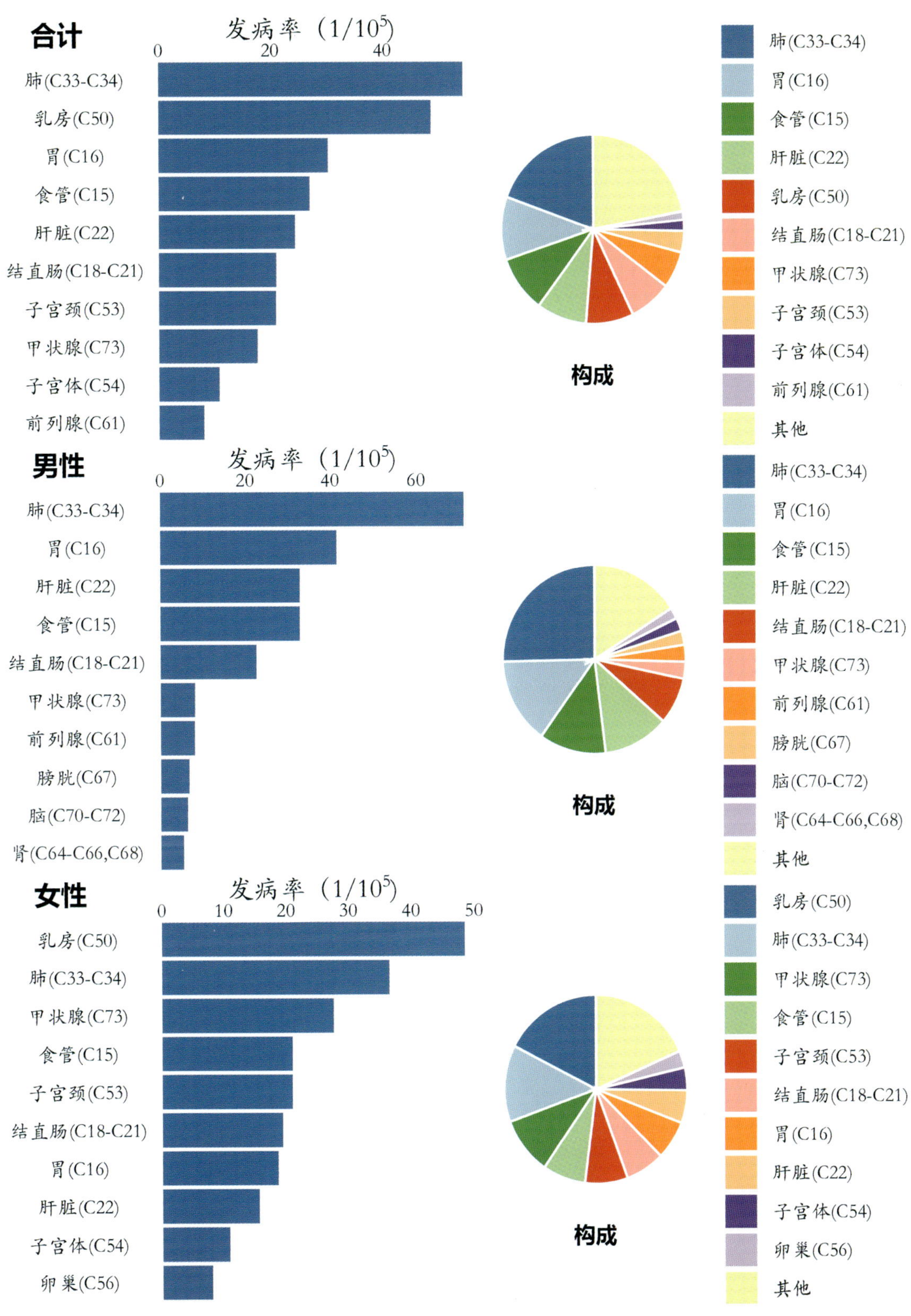

图 4-3 2020 年河南省肿瘤登记地区前 10 位恶性肿瘤发病率及发病构成

（四）河南省城市登记地区前 10 位恶性肿瘤发病情况

2020 年，河南省城市登记地区恶性肿瘤发病第 1 位的是乳腺癌，其次为肺癌、甲状腺癌、结直肠癌和胃癌，前 10 位恶性肿瘤占全部恶性肿瘤的 76.32%；男性恶性肿瘤发病第 1 位的是肺癌，其次为胃癌、肝癌、结直肠癌和食管癌，男性前 10 位恶性肿瘤占全部恶性肿瘤的 82.06%；女性恶性肿瘤发病第 1 位的是乳腺癌，其次为甲状腺癌、肺癌、结直肠癌和子宫颈癌，女性前 10 位恶性肿瘤占全部恶性肿瘤的 81.24 %。（表 4–5，图 4–4）

2.4 Incidence of the top 10 most common cancers in Henan urban areas

In Henan urban cancer registration areas in 2020, Breast cancer was the most common cancer, followed by cancers of Trachea, Bronchus & Lung, Thyroid Gland, Conlon, Rectum & Anus and Stomach. The 10 most common cancers accounted for 76.32% of all cancers. For males, Trachea, Bronchus & Lung cancer was the most common cancer followed by cancers of Stomach, Liver, Conlon, Rectum & Anus and Esophagus. The 10 most common cancers accounted for 82.06% of all cancers in males. For females, Breast cancer was the most common cancer followed by cancers of Thyroid Gland, Trachea, Bronchus & Lung, Conlon,Rectum & Anus and Cervix Uteri. The 10 most common cancers accounted for 81.24% of all cancers in females. (Table 4–5, Figure 4–4)

表 4–5　2020 年河南省城市肿瘤登记地区前 10 位恶性肿瘤发病情况

顺序	合计				男性				女性			
	癌种	发病率 ($1/10^5$)	构成 (%)	中标率 ($1/10^5$)	癌种	发病率 ($1/10^5$)	构成 (%)	中标率 ($1/10^5$)	癌种	发病率 ($1/10^5$)	构成 (%)	中标率 ($1/10^5$)
1	乳腺癌 (C50)	58.00	9.74	43.59	肺癌 (C33–C34)	73.03	24.50	48.86	乳腺癌 (C50)	58.00	19.41	43.59
2	肺癌 (C33–C34)	55.82	18.70	36.22	胃癌 (C16)	36.52	12.25	24.82	甲状腺癌 (C73)	43.86	14.68	37.58
3	甲状腺癌 (C73)	29.40	9.85	25.81	肝癌 (C22)	31.57	10.59	22.05	肺癌 (C33–C34)	38.68	12.94	24.71
4	结直肠癌 (C18–C21)	26.16	8.77	17.12	结直肠癌 (C18–C21)	29.15	9.78	19.87	结直肠癌 (C18–C21)	23.19	7.76	14.58
5	胃癌 (C16)	25.43	8.52	16.55	食管癌 (C15)	23.41	7.85	15.56	子宫颈癌 (C53)	19.91	6.66	14.98
6	肝癌 (C22)	22.15	7.42	14.81	甲状腺癌 (C73)	14.89	4.99	13.69	胃癌 (C16)	14.39	4.81	8.91
7	子宫颈癌 (C53)	19.91	3.34	14.98	前列腺癌 (C61)	12.34	4.14	7.69	肝癌 (C22)	12.78	4.28	7.87
8	食管癌 (C15)	17.99	6.03	11.31	膀胱癌 (C67)	9.16	3.07	5.99	食管癌 (C15)	12.58	4.21	7.33
9	前列腺癌 (C61)	12.34	2.06	7.69	肾及泌尿系统不明癌（C64–C66，C68）	7.30	2.45	5.20	子宫体癌 (C54)	11.27	3.77	8.04
10	子宫体癌 (C54)	11.27	1.89	8.04	恶性淋巴瘤 (C81–C85)	7.27	2.44	5.30	卵巢癌 (C56)	8.13	2.72	6.08

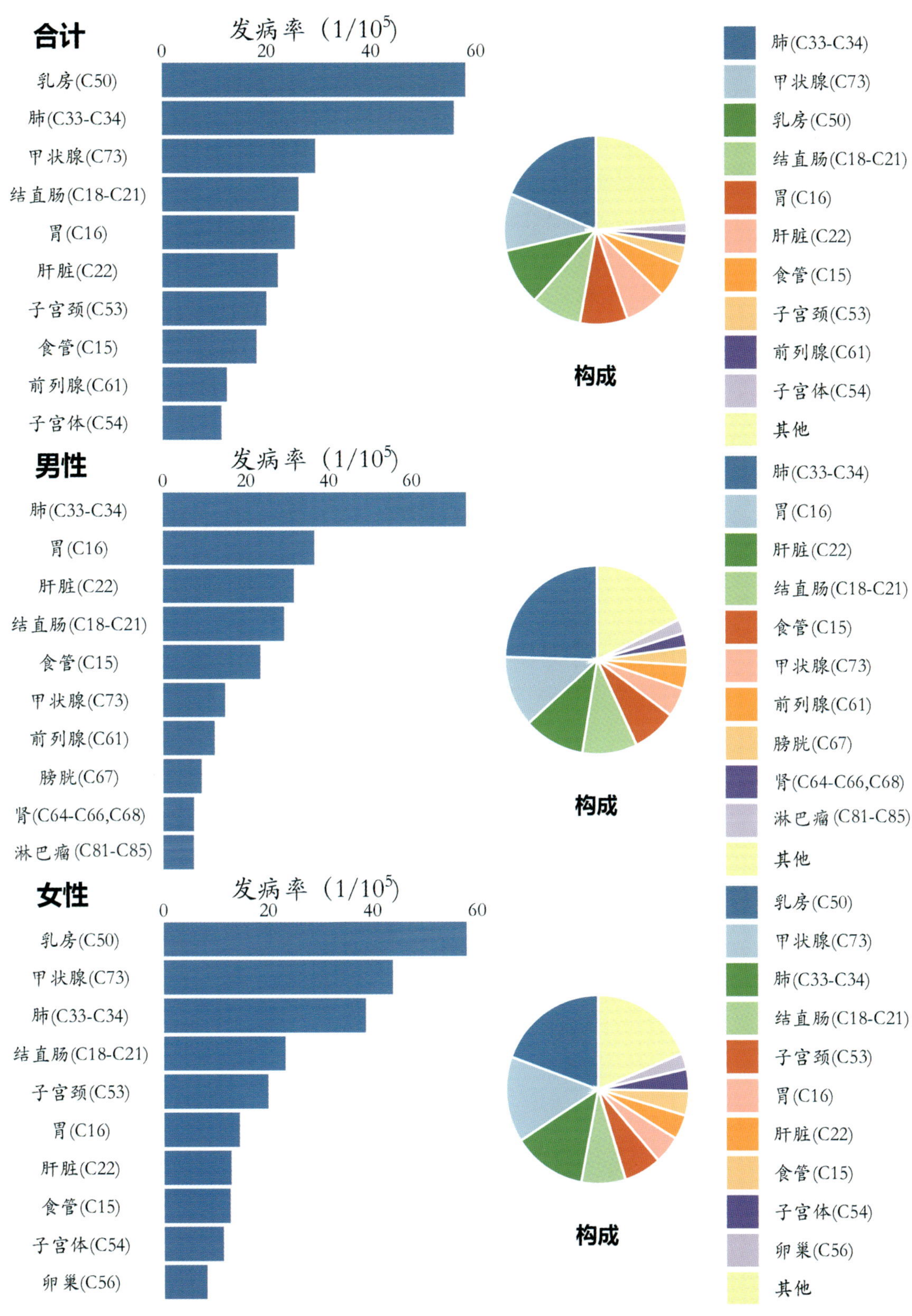

图 4-4 2020 年河南省城市登记地区前 10 位恶性肿瘤发病率及发病构成

（五）河南省农村登记地区前 10 位恶性肿瘤发病情况

2020 年，河南省农村肿瘤登记地区恶性肿瘤发病第 1 位的是肺癌，其次为乳腺癌、胃癌、食管癌和肝癌，前 10 位恶性肿瘤占全部恶性肿瘤的 79.02%；男性恶性肿瘤发病第 1 位是肺癌，其次为胃癌、食管癌、肝癌和结直肠癌，男性前 10 位恶性肿瘤占全部恶性肿瘤的 85.11 %；女性恶性肿瘤发病第 1 位是乳腺癌，其次为肺癌、食管癌、子宫颈癌和甲状腺癌，女性前 10 位恶性肿瘤占全部恶性肿瘤的 81.77 %。（表 4–6，图 4–5）

2.5 Incidence of the top 10 most common cancers in Henan rural areas

In Henan rural cancer registration areas in 2020, Trachea, Bronchus & Lung cancer was the most common cancer followed by cancers of Breast, Stomach, Esophagus and Liver. The 10 most common cancers accounted for 79.02% of all cancers. For males, Trachea, Bronchus & Lung cancer was the most common cancer followed by cancers of Stomach, Esophagus, Liver and Conlon,Rectum & Anus. The 10 most common cancers accounted for 85.11% of all cancers in males. For females, Breast cancer was the most common cancer followed by cancers of Trachea, Bronchus & Lung, Esophagus, Cervix Uteri and Thyroid Gland. The 10 most common cancers accounted for 81.77% of all cancers. (Table 4–6, Figure 4–5)

表 4–6 2020 年河南省农村登记地区前 10 位恶性肿瘤发病情况

顺序	合计				男性				女性			
	癌种	发病率 ($1/10^5$)	构成 (%)	中标率 ($1/10^5$)	癌种	发病率 ($1/10^5$)	构成 (%)	中标率 ($1/10^5$)	癌种	发病率 ($1/10^5$)	构成 (%)	中标率 ($1/10^5$)
1	肺癌 (C33–C34)	53.59	19.68	36.37	肺癌 (C33–C34)	70.43	25.72	50.75	乳腺癌 (C50)	44.76	16.54	35.96
2	乳腺癌 (C50)	44.76	7.97	35.96	胃癌 (C16)	43.44	15.87	31.29	肺癌 (C33–C34)	35.69	13.19	22.82
3	胃癌 (C16)	32.31	11.87	21.94	食管癌 (C15)	36.49	13.33	26.01	食管癌 (C15)	24.51	9.05	14.98
4	食管癌 (C15)	30.68	11.27	20.33	肝癌 (C22)	33.37	12.19	25.03	子宫颈癌 (C53)	21.46	7.93	16.99
5	肝癌 (C22)	25.35	9.31	17.96	结直肠癌 (C18–C21)	20.14	7.36	15.11	甲状腺癌 (C73)	20.97	7.75	18.40
6	子宫颈癌 (C53)	21.46	3.82	16.99	脑癌 (C70–C72)	6.60	2.41	5.48	胃癌 (C16)	20.47	7.56	13.08
7	结直肠癌 (C18–C21)	19.04	6.99	13.47	前列腺癌 (C61)	6.45	2.35	4.56	结直肠癌 (C18–C21)	17.88	6.61	11.88
8	甲状腺癌 (C73)	13.03	4.78	11.57	膀胱癌 (C67)	5.84	2.13	4.22	肝癌 (C22)	16.83	6.22	10.84
9	子宫体癌 (C54)	10.69	1.90	7.94	甲状腺癌 (C73)	5.56	2.03	5.07	子宫体癌 (C54)	10.69	3.95	7.94
10	卵巢癌 (C56)	8.03	1.43	6.52	肾及泌尿系统不明癌（C64–C66, C68）	4.70	1.72	3.63	卵巢癌 (C56)	8.03	2.97	6.52

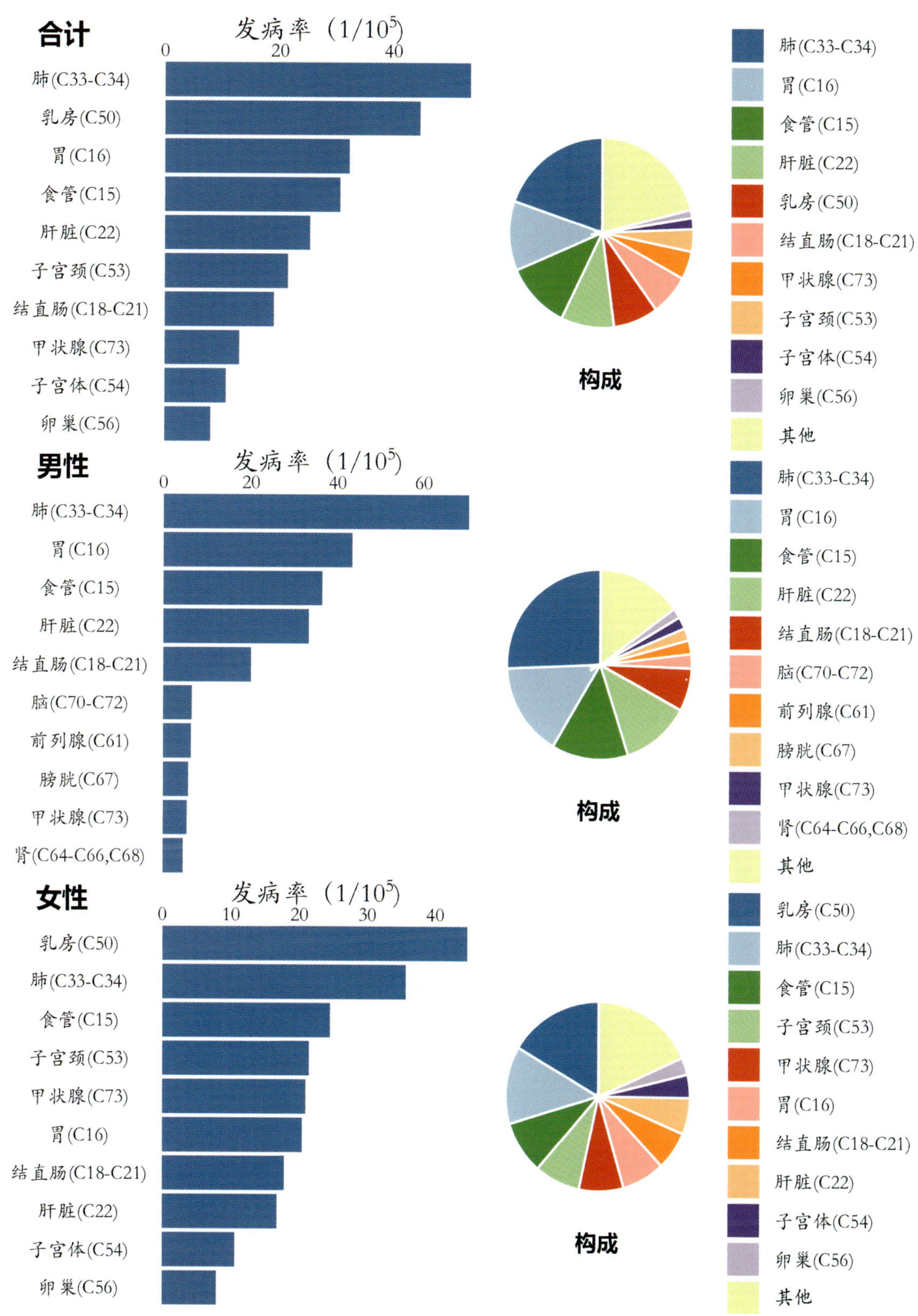

图 4-5 2020 年河南省农村登记地区前 10 位恶性肿瘤发病率及发病构成

三、恶性肿瘤死亡（ICD-10：C00–C96）

（一）恶性肿瘤死亡情况

2020 年，河南省肿瘤登记地区报告恶性肿瘤死亡病例数为 70 338 例（男性 43 276 例，女性 27 062 例），其中：城市地区恶性肿瘤死亡病例数为 19 697 例，占肿瘤登记地区全部的 28%；农村地区恶性肿瘤死亡病例数为 50 641 例，占肿瘤登记地区全部的 72%。

2020 年，河南省肿瘤登记地区恶性肿瘤死亡率为 163.02/10 万（男性 196.40/10 万，女性 128.19/10 万），中标率为 106.43/10 万，世标率为 106.68 /10 万，累积率（0~74 岁）12.12%。城市地区恶性肿瘤死亡率为 160.24 /10 万（男性 197.10/10 万，女性 123.54/10 万），中标率为 100.12/10 万，世标率 99.36/10 万，累积率（0~74 岁）为 11.06%；农村地区恶性肿瘤死亡率为 164.13/10 万（男性 196.13/10 万，女性 130.10/10 万），中标率为 109.03/10 万，世标率为 109.71/10 万，累积率（0~74 岁）为 12.55%。城市与农村相比，城市地区的男性和女性恶性肿瘤死亡率、中标率、世标率和累积率均低于农村地区。（表 4–7）

3. Cancer mortality（ICD–10:C00–C96）

3.1 Mortality of all cancer sites

The total number of cancer death reported in the Henan cancer registration areas in 2020 was 70,338 (Male: 43,276, Female: 27,062) with 19 697 (28%) were from urban areas and 50 641 (72%) from rural areas.

The mortality rate of all cancer sites was 163.02 per 100,000 population (196.40 per 100,000 population for males and 128.19 per 100,000 population for females). The ASR China was 106.43 per 100,000 population and ASR World was 106.68 per 100,000 population. The cumulative rate (0~74 years old) for both sexes was 12.12%.

The mortality rate of all cancers in urban areas was 160.24 per 100,000 population (197.10 per 100,000 population for males and 123.54 per 100,000 population for females). The ASR China was 100.12 per 100,000 population and ASR World was 99.36 per 100,000 population. The cumulative rate (0~74 years old) for both sexes was 11.06%.

The mortality rate of all cancer sites in rural areas was 164.13 per 100,000 population (196.13 per 100,000 population for males and 130.10 per 100,000 population for females). The ASR China was 109.03 per 100,000 population and ASR World was 109.71 per 100,000 population. The cumulative rate (0~74 years old) for both sex was 12.55%.

In urban areas, the crude incidence rates for both genders of all cancer sites were higher than those in rural areas. Whereas the ASR China, ASR World and cumulative rates in the urban areas were lower than in the rural areas. (Table 4–7)

表 4–7　2020 年河南省肿瘤登记地区恶性肿瘤（C00–C96）死亡主要指标

地区	性别	死亡数	死亡率（1/10⁵）	中标率（1/10⁵）	世标率（1/10⁵）	累积率 0~74(%)
全省	合计	70 338	163.02	106.43	106.68	12.12
	男性	43 276	196.40	137.37	137.58	15.79
	女性	27 062	128.19	78.15	78.31	8.59
城市地区	合计	19 697	160.24	100.12	99.36	11.06
	男性	12 088	197.10	130.05	128.55	14.69
	女性	7 609	123.54	73.09	72.90	7.68
农村地区	合计	50 641	164.13	109.03	109.71	12.55
	男性	31 188	196.13	140.32	141.28	16.23
	女性	19 453	130.10	80.29	80.59	8.96

（二）恶性肿瘤年龄别死亡率

河南省肿瘤登记地区 2020 年恶性肿瘤男性、女性年龄别死亡率随着年龄增长而增加。在 0~29 岁年龄组死亡率小于 10.00/10 万，此后略有升高，40~44 岁年龄组以后快速上升，到 85+ 年龄组死亡率达到最高值，死亡率为 1995.64/10 万。恶性肿瘤年龄别死亡率城乡比较，40 岁以前死亡率处于较低水平，城乡差别较小。在 45~79 岁年龄段城市死亡率低于农村，80 岁以后则呈现城市高于农村的特征。（表 4–8，图 4–6）

3.2 Age-specific mortality rate of all cancer sites

The age-specific cancer mortality rate of all sites in Henan increased with age. It was low at age group of 0~29, and increase sharply since 40 years old, and it reached the peak at age group of 85+. When assessing the mortality in urban and rural areas, the age-specific mortality rate was relatively low before 40 years old with less differences between the urban and rural areas. The mortality rates in urban areas were lower than those in urban areas at the age group of 45~79 years old and they were higher after 80 years old. (Table 4–8, Figure 4–6)

表 4–8　2020 年河南省肿瘤登记地区恶性肿瘤年龄别死亡率（1/10 万）

年龄组	全省			城市			农村		
	合计	男性	女性	合计	男性	女性	合计	男性	女性
合计	163.02	196.40	128.19	160.24	197.10	123.54	164.13	196.13	130.10
0–	0.89	0.43	1.40	2.35	1.50	3.27	0.31	0.00	0.65
1–	2.90	3.13	2.64	3.46	4.09	2.76	2.68	2.76	2.60
5–	3.63	3.64	3.62	3.26	3.22	3.30	3.76	3.78	3.74
10–	3.21	3.47	2.91	3.22	2.67	3.84	3.20	3.75	2.58
15–	3.10	3.58	2.57	2.58	3.13	1.98	3.29	3.74	2.79
20–	3.73	4.40	3.00	2.13	1.74	2.53	4.31	5.34	3.18
25–	4.49	4.63	4.34	3.01	3.76	2.30	5.08	4.95	5.22
30–	13.00	13.57	12.42	10.69	11.46	9.96	13.90	14.33	13.44
35–	17.69	20.38	14.88	14.64	18.21	11.25	18.99	21.24	16.53
40–	32.25	35.09	29.31	32.29	33.14	31.45	32.23	35.93	28.32
45–	68.19	78.00	58.13	64.64	70.42	58.88	69.81	81.36	57.79
50–	133.36	154.50	111.52	124.30	144.67	103.68	137.05	158.45	114.75
55–	226.09	280.72	170.98	216.61	284.59	149.34	230.04	279.13	180.11
60–	330.55	424.28	235.74	331.44	439.04	225.91	330.20	418.58	239.69
65–	651.27	859.11	447.75	579.76	785.82	386.07	678.88	886.60	472.23
70–	930.72	1 270.48	617.56	819.54	1 132.74	542.31	976.60	1 325.66	649.47
75–	1 194.17	1 609.86	830.79	1 017.44	1 358.03	734.00	1 273.44	1 718.58	875.66
80–	1 532.80	2 019.52	1 136.46	1 582.21	1 929.49	1 261.25	1 508.56	2 068.48	1 080.30
85–	1 995.64	2 640.80	1 583.41	2 224.67	2 939.58	1 708.68	1 901.68	2 504.80	1 535.44

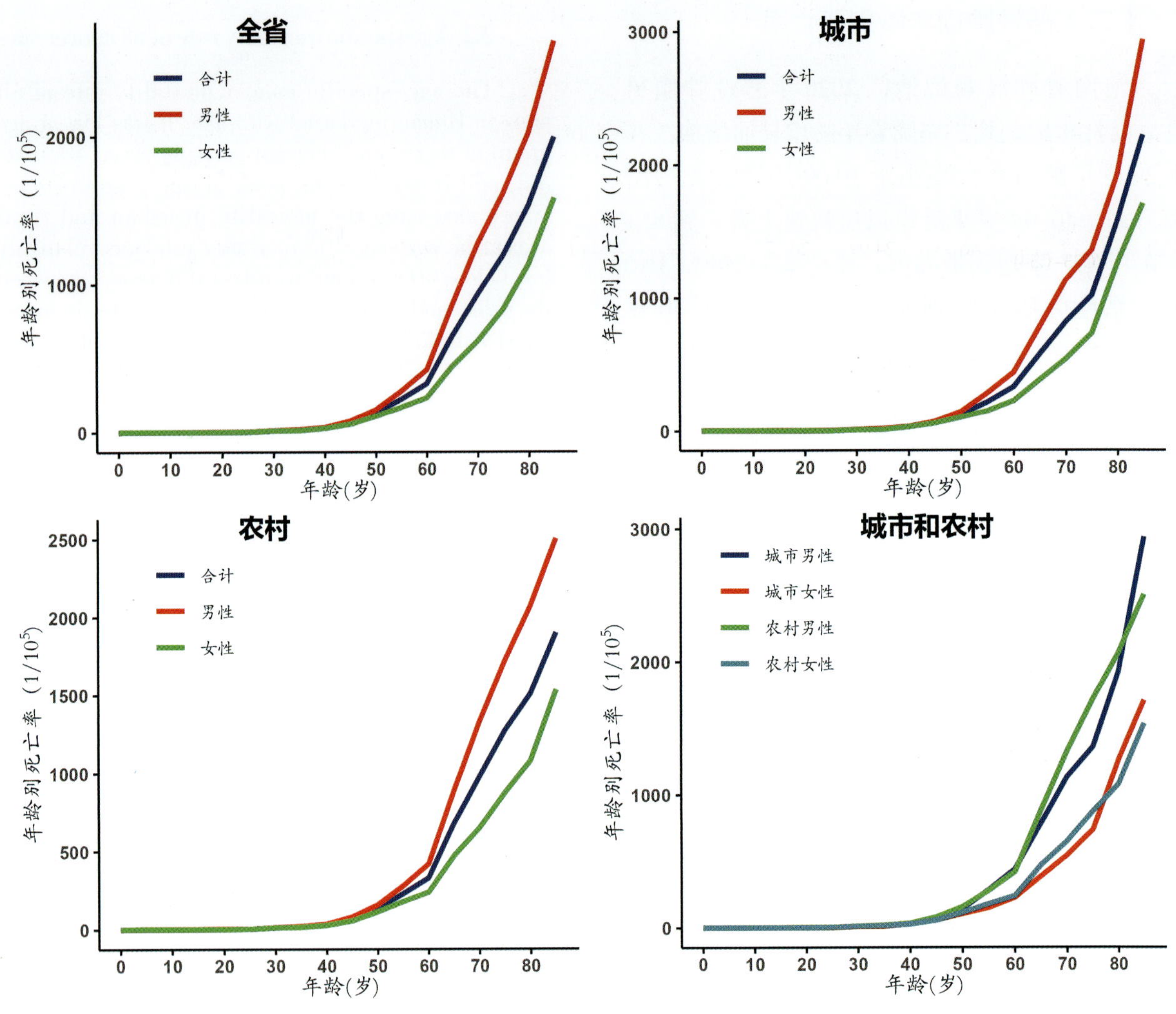

图 4-6　2020 年河南省肿瘤登记地区恶性肿瘤年龄别死亡率

（三）河南省前 10 位恶性肿瘤死亡情况

2020 年，河南省肿瘤登记地区恶性肿瘤死亡第 1 位的是肺癌，其次为胃癌、肝癌、食管癌和结直肠癌，前 10 位恶性肿瘤死亡病例数占全部恶性肿瘤死亡的 82.90%。男性恶性肿瘤死亡第 1 位的是肺癌，其次为胃癌、肝癌、食管癌和结直肠癌，男性前 10 位恶性肿瘤死亡病例数占男性全部恶性肿瘤死亡的 88.46%；女性恶性肿瘤死亡第 1 位的是肺癌，其次为食管癌、胃癌、肝癌和乳腺癌，女性前 10 位恶性肿瘤死亡病例数占女性全部恶性肿瘤死亡的 82.01%。（表 4–9，图 4–7）

3.3 Mortality of the top 10 leading causes of cancer death

In Henan cancer registration areas in 2020, Trachea, Bronchus & Lung cancer was the leading cause of cancer deaths followed by cancers of Stomach, Liver, Esophagus and Conlon,Rectum & Anus. The top 10 leading causes of cancer deaths accounted for 82.90% of all cancer deaths. For males, Trachea, Bronchus & Lung cancer was the leading cause of cancer deaths followed by cancers of Stomach, Liver, Esophagus and Conlon, Rectum & Anus, and the top 10 leading causes of cancer deaths accounted for 88.46% of all cancer deaths in males. For females, Trachea, Bronchus & Lung cancer was the leading cause of cancer death followed by cancers of Esophagus, Stomach, Liver and Breast, and the top 10 leading causes of cancer deaths accounted for 82.01% of all cancer deaths in females. (Table 4–9, Figure 4–7)

表 4-9　2020 年河南省肿瘤登记地区前 10 位恶性肿瘤死亡情况

顺序	合计				男性				女性			
	癌种	死亡率 ($1/10^5$)	构成 (%)	中标率 ($1/10^5$)	癌种	死亡率 ($1/10^5$)	构成 (%)	中标率 ($1/10^5$)	癌种	死亡率 ($1/10^5$)	构成 (%)	中标率 ($1/10^5$)
1	肺癌 (C33–C34)	40.73	24.99	26.17	肺癌 (C33–C34)	56.61	28.82	39.13	肺癌 (C33–C34)	24.16	18.85	14.26
2	胃癌 (C16)	23.78	14.59	15.24	胃癌 (C16)	32.74	16.67	22.70	食管癌 (C15)	15.88	12.39	8.96
3	肝癌 (C22)	21.37	13.11	14.41	肝癌 (C22)	28.78	14.65	20.72	胃癌 (C16)	14.43	11.26	8.37
4	食管癌 (C15)	21.14	12.97	13.25	食管癌 (C15)	26.18	13.33	17.93	肝癌 (C22)	13.64	10.64	8.25
5	结直肠癌 (C18–C21)	10.07	6.17	6.42	结直肠癌 (C18–C21)	10.96	5.58	7.58	乳腺癌 (C50)	10.06	7.84	6.79
6	乳腺癌 (C50)	10.06	3.02	6.79	脑癌 (C70–C72)	4.61	2.35	3.60	结直肠癌 (C18–C21)	9.13	7.12	5.37
7	子宫颈癌 (C53)	5.99	1.80	4.08	胰腺癌 (C25)	4.27	2.17	2.97	子宫颈癌 (C53)	5.99	4.67	4.08
8	脑癌 (C70–C72)	4.27	2.62	3.15	前列腺癌 (C61)	3.58	1.82	2.30	胆囊及其他癌 (C23–C24)	4.03	3.14	2.32
9	胰腺癌 (C25)	4.09	2.51	2.65	胆囊及其他癌 (C23–C24)	3.04	1.55	2.08	脑癌 (C70–C72)	3.93	3.06	2.70
10	前列腺癌 (C61)	3.58	1.12	2.30	恶性淋巴瘤 (C81–C85)	2.98	1.52	2.20	胰腺癌 (C25)	3.90	3.04	2.34

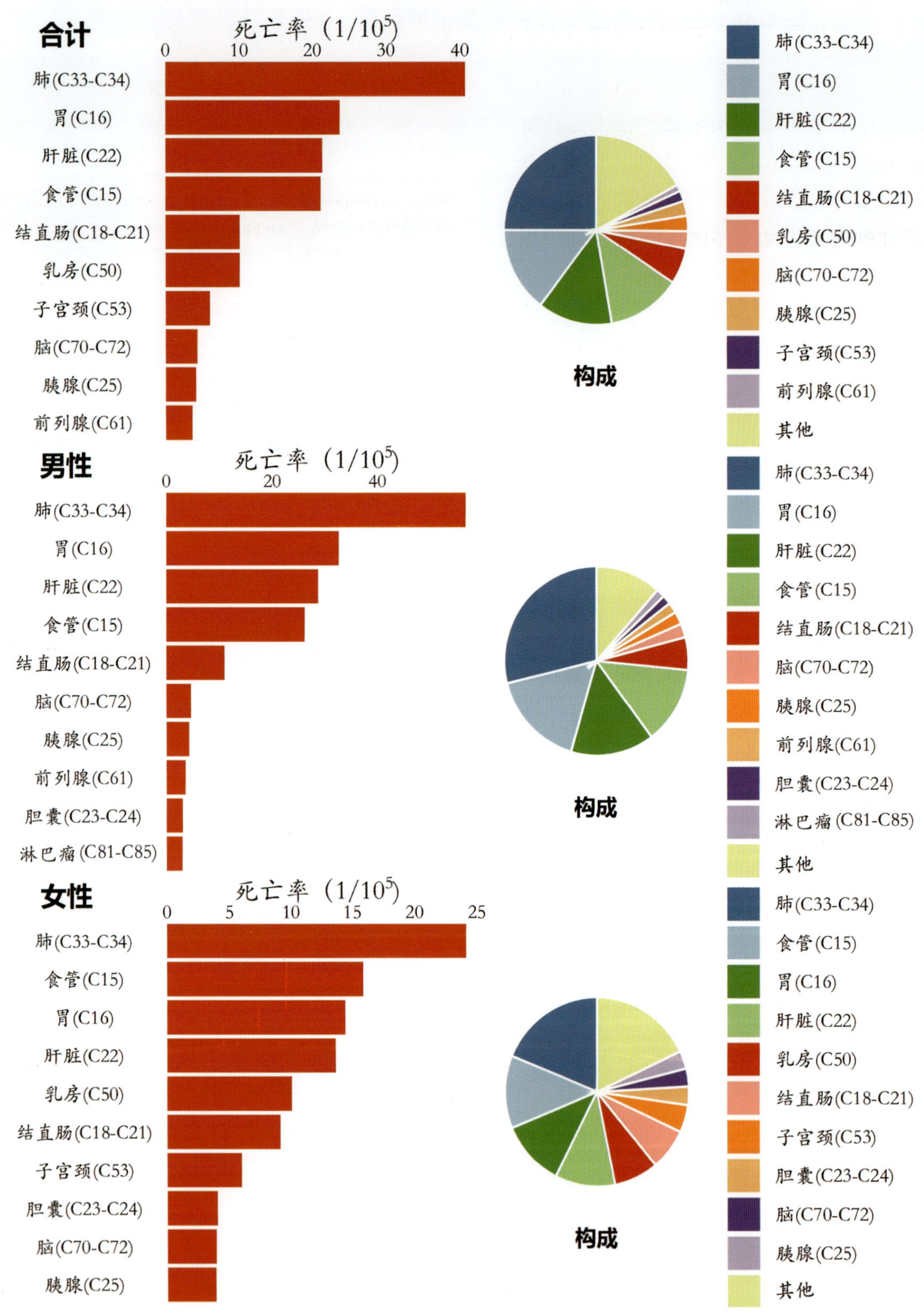

图 4–7　2020 年河南省肿瘤登记地区前 10 位恶性肿瘤死亡率及死亡构成

（四）河南省城市肿瘤登记地区前 10 位恶性肿瘤死亡情况

2020 年，河南省城市肿瘤登记地区恶性肿瘤死亡第 1 位的是肺癌，其次为肝癌、胃癌、食管癌和结直肠癌，前 10 位恶性肿瘤死亡病例数占全部恶性肿瘤死亡的 78.61%。男性恶性肿瘤死亡第 1 位的是肺癌，其次为肝癌、胃癌、食管癌和结直肠癌，男性前 10 位恶性肿瘤死亡病例数占男性全部恶性肿瘤死亡的 86.18%；女性恶性肿瘤死亡第 1 位的是肺癌，其次为肝癌、胃癌、乳腺癌和食管癌，女性前 10 位恶性肿瘤死亡病例数占女性全部恶性肿瘤死亡的 79.87%。（表 4-10，图 4-8）

3.4 Mortality of the top 10 leading causes of cancer death in Henan urban areas

In the urban areas of Henan cancer registration areas in 2020, Trachea, Bronchus & Lung cancer was the leading cause of cancer deaths, followed by cancers of Liver, Stomach, Esophagus and Conlon, Rectum & Anus. The top 10 leading causes of cancer deaths accounted for 78.61% of all cancer deaths. For males, Trachea, Bronchus & Lung cancer was the leading cause of cancer deaths, followed by cancers of Liver, Stomach, Esophagus and Conlon,Rectum & Anus, and the top 10 leading causes of cancer deaths accounted for 86.18% of all cancer deaths in males. For females, Trachea, Bronchus & Lung cancer was the leading cause of cancer death followed by cancers of Liver, Stomach, Breast and Esophagus, and the top 10 leading causes of cancer deaths accounted for 79.87% of all cancer deaths in females. (Table 4–10, Figure 4–8)

表 4–10 2020 年河南省城市肿瘤登记地区前 10 位恶性肿瘤死亡情况

顺序	合计				男性				女性			
	癌种	死亡率 ($1/10^5$)	构成 (%)	中标率 ($1/10^5$)	癌种	死亡率 ($1/10^5$)	构成 (%)	中标率 ($1/10^5$)	癌种	死亡率 ($1/10^5$)	构成 (%)	中标率 ($1/10^5$)
1	肺癌 (C33–C34)	40.73	25.42	24.73	肺癌 (C33–C34)	57.97	29.41	37.16	肺癌 (C33–C34)	23.58	19.08	13.48
2	肝癌 (C22)	19.95	12.45	12.95	肝癌 (C22)	27.65	14.03	18.87	肝癌 (C22)	12.27	9.94	7.34
3	胃癌 (C16)	19.47	12.15	11.90	胃癌 (C16)	27.44	13.92	17.89	胃癌 (C16)	11.53	9.33	6.47
4	食管癌 (C15)	15.08	9.41	8.98	食管癌 (C15)	19.84	10.07	12.72	乳腺癌 (C50)	11.51	9.32	7.45
5	结直肠癌 (C18–C21)	11.93	7.45	7.11	结直肠癌 (C18–C21)	13.88	7.04	8.79	食管癌 (C15)	10.34	8.37	5.55
6	乳腺癌 (C50)	11.51	3.60	7.45	前列腺癌 (C61)	5.53	2.80	3.10	结直肠癌 (C18–C21)	10.00	8.10	5.58
7	子宫颈癌 (C53)	5.70	1.78	3.78	胰腺癌 (C25)	5.49	2.79	3.56	子宫颈癌 (C53)	5.70	4.61	3.78
8	前列腺癌 (C61)	5.53	1.72	3.10	脑癌 (C70–C72)	4.55	2.31	3.37	胰腺癌 (C25)	5.21	4.22	2.95
9	胰腺癌 (C25)	5.35	3.34	3.25	白血病 (C91–C95)	3.78	1.92	2.77	胆囊及其他癌 (C23–C24)	4.40	3.56	2.39
10	卵巢癌 (C56)	4.12	1.29	2.58	胆囊及其他癌 (C23–C24)	3.73	1.89	2.36	卵巢癌 (C56)	4.12	3.34	2.58

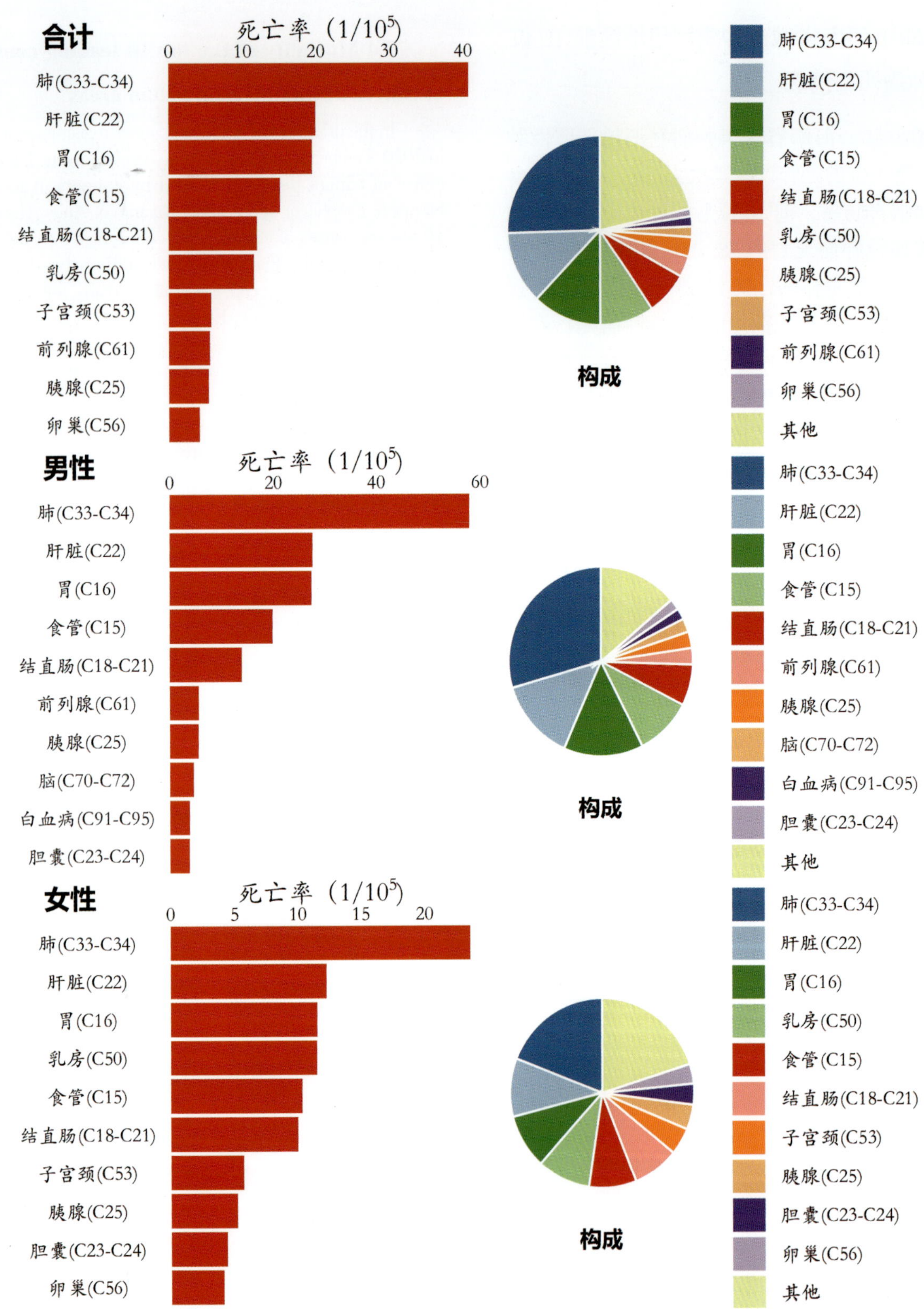

图 4-8 2020 年河南省城市肿瘤登记地区前 10 位恶性肿瘤死亡率及死亡构成

（五）河南省农村肿瘤登记地区前 10 位恶性肿瘤死亡情况

2020 年，河南省农村肿瘤登记地区恶性肿瘤死亡第 1 位的是肺癌，其次为胃癌、食管癌、肝癌和乳腺癌，前 10 位恶性肿瘤死亡病例数占全部恶性肿瘤死亡的 85.22%。男性恶性肿瘤死亡第 1 位的是肺癌，其次为胃癌、肝癌、食管癌和结直肠癌，男性前 10 位恶性肿瘤死亡病例数占男性全部恶性肿瘤死亡的 89.37%；女性恶性肿瘤死亡第 1 位的是肺癌，其次为食管癌、胃癌、肝癌和乳腺癌，女性前 10 位恶性肿瘤死亡病例数占女性全部恶性肿瘤死亡的 83.13%。（表 4–11，图 4–9）

3.5 Mortality of the top 10 leading causes of cancer death in Henan rural areas

In the rural areas of Henan cancer registration areas in 2020, Trachea, Bronchus & Lung cancer was the leading cause of cancer deaths, followed by cancers of Stomach, Esophagus, Liver and Breast. The top 10 leading causes of cancer deaths accounted for 85.22% of all cancer deaths. For males, Trachea, Bronchus & Lung cancer was the leading cause of cancer deaths, followed by cancers of Stomach, Liver, Esophagus and Conlon, Rectum & Anus, and the top 10 leading causes of cancer deaths accounted for 89.37% of all cancer deaths in males. For females, Trachea, Bronchus & Lung cancer was the leading cause of cancer death followed by cancers of Esophagus, Stomach, Liver and Breast, and the top 10 leading causes of cancer deaths accounted for 83.13% of all cancer deaths in females. (Table 4–11, Figure 4–9)

表 4–11　2020 年河南省农村肿瘤登记地区前 10 位恶性肿瘤死亡情况

顺序	合计				男性				女性			
	癌种	死亡率 ($1/10^5$)	构成 (%)	中标率 ($1/10^5$)	癌种	死亡率 ($1/10^5$)	构成 (%)	中标率 ($1/10^5$)	癌种	死亡率 ($1/10^5$)	构成 (%)	中标率 ($1/10^5$)
1	肺癌 (C33–C34)	40.73	24.82	26.76	肺癌 (C33–C34)	56.08	28.59	39.91	肺癌 (C33–C34)	24.40	18.76	14.59
2	胃癌 (C16)	25.50	15.53	16.63	胃癌 (C16)	34.78	17.73	24.72	食管癌 (C15)	18.16	13.96	10.40
3	食管癌 (C15)	23.56	14.35	15.06	肝癌 (C22)	29.21	14.89	21.48	胃癌 (C16)	15.62	12.01	9.16
4	肝癌 (C22)	21.94	13.37	15.02	食管癌 (C15)	28.63	14.60	20.17	肝癌 (C22)	14.21	10.92	8.64
5	乳腺癌 (C50)	9.46	2.79	6.50	结直肠癌 (C18–C21)	9.84	5.01	7.07	乳腺癌 (C50)	9.46	7.27	6.50
6	结直肠癌 (C18–C21)	9.32	5.68	6.13	脑癌 (C70–C72)	4.63	2.36	3.69	结直肠癌 (C18–C21)	8.77	6.74	5.28
7	子宫颈癌 (C53)	6.11	1.80	4.20	胰腺癌 (C25)	3.80	1.94	2.73	子宫颈癌 (C53)	6.11	4.70	4.20
8	脑癌 (C70–C72)	4.40	2.68	3.30	前列腺癌 (C61)	2.83	1.44	1.94	脑癌 (C70–C72)	4.17	3.20	2.88
9	胰腺癌 (C25)	3.59	2.19	2.39	胆囊及其他癌 (C23–C24)	2.77	1.41	1.96	胆囊及其他癌 (C23–C24)	3.88	2.98	2.29
10	胆囊及其他癌 (C23–C24)	3.31	2.01	2.13	恶性淋巴瘤 (C81–C85)	2.75	1.40	2.09	胰腺癌 (C25)	3.36	2.59	2.08

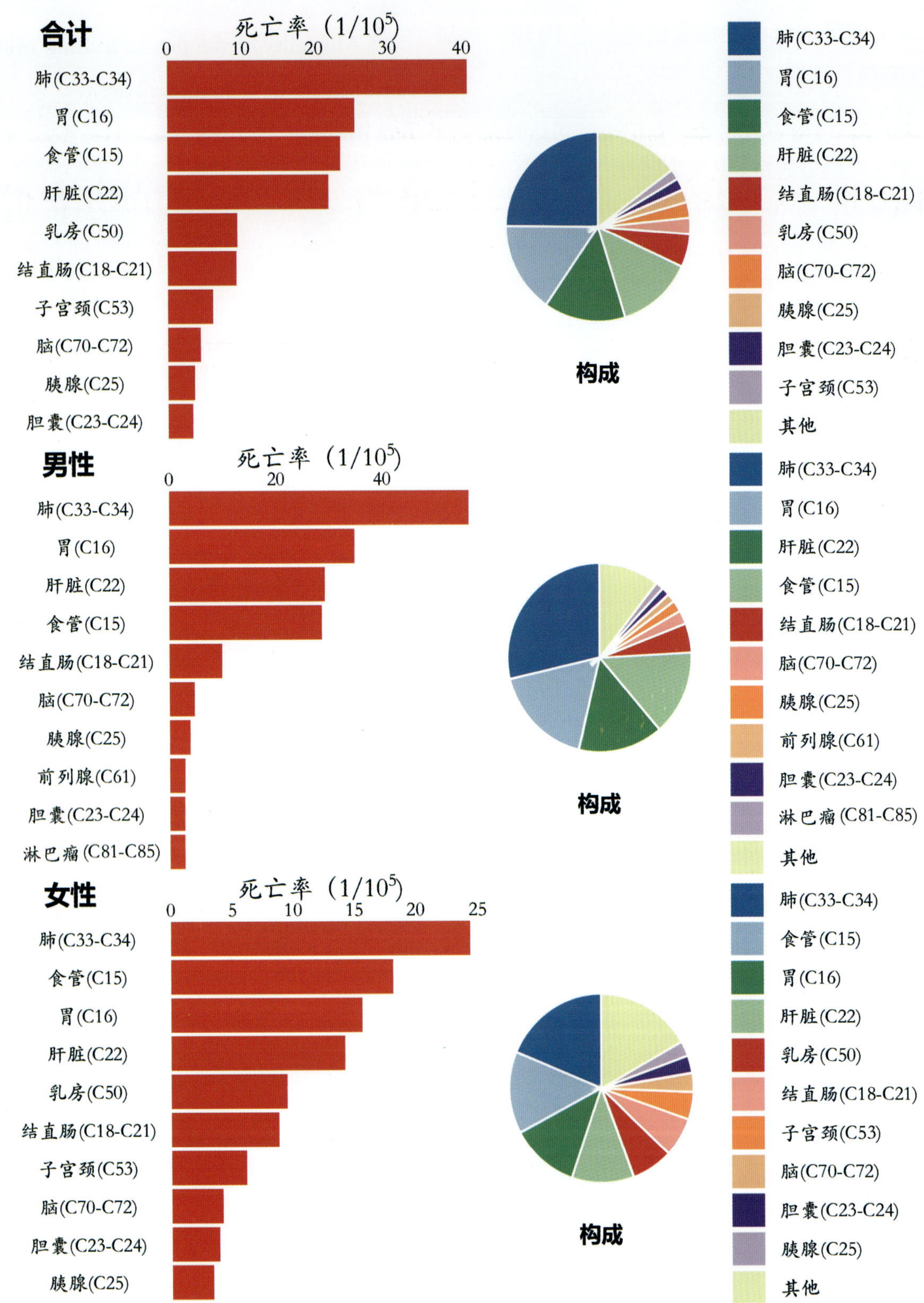

图 4-9 河南省农村肿瘤登记地区前 10 位恶性肿瘤死亡率及死亡构成

第五章　各部位恶性肿瘤发病与死亡情况

Chapter 5　Incidence and mortality of each kind of cancers

一、口腔

2020 年，河南省肿瘤登记地区口腔癌的发病率为 3.30/10 万，中标率为 2.41/10 万，世标率为 2.34/10 万，发病例数占全部癌症新发病例数的 1.18%；其中，男性和女性发病率分别为 4.04/10 万和 2.53/10 万，城市地区和农村地区发病率分别为 3.96/10 万和 3.04/10 万；中标发病率呈现男性高于女性、城市地区高于农村地区的特点，男性中标发病率是女性的 1.69 倍，城市地区中标发病率是农村地区的 1.19 倍。同期，口腔癌的死亡率为 1.46/10 万，中标率为 0.96/10 万，世标率为 0.95/10 万，死亡病例数占全部癌症死亡病例数的 0.90%；其中，男性和女性死亡率分别为 1.80/10 万和 1.10/10 万，城市地区和农村地区死亡率分别为 1.73/10 万和 1.35/10 万；中标死亡率呈现男性高于女性、城市地区高于农村地区的特点，男性中标死亡率是女性的 1.85 倍，城市地区中标死亡率是农村地区的 1.18 倍。（表 5-1）

1. Oral cavity & pharynx

In 2020, there were 1424 new cases diagnosed as oral cavity & pharynx cancer in registration areas of Henan Province, China (890 males and 534 females, 487 in urban areas and 937 in rural areas), accounting for 1.18% of new cases of all cancers. The crude incidence rate was 3.30 per 100,000, with the ASR China 2.41 per 100,000 and the ASR World 2.34 per 100,000, respectively. Subgroup analysis showed that the incidence of ASR China was 1.69 times in males as that in females, and it was 1.19 times in urban areas as that in rural areas. The cumulative incidence rate for subjects aged 0 to 74 years was 0.27%. (Table 5-1)

A total of 630 cases died of oral cavity & pharynx cancer in 2020 (397 males and 233 females, 213 in urban areas and 417 in rural areas), accounting for 0.90% of all cancer deaths. The crude mortality rate was 1.46 per 100,000, with the ASR China of 0.96 per 100,000 and the ASR World of 0.95 per 100,000, respectively. Subgroup analysis showed that the mortality of ASR China was 1.85 times in males as that in females, and it was 1.18 times in urban areas as that in rural areas. The cumulative mortality rate for subjects aged 0 to 74 years was 0.11%. (Table 5-1)

表 5-1　2020 年河南省肿瘤登记地区口腔癌发病与死亡情况

地区	性别	病例数	粗率（1/10^5）	构成（%）	中标率（1/10^5）	世标率（1/10^5）	累积率 0～74（%）
发病							
全省	合计	1 424	3.30	1.18	2.41	2.34	0.27
	男性	890	4.04	1.44	3.04	2.97	0.35
	女性	534	2.53	0.91	1.80	1.73	0.19
城市地区	合计	487	3.96	1.33	2.72	2.69	0.31
	男性	321	5.23	1.76	3.64	3.67	0.43
	女性	166	2.70	0.90	1.85	1.77	0.20
农村地区	合计	937	3.04	1.12	2.28	2.19	0.25
	男性	569	3.58	1.31	2.79	2.68	0.32
	女性	368	2.46	0.91	1.78	1.71	0.19

续表

地区	性别	病例数	粗率 (1/10⁵)	构成 (%)	中标率 (1/10⁵)	世标率 (1/10⁵)	累积率 0～74 (%)
死亡							
全省	合计	630	1.46	0.90	0.96	0.95	0.11
	男性	397	1.80	0.92	1.26	1.27	0.14
	女性	233	1.10	0.86	0.68	0.66	0.07
城市地区	合计	213	1.73	1.08	1.07	1.09	0.12
	男性	134	2.18	1.11	1.41	1.48	0.17
	女性	79	1.28	1.04	0.76	0.75	0.07
农村地区	合计	417	1.35	0.82	0.91	0.89	0.10
	男性	263	1.65	0.84	1.20	1.18	0.13
	女性	154	1.03	0.79	0.65	0.62	0.07

口腔癌年龄别发病率在 0~39 岁年龄段处于较低水平，40 岁以后快速上升，在 80 岁达到峰值；年龄别死亡率在 0~49 岁年龄段处于较低水平，50 岁以后快速上升，在 85 岁达到峰值；年龄别发病率和死亡率均呈现男性高于女性的特点；城市地区和农村地区年龄别率虽然有一定差异，但是总体趋势类同。（图 5–1a）

在 14 个城市肿瘤登记地区中，男性口腔癌标化发病率最高的是鹤壁市城区（6.01/10 万），其次是漯河市城区（4.99/10 万）和许昌市魏都区（4.87/10 万）；女性标化发病率最高的是鹤壁市城区（5.21/10 万），其次是南阳市卧龙区（3.32/10 万）和济源市（3.00/10 万）。男性标化死亡率最高的是南阳市卧龙区（2.71/10 万），其次是济源市（2.39/10 万）和鹤壁市城区（2.24/10 万）；女性标化死亡率最高的是鹤壁市城区（2.13/10 万），其次是南阳市卧龙区（1.56/10 万）和许昌市魏都区（1.49/10 万）。（图 5–1b）

The age-specific incidence of oral cavity & pharynx cancer was low at age group of 0~39, and it started increasing sharply at age group of 40, it reached the peak at age of 80. The age specific mortality was low at age group of 0~49, and it started increasing sharply at age group of 50, it reached the peak at age of 85. Age specific incidence and mortality were all higher in males than in females, The change pattern of age specific incidence and mortality were similar in urban areas and rural areas. (Figure 5–1a)

Among the 14 urban cancer registries, the ASR China incidence rate of oral cavity & pharynx cancer in males was the highest in Hebi City (6.01 per 100,000) followed by Luohe City (4.99 per 100,000), and Xuchang Weidu District (4.87 per 100,000). For females, it was the highest in Hebi City (5.21 per 100,000), followed by Nanyang Wolong District (3.32 per 100,000), and Jiyuan City (3.00 per 100,000). The ASR China mortality rate of oral cavity & pharynx cancer in males was the highest in Nanyang Wolong District (2.71 per 100,000) followed by Jiyuan City (2.39 per 100,000), and Hebi City (2.24 per 100,000). For females, it was the highest in Hebi City (2.13 per 100,000), followed by Nanyang Wolong District (1.56 per 100,000), and Xuchang Weidu District (1.49 per 100,000). (Figure 5–1b)

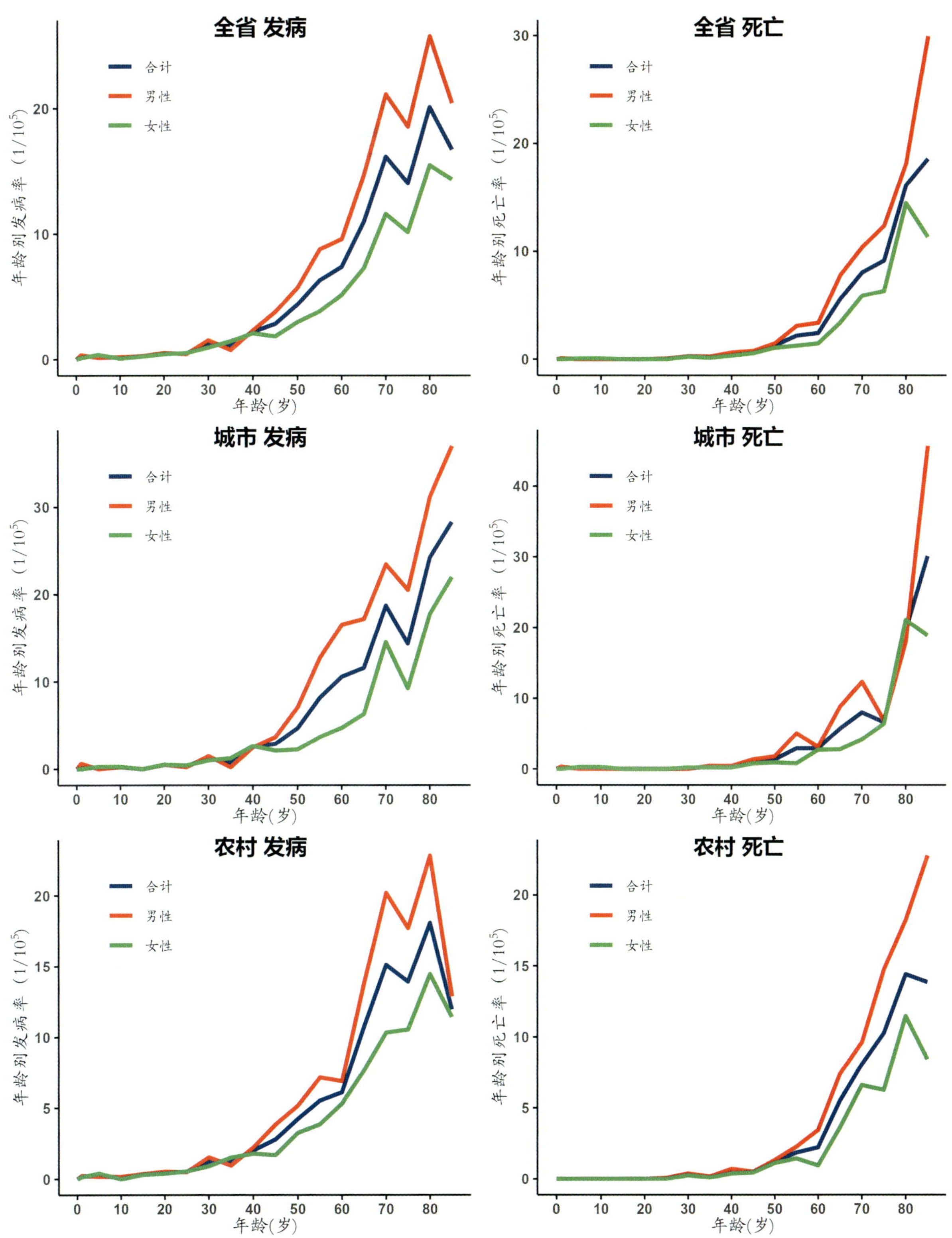

图 5-1a　2020 年河南省肿瘤登记地区口腔癌年龄别发病率和死亡率

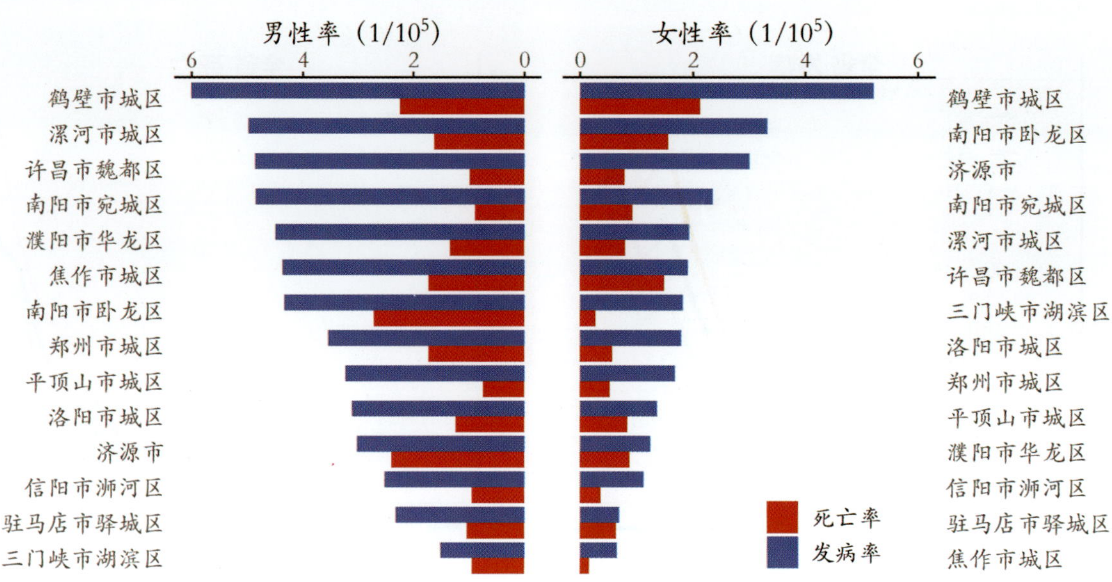

图 5-1b　2020 年河南省城市肿瘤登记地区口腔癌发病率和死亡率

在 41 个农村肿瘤登记地区中，男性口腔癌标化发病率最高的是范县（7.68/10 万），其次是内乡县（4.75/10 万）和汝阳县（4.73/10 万）；女性标化发病率最高的是郸城县（5.58/10 万），其次是范县（4.34/10 万）和栾川县（3.39/10 万）。男性标化死亡率最高的是浚县（3.96/10 万），其次是内乡县（3.19/10 万）和新野县（2.97/10 万）；女性标化死亡率最高的是浚县（2.62/10 万），其次是郸城县（2.35/10 万）和临颍县（1.62/10 万）。（图 5-1c）

Among the 41 rural cancer registries, the ASR China incidence rate of oral cavity & pharynx cancer in males was the highest in Fan County (7.68 per 100,000) followed by Neixiang County (4.75 per 100,000), and Ruyang County (4.73 per 100,000). For females, it was the highest in Dancheng County (5.58 per 100,000), followed by Fan County (4.34 per 100,000), and Luanchuan County (3.39 per 100,000). The ASR China mortality rate of oral cavity & pharynx cancer in males was the highest in Xun County (3.96 per 100,000) followed by Neixiang County (3.19 per 100,000), and Xinye County (2.97 per 100,000). For females, it was the highest in Xun County (2.62 per 100,000), followed by Dancheng County (2.35 per 100,000), and Linying County (1.62 per 100,000). (Figure 5–1c)

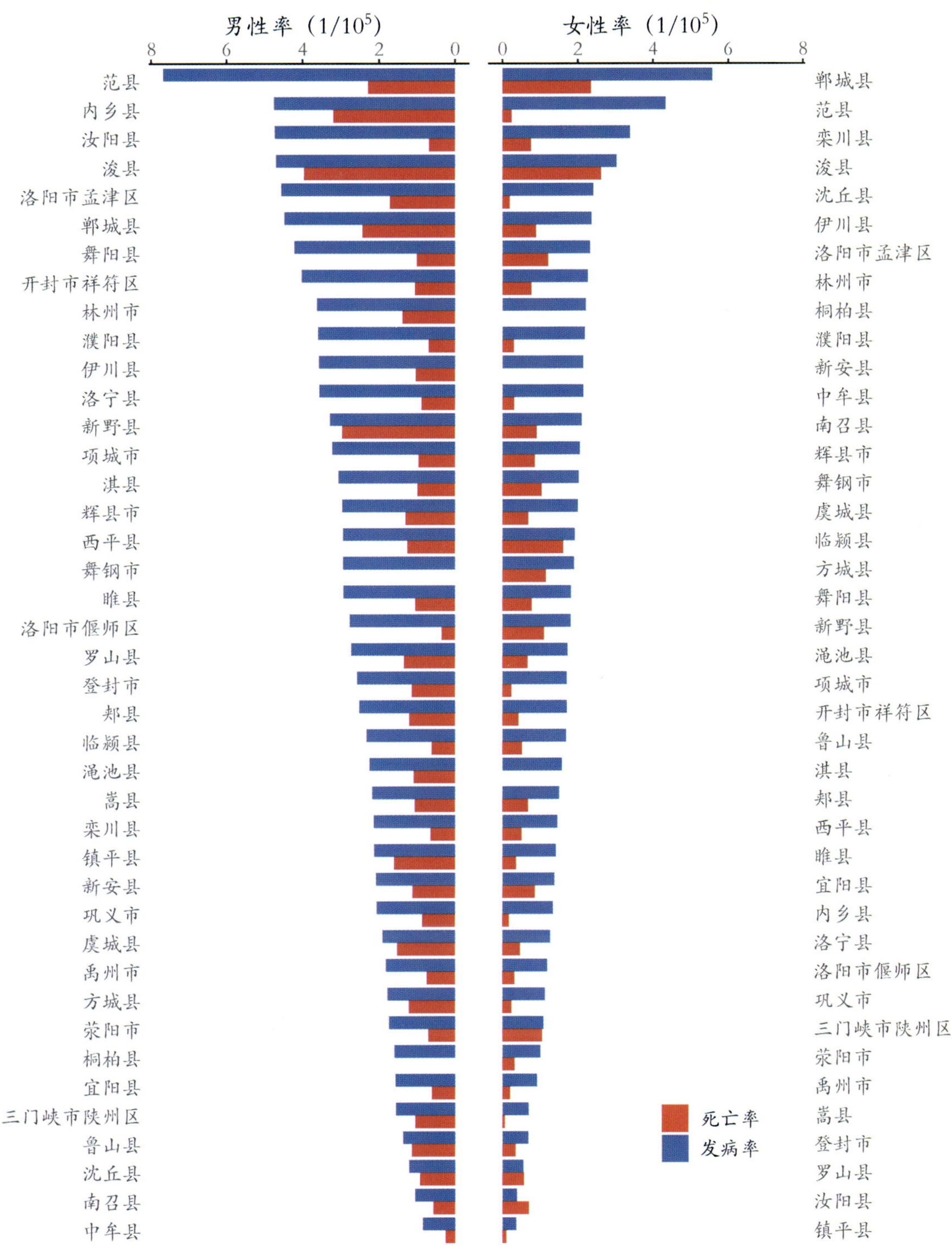

图 5-1c　2020 年河南省农村肿瘤登记地区口腔癌发病率和死亡率

二、鼻咽

2020 年，河南省肿瘤登记地区鼻咽癌的发病率为 0.97/10 万，中标率为 0.74/10 万，世标率为 0.72/10 万，发病例数占全部癌症新发病例数的 0.35%；其中，男性和女性发病率分别为 1.29/10 万和 0.63/10 万，城市地区和农村地区发病率分别为 0.87/10 万和 1.01/10 万；中标发病率呈现男性高于女性、农村地区高于城市地区的特点，男性中标发病率是女性的 2.20 倍，农村地区中标发病率是城市地区的 1.22 倍。同期，鼻咽癌的死亡率为 0.52/10 万，中标率为 0.36/10 万，世标率为 0.35/10 万，死亡病例数占全部癌症死亡病例数的 0.32%；其中，男性和女性死亡率分别为 0.69/10 万和 0.34/10 万，城市地区和农村地区死亡率分别为 0.53/10 万和 0.51/10 万；中标死亡率呈现男性高于女性、农村地区与城市地区相当的特点，男性中标死亡率是女性的 2.17 倍，农村地区中标死亡率和城市地区持平。（表 5-2）

2. Nasopharynx

In 2020, there were 418 new cases diagnosed as nasopharynx cancer in registration areas of Henan Province, China (285 males and 133 females, 107 in urban areas and 311 in rural areas), accounting for 0.35% of new cases of all cancers. The crude incidence rate was 0.97 per 100,000, with the ASR China 0.74 per 100,000 and the ASR World 0.72 per 100,000, respectively. Subgroup analysis showed that the incidence of ASR China was 2.20 times in males as that in females, and it was 1.22 times in rural areas as that in urban areas. The cumulative incidence rate for subjects aged 0 to 74 years was 0.08%. (Table 5-2)

A total of 223 cases died of nasopharynx cancer in 2020 (151 males and 72 females, 65 in urban areas and 158 in rural areas), accounting for 0.32% of all cancer deaths. The crude mortality rate was 0.52 per 100,000, with the ASR China of 0.36 per 100,000 and the ASR World of 0.35 per 100,000, respectively. Subgroup analysis showed that the mortality of ASR China was 2.17 times in males as that in females, and it was similar in urban areas as that in rural areas. The cumulative mortality rate for subjects aged 0 to 74 years was 0.04%. (Table 5-2)

表 5-2　2020 年河南省肿瘤登记地区鼻咽癌发病与死亡情况

地区	性别	病例数	粗率（1/10⁵）	构成（%）	中标率（1/10⁵）	世标率（1/10⁵）	累积率 0~74（%）
发病							
全省	合计	418	0.97	0.35	0.74	0.72	0.08
	男性	285	1.29	0.46	1.01	0.99	0.11
	女性	133	0.63	0.23	0.46	0.44	0.05
城市地区	合计	107	0.87	0.29	0.64	0.63	0.07
	男性	79	1.29	0.43	0.95	0.94	0.11
	女性	28	0.45	0.15	0.34	0.32	0.04
农村地区	合计	311	1.01	0.37	0.78	0.75	0.09
	男性	206	1.30	0.47	1.04	1.01	0.11
	女性	105	0.70	0.26	0.51	0.50	0.06
死亡							
全省	合计	223	0.52	0.32	0.36	0.35	0.04
	男性	151	0.69	0.35	0.50	0.50	0.06
	女性	72	0.34	0.27	0.23	0.21	0.02
城市地区	合计	65	0.53	0.33	0.36	0.36	0.04
	男性	47	0.77	0.39	0.53	0.53	0.06
	女性	18	0.29	0.24	0.20	0.19	0.02
农村地区	合计	158	0.51	0.31	0.36	0.35	0.04
	男性	104	0.65	0.33	0.49	0.48	0.06
	女性	54	0.36	0.28	0.24	0.22	0.02

鼻咽癌年龄别发病率在0~29岁年龄段处于较低水平，30岁以后快速上升，在70岁达到峰值；年龄别死亡率在0~39岁年龄段处于较低水平，40岁以后快速上升，在85岁达到峰值；年龄别发病率和死亡率均呈现男性高于女性的特点；城市地区和农村地区年龄别率虽然有一定差异，但是总体趋势类同。（图5-2a）

The age specific incidence of nasopharynx cancer was low at age group of 0~29, and it started increasing sharply at age group of 30, it reached the peak at age of 70. The age specific mortality was low at age group of 0~39, and it started increasing sharply at age group of 40, it reached the peak at age of 85. Age specific incidence and mortality were all higher in males than in females. The change pattern of age specific incidence and mortality were similar in urban areas and rural areas. (Figure 5-2a)

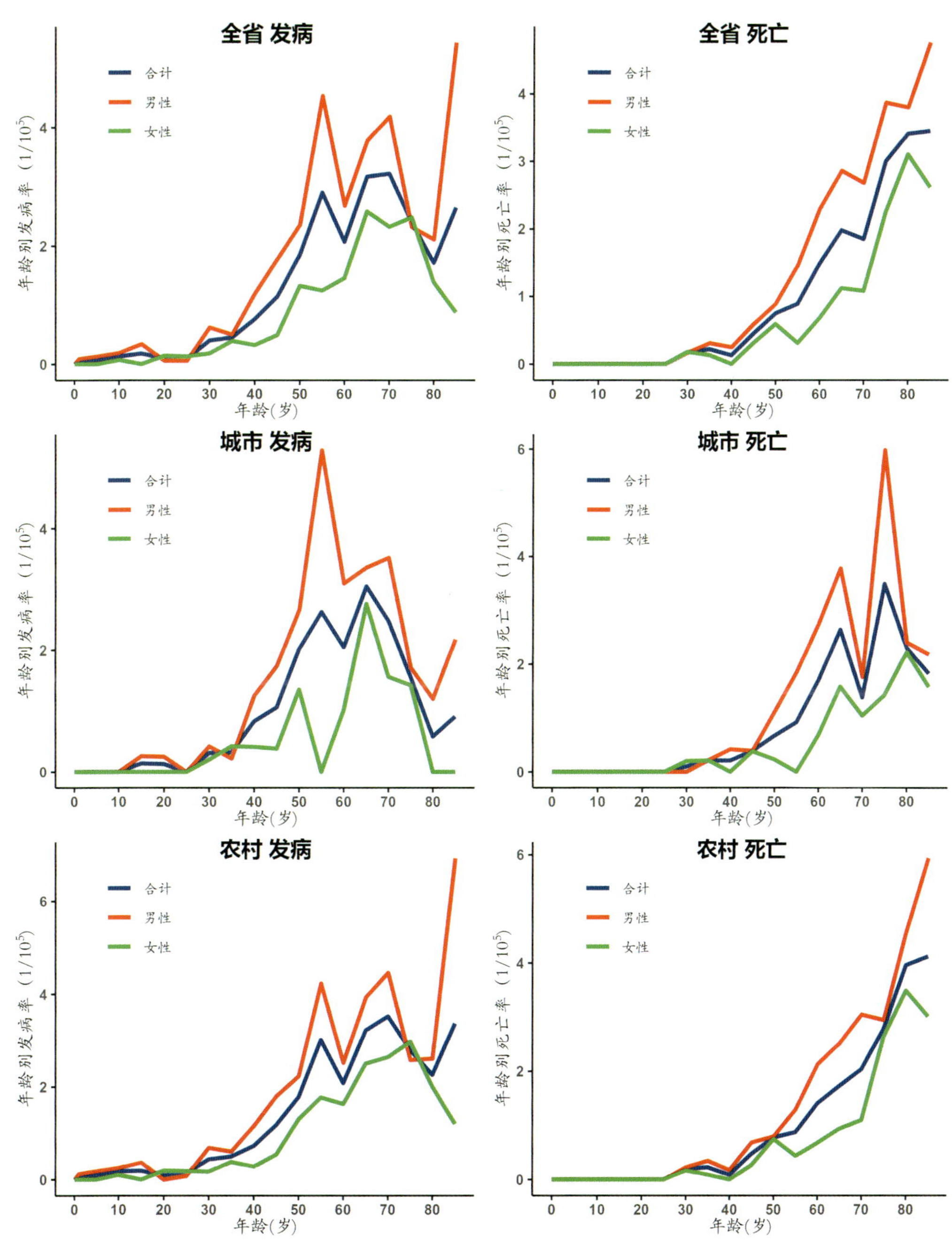

图5-2a 2020年河南省肿瘤登记地区鼻咽癌年龄别发病率和死亡率

在14个城市肿瘤登记地区中，男性鼻咽癌标化发病率最高的是南阳市宛城区（2.49/10万），其次是信阳市浉河区（1.78/10万）和许昌市魏都区（1.57/10万）；女性标化发病率最高的是信阳市浉河区（1.14/10万），其次是濮阳市华龙区（1.01/10万）和许昌市魏都区（0.76/10万）。男性标化死亡率最高的是信阳市浉河区(1.49/10万)，其次是许昌市魏都区（1.37/10万）和南阳市卧龙区（0.7/10万）；女性标化死亡率最高的是信阳市浉河区（1/10万），其次是濮阳市华龙区（0.68/10万）和郑州市城区（0.40/10万）。（图5-2b）

Among the 14 urban cancer registries, the ASR China incidence rate of nasopharynx cancer in males was the highest in Nanyang Wancheng District (2.49 per 100,000) followed by Xinyang Shihe District (1.78 per 100,000), and Xuchang Weidu District (1.57 per 100,000). For females, it was the highest in Xinyang Shihe District (1.14 per 100,000), followed by Puyang Hualong District (1.01 per 100,000), and Xuchang Weidu District (0.76 per 100,000). The ASR China mortality rate of nasopharynx cancer in males was the highest in Xinyang Shihe District (1.49 per 100,000) followed by Xuchang Weidu District (1.37 per 100,000), and Nanyang Wolong District (0.70 per 100,000). For females, it was the highest in Xinyang Shihe District (1 per 100,000), followed by Puyang Hualong District (0.68 per 100,000), and Zhengzhou City (0.40 per 100,000). (Figure 5-2b)

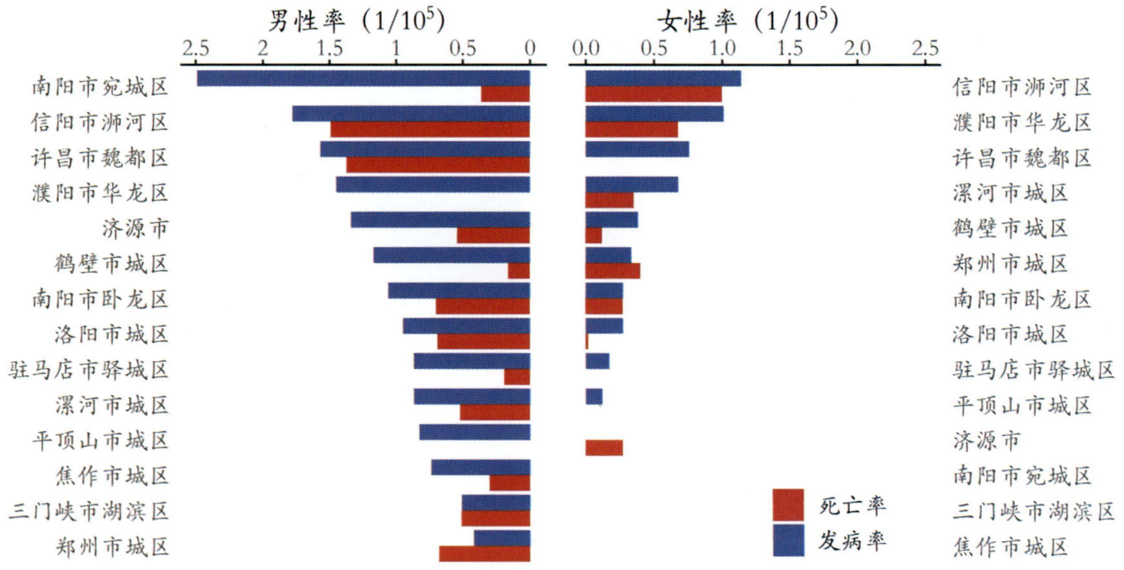

图5-2b　2020年河南省城市肿瘤登记地区鼻咽癌发病率和死亡率

在41个农村肿瘤登记地区中，男性鼻咽癌标化发病率最高的是罗山县（3.28/10万），其次是南召县（3.17/10万）和桐柏县（3.12/10万）；女性标化发病率最高的是范县（1.52/10万），其次是罗山县（1.46/10万）和郸城县（1.19/10万）。男性标化死亡率最高的是汝阳县（1.50/10万），其次是栾川县(1.26/10万)和罗山县(1.10/10万)；女性标化死亡率最高的是桐柏县（1.25/10万），其次是舞钢市(0.86/10万)和新野县(0.78/10万)。（图5-2c）

Among the 41 rural cancer registries, the ASR China incidence rate of nasopharynx cancer in males was the highest in Luoshan District (3.28 per 100, 000) followed by Nanzhao County (3.17 per 100,000), and Tongbai County (3.12 per 100,000). For females, it was the highest in Fan County (1.52 per 100,000), followed by Luoshan County (1.46 per 100,000), and Dancheng County (1.19 per 100,000). The ASR China mortality rate of nasopharynx cancer in males was the highest in Ruyang County (1.50 per 100,000) followed by Luanchuan County (1.26 per 100,000), and Luoshan County (1.10 per 100,000). For females, it was the highest in Tongbai County (1.25 per 100 ,000), followed by Wugang City (0.86 per 100,000), and Xinye County (0.78 per 100,000). (Figure 5-2c)

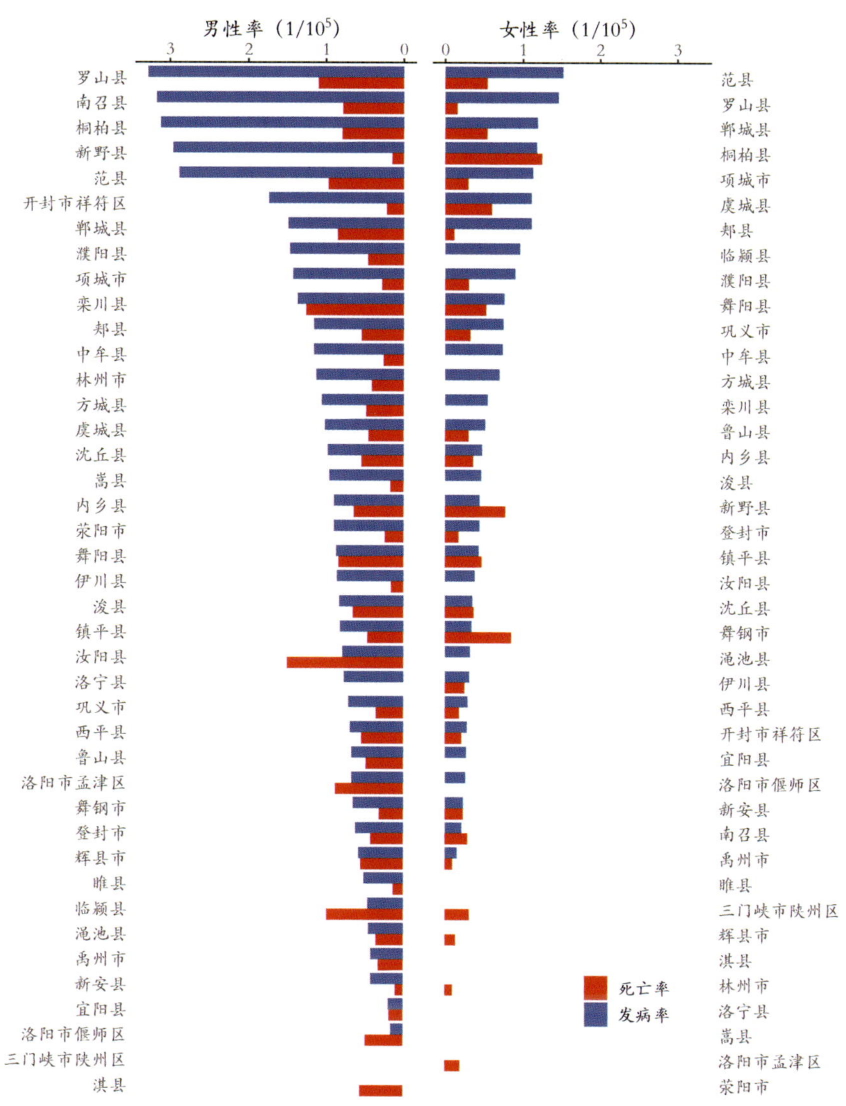

图 5-2c　2020 年河南省农村肿瘤登记地区鼻咽癌发病率和死亡率

三、食管

2020 年，河南省肿瘤登记地区食管癌的发病率为 27.07/10 万，中标率为 17.68/10 万，世标率为 17.79/10 万，发病例数占全部癌症新发病例数的 9.68%；其中，男性和女性发病率分别为 32.85/10 万和 21.03/10 万，城市地区和农村地区发病率分别为 17.99/10 万和 30.68/10 万；中标发病率呈现男性高于女性、农村地区高于城市地区的特点，男性中标发病率是女性的 1.81 倍，农村地区中标发病率是城市地区的 1.80 倍。同期，食管癌的死亡率为 21.14/10 万，中标率为 13.25/10 万，世标率为 13.20/10 万，死亡病例数

3. Esophagus

In 2020, there were 11678 new cases diagnosed as esophagus cancer in registration areas of Henan Province, China (7239 males and 4439 females, 2211 in urban areas and 9467 in rural areas), accounting for 9.68% of new cases of all cancers. The crude incidence rate was 27.07 per 100,000, with the ASR China 17.68 per 100,000 and the ASR World 17.79 per 100,000, respectively. Subgroup analysis showed that the incidence of ASR China was 1.81 times in males as that in females, and it was 1.80 times in rural areas as that in urban areas. The cumulative incidence rate for subjects aged 0 to 74 years was 2.28%. (Table 5–3)

A total of 9122 cases died of esophagus cancer in 2020 (5769 males and 3353 females, 1854 in urban areas and 7268 in rural areas), accounting for 12.97% of all cancer deaths. The crude mortality rate was 21.14

占全部癌症死亡病例数的 12.97%；其中，男性和女性死亡率分别为 26.18/10 万和 15.88/10 万，城市地区和农村地区死亡率分别为 15.08/10 万和 23.56/10 万；中标死亡率呈现男性高于女性、农村地区高于城市地区的特点，男性中标死亡率是女性的 2.00 倍，农村地区中标死亡率是城市地区的 1.68 倍。（表 5–3）

per 100,000, with the ASR China of 13.25 per 100,000 and the ASR World of 13.20 per 100,000, respectively. Subgroup analysis showed that the mortality of ASR China was 2.00 times in males as that in females, and it was 1.68 times in rural areas as that in urban areas. The cumulative mortality rate for subjects aged 0 to 74 years was 1.5%. (Table 5–3)

表 5–3 2020 年河南省肿瘤登记地区食管癌发病与死亡情况

地区	性别	病例数	粗率（$1/10^5$）	构成（%）	中标率（$1/10^5$）	世标率（$1/10^5$）	累积率 0 ~ 74（%）
发病							
全省	合计	11 678	27.07	9.68	17.68	17.79	2.28
	男性	7 239	32.85	11.71	22.95	23.14	2.99
	女性	4 439	21.03	7.54	12.71	12.74	1.59
城市地区	合计	2 211	17.99	6.03	11.31	11.43	1.47
	男性	1 436	23.41	7.85	15.56	15.79	2.03
	女性	775	12.58	4.21	7.33	7.33	0.94
农村地区	合计	9 467	30.68	11.27	20.33	20.42	2.61
	男性	5 803	36.49	13.33	26.01	26.16	3.37
	女性	3 664	24.51	9.05	14.98	15.00	1.86
死亡							
全省	合计	9 122	21.14	12.97	13.25	13.20	1.50
	男性	5 769	26.18	13.33	17.93	17.88	2.07
	女性	3 353	15.88	12.39	8.96	8.93	0.96
城市地区	合计	1 854	15.08	9.41	8.98	9.05	1.02
	男性	1 217	19.84	10.07	12.72	12.90	1.53
	女性	637	10.34	8.37	5.55	5.54	0.55
农村地区	合计	7 268	23.56	14.35	15.06	14.94	1.69
	男性	4 552	28.63	14.60	20.17	19.99	2.28
	女性	2 716	18.16	13.96	10.40	10.35	1.13

食管癌年龄别发病率在 0~39 岁年龄段处于较低水平，40 岁以后快速上升，在 85 岁达到峰值；年龄别死亡率在 0~49 岁年龄段处于较低水平，50 岁以后快速上升，在 85 岁达到峰值；年龄别发病率和死亡率均呈现男性高于女性的特点；城市地区和农村地区年龄别率虽然有一定差异，但是总体趋势类同。（图 5-3a）

在 14 个城市肿瘤登记地区中，男性食管癌标化发病率最高的是南阳市卧龙区（34.47/10 万），其次是济源市（31.92/10 万）和鹤壁市城区（29.66/10 万）；女性标化发病率最高的是鹤壁市城区（16.94/10 万），其次是济源市（16.74/10 万）和南阳市卧龙区（14.61/10 万）。男性标化死亡率最高的是南阳市卧龙区（32.14/10 万），其次是济源市（29.94/10 万）和鹤壁市城区（24.15/10 万）；女性标化死亡率最高的是南阳市卧龙区（14.57/10 万），其次是济源市（14.08/10 万）和鹤壁市城区（11.30/10 万）。（图 5-3b）

在 41 个农村肿瘤登记地区中，男性食管癌标化发病率最高的是淇县（79.92/10 万），其次是林州市（50.98/10 万）和洛宁县（47.97/10 万）；女性标化发病率最高的是淇县（52.01/10 万），其次是林州市（33.42/10 万）和浚县（31.98/10 万）。男性标化死亡率最高的是淇县（44.92/10 万），其次是洛宁县（44.3/10 万）和林州市（42.01/10 万）；女性标化死亡率最高的是林州市（28.41/10 万），其次是嵩县（23.36/10 万）和洛宁县（20.07/10 万）。（图 5-3c）

The age specific incidence of esophagus cancer was low at age group of 0~39, and it started increasing sharply at age group of 40, it reached the peak at age of 85. The age specific mortality was low at age group of 0~49, and it started increasing sharply at age group of 50, it reached the peak at age of 85. Age specific incidence and mortality were all higher in males than in females, The change pattern of age specific incidence and mortality were similar in urban areas and rural areas. (Figure 5-3a)

Among the 14 urban cancer registries, the ASR China incidence rate of esophagus cancer in males was the highest in Nanyang Wolong District (34.47 per 100,000) followed by Jiyuan City (31.92 per 100,000), and Hebi City (29.66 per 100,000). For females, it was the highest in Hebi City (16.94 per 100,000), followed by Jiyuan City (16.74 per 100,000), and Nanyang Wolong District (14.61 per 100,000). The ASR China mortality rate of esophagus cancer in males was the highest in Nanyang Wolong District (32.14 per 100,000) followed by Jiyuan City (29.94 per 100,000), and Hebi City (24.15 per 100,000). For females, it was the highest in Nanyang Wolong District (14.57 per 100,000), followed by Jiyuan City (14.08 per 100,000), and Hebi City (11.3 per 100,000). (Figure 5-3b)

Among the 41 rural cancer registries, the ASR China incidence rate of esophagus cancer in males was the highest in Qi County (79.92 per 100,000) followed by Linzhou City (50.98 per 100,000), and Luoning County (47.97 per 100,000). For females, it was the highest in Qi County (52.01 per 100,000), followed by Linzhou City (33.42 per 100,000), and Xun County (31.98 per 100,000). The ASR China mortality rate of esophagus cancer in males was the highest in Qi County (44.92 per 100,000) followed by Luoning County (44.30 per 100,000), and Linzhou City (42.01 per 100,000). For females, it was the highest in Linzhou City (28.41 per 100,000), followed by Song County (23.36 per 100,000), and Luoning County (20.07 per 100,000). (Figure 5-3c)

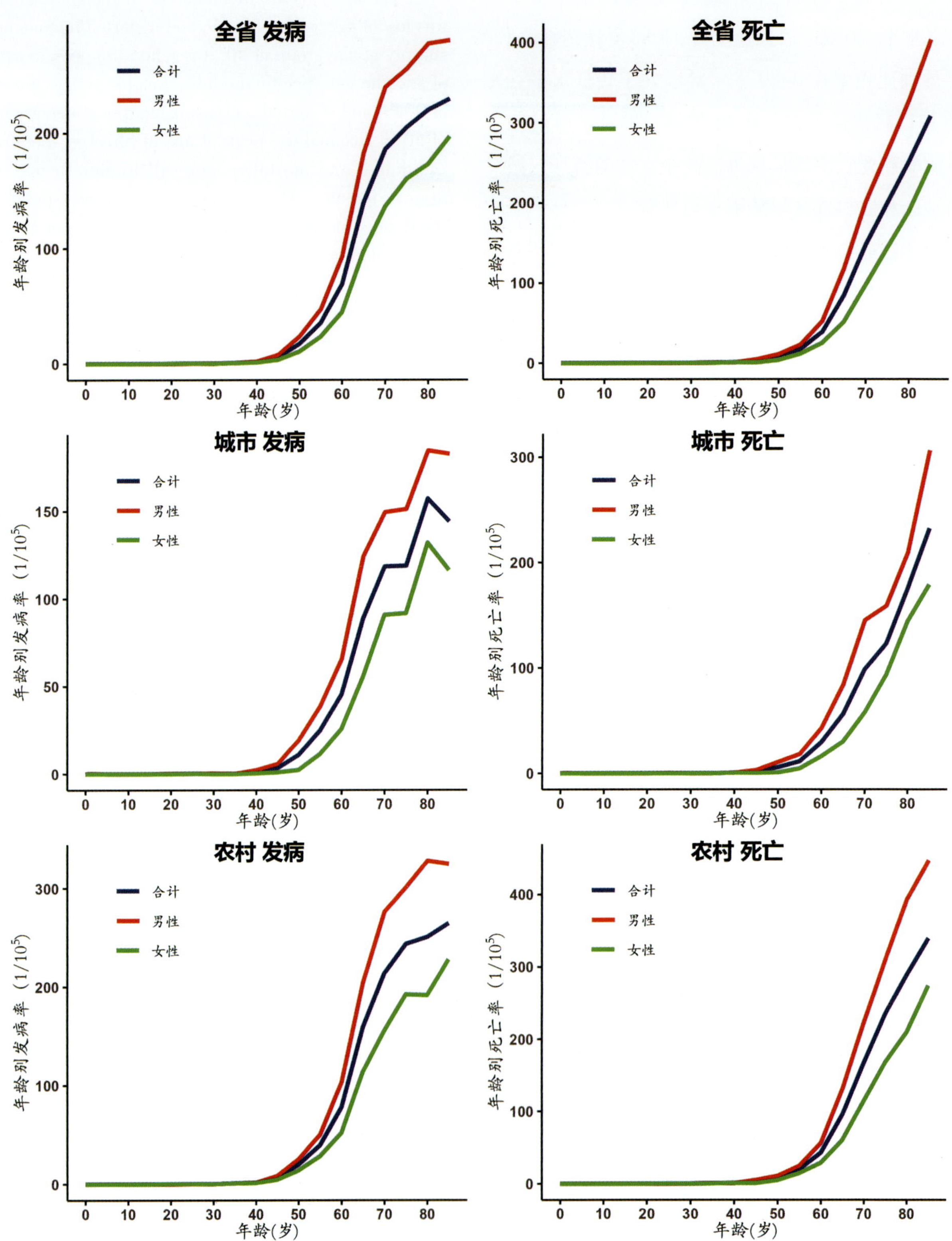

图 5-3a　2020 年河南省肿瘤登记地区食管癌年龄别发病率和死亡率

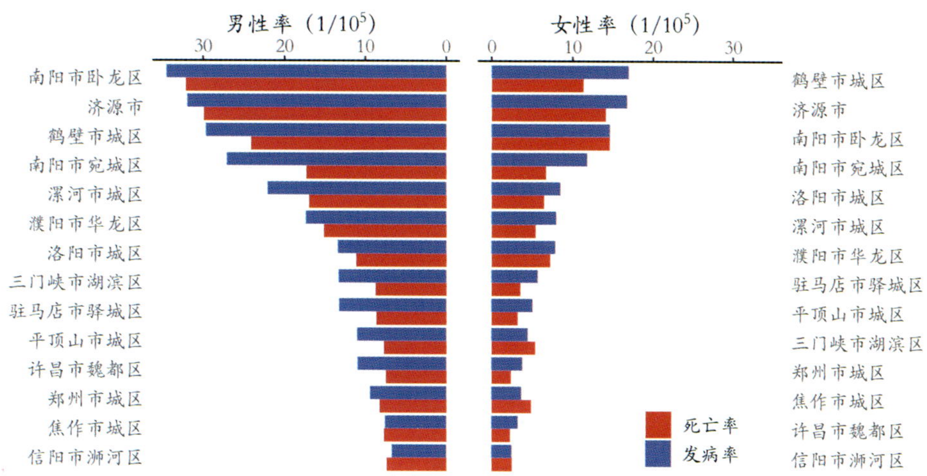

图 5-3b　2020 年河南省城市肿瘤登记地区食管癌发病率和死亡率

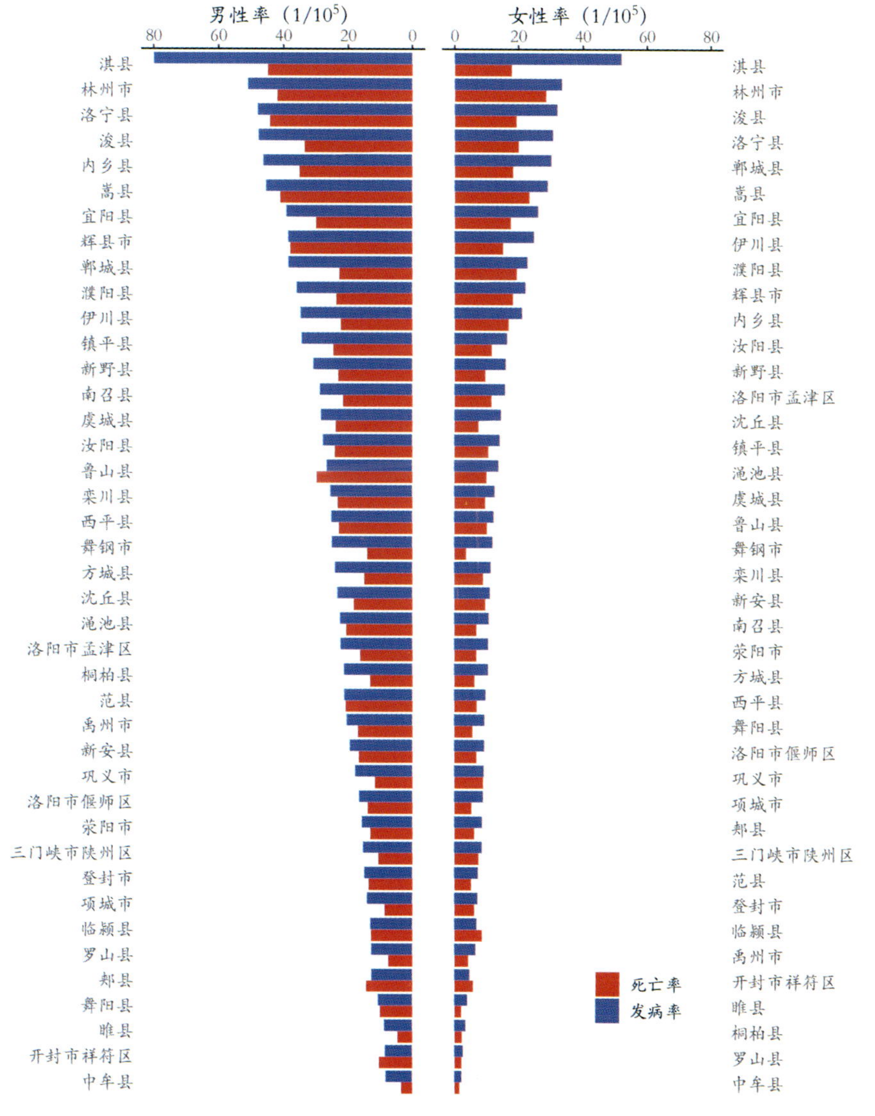

图 5-3c　2020 年河南省农村肿瘤登记地区食管癌发病率和死亡率

2020 年，河南省肿瘤登记地区食管癌发病病例中有确切解剖学亚部位信息的占 48.12%，亚部位未特指的占 51.88%。在有亚部位信息的食管病例中，颈部占 15.70%，胸部占 26.10%，腹部占 4.42%，上段占 14.92%，中段占 23.10%，下段占 10.96%，交搭跨越占 4.8%。（图 5-3d）

About 48.12% of the esophagus cancer had specific subsite. Among those cases, cervical accounted for 15.70%, thoracic accounted for 26.10%, abdominal accounted for 4.42%, upper accounted for 14.92%, middle accounted for 23.10%, lower accounted for 10.96%, and overlapping accounted for 4.8%. (Figure 5-3d)

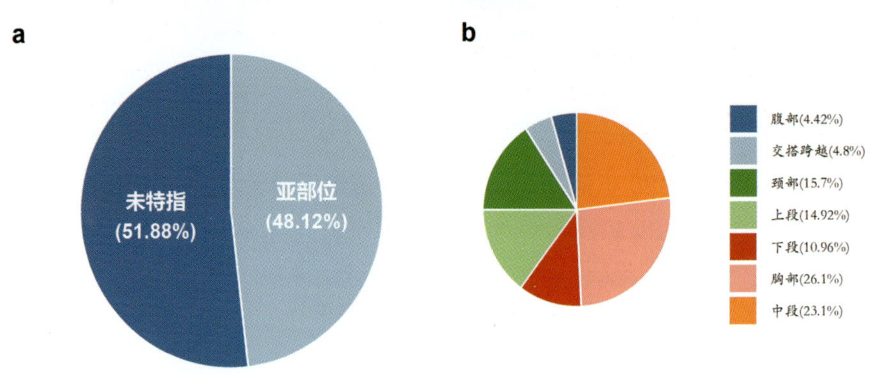

图 5-3d 2020 年河南省肿瘤登记地区食管癌发病病例亚部位构成

2020 年，河南省肿瘤登记地区食管癌发病病例中有明确组织病理学分型的占 68.67%，组织学类型未特指的占 31.33%。在有组织病理学分型的食管病例中，鳞状细胞癌占 51.75%，腺癌占 6.45%，腺鳞癌占 1.02%，其他占 40.77%。（图 5-3e）

About 68.67% of the esophagus cancer had morphological verification. Among those cases, Squamous cell accounted for 51.75%, Adenocarcinoma accounted for 6.45%, Adenosquamous accounted for 1.02%, and Others accounted for 40.77%. (Figure 5-3e)

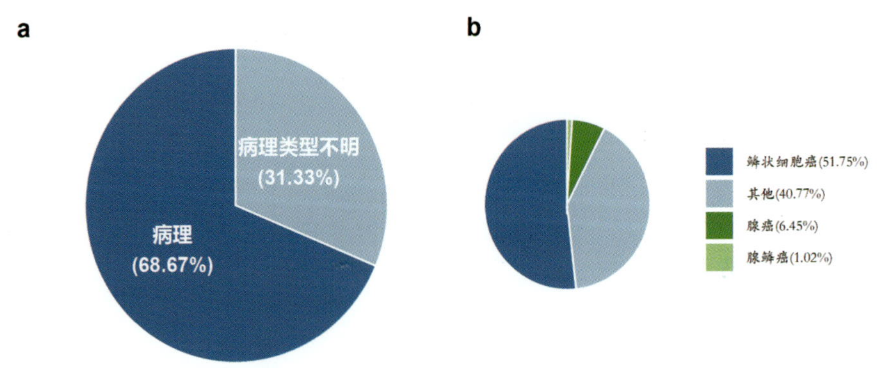

图 5-3e 2020 年河南省肿瘤登记地区食管癌发病病例形态学构成

四、胃

2020年，河南省肿瘤登记地区胃癌的发病率为30.35/10万，中标率为20.34/10万，世标率为20.36/10万，发病例数占全部癌症新发病例数的10.85%；其中，男性和女性发病率分别为41.51/10万和18.70/10万，城市地区和农村地区发病率分别为25.43/10万和32.31/10万；中标发病率呈现男性高于女性、农村地区高于城市地区的特点，男性中标发病率是女性的2.48倍，农村地区中标发病率是城市地区的1.33倍。同期，胃癌的死亡率为23.78/10万，中标率为15.24/10万，世标率为15.19/10万，死亡病例数占全部癌症死亡病例数的14.59%；其中，男性和女性死亡率分别为32.74/10万和14.43/10万，城市地区和农村地区死亡率分别为19.47/10万和25.50/10万；中标死亡率呈现男性高于女性、农村地区高于城市地区的特点，男性中标死亡率是女性的2.71倍，农村地区中标死亡率是城市地区的1.40倍。（表5-4）

4. Stomach

In 2020, there were 13,094 new cases diagnosed as stomach cancer in registration areas of Henan Province, China (9,147 males and 3,947 females, 3,126 in urban areas and 9,968 in rural areas), accounting for 10.85% of new cases of all cancers. The crude incidence rate was 30.35 per 100,000, with the ASR China 20.34 per 100,000 and the ASR World 20.36 per 100,000, respectively. Subgroup analysis showed that the incidence of ASR China was 2.48 times in males as that in females, and it was 1.33 times in rural areas as that in urban areas. The cumulative incidence rate for subjects aged 0 to 74 years was 2.57%. (Table 5–4)

A total of 10,260 cases died of stomach cancer in 2020 (7,214 males and 3,046 females, 2,393 in urban areas and 7,867 in rural areas), accounting for 14.59% of all cancer deaths. The crude mortality rate was 23.78 per 100,000, with the ASR China of 15.24 per 100,000 and the ASR World of 15.19 per 100,000, respectively. Subgroup analysis showed that the mortality of ASR China was 2.71 times in males as that in females, and it was 1.40 times in rural areas as that in urban areas. The cumulative mortality rate for subjects aged 0 to 74 years was 1.77%. (Table 5–4)

表5-4 2020年河南省肿瘤登记地区胃癌发病与死亡情况

地区	性别	病例数	粗率（1/10^5）	构成（%）	中标率（1/10^5）	世标率（1/10^5）	累积率 0～74（%）
发病							
全省	合计	13 094	30.35	10.85	20.34	20.36	2.57
	男性	9 147	41.51	14.80	29.37	29.52	3.82
	女性	3 947	18.70	6.70	11.84	11.71	1.36
城市地区	合计	3 126	25.43	8.52	16.55	16.64	2.14
	男性	2 240	36.52	12.25	24.82	25.03	3.33
	女性	886	14.39	4.81	8.91	8.88	1.02
农村地区	合计	9 968	32.31	11.87	21.94	21.91	2.74
	男性	6 907	43.44	15.87	31.29	31.40	4.01
	女性	3 061	20.47	7.56	13.08	12.90	1.49

续表

地区	性别	病例数	粗率（1/10^5）	构成（%）	中标率（1/10^5）	世标率（1/10^5）	累积率 0～74（%）
死亡							
全省	合计	10 260	23.78	14.59	15.24	15.19	1.77
	男性	7 214	32.74	16.67	22.70	22.62	2.70
	女性	3 046	14.43	11.26	8.37	8.36	0.87
城市地区	合计	2 393	19.47	12.15	11.90	11.89	1.36
	男性	1 683	27.44	13.92	17.89	17.93	2.16
	女性	710	11.53	9.33	6.47	6.41	0.62
农村地区	合计	7 867	25.50	15.53	16.63	16.56	1.93
	男性	5 531	34.78	17.73	24.72	24.57	2.91
	女性	2 336	15.62	12.01	9.16	9.17	0.98

胃癌年龄别发病率在 0~39 岁年龄段处于较低水平，40 岁以后快速上升，在 85 岁达到峰值；年龄别死亡率在 0~49 岁年龄段处于较低水平，50 岁以后快速上升，在 85 岁达到峰值；年龄别发病率和死亡率均呈现男性高于女性的特点；城市地区和农村地区年龄别率虽然有一定差异，但是总体趋势类同。（图 5-4a）

在 14 个城市肿瘤登记地区中，男性胃癌标化发病率最高的是济源市（87.78/10 万），其次是南阳市卧龙区（48.79/10 万）和南阳市宛城区（46.52/10 万）；女性标化发病率最高的是济源市（27.08/10 万），其次是南阳市宛城区（16.35/10 万）和南阳市卧龙区（14.65/10 万）。男性标化死亡率最高的是济源市（69.92/10 万），其次是南阳市卧龙区（42.81/10 万）和南阳市宛城区（32.44/10 万）；女性标化死亡率最高的是济源市（24.73/10 万），其次是南阳市卧龙区（16.99/10 万）和南阳市宛城区（9.81/10 万）。（图 5-4b）

The age specific incidence of stomach cancer was low at age group of 0~39, and it started increasing sharply at age group of 40, it reached the peak at age of 85. The age specific mortality was low at age group of 0~49, and it started increasing sharply at age group of 50, it reached the peak at age of 85. Age specific incidence and mortality were all higher in males than in females, The change pattern of age specific incidence and mortality were similar in urban areas and rural areas. (Figure 5–4a)

Among the 14 urban cancer registries, the ASR China incidence rate of stomach cancer in males was the highest in Jiyuan City (87.78 per 100,000) followed by Nanyang Wolong District (48.79 per 100,000), and Nanyang Wancheng District (46.52 per 100,000). For females, it was the highest in Jiyuan City (27.08 per 100,000), followed by Nanyang Wancheng District (16.35 per 100,000), and Nanyang Wolong District (14.65 per 100,000). The ASR China mortality rate of stomach cancer in males was the highest in Jiyuan City (69.92 per 100,000) followed by Nanyang Wolong District (42.81 per 100,000), and Nanyang Wancheng District (32.44 per 100,000). For females, it was the highest in Jiyuan City (24.73 per 100,000), followed by Nanyang Wolong District (16.99 per 100,000), and Nanyang Wancheng District (9.81 per 100,000). (Figure 5–4b)

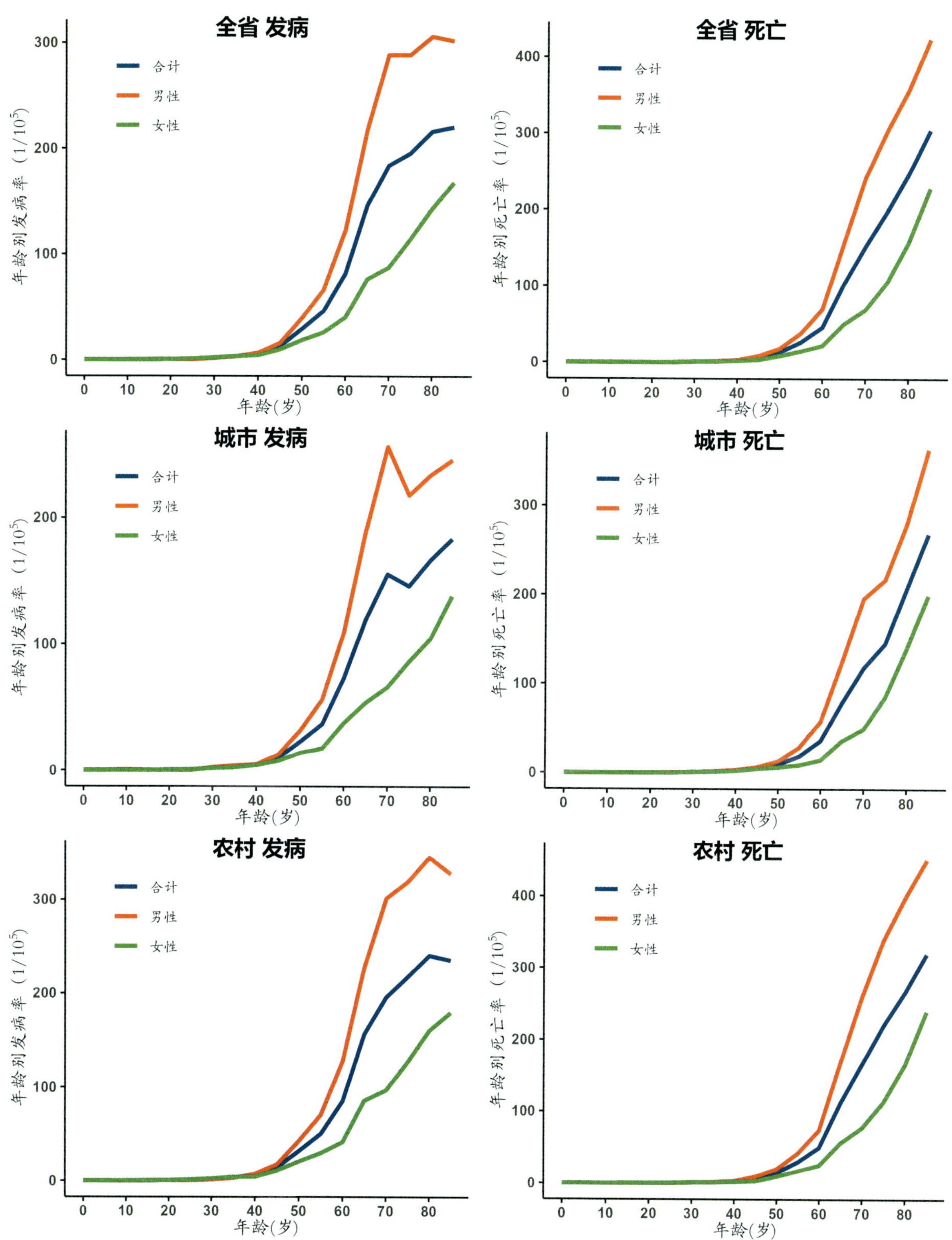

图 5-4a　2020 年河南省肿瘤登记地区胃癌年龄别发病率和死亡率

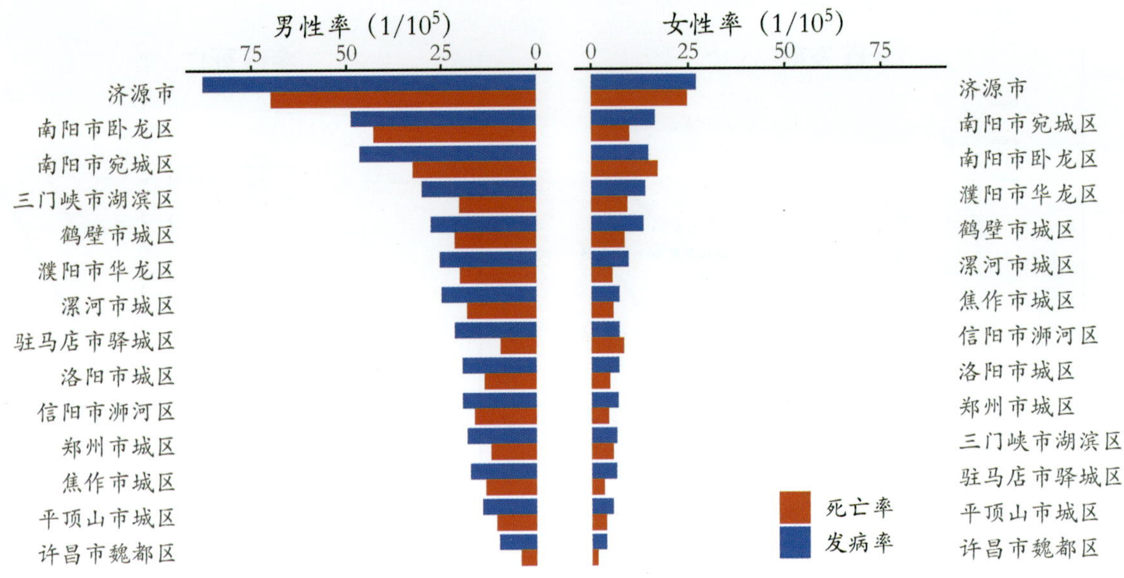

图 5-4b　2020 年河南省城市肿瘤登记地区胃癌发病率和死亡率

在 41 个农村肿瘤登记地区中，男性胃癌标化发病率最高的是南召县（70.19/10 万），其次是林州市（65.11/10 万）和内乡县（51.41/10 万）；女性标化发病率最高的是林州市（30.67/10 万），其次是郸城县（29.55/10 万）和淇县（23.00/10 万）。男性标化死亡率最高的是南召县（59.28/10 万），其次是林州市（53.84/10 万）和嵩县（39.65/10 万）；女性标化死亡率最高的是林州市（19.37/10 万），其次是南召县（16.02/10 万）和郸城县（15.96/10 万）。（图 5-4c）

2020 年，河南省肿瘤登记地区胃癌发病病例中有确切解剖学亚部位信息的占 57.82%，亚部位未特指的占 42.18%。在有亚部位信息的胃病例中，贲门占 52.97%，胃底占 12.17%，胃体占 14.56%，胃窦占 7.49%，胃幽门占 1.91%，胃小弯占 4.96%，胃大弯占 0.95%，交搭跨越占 4.99%。（图 5-4d）

Among the 41 rural cancer registries, the ASR China incidence rate of stomach cancer in males was the highest in Nanzhao County (70.19 per 100,000) followed by Linzhou City (65.11 per 100,000), and Neixiang County (51.41 per 100,000). For females, it was the highest in Linzhou City (30.67 per 100,000), followed by Dancheng County (29.55 per 100,000), and Qi County (23.00 per 100,000). The ASR China mortality rate of stomach cancer in males was the highest in Nanzhao County (59.28 per 100,000) followed by Linzhou City (53.84 per 100,000), and Song County (39.65 per 100,000). For females, it was the highest in Linzhou City (19.37 per 100,000), followed by Nanzhao County (16.02 per 100,000), and Dancheng County (15.96 per 100,000). (Figure 5-4c)

About 57.82% of the stomach cancer had specific subsite. Among those cases, cardia accounted for 52.97%, fundus accounted for 12.17%, body accounted for 14.56%, pylorus antrum accounted for 7.49%, pylorus accounted for 1.91%, lesser cuvature accounted for 4.96%, greater cuvature accounted for 0.95%, and overlapping accounted for 4.99%. (Figure 5-4d)

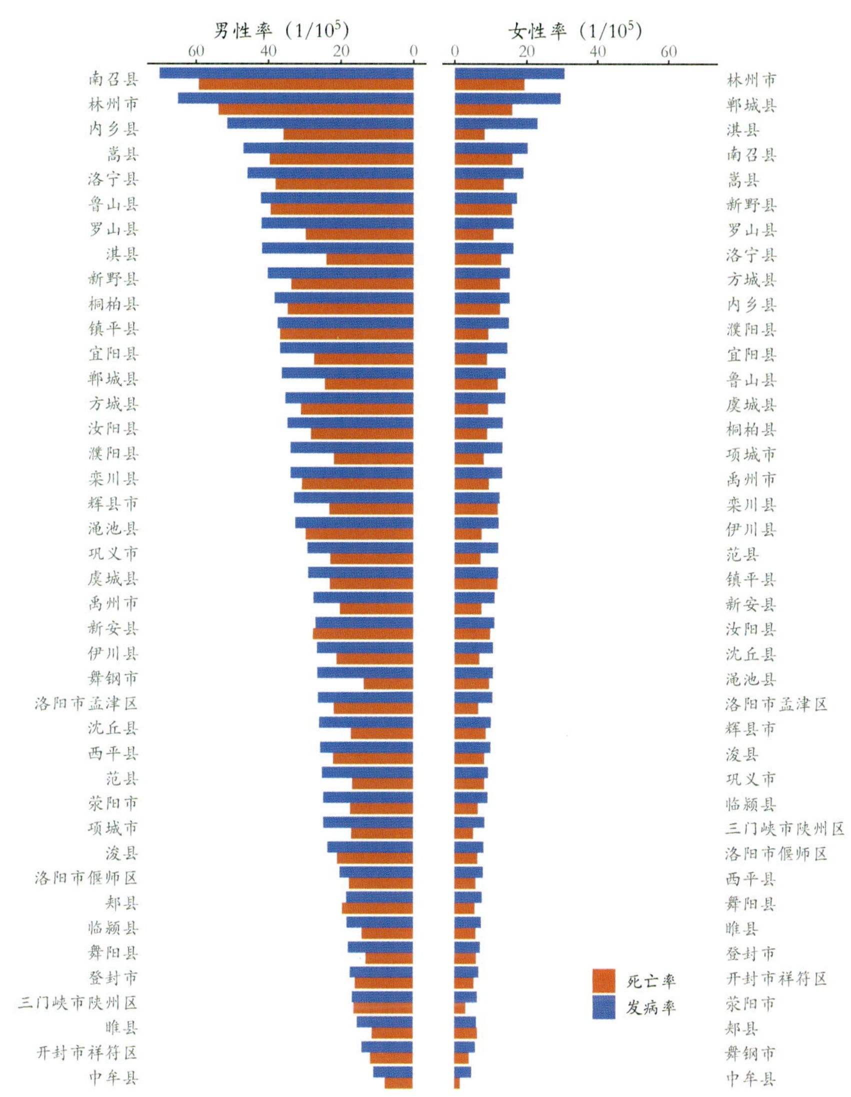

图 5-4c　2020 年河南省农村肿瘤登记地区胃癌发病率和死亡率

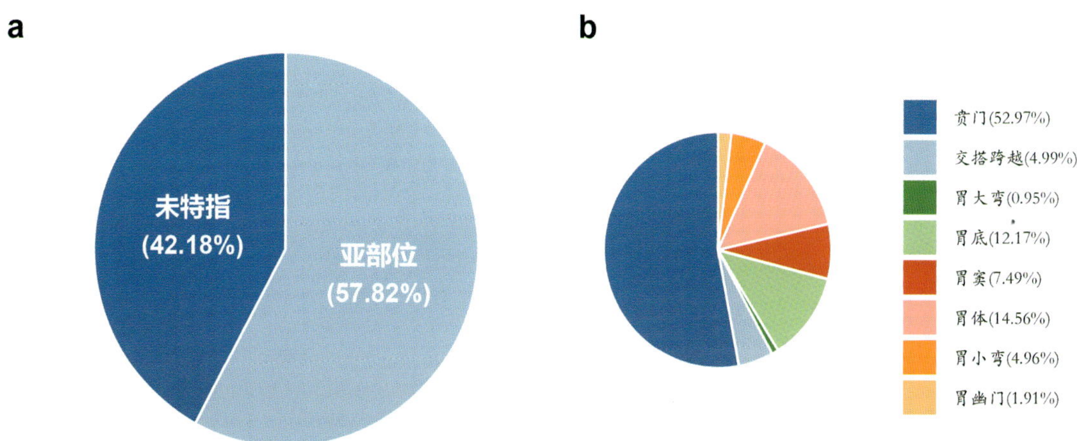

图 5-4d　2020 年河南省肿瘤登记地区胃癌发病病例亚部位构成

2020 年，河南省肿瘤登记地区胃癌发病病例中有明确组织病理学分型的占 65.58%，组织学类型未特指的占 34.42%。在有组织病理学分型的胃癌病例中，鳞状细胞癌占 3.00%，腺癌占 50.11%，腺鳞癌占 0.20%，类癌占 0.52%，其他占 46.17%。（图 5-4e）

About 65.58% of the stomach cancer had morphological verification. Among those cases, Squamous cell accounted for 3%, Adenocarcinoma accounted for 50.11%, Adenosquamous accounted for 0.2%, Carcinoid accounted for 0.52%, and others accounted for 46.17%. (Figure 5-4e)

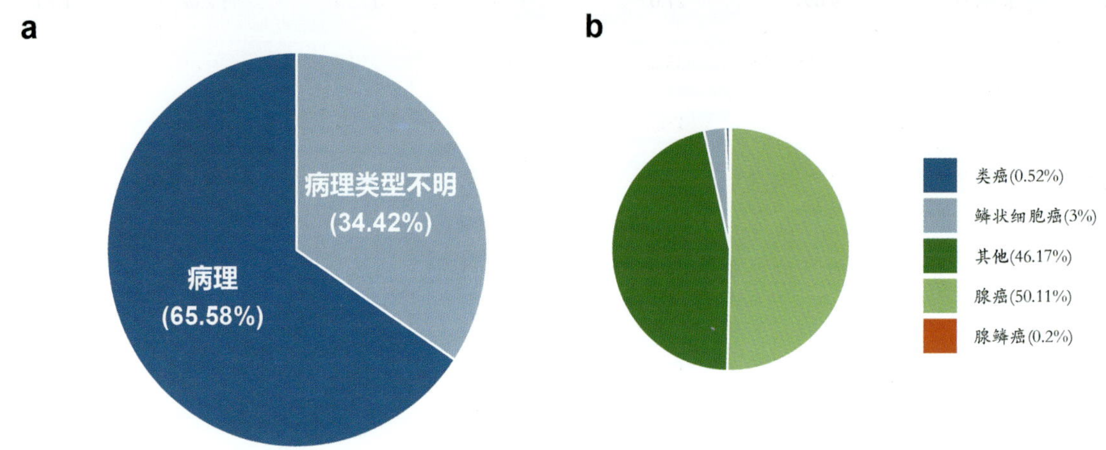

图 5-4e 2020 年河南省肿瘤登记地区胃癌发病病例形态学构成

五、结直肠

2020 年，河南省肿瘤登记地区结直肠癌的发病率为 21.07/10 万，中标率为 14.56/10 万，世标率为 14.36/10 万，发病例数占全部癌症新发病例数的 7.53%；其中，男性和女性发病率分别为 22.65/10 万和 19.43/10 万，城市地区和农村地区发病率分别为 26.16/10 万和 19.04/10 万；中标发病率呈现男性高于女性、城市地区高于农村地区的特点，男性中标发病率是女性的 1.30 倍，城市地区中标发病率是农村地区的 1.27 倍。同期，结直肠癌的死亡率为 10.07/10 万，中标率为 6.42/10 万，世标率为 6.39/10 万，死亡病例数占全部癌症死亡病例数的 6.17%；其中，男性和女性死亡率分别为 10.96/10 万和 9.13/10 万，城市地区和农村地区死亡率分别为 11.93/10 万和 9.32/10 万；中标死亡率呈现男性高于女性、城市地区高于农村地区的特点，男性中标死亡率是女性的 1.41 倍，城市地区中标死亡率是农村地区的 1.16 倍。（表 5-5）

5. Colorectum

In 2020, there were 9,091 new cases diagnosed as colon rectum cancer in registration areas of Henan Province, China (4,990 males and 4,101 females, 3,216 in urban areas and 5,875 in rural areas), accounting for 7.53% of new cases of all cancers. The crude incidence rate was 21.07 per 100,000, with the ASR China 14.56 per 100,000 and the ASR World 14.36 per 100,000, respectively. Subgroup analysis showed that the incidence of ASR China was 1.30 times in males as that in females, and it was 1.27 times in urban areas as that in rural areas. The cumulative incidence rate for subjects aged 0 to 74 years was 1.75%. (Table 5-5)

A total of 4,343 cases died of colon rectum cancer in 2020 (2,415 males and 1,928 females, 1,467 in urban areas and 2,876 in rural areas), accounting for 6.17% of all cancer deaths. The crude mortality rate was 10.07 per 100,000, with the ASR China of 6.42 per 100,000 and the ASR World of 6.39 per 100,000, respectively. Subgroup analysis showed that the mortality of ASR China was 1.41 times in males as that in females, and it was 1.16 times in urban areas as that in rural areas. The cumulative mortality rate for subjects aged 0 to 74 years was 0.67%. (Table 5-5)

表 5–5　2020 年河南省肿瘤登记地区结直肠癌发病与死亡情况

地区	性别	病例数	粗率（1/10^5）	构成（%）	中标率（1/10^5）	世标率（1/10^5）	累积率 0～74（%）
发病							
全省	合计	9 091	21.07	7.53	14.56	14.36	1.75
	男性	4 990	22.65	8.07	16.53	16.24	1.99
	女性	4 101	19.43	6.97	12.69	12.57	1.52
城市地区	合计	3 216	26.16	8.77	17.12	17.04	2.05
	男性	1 788	29.15	9.78	19.87	19.75	2.41
	女性	1 428	23.19	7.76	14.58	14.53	1.72
农村地区	合计	5 875	19.04	6.99	13.47	13.24	1.63
	男性	3 202	20.14	7.36	15.11	14.77	1.82
	女性	2 673	17.88	6.61	11.88	11.76	1.44
死亡							
全省	合计	4 343	10.07	6.17	6.42	6.39	0.67
	男性	2 415	10.96	5.58	7.58	7.55	0.80
	女性	1 928	9.13	7.12	5.37	5.34	0.55
城市地区	合计	1 467	11.93	7.45	7.11	7.18	0.71
	男性	851	13.88	7.04	8.79	8.94	0.93
	女性	616	10.00	8.10	5.58	5.61	0.52
农村地区	合计	2 876	9.32	5.68	6.13	6.06	0.65
	男性	1 564	9.84	5.01	7.07	6.97	0.75
	女性	1 312	8.77	6.74	5.28	5.24	0.56

结直肠癌年龄别发病率在 0~34 岁年龄段处于较低水平，35 岁以后快速上升，在 80 岁达到峰值；年龄别死亡率在 0~49 岁年龄段处于较低水平，50 岁以后快速上升，在 85 岁达到峰值；年龄别发病率和死亡率均呈现男性高于女性的特点；城市地区和农村地区年龄别率虽然有一定差异，但是总体趋势类同。（图 5-5a）

在 14 个城市肿瘤登记地区中，男性结直肠癌标化发病率最高的是濮阳市华龙区（29.51/10 万），其次是漯河市城区（25.72/10 万）和郑州市城区（25.02/10 万）；女性标化发病率最高的是濮阳市华龙区（19.32/10 万），其次是漯河市城区（18.62/10 万）和济源市（17.20/10 万）。男性标化死亡率最高的是濮阳市华龙区(13.87/10 万），其次是南阳市卧龙区（11.92/10 万）和济源市（11.42/10 万）；女性标化死亡率最高的是濮阳市华龙区（10.32/10 万），其次是南阳市卧龙区（8.95/10 万）和济源市（7.96/10 万）。（图 5-5b）

在 41 个农村肿瘤登记地区中，男性结直肠癌标化发病率最高的是罗山县（22.49/10 万），其次是濮阳县（21.41/10 万）和桐柏县（21.26/10 万）；女性标化发病率最高的是郸城县（18.76/10 万），其次是虞城县（18.41/10 万）和开封市祥符区（15.36/10 万）。男性标化死亡率最高的是虞城县(12.31/10万),其次是桐柏县(11.62/10万)和方城县（11.07/10 万）；女性标化死亡率最高的是郸城县(9.74/10 万),其次是虞城县(9.01/10 万）和中牟县（8.47/10 万）。（图 5-5c）

The age specific incidence of colon rectum cancer was low at age group of 0~34, and it started increasing sharply at age group of 35, it reached the peak at age of 80. The age specific mortality was low at age group of 0~49, and it started increasing sharply at age group of 50, it reached the peak at age of 85. Age specific incidence and mortality were all higher in males than in females, The change pattern of age specific incidence and mortality were similar in urban areas and rural areas. (Figure 5-5a)

Among the 14 urban cancer registries, the ASR China incidence rate of colon rectum cancer in males was the highest in Puyang Hualong District (29.51 per 100,000) followed by Luohe City (25.72 per 100,000), and Zhengzhou City (25.02 per 100,000). For females, it was the highest in Puyang Hualong District (19.32 per 100,000), followed by Luohe City (18.62 per 100,000), and Jiyuan City (17.20 per 100,000). The ASR China mortality rate of colon rectum cancer in males was the highest in Puyang Hualong District (13.87 per 100,000) followed by Nanyang Wolong District (11.92 per 100,000), and Jiyuan City (11.42 per 100,000). For females, it was the highest in Puyang Hualong District (10.32 per 100,000), followed by Nanyang Wolong District (8.95 per 100,000), and Jiyuan City (7.96 per 100,000). (Figure 5-5b)

Among the 41 rural cancer registries, the ASR China incidence rate of colon rectum cancer in males was the highest in Luoshan County (22.49 per 100,000) followed by Puyang County (21.41 per 100,000), and Tongbai County (21.26 per 100,000). For females, it was the highest in Dancheng County (18.76 per 100,000), followed by Yucheng County (18.41 per 100,000), and Kaifeng Xiangfu District (15.36 per 100,000). The ASR China mortality rate of colon rectum cancer in males was the highest in Yucheng County (12.31 per 100,000) followed by Tongbai County (11.62 per 100,000), and Fangcheng County (11.07 per 100,000). For females, it was the highest in Dancheng County (9.74 per 100,000), followed by Yucheng County (9.01 per 100,000), and Zhongmu County (8.47 per 100,000). (Figure 5-5c)

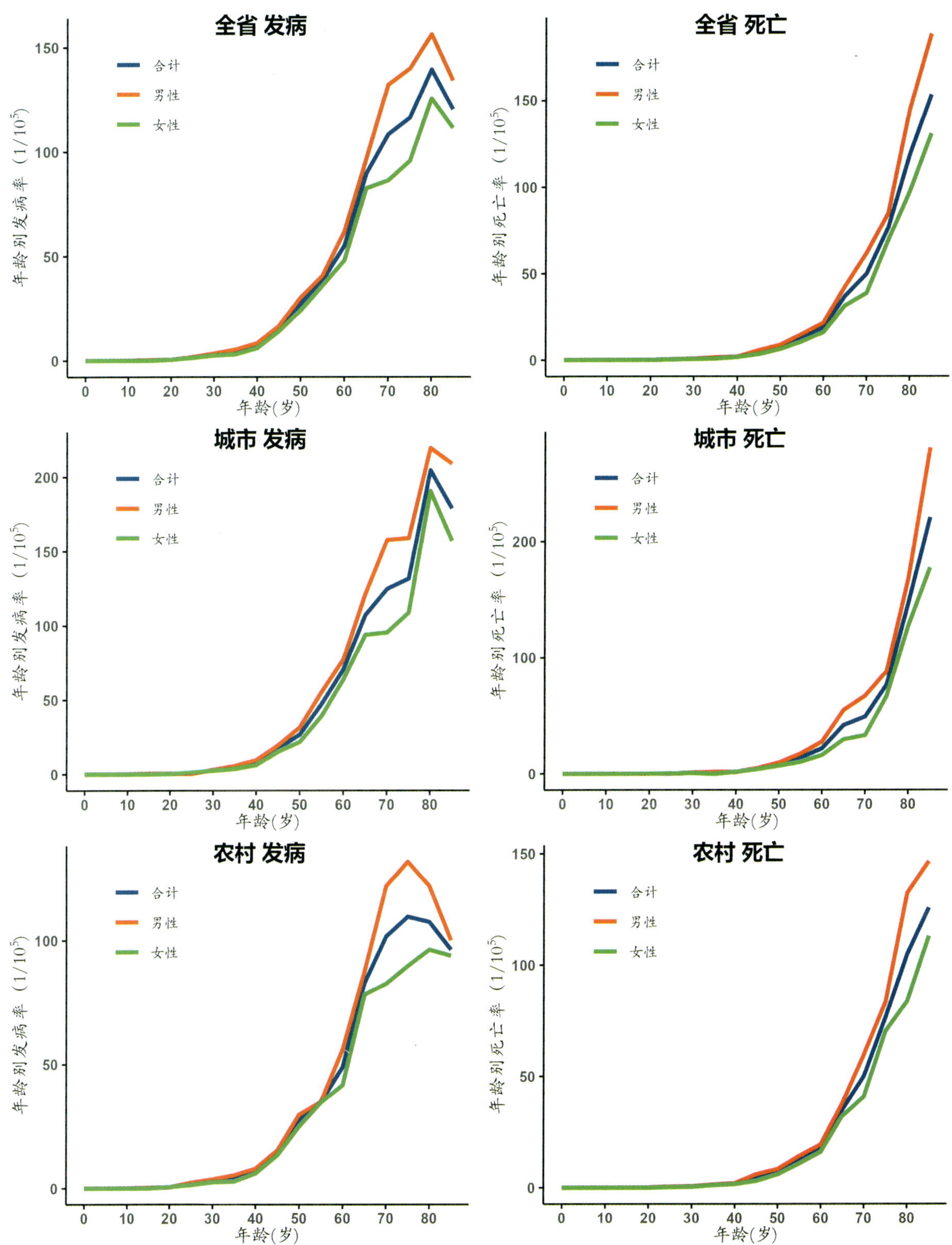

图 5-5a　2020 年河南省肿瘤登记地区结直肠癌年龄别发病率和死亡率

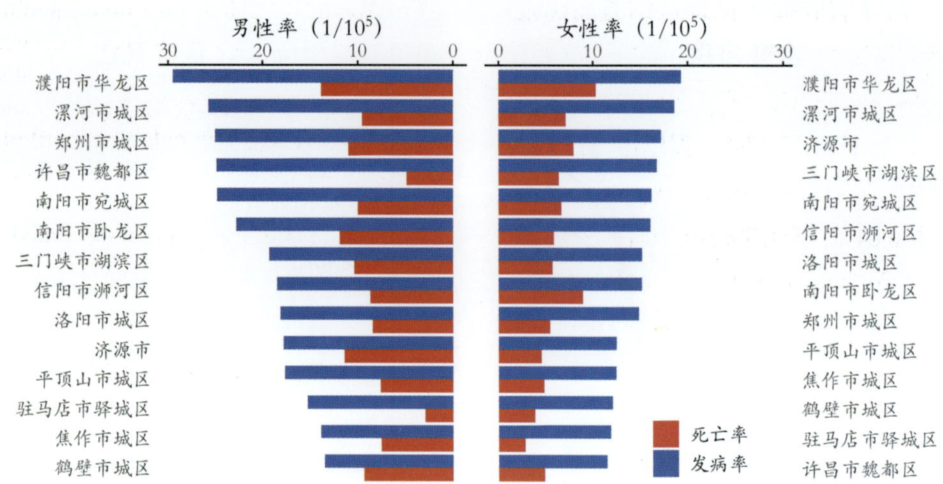

图 5-5b　2020 年河南省城市肿瘤登记地区结直肠癌发病率和死亡率

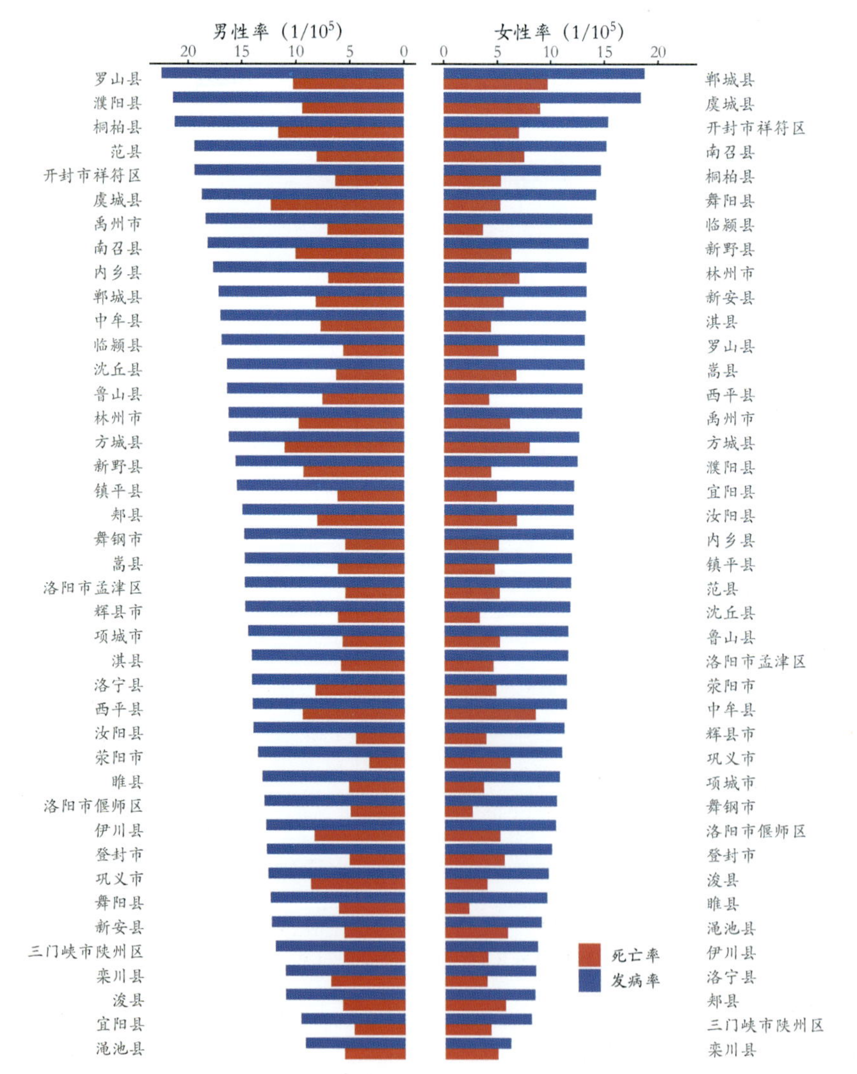

图 5-5c　2020 年河南省农村肿瘤登记地区结直肠癌发病率和死亡率

2020 年，河南省肿瘤登记地区结直肠癌发病病例中有确切解剖学亚部位信息的占 31.72%，亚部位未特指的占 68.28%。在有亚部位信息的结直肠病例中，盲肠占 13.47%，阑尾占 3.84%，升结肠占 19.80%，结肠肝曲占 4.31%，横结肠占 7.92%，脾曲占 0.64%，降结肠占 6.10%，乙状结肠占 27.70%，交搭跨越占 16.22%。（图 5–5d）

About 31.72% of the colon rectum cancer had specific subsite. Among those cases, caecum accounted for 13.47%, appendix accounted for 3.84%, ascending colon accounted for 19.80%, hepatic flexure accounted for 4.31%, transverse colon accounted for 7.92%, splenic flexure accounted for 0.64%, descending colon accounted for 6.10%, sigmoid colon accounted for 27.70%, and overlapping accounted for 16.22%. (Figure 5–5d)

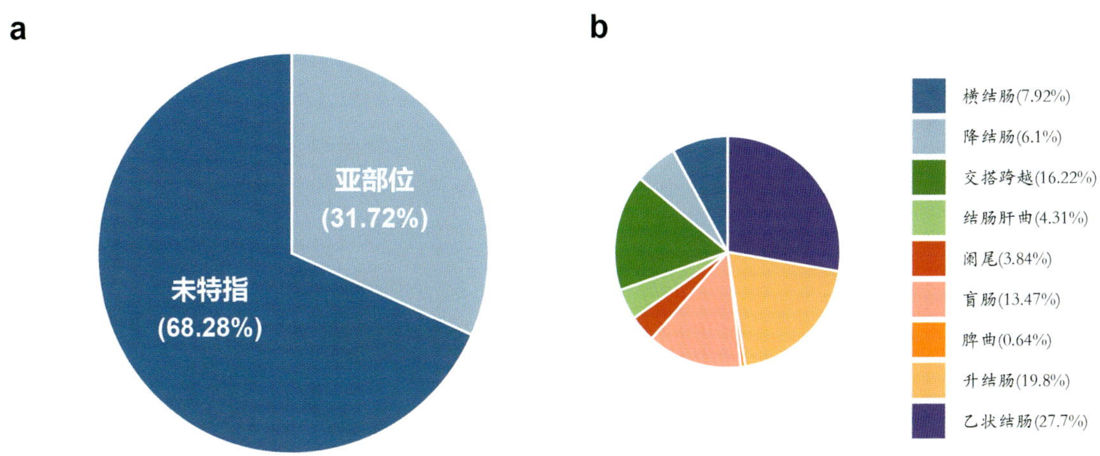

图 5–5d　2020 年河南省肿瘤登记地区结直肠癌发病病例亚部位构成

六、肝

2020 年，河南省肿瘤登记地区肝癌的发病率为 24.44/10 万，中标率为 17.03/10 万，世标率为 16.94/10 万，发病例数占全部癌症新发病例数的 8.74%；其中，男性和女性发病率分别为 32.87/10 万和 15.65/10 万，城市地区和农村地区发病率分别为 22.15/10 万和 25.35/10 万；中标发病率呈现男性高于女性、农村地区高于城市地区的特点，男性中标发病率是女性的 2.43 倍，农村地区中标发病率是城市地区的 1.21 倍。同期，肝癌的死亡率为 21.37/10 万，中标率为 14.41/10 万，世标率为 14.41/10 万，死亡病例数占全部癌症死亡病例数的 13.11%；其中，男性和女性死亡率分别为

6. Liver

In 2020, there were 10,545 new cases diagnosed as liver cancer in registration areas of Henan Province, China (7,242 males and 3,303 females, 2,723 in urban areas and 7,822 in rural areas), accounting for 8.74% of new cases of all cancers. The crude incidence rate was 24.44 per 100,000, with the ASR China 17.03 per 100,000 and the ASR World 16.94 per 100,000, respectively. Subgroup analysis showed that the incidence of ASR China was 2.43 times in males as that in females, and it was 1.21 times in rural areas as that in urban areas. The cumulative incidence rate for subjects aged 0 to 74 years was 2.04%. (Table 5–6)

A total of 9,221 cases died of liver cancer in 2020 (6,341 males and 2,880 females, 2,452 in urban areas and 6,769 in rural areas), accounting for 13.11% of all cancer deaths. The crude mortality rate was 21.37 per 100,000, with the ASR China of

28.78/10 万和 13.64/10 万，城市地区和农村地区死亡率分别为 19.95/10 万和 21.94/10 万；中标死亡率呈现男性高于女性、农村地区高于城市地区的特点，男性中标死亡率是女性的 2.51 倍，农村地区中标死亡率是城市地区的 1.16 倍。（表 5–6）

14.41 per 100,000 and the ASR World of 14.41 per 100,000, respectively. Subgroup analysis showed that the mortality of ASR China was 2.51 times in males as that in females, and it was 1.16 times in rural areas as that in urban areas. The cumulative mortality rate for subjects aged 0 to 74 years was 1.70%. (Table 5–6)

表 5–6　2020 年河南省肿瘤登记地区肝癌发病与死亡情况

地区	性别	病例数	粗率（1/10^5）	构成（%）	中标率（1/10^5）	世标率（1/10^5）	累积率 0～74（%）
发病							
全省	合计	10 545	24.44	8.74	17.03	16.94	2.04
	男性	7 242	32.87	11.71	24.17	24.03	2.90
	女性	3 303	15.65	5.61	9.95	9.93	1.20
城市地区	合计	2 723	22.15	7.42	14.81	14.82	1.78
	男性	1 936	31.57	10.59	22.05	22.03	2.63
	女性	787	12.78	4.28	7.87	7.92	0.95
农村地区	合计	7 822	25.35	9.31	17.96	17.82	2.15
	男性	5 306	33.37	12.19	25.03	24.82	3.00
	女性	2 516	16.83	6.22	10.84	10.78	1.30
死亡							
全省	合计	9 221	21.37	13.11	14.41	14.41	1.70
	男性	6 341	28.78	14.65	20.72	20.68	2.46
	女性	2 880	13.64	10.64	8.25	8.30	0.94
城市地区	合计	2 452	19.95	12.45	12.95	13.05	1.52
	男性	1 696	27.65	14.03	18.87	18.96	2.21
	女性	756	12.27	9.94	7.34	7.45	0.87
农村地区	合计	6 769	21.94	13.37	15.02	14.98	1.76
	男性	4 645	29.21	14.89	21.48	21.38	2.55
	女性	2 124	14.21	10.92	8.64	8.67	0.98

肝癌年龄别发病率在 0~29 岁年龄段处于较低水平，30 岁以后快速上升，在 85 岁达到峰值；年龄别死亡率在 0~39 岁年龄段处于较低水平，40 岁以后快速上升，在 85 岁达到峰值；年龄别发病率和死亡率均呈现男性高于女性的特点；城市地区和农村地区年龄别率虽然有一定差异，但是总体趋势类同。（图 5–6a）

The age specific incidence of liver cancer was low at age group of 0~29, and it started increasing sharply at age group of 30, it reached the peak at age of 85. The age specific mortality was low at age group of 0~39, and it started increasing sharply at age group of 40, it reached the peak at age of 85. Age specific incidence and mortality were all higher in males than in females, The change pattern of age specific incidence and mortality were similar in urban areas and rural areas. (Figure 5–6a)

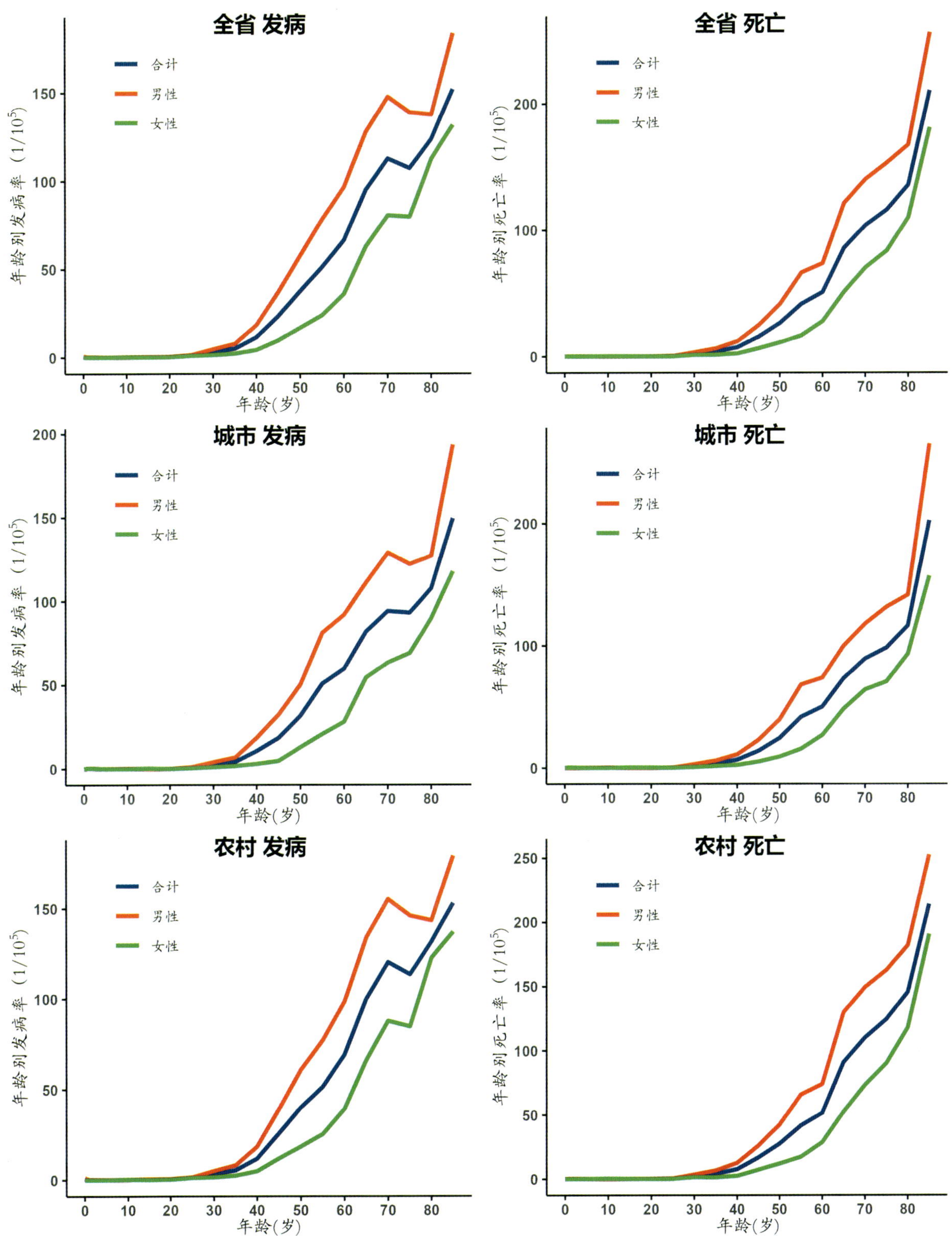

图 5-6a　2020 年河南省肿瘤登记地区肝癌年龄别发病率和死亡率

在 14 个城市肿瘤登记地区中，男性肝癌标化发病率最高的是漯河市城区（36.56/10 万），其次是南阳市卧龙区（31.25/10 万）和南阳市宛城区（30.55/10 万）；女性标化发病率最高的是济源市（15.56/10 万），其次是漯河市城区（13.14/10 万）和南阳市宛城区（11.84/10 万）。男性标化死亡率最高的是漯河市城区（31.64/10 万），其次是南阳市卧龙区（26.89/10 万）和济源市（26.81/10 万）；女性标化死亡率最高的是济源市（13.92/10 万），其次是濮阳市华龙区（11.76/10 万）和漯河市城区（11.50/10 万）。（图 5-6b）

Among the 14 urban cancer registries, the ASR China incidence rate of liver cancer in males was the highest in Luohe City (36.56 per 100,000) followed by Nanyang Wolong District (31.25 per 100,000), and Nanyang Wancheng District (30.55 per 100,000). For females, it was the highest in Jiyuan City (15.56 per 100,000), followed by Luohe City (13.14 per 100,000), and Nanyang Wancheng District (11.84 per 100,000). The ASR China mortality rate of liver cancer in males was the highest in Luohe City (31.64 per 100,000) followed by Nanyang Wolong District (26.89 per 100,000), and Jiyuan City (26.81 per 100,000). For females, it was the highest in Jiyuan City (13.92 per 100,000), followed by Puyang Hualong District (11.76 per 100,000), and Luohe City (11.50 per 100,000). (Figure 5-6b)

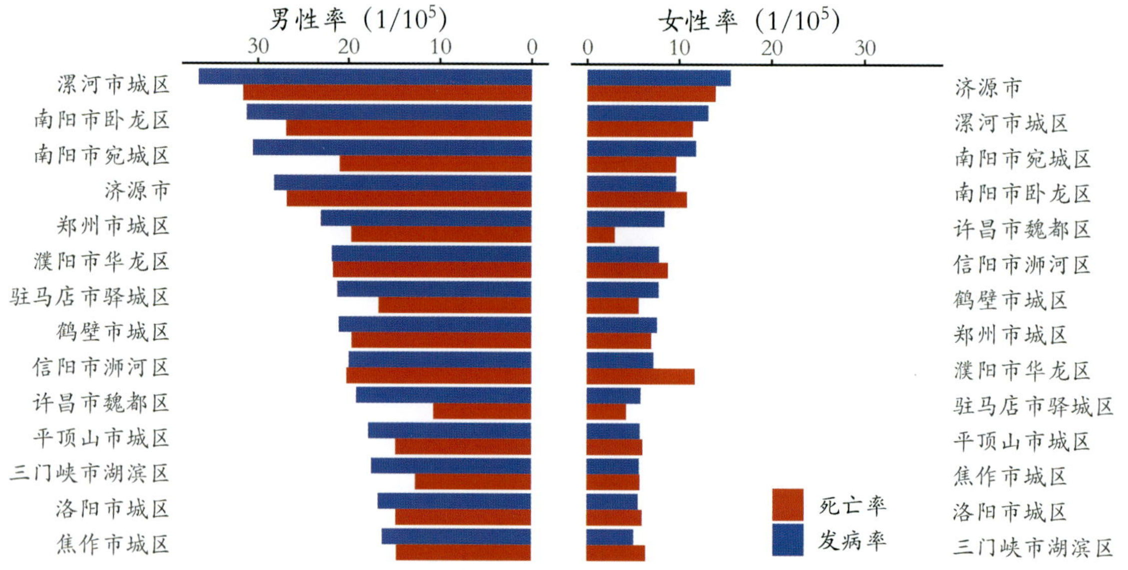

图 5-6b　2020 年河南省城市肿瘤登记地区肝癌发病率和死亡率

在 41 个农村肿瘤登记地区中，男性肝癌标化发病率最高的是睢县（43.22/10 万），其次是禹州市（41.03/10 万）和中牟县（40.52/10 万）；女性标化发病率最高的是郸城县（26.68/10 万），其次是禹州市（21.26/10 万）和睢县（18.73/10 万）。男性标化死亡率最高的是禹州市（36.98/10 万），其次是桐柏县（36.88/10 万）和睢县（36.33/10 万）；女性标化死亡率最高的是郸城县（19.12/10 万），其次是禹州市（18.96/10 万）和睢县（14.22/10 万）。（图 5-6c）

Among the 41 rural cancer registries, the ASR China incidence rate of liver cancer in males was the highest in Sui County (43.22 per 100,000) followed by Yuzhou City (41.03 per 100,000), and Zhongmu County (40.52 per 100,000). For females, it was the highest in Dancheng County (26.68 per 100,000), followed by Yuzhou City (21.26 per 100,000), and Sui County (18.73 per 100,000). The ASR China mortality rate of liver cancer in males was the highest in Yuzhou City (36.98 per 100,000) followed by Tongbai County (36.88 per 100,000), and Sui County (36.33 per 100,000). For females, it was the highest in Dancheng County (19.12 per 100,000), followed by Yuzhou City (18.96 per 100,000), and Sui County (14.22 per 100,000). (Figure 5-6c)

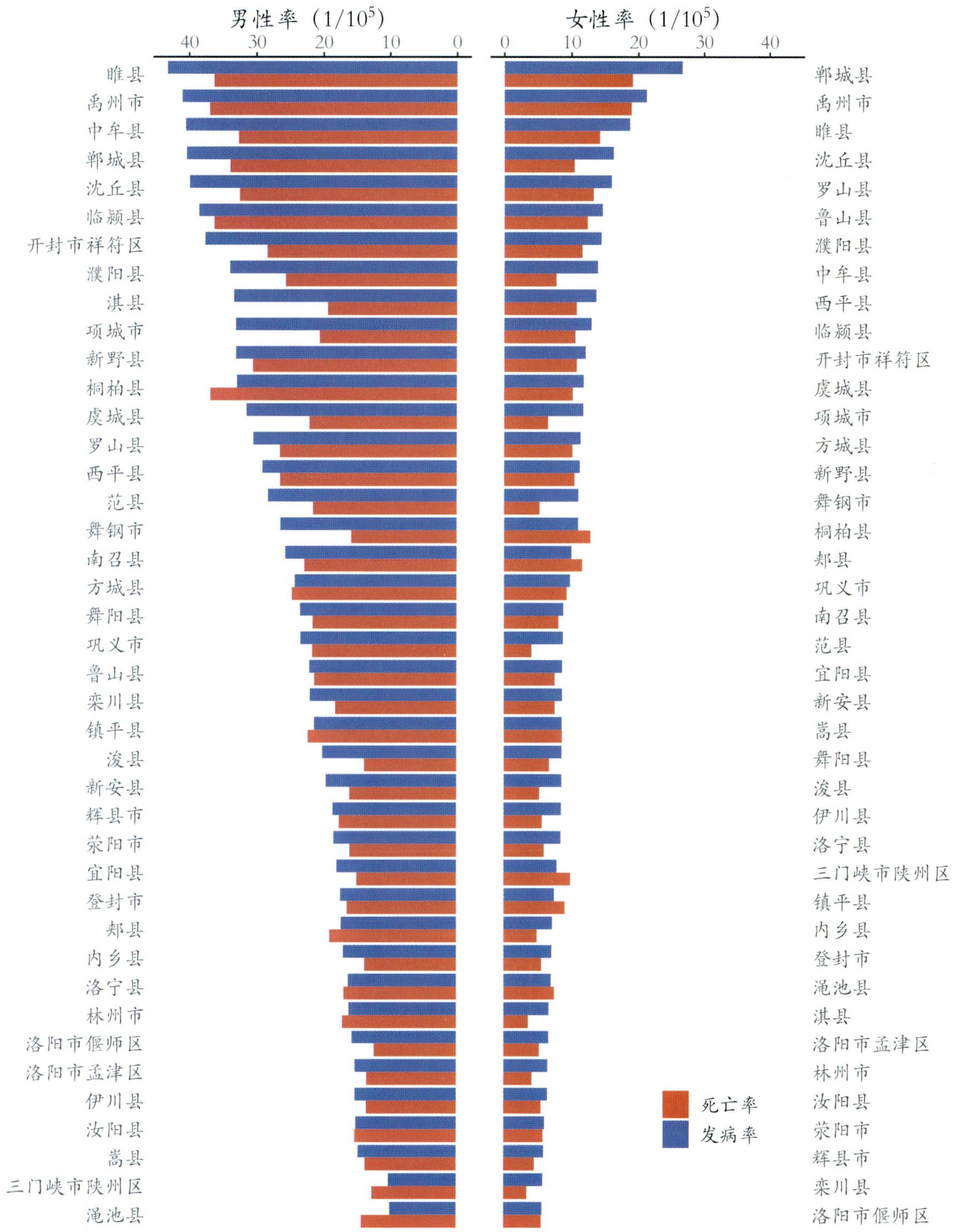

图 5-6c　2020 年河南省农村肿瘤登记地区肝癌发病率和死亡率

七、胆囊

2020 年，河南省肿瘤登记地区胆囊癌的发病率为 4.40/10 万，中标率为 2.87/10 万，世标率为 2.88/10 万，发病例数占全部癌症新发病例数的 1.57%；其中，男性和女性发病率分别为 3.91/10 万和 4.91/10 万，城市地区和农村地区发病率分别为 5.10/10 万和 4.12/10 万；中标发病率呈现女性高于男性、城市地区高于农村地区的特点，女性中标发病率是男性的 1.08 倍，城市地区中标发病率是农村地区的 1.13 倍。同期，胆囊癌的死亡率为 3.52/10 万，中标率为 2.21/10 万，世标率为 2.24/10 万，死亡病例数占全部癌症死亡病例数的 2.16%；其中，男性和女性死亡率分别为 3.04/10 万和 4.03/10 万，城市地区和农村地区死亡率分别为 4.07/10 万和 3.31/10 万；中标死亡率呈现女性高于男性、城市地区高于农村地区的特点，女性中标死亡率是男性的 1.12 倍，城市地区中标死亡率是农村地区的 1.12 倍。（表 5–7）

7. Gallbladder

In 2020, there were 1,898 new cases diagnosed as gallbladder cancer in registration areas of Henan Province, China (862 males and 1,036 females, 627 in urban areas and 1,271 in rural areas), accounting for 1.57% of new cases of all cancers. The crude incidence rate was 4.40 per 100,000, with the ASR China 2.87 per 100,000 and the ASR World 2.88 per 100,000, respectively. Subgroup analysis showed that the incidence of ASR China was 1.08 times in females as that in males, and it was 1.13 times in urban areas as that in rural areas. The cumulative incidence rate for subjects aged 0 to 74 years was 0.34%. (Table 5–7)

A total of 1,520 cases died of gallbladder cancer in 2020 (669 males and 851 females, 500 in urban areas and 1,020 in rural areas), accounting for 2.16% of all cancer deaths. The crude mortality rate was 3.52 per 100,000, with the ASR China of 2.21 per 100,000 and the ASR World of 2.24 per 100,000, respectively. Subgroup analysis showed that the mortality of ASR China was 1.12 times in females as that in males, and it was 1.12 times in urban areas as that in rural areas. The cumulative mortality rate for subjects aged 0 to 74 years was 0.25%. (Table 5–7)

表 5–7　2020 年河南省肿瘤登记地区胆囊癌发病与死亡情况

地区	性别	病例数	粗率 ($1/10^5$)	构成 (%)	中标率 ($1/10^5$)	世标率 ($1/10^5$)	累积率 0 ~ 74 (%)
发病							
全省	合计	1 898	4.40	1.57	2.87	2.88	0.34
	男性	862	3.91	1.39	2.76	2.76	0.33
	女性	1 036	4.91	1.76	2.98	2.99	0.35
城市地区	合计	627	5.10	1.71	3.12	3.15	0.36
	男性	301	4.91	1.65	3.21	3.29	0.38
	女性	326	5.29	1.77	3.03	3.01	0.33
农村地区	合计	1 271	4.12	1.51	2.76	2.77	0.34
	男性	561	3.53	1.29	2.57	2.54	0.31
	女性	710	4.75	1.75	2.95	2.98	0.36

续表

地区	性别	病例数	粗率（1/10^5）	构成（%）	中标率（1/10^5）	世标率（1/10^5）	累积率 0～74（%）
死亡							
全省	合计	1 520	3.52	2.16	2.21	2.24	0.25
	男性	669	3.04	1.55	2.08	2.11	0.25
	女性	851	4.03	3.14	2.32	2.34	0.26
城市地区	合计	500	4.07	2.54	2.38	2.44	0.26
	男性	229	3.73	1.89	2.36	2.46	0.28
	女性	271	4.40	3.56	2.39	2.42	0.24
农村地区	合计	1 020	3.31	2.01	2.13	2.15	0.25
	男性	440	2.77	1.41	1.96	1.96	0.24
	女性	580	3.88	2.98	2.29	2.31	0.27

胆囊癌年龄别发病率在0~39岁年龄段处于较低水平，40岁以后快速上升，在85岁达到峰值；年龄别死亡率在0~49岁年龄段处于较低水平，50岁以后快速上升，在85岁达到峰值；年龄别发病率和死亡率均呈现男性高于女性的特点；城市地区和农村地区年龄别率虽然有一定差异，但是总体趋势类同。（图5-7a）

在14个城市肿瘤登记地区中，男性胆囊癌标化发病率最高的是三门峡市湖滨区（6.64/10万），其次是鹤壁市城区（5.02/10万）和漯河市城区（4.49/10万）；女性标化发病率最高的是三门峡市湖滨区（5.52/10万），其次是济源市（5.51/10万）和许昌市魏都区（5.39/10万）。男性标化死亡率最高的是漯河市城区（3.59/10万），其次是济源市（3.21/10万）和郑州市城区（3.10/10万）；女性标化死亡率最高的是三门峡市湖滨区（4.82/10万），其次是漯河市城区（3.55/10万）和济源市（3.43/10万）。（图5-7b）

The age specific incidence of gallbladder cancer was low at age group of 0~39, and it started increasing sharply at age group of 40, it reached the peak at age of 85. The age specific mortality was low at age group of 0~49, and it started increasing sharply at age group of 50, it reached the peak at age of 85. Age specific incidence and mortality were all higher in males than in females, The change pattern of age specific incidence and mortality were similar in urban areas and rural areas. (Figure 5-7a)

Among the 14 urban cancer registries, the ASR China incidence rate of gallbladder cancer in males was the highest in Sanmenxia Hubin District (6.64 per 100,000) followed by Hebi City (5.02 per 100,000), and Luohe City (4.49 per 100,000). For females, it was the highest in Sanmenxia Hubin District (5.52 per 100,000), followed by Jiyuan City (5.51 per 100,000), and Xuchang Weidu District (5.39 per 100,000). The ASR China mortality rate of gallbladder cancer in males was the highest in Luohe City (3.59 per 100,000) followed by Jiyuan City (3.21 per 100,000), and Zhengzhou City (3.10 per 100,000). For females, it was the highest in Sanmenxia Hubin District (4.82 per 100,000), followed by Luohe City (3.55 per 100,000), and Jiyuan City (3.43 per 100,000). (Figure 5-7b)

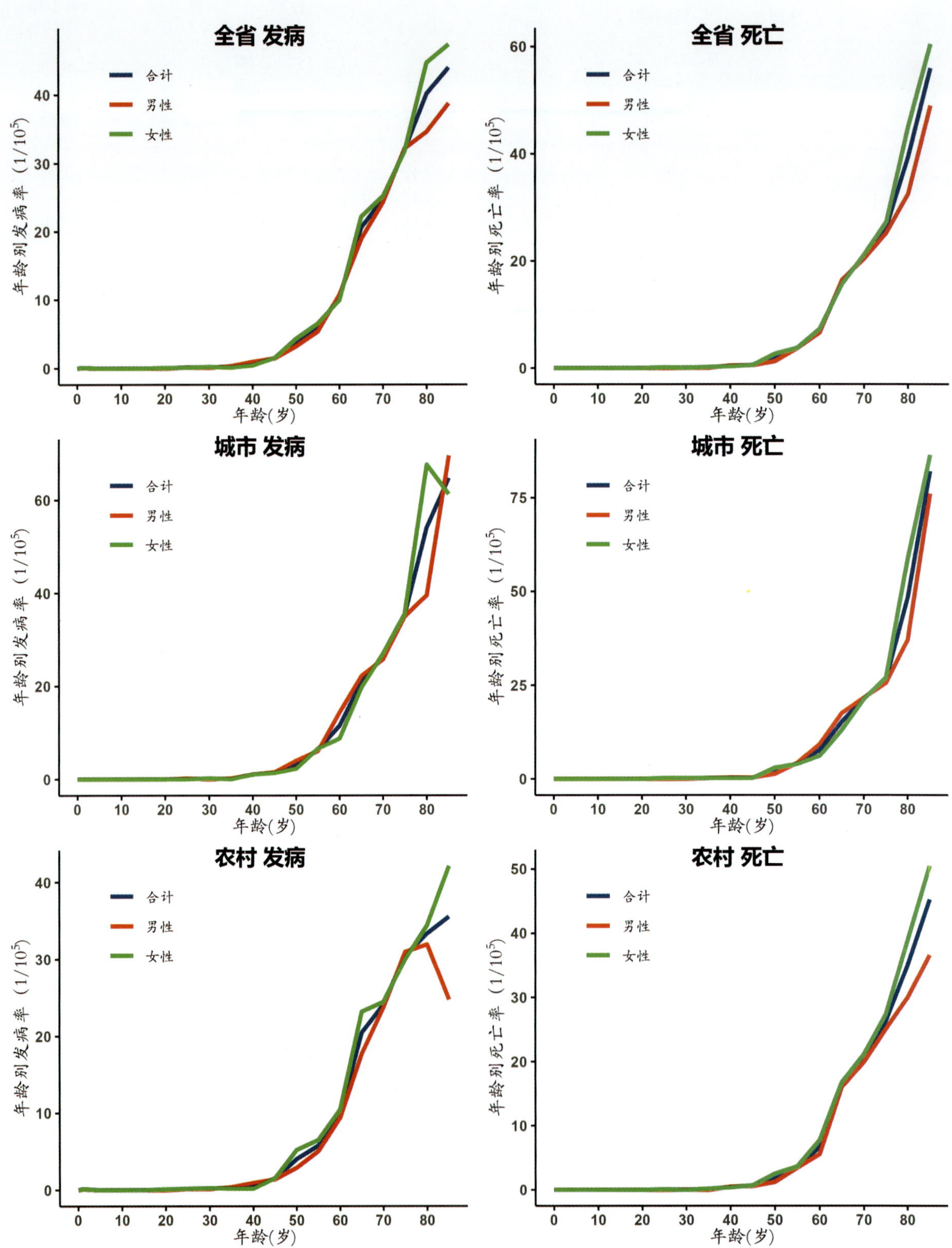

图 5-7a　2020 年河南省肿瘤登记地区胆囊癌年龄别发病率和死亡率

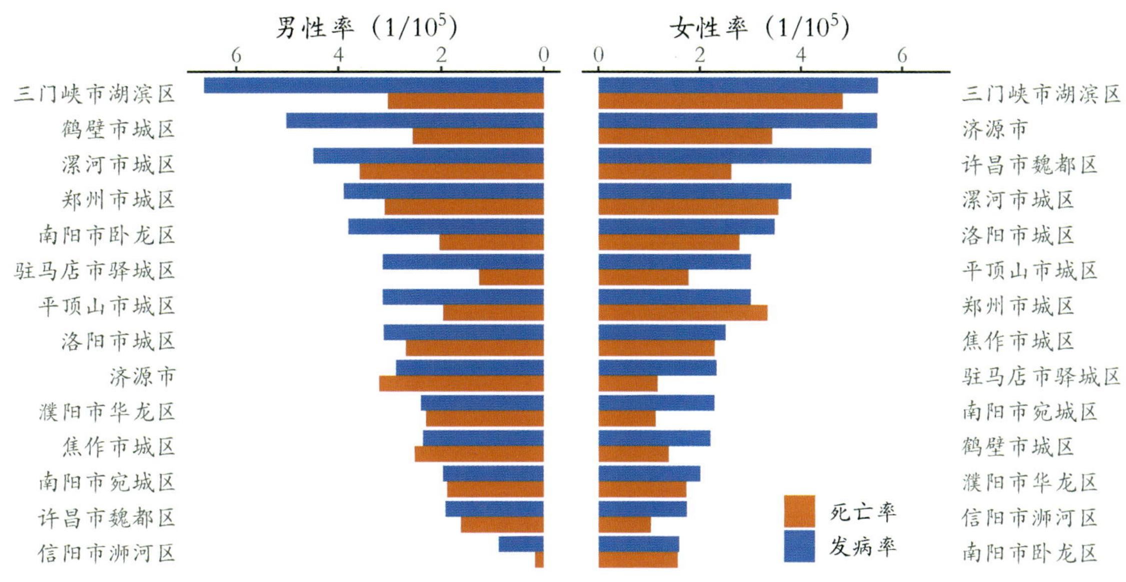

图 5-7b　2020 年河南省城市肿瘤登记地区胆囊癌发病率和死亡率

在 41 个农村肿瘤登记地区中，男性胆囊癌标化发病率最高的是洛宁县（7.76/10 万），其次是开封市祥符区（5.05/10 万）和西平县（4.91/10 万）；女性标化发病率最高的是洛宁县（8.88/10 万），其次是三门峡市陕州区（7.04/10 万）和宜阳县（5.44/10 万）。男性标化死亡率最高的是开封市祥符区（7.24/10 万），其次是西平县（6.08/10 万）和洛宁县（6.04/10 万）；女性标化死亡率最高的是三门峡市陕州区（6.55/10 万），其次是洛宁县（6.43/10 万）和西平县（5.39/10 万）。（图 5-7c）

Among the 41 rural cancer registries, the ASR China incidence rate of gallbladder cancer in males was the highest in Luoning County (7.76 per 100,000) followed by Kaifeng Xiangfu District (5.05 per 100,000), and Xiping County (4.91 per 100,000). For females, it was the highest in Luoning County (8.88 per 100,000), followed by Sanmenxia Shanzhou District (7.04 per 100,000), and Yiyang County (5.44 per 100,000). The ASR China mortality rate of gallbladder cancer in males was the highest in Kaifeng Xiangfu District (7.24 per 100,000) followed by Xiping County (6.08 per 100,000), and Luoning County (6.04 per 100,000). For females, it was the highest in Sanmenxia Shanzhou District (6.55 per 100,000), followed by Luoning County (6.43 per 100,000), and Xiping County (5.39 per 100,000). (Figure 5-7c)

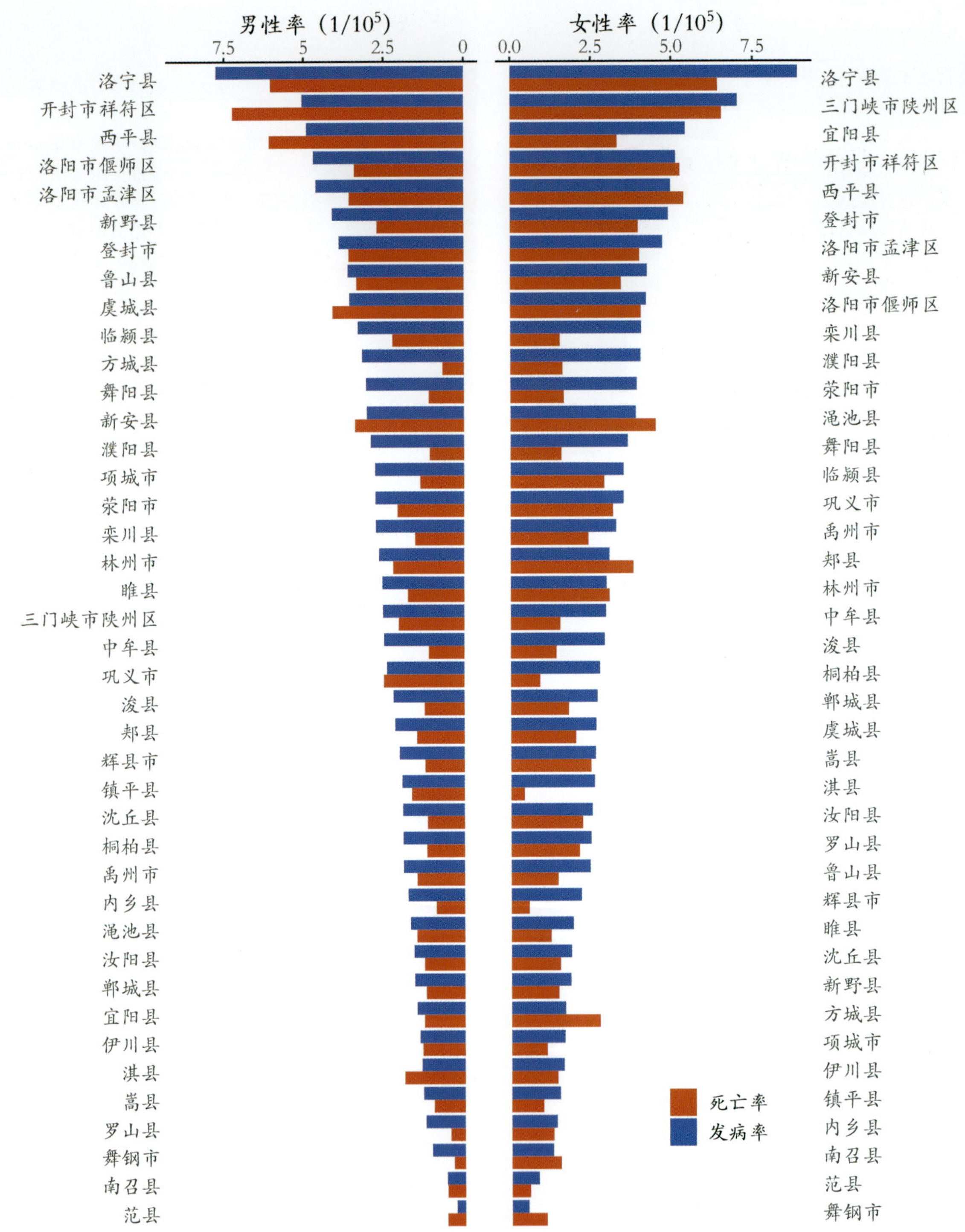

图 5-7c　2020 年河南省农村肿瘤登记地区胆囊癌发病率和死亡率

八、胰腺

2020 年，河南省肿瘤登记地区胰腺癌的发病率为 4.85/10 万，中标率为 3.26/10 万，世标率为 3.24/10 万，发病例数占全部癌症新发病例数的 1.73%；其中，男性和女性发病率分别为 5.02/10 万和 4.68/10 万，城市地区和农村地区发病率分别为 6.16/10 万和 4.33/10 万；中标发病率呈现男性高于女性、城市地区高于农村地区的特点，男性中标发病率是女性的 1.23 倍，城市地区中标发病率是农村地区的 1.29 倍。同期，胰腺癌的死亡率为 4.09/10 万，中标率为 2.65/10 万，世标率为 2.66/10 万，死亡病例数占全部癌症死亡病例数的 2.51%；其中，男性和女性死亡率分别为 4.27/10 万和 3.90/10 万，城市地区和农村地区死亡率分别为 5.35/10 万和 3.59/10 万；中标死亡率呈现男性高于女性、城市地区高于农村地区的特点，男性中标死亡率是女性的 1.27 倍，城市地区中标死亡率是农村地区的 1.36 倍。（表 5–8）

8. Pancreas

In 2020, there were 2,093 new cases diagnosed as pancreas cancer in registration areas of Henan Province, China (1,106 males and 987 females, 757 in urban areas and 1,336 in rural areas), accounting for 1.73% of new cases of all cancers. The crude incidence rate was 4.85 per 100,000, with the ASR China 3.26 per 100,000 and the ASR World 3.24 per 100,000, respectively. Subgroup analysis showed that the incidence of ASR China was 1.23 times in males as that in females, and it was 1.29 times in urban areas as that in rural areas. The cumulative incidence rate for subjects aged 0 to 74 years was 0.39%. (Table 5–8)

A total of 1765 cases died of pancreas cancer in 2020 (941 males and 824 females, 658 in urban areas and 1107 in rural areas), accounting for 2.51% of all cancer deaths. The crude mortality rate was 4.09 per 100,000, with the ASR China of 2.65 per 100,000 and the ASR World of 2.66 per 100,000, respectively. Subgroup analysis showed that the mortality of ASR China was 1.27 times in males as that in females, and it was 1.36 times in urban areas as that in rural areas. The cumulative mortality rate for subjects aged 0 to 74 years was 0.31%. (Table 5–8)

表 5–8　2020 年河南省肿瘤登记地区胰腺癌发病与死亡情况

地区	性别	病例数	发病率（$1/10^5$）	构成（%）	中标率（$1/10^5$）	世标率（$1/10^5$）	累积率 0～74（%）
发病							
全省	合计	2 093	4.85	1.73	3.26	3.24	0.39
	男性	1 106	5.02	1.79	3.60	3.59	0.44
	女性	987	4.68	1.68	2.93	2.91	0.33
城市地区	合计	757	6.16	2.06	3.87	3.89	0.45
	男性	399	6.51	2.18	4.32	4.38	0.54
	女性	358	5.81	1.95	3.43	3.41	0.37
农村地区	合计	1 336	4.33	1.59	3.00	2.97	0.36
	男性	707	4.45	1.62	3.30	3.25	0.41
	女性	629	4.21	1.55	2.71	2.69	0.32

续表

地区	性别	病例数	粗率（1/10^5）	构成（%）	中标率（1/10^5）	世标率（1/10^5）	累积率 0~74（%）
死亡							
全省	合计	1 765	4.09	2.51	2.65	2.66	0.31
	男性	941	4.27	2.17	2.97	2.99	0.36
	女性	824	3.90	3.04	2.34	2.34	0.26
城市地区	合计	658	5.35	3.34	3.25	3.30	0.37
	男性	337	5.49	2.79	3.56	3.63	0.42
	女性	321	5.21	4.22	2.95	2.97	0.31
农村地区	合计	1 107	3.59	2.19	2.39	2.38	0.29
	男性	604	3.80	1.94	2.73	2.72	0.33
	女性	503	3.36	2.59	2.08	2.07	0.24

胰腺癌年龄别发病率在 0~39 岁年龄段处于较低水平，40 岁以后快速上升，在 85 岁达到峰值；年龄别死亡率在 0~39 岁年龄段处于较低水平，40 岁以后快速上升，在 85 岁达到峰值；年龄别发病率和死亡率均呈现男性高于女性的特点；城市地区和农村地区年龄别率虽然有一定差异，但是总体趋势类同。（图 5–8a）

在 14 个城市肿瘤登记地区中，男性胰腺癌标化发病率最高的是郑州市城区（7.16/10 万），其次是三门峡市湖滨区（5.53/10 万）和濮阳市华龙区（5.45/10 万）；女性标化发病率最高的是郑州市城区（5.11/10 万），其次是许昌市魏都区（4.53/10 万）和信阳市浉河区（4.50/10 万）。男性标化死亡率最高的是濮阳市华龙区（6.79/10 万），其次是郑州市城区（4.73/10 万）和许昌市魏都区（4.64/10 万）；女性标化死亡率最高的是濮阳市华龙区（4.49/10 万），其次是济源市（4.31/10 万）和信阳市浉河区（3.78/10 万）。（图 5–8b）

The age specific incidence of pancreas cancer was low at age group of 0~39, and it started increasing sharply at age group of 40, it reached the peak at age of 85. The age specific mortality was low at age group of 0~39, and it started increasing sharply at age group of 40, it reached the peak at age of 85. Age specific incidence and mortality were all higher in males than in females, The change pattern of age specific incidence and mortality were similar in urban areas and rural areas. (Figure 5–8a)

Among the 14 urban cancer registries, the ASR China incidence rate of pancreas cancer in males was the highest in Zhengzhou City (7.16 per 100,000) followed by Sanmenxia Hubin District (5.53 per 100,000), and Puyang Hualong District (5.45 per 100,000). For females, it was the highest in Zhengzhou City (5.11 per 100,000), followed by Xuchang Weidu District (4.53 per 100,000), and Xinyang Shihe District (4.50 per 100,000). The ASR China mortality rate of pancreas cancer in males was the highest in Puyang Hualong District (6.79 per 100,000) followed by Zhengzhou City (4.73 per 100,000), and Xuchang Weidu District (4.64 per 100,000). For females, it was the highest in Puyang Hualong District (4.49 per 100,000), followed by Jiyuan City (4.31 per 100,000), and Xinyang Shihe District (3.78 per 100,000). (Figure 5–8b)

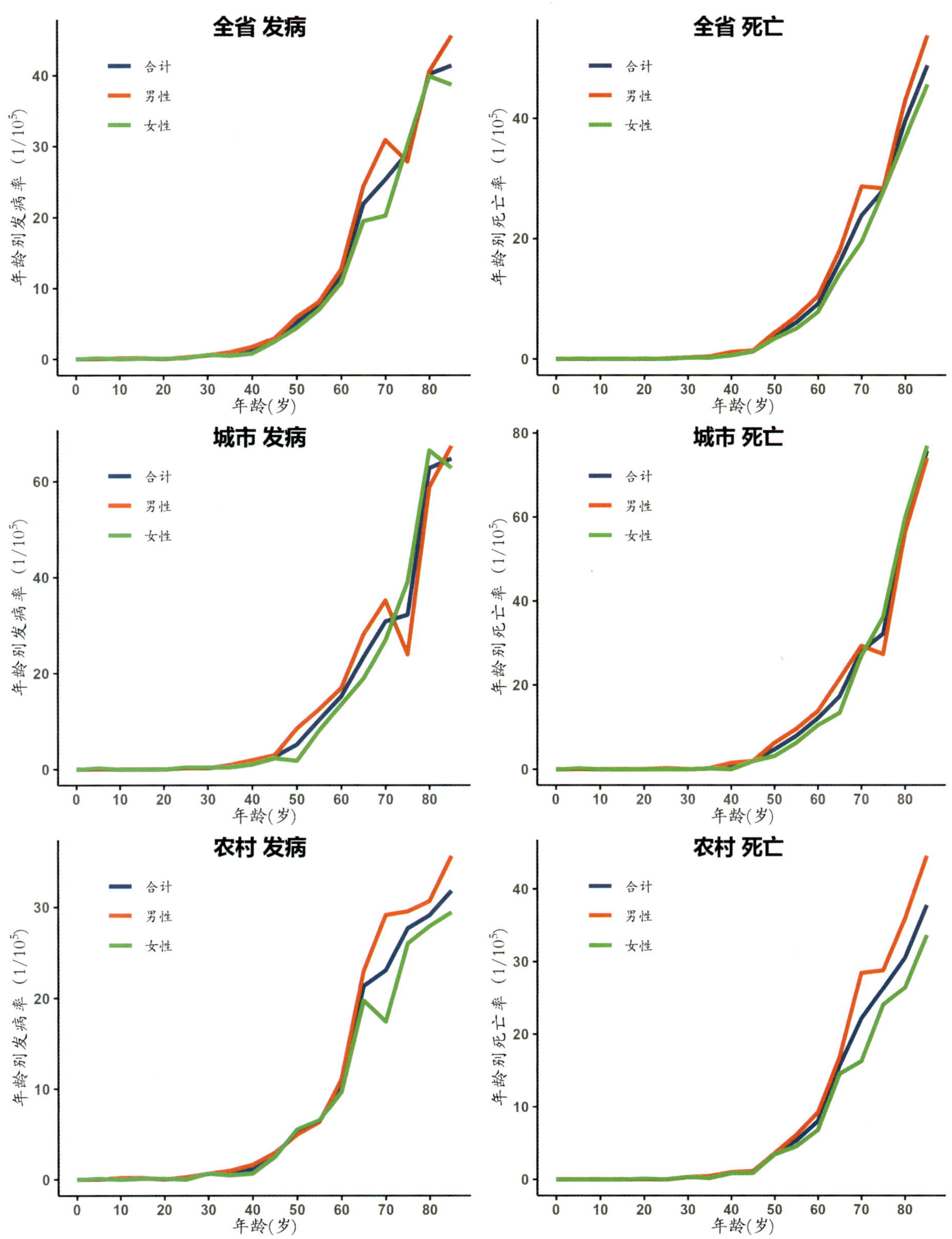

图 5-8a　2020 年河南省肿瘤登记地区胰腺癌年龄别发病率和死亡率

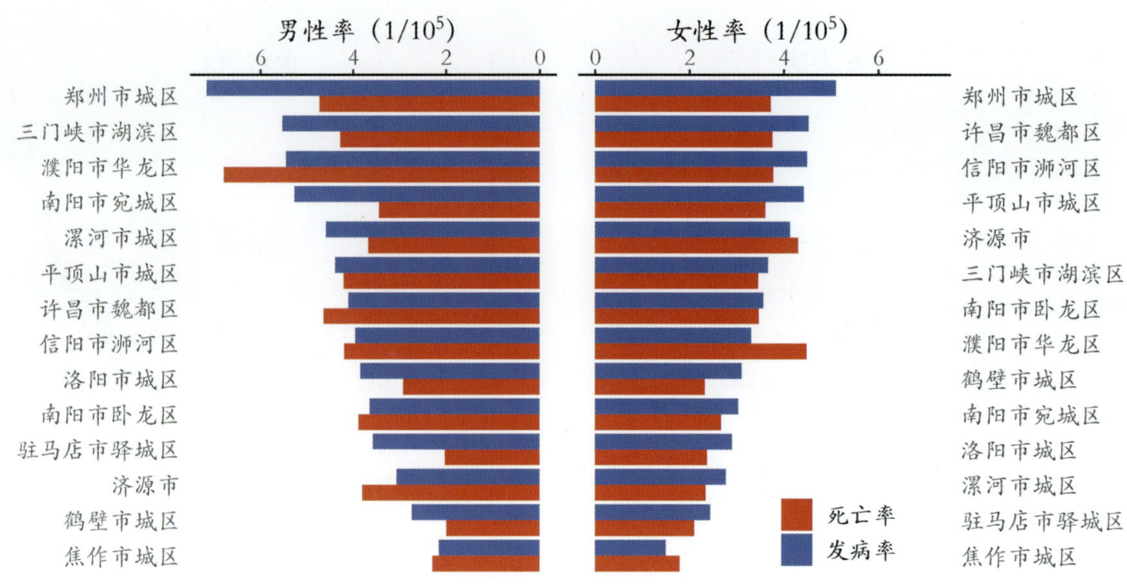

图 5–8b　2020 年河南省城市肿瘤登记地区胰腺癌发病率和死亡率

在 41 个农村肿瘤登记地区中，男性胰腺癌标化发病率最高的是开封市祥符区（6.46/10 万），其次是范县（6.28/10 万）和濮阳县（5.74/10 万）；女性标化发病率最高的是范县（6.36/10 万），其次是中牟县（4.94/10 万）和桐柏县（4.92/10 万）。男性标化死亡率最高的是三门峡市陕州区（6.12/10 万），其次是开封市祥符区（4.81/10 万）和濮阳县（4.49/10 万）；女性标化死亡率最高的是桐柏县（3.68/10 万），其次是开封市祥符区（3.58/10 万）和西平县（3.51/10 万）。（图 5–8c）

2020 年，河南省肿瘤登记地区胰腺癌发病病例中有确切解剖学亚部位信息的占 41.71%，亚部位未特指的占 58.29%。在有亚部位信息的胰腺病例中，胰头占 50.03%，胰体占 20.95%，胰尾占 6.51%，胰管占 2.05%，内分泌占 14.01%，其他部位占 4.65%，交搭跨越占 1.80%。（图 5–8d）

Among the 41 rural cancer registries, the ASR China incidence rate of pancreas cancer in males was the highest in Kaifeng Xiangfu District (6.46 per 100,000) followed by Fan County (6.28 per 100,000), and Puyang County (5.74 per 100,000). For females, it was the highest in Fan County (6.36 per 100,000), followed by Zhongmu County (4.94 per 100,000), and Tongbai County (4.92 per 100,000). The ASR China mortality rate of pancreas cancer in males was the highest in Sanmenxia Shanzhou District (6.12 per 100,000) followed by Kaifeng Xiangfu District (4.81 per 100,000), and Puyang County (4.49 per 100,000). For females, it was the highest in Tongbai County (3.68 per 100,000), followed by Kaifeng Xiangfu District (3.58 per 100,000), and Xiping County (3.51 per 100,000). (Figure 5–8c)

About 41.71% of the pancreas cancer had specific subsite. Among those cases, head accounted for 50.03%, body accounted for 20.95%, tail accounted for 6.51%, pancreatic accounted for 2.05%, endocrine accounted for 14.01%, other parts accounted for 4.65%, and overlapping accounted for 1.80%. (Figure 5–8d)

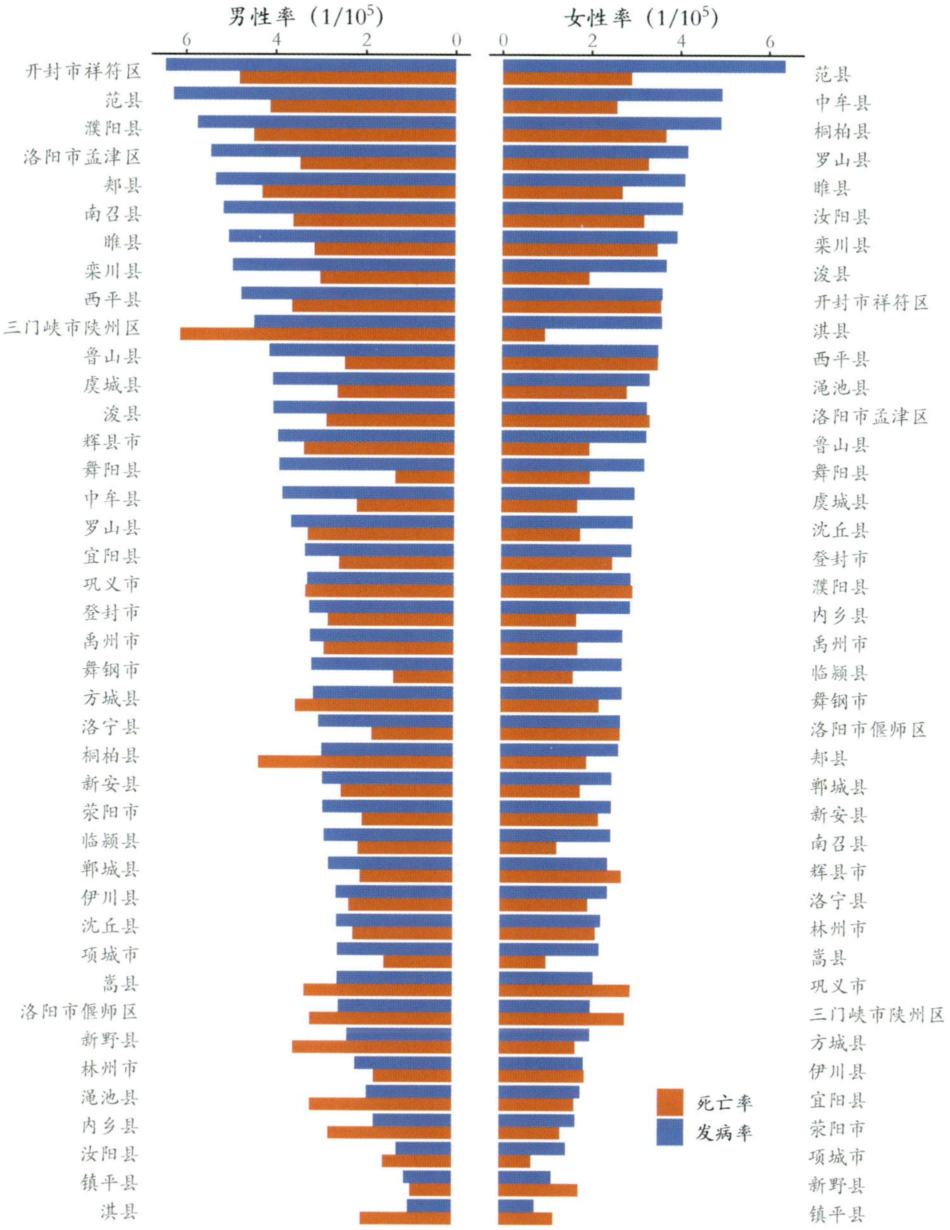

男性率（$1/10^5$）

6 4 2 0

开封市祥符区
范县
濮阳县
洛阳市孟津区
郏县
南召县
睢县
栾川县
西平县
三门峡市陕州区
鲁山县
虞城县
浚县
辉县市
舞阳县
中牟县
罗山县
宜阳县
巩义市
登封市
禹州市
舞钢市
方城县
洛宁县
桐柏县
新安县
荥阳市
临颍县
郸城县
伊川县
沈丘县
项城市
嵩县
洛阳市偃师区
新野县
林州市
渑池县
内乡县
汝阳县
镇平县
淇县

女性率（$1/10^5$）

0 2 4 6

范县
中牟县
桐柏县
罗山县
睢县
汝阳县
栾川县
浚县
开封市祥符区
淇县
西平县
渑池县
洛阳市孟津区
鲁山县
舞阳县
虞城县
沈丘县
登封市
濮阳县
内乡县
禹州市
临颍县
舞钢市
洛阳市偃师区
郏县
郸城县
新安县
南召县
辉县市
洛宁县
林州市
嵩县
巩义市
三门峡市陕州区
方城县
伊川县
宜阳县
荥阳市
项城市
新野县
镇平县

死亡率
发病率

图 5-8c　2020 年河南省农村肿瘤登记地区胰腺癌发病率和死亡率

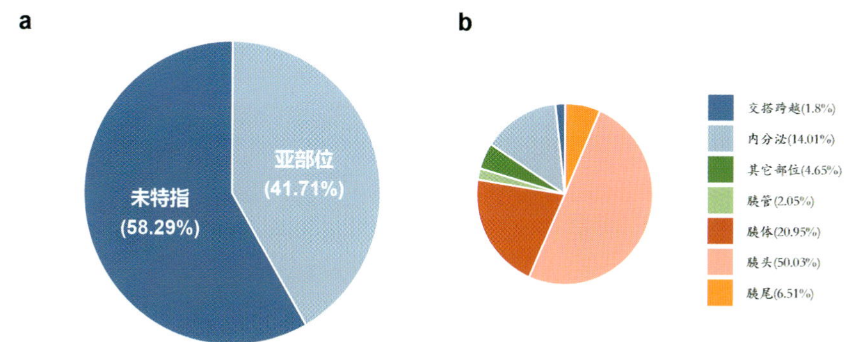

图 5-8d　2020 年河南省肿瘤登记地区胰腺癌发病病例亚部位构成

九、喉

2020 年，河南省肿瘤登记地区喉癌的发病率为 1.42/10 万，中标率为 0.98/10 万，世标率为 0.99/10 万，发病例数占全部癌症新发病例数的 0.51%；其中，男性和女性发病率分别为 2.46/10 万和 0.34/10 万，城市地区和农村地区发病率分别为 1.71/10 万和 1.31/10 万；中标发病率呈现男性高于女性、城市地区高于农村地区的特点，男性中标发病率是女性的 7.70 倍，城市地区中标发病率是农村地区的 1.23 倍。同期，喉癌的死亡率为 0.73/10 万，中标率为 0.47/10 万，世标率为 0.48/10 万，死亡病例数占全部癌症死亡病例数的 0.45%；其中，男性和女性死亡率分别为 1.25/10 万和 0.19/10 万，城市地区和农村地区死亡率分别为 0.89/10 万和 0.67/10 万；中标死亡率呈现男性高于女性、城市地区高于农村地区的特点，男性中标死亡率是女性的 7.91 倍，城市地区中标死亡率是农村地区的 1.27 倍。（表 5–9）

喉癌年龄别发病率在 0~39 岁年龄段处于较低水平，40 岁以后快速上升，在 75 岁达到峰值；年龄别死亡率在 0~54 岁年龄段处于较低水平，55 岁以后快速上升，在 85 岁达到峰值；年龄别发病率和死亡率均呈现男性高于女性的特点；城市地区和农村地区年龄别率虽然有一定差异，但是总体趋势类同。（图 5–9a）

9. Larynx

In 2020, there were 614 new cases diagnosed as larynx cancer in registration areas of Henan Province, China (542 males and 72 females, 210 in urban areas and 404 in rural areas), accounting for 0.51% of new cases of all cancers. The crude incidence rate was 1.42 per 100,000, with the ASR China 0.98 per 100,000 and the ASR World 0.99 per 100,000, respectively. Subgroup analysis showed that the incidence of ASR China was 7.70 times in males as that in females, and it was 1.23 times in urban areas as that in rural areas. The cumulative incidence rate for subjects aged 0 to 74 years was 0.13%. (Table 5–9)

A total of 317 cases died of larynx cancer in 2020 (276 males and 41 females, 110 in urban areas and 207 in rural areas), accounting for 0.45% of all cancer deaths. The crude mortality rate was 0.73 per 100,000, with the ASR China of 0.47 per 100,000 and the ASR World of 0.48 per 100,000, respectively. Subgroup analysis showed that the mortality of ASR China was 7.91 times in males as that in females, and it was 1.27 times in urban areas as that in rural areas. The cumulative mortality rate for subjects aged 0 to 74 years was 0.06%. (Table 5–9)

The age specific incidence of larynx cancer was low at age group of 0~39, and it started increasing sharply at age group of 40, it reached the peak at age of 75. The age specific mortality was low at age group of 0~54, and it started increasing sharply at age group of 55, it reached the peak at age of 85. Age specific incidence and mortality were all higher in males than in females, The change pattern of age specific incidence and mortality were similar in urban areas and rural areas. (Figure 5–9a)

表 5-9　2020 年河南省肿瘤登记地区喉癌发病与死亡情况

地区	性别	病例数	粗率（1/10^5）	构成（%）	中标率（1/10^5）	世标率（1/10^5）	累积率 0～74（%）
发病							
全省	合计	614	1.42	0.51	0.98	0.99	0.13
	男性	542	2.46	0.88	1.77	1.78	0.23
	女性	72	0.34	0.12	0.23	0.23	0.03
城市地区	合计	210	1.71	0.57	1.13	1.15	0.14
	男性	193	3.15	1.06	2.14	2.18	0.27
	女性	17	0.28	0.09	0.18	0.19	0.02
农村地区	合计	404	1.31	0.48	0.92	0.92	0.12
	男性	349	2.19	0.80	1.61	1.62	0.21
	女性	55	0.37	0.14	0.24	0.24	0.03
死亡							
全省	合计	317	0.73	0.45	0.47	0.48	0.06
	男性	276	1.25	0.64	0.87	0.87	0.10
	女性	41	0.19	0.15	0.11	0.12	0.01
城市地区	合计	110	0.89	0.56	0.56	0.57	0.07
	男性	101	1.65	0.84	1.09	1.09	0.14
	女性	9	0.15	0.12	0.07	0.08	0.01
农村地区	合计	207	0.67	0.41	0.44	0.44	0.05
	男性	175	1.10	0.56	0.78	0.78	0.09
	女性	32	0.21	0.16	0.12	0.13	0.01

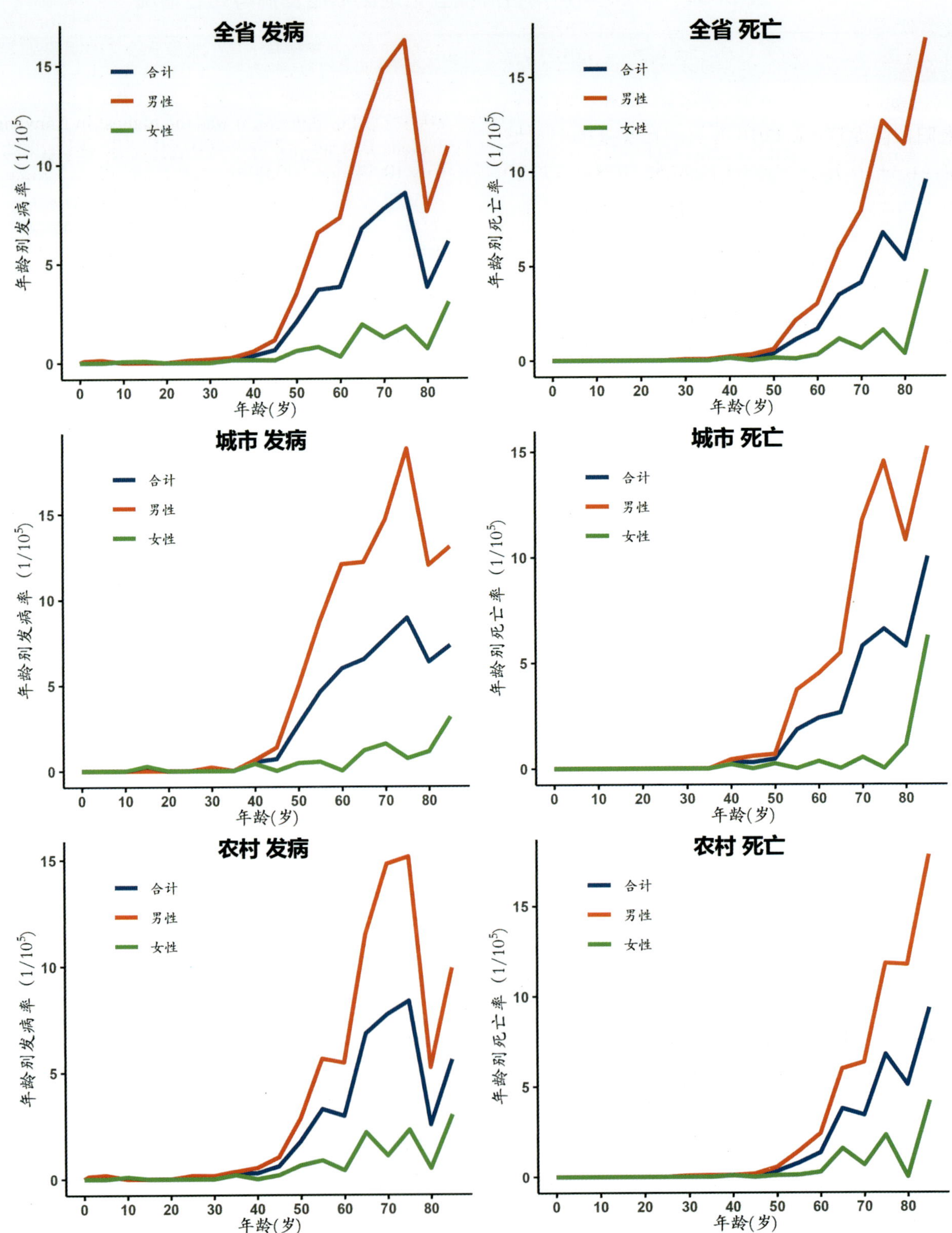

图 5-9a　2020 年河南省肿瘤登记地区喉癌年龄别发病率和死亡率

在 14 个城市肿瘤登记地区中，男性喉癌标化发病率最高的是南阳市卧龙区（3.28/10 万），其次是许昌市魏都区（3.15/10 万）和郑州市城区（3.06/10 万）；女性标化发病率最高的是南阳市卧龙区（0.83/10 万），其次是鹤壁市城区（0.54/10 万）和驻马店市驿城区（0.29/10 万）。男性标化死亡率最高的是三门峡市湖滨区（3.17/10 万），其次是郑州市城区（1.89/10 万）和南阳市卧龙区（1.49/10 万）；女性标化死亡率最高的是三门峡市湖滨区（0.49/10 万），其次是信阳市浉河区（0.45/10 万）和济源市（0.28/10 万）。（图 5-9b）

Among the 14 urban cancer registries, the ASR China incidence rate of larynx cancer in males was the highest in Nanyang Wolong District (3.28 per 100,000) followed by Xuchang Weidu District (3.15 per 100,000), and Zhengzhou City (3.06 per 100,000). For females, it was the highest in Nanyang Wolong District (0.83 per 100,000), followed by Hebi City (0.54 per 100,000), and Zhumadian Yicheng District (0.29 per 100,000). The ASR China mortality rate of larynx cancer in males was the highest in Sanmenxia Hubin District (3.17 per 100,000) followed by Zhengzhou City (1.89 per 100,000), and Nanyang Wolong District (1.49 per 100,000). For females, it was the highest in Sanmenxia Hubin District (0.49 per 100,000), followed by Xinyang Shihe District (0.45 per 100,000), and Jiyuan City (0.28 per 100,000). (Figure 5-9b)

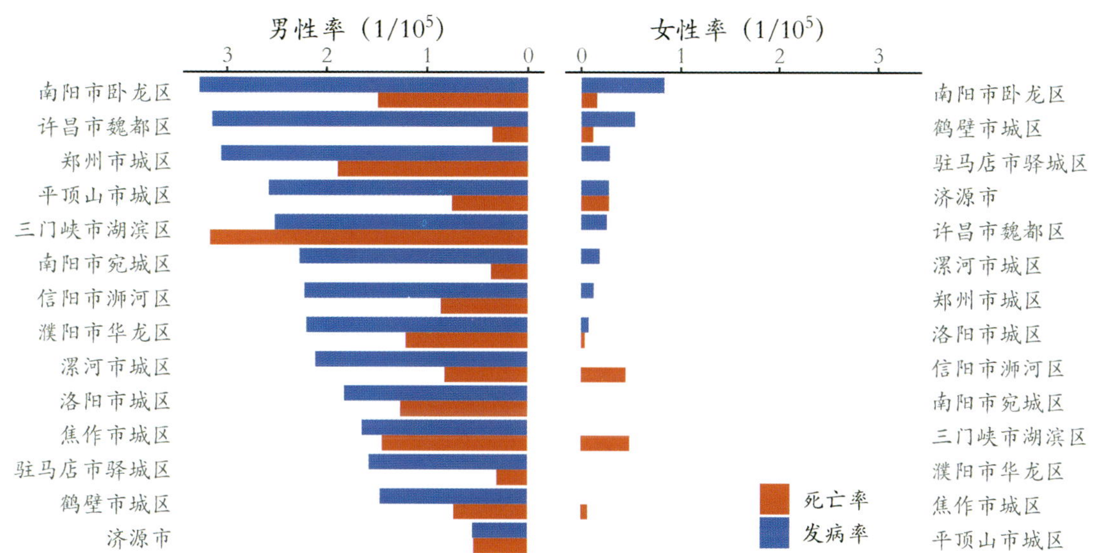

图 5-9b　2020 年河南省城市肿瘤登记地区喉癌发病率和死亡率

在 41 个农村肿瘤登记地区中，男性喉癌标化发病率最高的是范县（5.01/10 万），其次是濮阳县（3.27/10 万）和开封市祥符区（2.98/10 万）；女性标化发病率最高的是郸城县（1.52/10 万），其次是淇县（1.06/10 万）和内乡县（0.90/10 万）。男性标化死亡率最高的是濮阳县（2.94/10 万），其次是郏县（2.26/10 万）和郸城县（1.70/10 万）；女性标化死亡率最高的是郸城县（0.95/10 万），其次是淇县（0.80/10 万）和西平县（0.44/10 万）。（图 5-9c）

Among the 41 rural cancer registries, the ASR China incidence rate of larynx cancer in males was the highest in Fan County (5.01 per 100,000) followed by Puyang County (3.27 per 100,000), and Kaifeng Xiangfu District (2.98 per 100,000). For females, it was the highest in Dancheng County (1.52 per 100,000), followed by Qi County (1.06 per 100,000), and Neixiang County (0.90 per 100,000). The ASR China mortality rate of larynx cancer in males was the highest in Puyang County (2.94 per 100,000) followed by Jia County (2.26 per 100,000), and Dancheng County (1.70 per 100,000). For females, it was the highest in Dancheng County (0.95 per 100,000), followed by Qi County (0.80 per 100,000), and Xiping County (0.44 per 100,000). (Figure 5-9c)

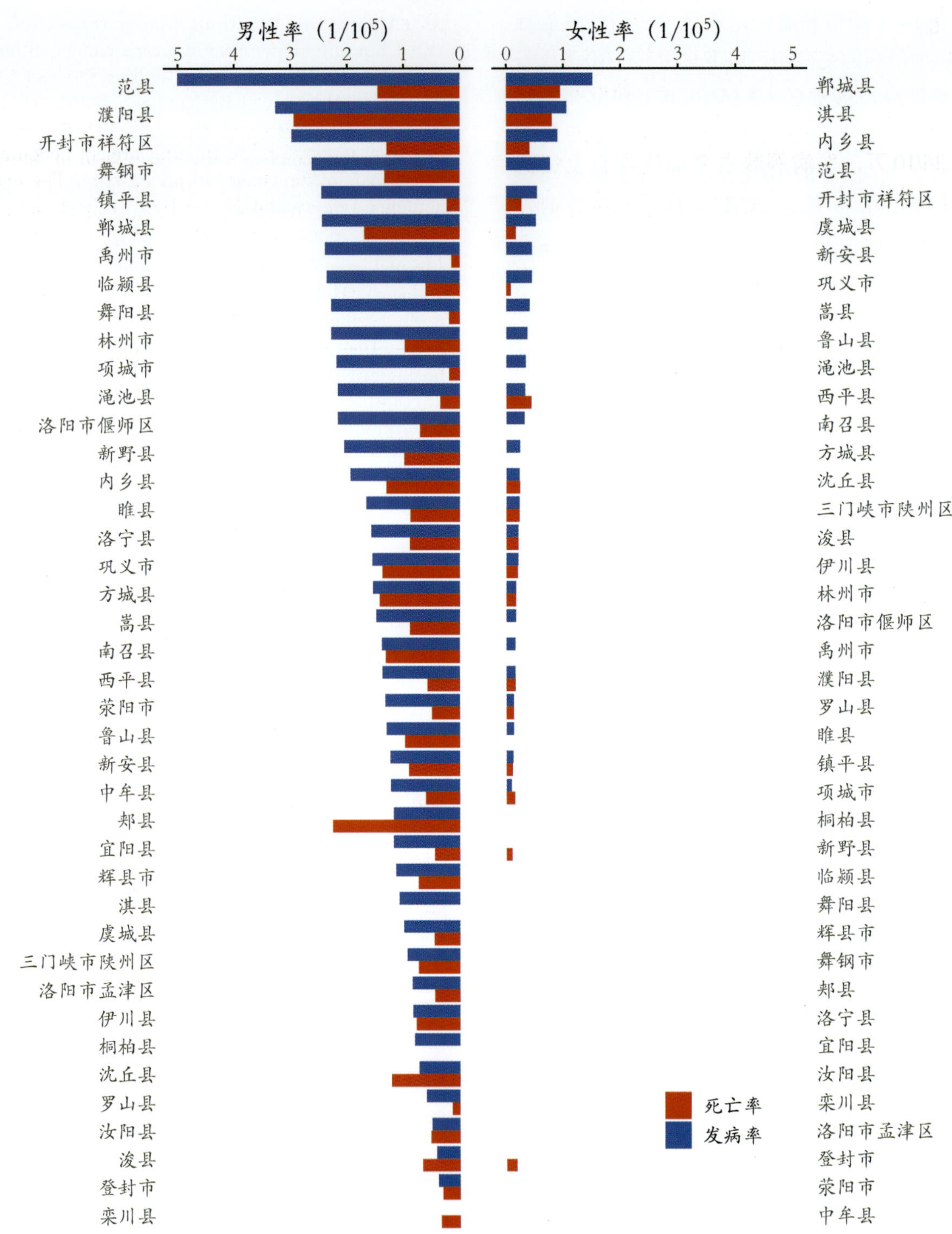

图 5-9c 2020 年河南省农村肿瘤登记地区喉癌发病率和死亡率

十、肺

2020 年，河南省肿瘤登记地区肺癌的发病率为 54.23/10 万，中标率为 36.31/10 万，世标率为 36.36/10 万，发病例数占全部癌症新发病例数的 19.39%；其中，男性和女性发病率分别为 71.15/10 万和 36.56/10 万，城市地区和农村地区发病率分别为 55.82/10 万和 53.59/10 万；中标发病率呈现男性高于女性、农村地区高于城市地区的特点，男性中标发病率是女性的 2.14 倍，农村地区中标发病率和城市地区基本持平。同期，肺癌的死亡率为 40.73/10 万，中标率为 26.17/10 万，世标率为 26.23/10 万，死亡病例数占全部癌症死亡病例数的 24.99%；其中，男性和女性死亡率分别为 56.61/10 万和 24.16/10 万，城市地区和农村地区死亡率分别为 40.73/10 万和 40.73/10 万；中标死亡率呈现男性高于女性、农村地区高于城市地区的特点，男性中标死亡率是女性的 2.74 倍，农村地区中标死亡率是城市地区的 1.08 倍。（表 5–10）

10. Lung

In 2020, there were 23,397 new cases diagnosed as lung cancer in registration areas of Henan Province, China (15,678 males and 7,719 females, 6,861 in urban areas and 16,536 in rural areas), accounting for 19.39% of new cases of all cancers. The crude incidence rate was 54.23 per 100,000, with the ASR China 36.31 per 100,000 and the ASR World 36.36 per 100,000, respectively. Subgroup analysis showed that the incidence of ASR China was 2.14 times in males as that in females, and it was similar in rural areas as that in urban areas. The cumulative incidence rate for subjects aged 0 to 74 years was 4.51%. (Table 5–10)

A total of 17,574 cases died of lung cancer in 2020 (12,473 males and 5,101 females, 5,007 in urban areas and 12,567 in rural areas), accounting for 24.99% of all cancer deaths. The crude mortality rate was 40.73 per 100,000, with the ASR China of 26.17 per 100,000 and the ASR World of 26.23 per 100,000, respectively. Subgroup analysis showed that the mortality of ASR China was 2.74 times in males as that in females, and it was 1.08 times in rural areas as that in urban areas. The cumulative mortality rate for subjects aged 0 to 74 years was 3.08%. (Table 5–10)

表 5–10 2020 年河南省肿瘤登记地区肺癌发病与死亡情况

地区	性别	病例数	发病率（1/10^5）	构成（%）	中标率（1/10^5）	世标率（1/10^5）	累积率 0 ~ 74（%）
死亡							
全省	合计	23 397	54.23	19.39	36.31	36.36	4.51
	男性	15 678	71.15	25.36	50.17	50.37	6.35
	女性	7 719	36.56	13.11	23.39	23.29	2.75
城市地区	合计	6 861	55.82	18.70	36.22	36.44	4.49
	男性	4 479	73.03	24.50	48.86	49.54	6.29
	女性	2 382	38.68	12.94	24.71	24.52	2.82
农村地区	合计	16 536	53.59	19.68	36.37	36.34	4.52
	男性	11 199	70.43	25.72	50.75	50.74	6.37
	女性	5 337	35.69	13.19	22.82	22.77	2.72

续表

地区	性别	病例数	发病率 (1/10^5)	构成（%）	中标率 (1/10^5)	世标率 (1/10^5)	累积率 0 ~ 74（%）
死亡							
全省	合计	17 574	40.73	24.99	26.17	26.23	3.08
	男性	12 473	56.61	28.82	39.13	39.19	4.62
	女性	5 101	24.16	18.85	14.26	14.36	1.60
城市地区	合计	5 007	40.73	25.42	24.73	25.00	2.84
	男性	3 555	57.97	29.41	37.16	37.67	4.34
	女性	1 452	23.58	19.08	13.48	13.57	1.45
农村地区	合计	12 567	40.73	24.82	26.76	26.73	3.17
	男性	8 918	56.08	28.59	39.91	39.78	4.72
	女性	3 649	24.40	18.76	14.59	14.69	1.66

肺癌年龄别发病率在 0~39 岁年龄段处于较低水平，40 岁以后快速上升，在 85 岁达到峰值；年龄别死亡率在 0~44 岁年龄段处于较低水平，45 岁以后快速上升，在 85 岁达到峰值；年龄别发病率和死亡率均呈现男性高于女性的特点；城市地区和农村地区年龄别率虽然有一定差异，但是总体趋势类同。（图 5–10a）

在 14 个城市肿瘤登记地区中，男性肺癌标化发病率最高的是漯河市城区（71.99/10 万），其次是南阳市宛城区（59.03/10 万）和濮阳市华龙区（58.99/10 万）；女性标化发病率最高的是濮阳市华龙区（35.75/10 万），其次是郑州市城区（34.40/10 万）和平顶山市城区（29.51/10 万）。男性标化死亡率最高的是濮阳市华龙区（69.24/10 万），其次是漯河市城区（59.41/10 万）和三门峡市湖滨区（48.81/10 万）；女性标化死亡率最高的是濮阳市华龙区（30.61/10 万），其次是南阳市卧龙区（19.94/10 万）和漯河市城区（18.42/10 万）。（图 5–10b）

The age specific incidence of lung cancer was low at age group of 0~39, and it started increasing sharply at age group of 40, it reached the peak at age of 85. The age specific mortality was low at age group of 0~44, and it started increasing sharply at age group of 45, it reached the peak at age of 85. Age specific incidence and mortality were all higher in males than in females, The change pattern of age specific incidence and mortality were similar in urban areas and rural areas. (Figure 5–10a)

Among the 14 urban cancer registries, the ASR China incidence rate of lung cancer in males was the highest in Luohe City (71.99 per 100,000) followed by Nanyang Wancheng District (59.03 per 100,000), and Puyang Hualong District (58.99 per 100,000). For females, it was the highest in Puyang Hualong District (35.75 per 100,000), followed by Zhengzhou City (34.40 per 100,000), and Pingdingshan City (29.51 per 100,000). The ASR China mortality rate of lung cancer in males was the highest in Puyang Hualong District (69.24 per 100,000) followed by Luohe City (59.41 per 100,000), and Sanmenxia Hubin District (48.81 per 100,000). For females, it was the highest in Puyang Hualong District (30.61 per 100,000), followed by Nanyang Wolong District (19.94 per 100,000), and Luohe City (18.42 per 100,000). (Figure 5–10b)

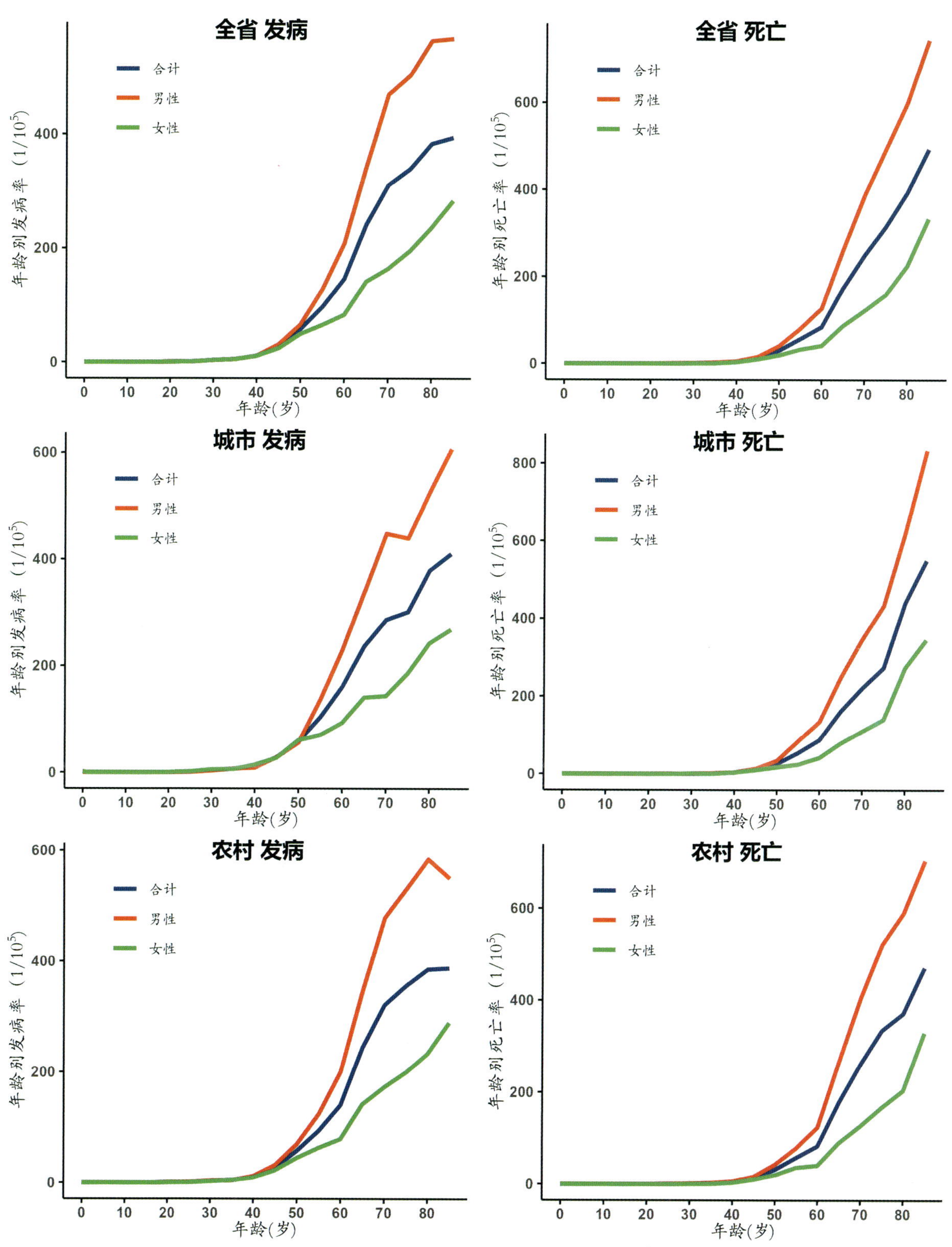

图 5-10a　2020 年河南省肿瘤登记地区肺癌年龄别发病率和死亡率

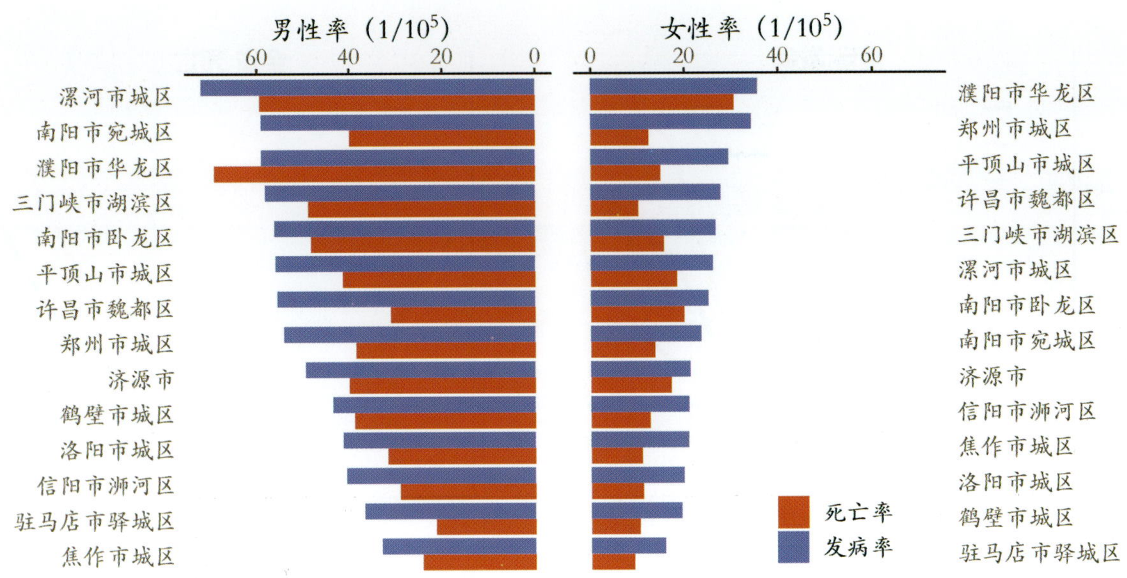

图 5-10b　2020 年河南省城市肿瘤登记地区肺癌发病率和死亡率

在 41 个农村肿瘤登记地区中，男性肺癌标化发病率最高的是禹州市（116.22/10 万），其次是濮阳县（100.21/10 万）和范县（76.11/10 万）；女性标化发病率最高的是濮阳县（42.09/10 万），其次是禹州市（40.71/10 万）和中牟县（34.28/10 万）。男性标化死亡率最高的是禹州市（101.04/10 万），其次是濮阳县（76.69/10 万）和范县（63.49/10 万）；女性标化死亡率最高的是禹州市（29.85/10 万），其次是濮阳县（25.95/10 万）和郏县（23.85/10 万）。（图 5-10c）

2020 年，河南省肿瘤登记地区肺癌发病病例中有确切解剖学亚部位信息的占 40.80%，亚部位未特指的占 59.20%。在有亚部位信息的肺病例中，气管占 0.57%，主支气管占 12.93%，上叶占 46.29%，中叶占 15.34%，下叶占 22.75%，交搭跨越占 2.12%。（图 5-10d）

Among the 41 rural cancer registries, the ASR China incidence rate of lung cancer in males was the highest in Yuzhou City (116.22 per 100,000) followed by Puyang County (100.21 per 100,000), and Fan County (76.11 per 100,000). For females, it was the highest in Puyang County (42.09 per 100,000), followed by Yuzhou City (40.71 per 100,000), and Zhongmu County (34.28 per 100,000). The ASR China mortality rate of lung cancer in males was the highest in Yuzhou City (101.04 per 100,000) followed by Puyang County (76.69 per 100,000), and Fan County (63.49 per 100,000). For females, it was the highest in Yuzhou City (29.85 per 100,000), followed by Puyang County (25.95 per 100,000), and Jia County (23.85 per 100,000). (Figure 5-10c)

About 40.80% of the lung cancer had specific subsite. Among those cases, trachea accounted for 0.57%, main bronchus accounted for 12.93%, upper lobe accounted for 46.29%, middle lobe accounted for 15.34%, lower lobe accounted for 22.75%, and overlapping accounted for 2.12%. (Figure 5-10d)

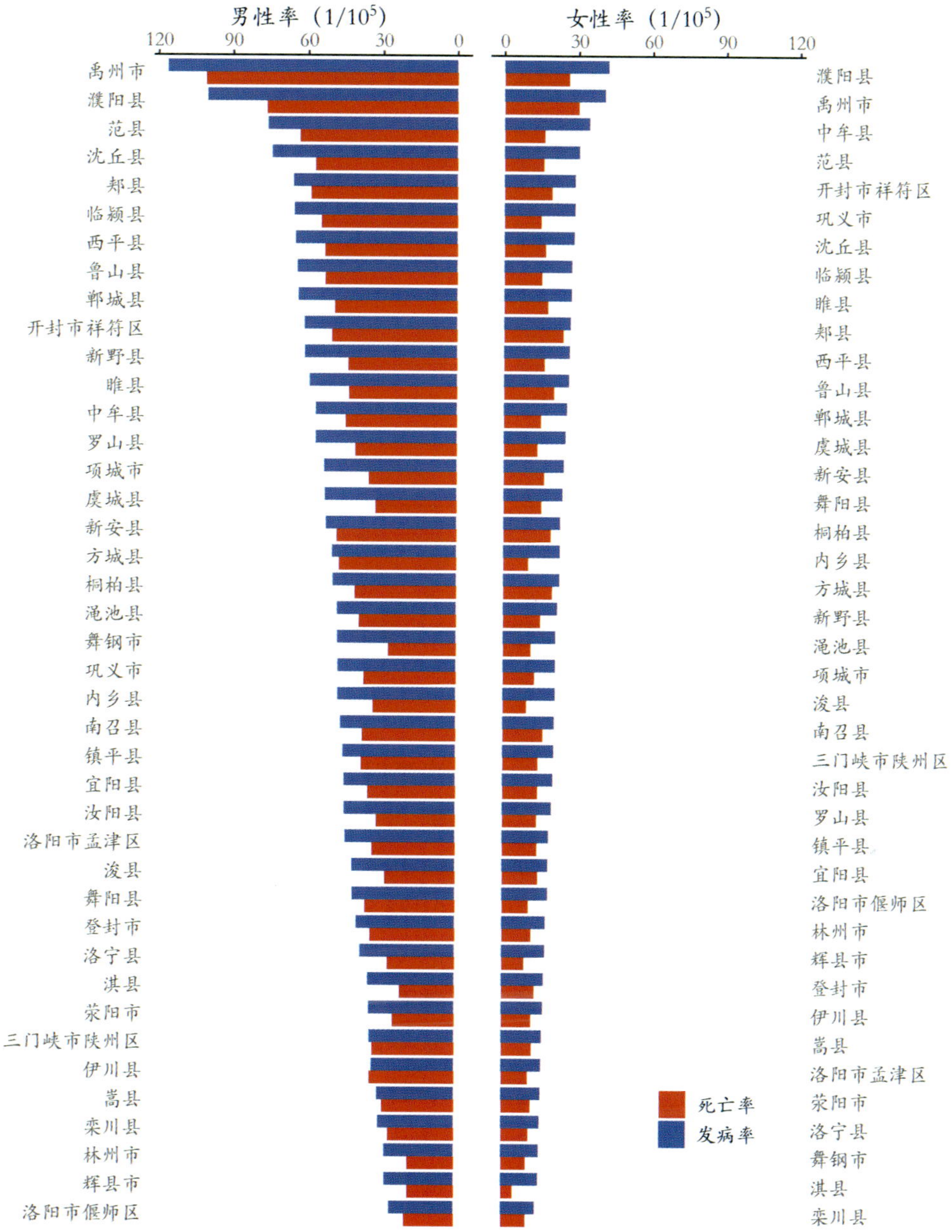

图 5-10c　2020 年河南省农村肿瘤登记地区肺癌发病率和死亡率

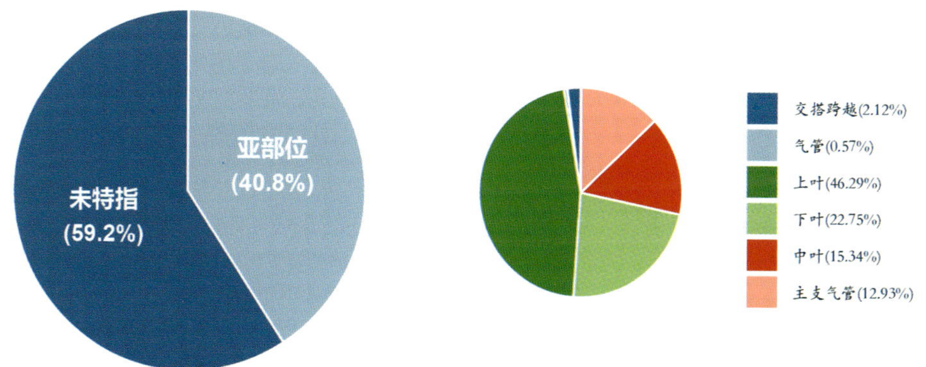

图 5-10d　2020 年河南省肿瘤登记地区肺癌发病病例亚部位构成

2020 年，河南省肿瘤登记地区肺癌发病病例中有明确组织病理学分型的占 60.89%，组织学类型未特指的占 39.11%。在有组织病理学分型的肺病例中，鳞状细胞癌占 13.11%，腺癌占 30.25%，腺鳞癌占 0.68%，小细胞癌占 6.79%，大细胞癌占 0.15%，其他占 49.02%。（图 5-10e）

About 60.89% of the lung cancer had morphological verification. Among those cases, Squamous cell accounted for 13.11%, Adenocarcinoma accounted for 30.25%, Adenosquamous accounted for 0.68%, Small cell accounted for 6.79%, Large cell accounted for 0.15%, and others accounted for 49.02%. (Figure 5-10e)

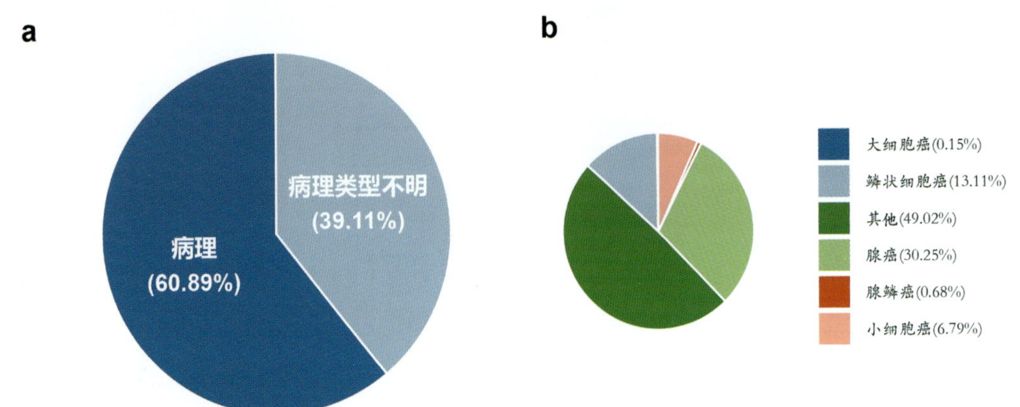

图 5-10e　2020 年河南省肿瘤登记地区肺癌发病病例形态学构成

十一、骨

2020 年，河南省肿瘤登记地区骨癌的发病率为 2.07/10 万，中标率为 1.67/10 万，世标率为 1.66/10 万，发病例数占全部癌症新发病例数的 0.74%；其中，男性和女性发病率分别为 2.23/10 万和 1.90/10 万，城市地区和农村地区发病率分别为 1.69/10 万和 2.22/10 万；中标发病率呈现男性高于女性、农村地区高于城市地区的特点，男性中标发病率是女性的 1.23 倍，农村地区中标发病率是城市地区的 1.37 倍。同期，骨癌的死亡率为 1.26/10 万，中标率为 0.90/10 万，世标率为 0.89/10 万，死亡病例数占全部癌症死亡病例数的 0.77%；其中，男性和女性死亡率分别为 1.51/10 万和 1.00/10 万，城市地区和农村地区死亡率分别为 1.00/10 万和 1.36/10 万；中标死亡率呈现男性高于女性、农村地区高于城市地区的特点，男性中标死亡率是女性的 1.74 倍，农村地区中标死亡率是城市地区的 1.52 倍。（表 5-11）

11. Bone

In 2020, there were 893 new cases diagnosed as bone cancer in registration areas of Henan Province, China (491 males and 402 females, 208 in urban areas and 685 in rural areas), accounting for 0.74% of new cases of all cancers. The crude incidence rate was 2.07 per 100,000, with the ASR China 1.67 per 100,000 and the ASR World 1.66 per 100,000, respectively. Subgroup analysis showed that the incidence of ASR China was 1.23 times in males as that in females, and it was 1.37 times in rural areas as that in urban areas. The cumulative incidence rate for subjects aged 0 to 74 years was 0.17%. (Table 5-11)

A total of 544 cases died of bone cancer in 2020 (333 males and 211 females, 123 in urban areas and 421 in rural areas), accounting for 0.77% of all cancer deaths. The crude mortality rate was 1.26 per 100,000, with the ASR China of 0.90 per 100,000 and the ASR World of 0.89 per 100,000, respectively. Subgroup analysis showed that the mortality of ASR China was 1.74 times in males as that in females, and it was 1.52 times in rural areas as that in urban areas. The cumulative mortality rate for subjects aged 0 to 74 years was 0.09%. (Table 5-11)

表 5-11　2020 年河南省肿瘤登记地区骨癌发病与死亡情况

地区	性别	病例数	发病率 (1/10^5)	构成 (%)	中标率 (1/10^5)	世标率 (1/10^5)	累积率 0~74 (%)
发病							
全省	合计	893	2.07	0.74	1.67	1.66	0.17
	男性	491	2.23	0.79	1.84	1.86	0.18
	女性	402	1.90	0.68	1.50	1.45	0.15
城市地区	合计	208	1.69	0.57	1.32	1.35	0.13
	男性	124	2.02	0.68	1.57	1.59	0.16
	女性	84	1.36	0.46	1.10	1.13	0.10
农村地区	合计	685	2.22	0.82	1.81	1.78	0.18
	男性	367	2.31	0.84	1.94	1.96	0.19
	女性	318	2.13	0.79	1.67	1.59	0.17
死亡							
全省	合计	544	1.26	0.77	0.90	0.89	0.09
	男性	333	1.51	0.77	1.15	1.14	0.12
	女性	211	1.00	0.78	0.66	0.66	0.07
城市地区	合计	123	1.00	0.62	0.66	0.67	0.07
	男性	72	1.17	0.60	0.83	0.84	0.10
	女性	51	0.83	0.67	0.50	0.51	0.04
农村地区	合计	421	1.36	0.83	1.00	0.99	0.10
	男性	261	1.64	0.84	1.28	1.27	0.13
	女性	160	1.07	0.82	0.72	0.72	0.08

骨癌年龄别发病率在 0~39 岁年龄段处于较低水平，40 岁以后快速上升，在 80 岁达到峰值；年龄别死亡率在 0~49 岁年龄段处于较低水平，50 岁以后快速上升，在 85 岁达到峰值；年龄别发病率和死亡率均呈现男性高于女性的特点；城市地区和农村地区年龄别率虽然有一定差异，但是总体趋势类同。（图 5-11a）

在 14 个城市肿瘤登记地区中，男性骨癌标化发病率最高的是济源市（3.51/10 万），其次是漯河市城区（3.01/10 万）和信阳市浉河区（2.56/10 万）；女性标化发病率最高的是信阳市浉河区（2.55/10 万），其次是鹤壁市城区（2.15/10 万）和郑州市城区（2.02/10 万）。男性标化死亡率最高的是南阳市卧龙区（2.07/10 万），其次是南阳市宛城区（1.83/10 万）和漯河市城区（1.43/10 万）；女性标化死亡率最高的是济源市（0.81/10 万），其次是南阳市宛城区（0.67/10 万）和鹤壁市城区（0.64/10 万）。（图 5-11b）

在 41 个农村肿瘤登记地区中，男性骨癌标化发病率最高的是临颍县（5.87/10 万），其次是方城县（5.45/10 万）和禹州市（3.96/10 万）；女性标化发病率最高的是方城县（4.36/10 万），其次是栾川县（4.29/10 万）和范县（4.01/10 万）。男性标化死亡率最高的是罗山县（2.96/10 万），其次是禹州市（2.75/10 万）和嵩县（2.64/10 万）；女性标化死亡率最高的是罗山县（1.66/10 万），其次是禹州市（1.64/10 万）和林州市（1.58/10 万）。（图 5-11c）

The age specific incidence of bone cancer was low at age group of 0~39, and it started increasing sharply at age group of 40, it reached the peak at age of 80. The age specific mortality was low at age group of 0~49, and it started increasing sharply at age group of 50, it reached the peak at age of 85. Age specific incidence and mortality were all higher in males than in females, The change pattern of age specific incidence and mortality were similar in urban areas and rural areas. (Figure 5-11-a)

Among the 14 urban cancer registries, the ASR China incidence rate of bone cancer in males was the highest in Jiyuan City (3.51 per 100,000) followed by Luohe City (3.01 per 100,000), and Xinyang Shihe District (2.56 per 100,000). For females, it was the highest in Xinyang Shihe District (2.55 per 100,000), followed by Hebi City (2.15 per 100,000), and Zhengzhou City (2.02 per 100,000). The ASR China mortality rate of bone cancer in males was the highest in Nanyang Wolong District (2.07 per 100,000) followed by Nanyang Wancheng District (1.83 per 100,000), and Luohe City (1.43 per 100,000). For females, it was the highest in Jiyuan City (0.81 per 100,000), followed by Nanyang Wancheng District (0.67 per 100,000), and Hebi City (0.64 per 100,000). (Figure 5-11b)

Among the 41 rural cancer registries, the ASR China incidence rate of bone cancer in males was the highest in Linying County (5.87 per 100,000) followed by Fangcheng County (5.45 per 100,000), and Yuzhou City (3.96 per 100,000). For females, it was the highest in Fangcheng County (4.36 per 100,000), followed by Luanchuan County (4.29 per 100,000), and Fan County (4.01 per 100,000). The ASR China mortality rate of bone cancer in males was the highest in Luoshan County (2.96 per 100,000) followed by Yuzhou City (2.75 per 100,000), and Song County (2.64 per 100,000). For females, it was the highest in Luoshan County (1.66 per 100,000), followed by Yuzhou City (1.64 per 100,000), and Linzhou City (1.58 per 100,000). (Figure 5-11c)

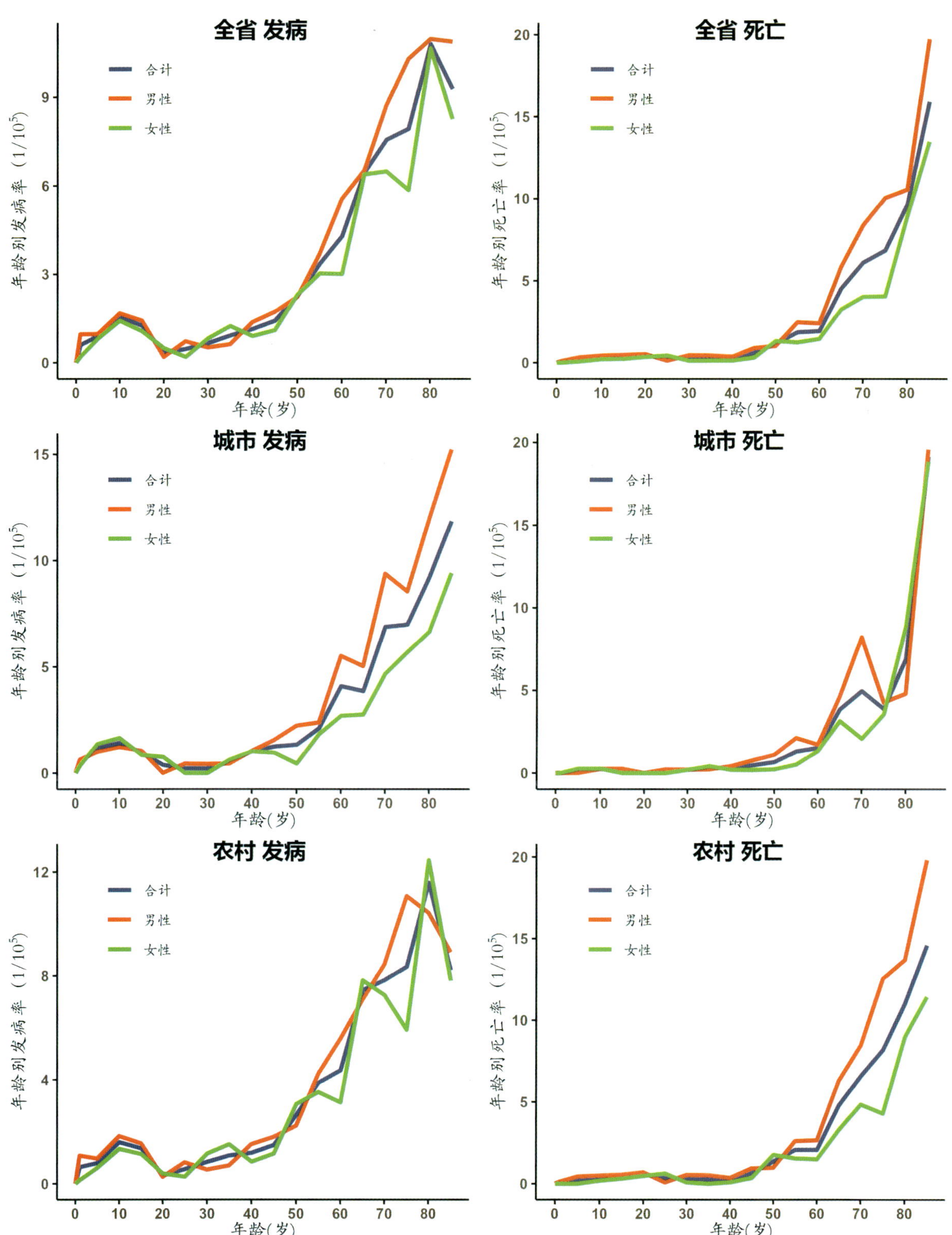

图 5-11a 2020 年河南省肿瘤登记地区骨癌年龄别发病率和死亡率

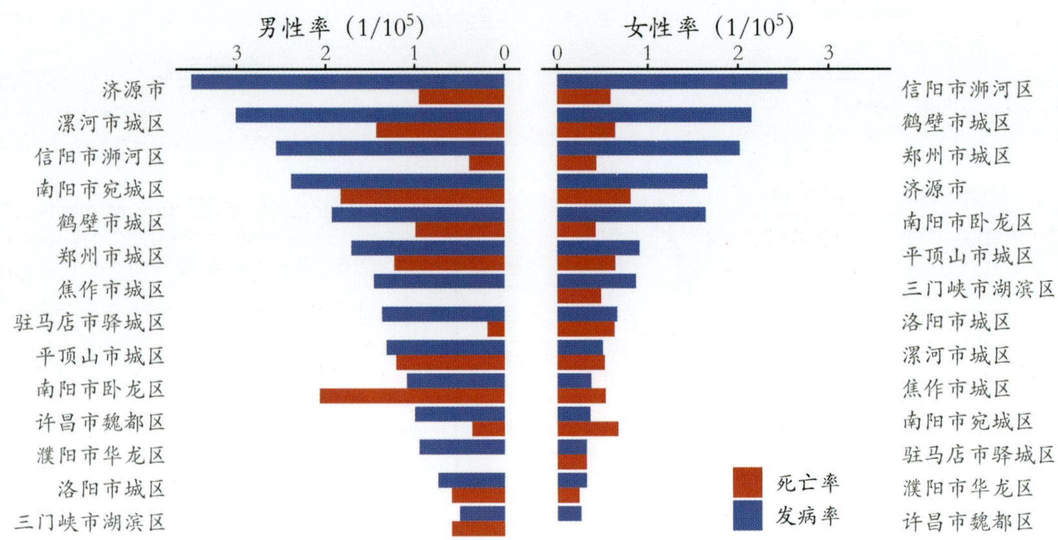

图 5-11b　2020 年河南省城市肿瘤登记地区骨癌发病率和死亡率

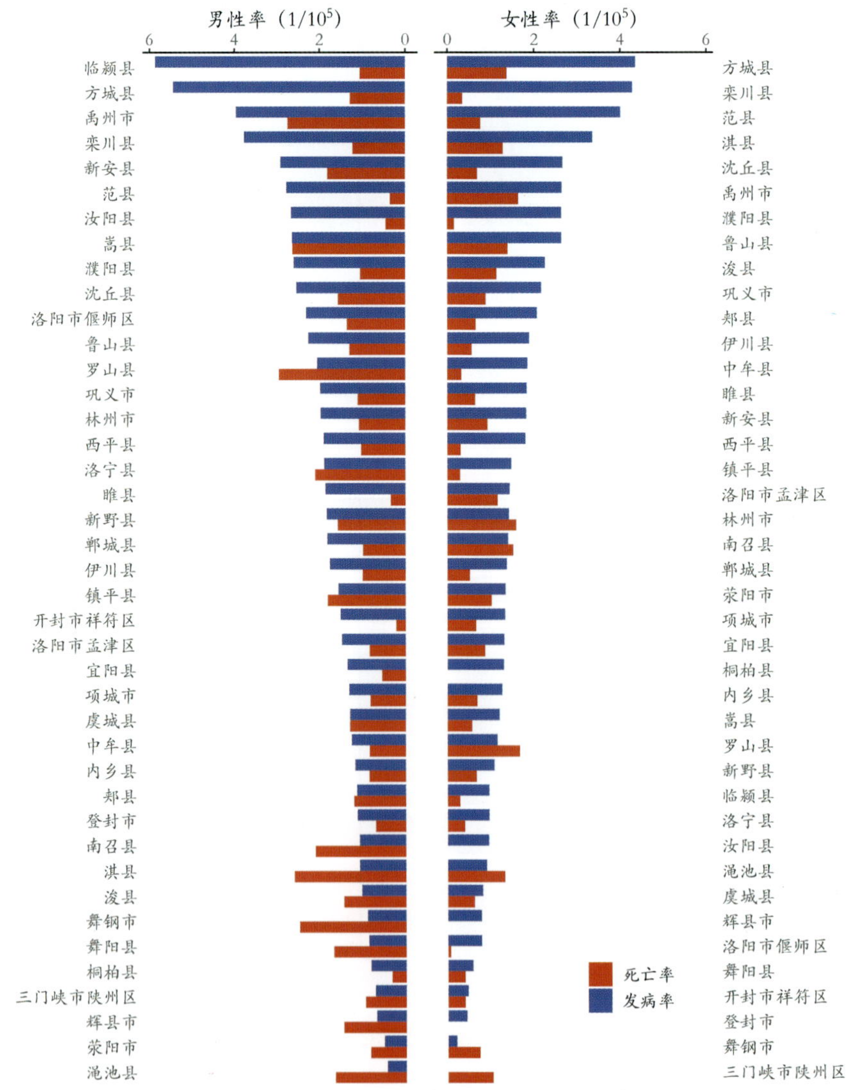

图 5-11c　2020 年河南省农村肿瘤登记地区骨癌发病率和死亡率

十二、女性乳腺

2020 年，河南省肿瘤登记地区女性乳腺癌的发病率为 48.62/10 万，中标率为 38.26/10 万，世标率为 35.55/10 万，发病例数占全部癌症新发病例数的 8.50%；其中，城市地区和农村地区发病率分别为 58.00/10 万和 44.76/10 万；中标发病率呈现城市地区高于农村地区的特点，城市地区中标发病率是农村地区的 1.21 倍。同期，女性乳腺癌的死亡率为 10.06/10 万，中标率为 6.79/10 万，世标率为 6.71/10 万，死亡病例数占全部癌症死亡病例数的 3.02%；其中，城市地区和农村地区死亡率分别为 11.51/10 万和 9.46/10 万；中标死亡率呈现城市地区高于农村地区的特点，城市地区中标死亡率是农村地区的 1.15 倍。（表 5–12）

12. Female breast

In 2020, there were 10,265 new cases diagnosed as female breast cancer in registration areas of Henan Province, China (3,572 in urban areas and 6,693 in rural areas), accounting for 8.50% of new cases of all cancers. The crude incidence rate was 48.62 per 100,000, with the ASR China 38.26 per 100,000 and the ASR World 35.55 per 100,000, respectively. Subgroup analysis showed that the incidence of ASR China was 1.21 times in urban areas as that in rural areas. The cumulative incidence rate for subjects aged 0 to 74 years was 3.82%. (Table 5–12)

A total of 2,123 cases died of female breast cancer in 2020 (709 in urban areas and 1,414 in rural areas), accounting for 3.02% of all cancer deaths. The crude mortality rate was 10.06 per 100,000, with the ASR China 6.79 per 100,000 and the ASR World 6.71 per 100,000, respectively. Subgroup analysis showed that the mortality of ASR China was 1.15 times in urban areas as that in rural areas. The cumulative mortality rate for subjects aged 0 to 74 years was 0.78%. (Table 5–12)

表 5–12　2020 年河南省肿瘤登记地区女性乳腺癌发病与死亡情况

地区	病例数	发病率（1/10^5）	构成（%）	中标率（1/10^5）	世标率（1/10^5）	累积率 0～74（%）
发病						
全省	10 265	48.62	8.50	38.26	35.55	3.82
城市地区	3 572	58.00	9.74	43.59	40.77	4.43
农村地区	6 693	44.76	7.97	35.96	33.30	3.57
死亡						
全省	2 123	10.06	3.02	6.79	6.71	0.78
城市地区	709	11.51	3.60	7.45	7.33	0.80
农村地区	1 414	9.46	2.79	6.50	6.44	0.77

女性乳腺癌年龄别发病率在 0~19 岁年龄段处于较低水平，20 岁以后快速上升，在 50 岁达到峰值；年龄别死亡率在 0~39 岁年龄段处于较低水平，40 岁以后快速上升，在 85 岁达到峰值；城市地区和农村地区年龄别率虽然有一定差异，但是总体趋势类同。（图 5–12a）

The age specific incidence of female breast cancer was low at age group of 0~19, and it started increasing sharply at age group of 20, it reached the peak at age of 50. The age specific mortality was low at age group of 0~39, and it started increasing sharply at age group of 40, it reached the peak at age of 85. The change pattern of age specific incidence and mortality were similar in urban areas and rural areas. (Figure 5–12a)

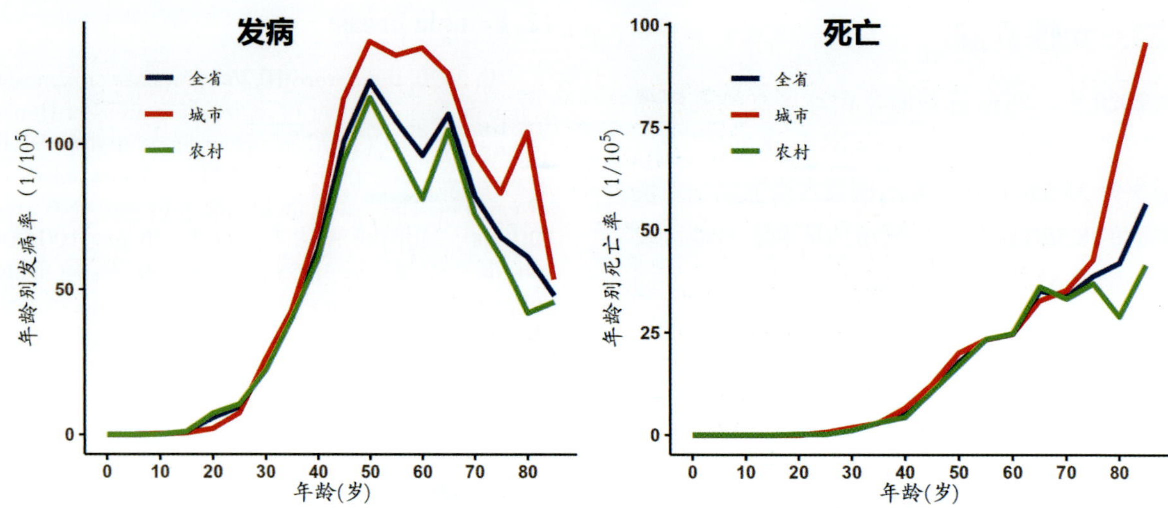

图 5-12a 2020 年河南省肿瘤登记地区女性乳腺癌年龄别发病率和死亡率

在 14 个城市肿瘤登记地区中，女性乳腺癌标化发病率最高的是许昌市魏都区（68.90/10 万），其次是濮阳市华龙区（63.41/10 万）和南阳市宛城区（58.64/10 万）；标化死亡率最高的是漯河市城区（12.89/10 万），其次是濮阳市华龙区（12.57/10 万）和南阳市卧龙区（10.67/10 万）。（图 5-12b）

Among the 14 urban cancer registries, the ASR China incidence rate of female breast was the highest in Xuchang Weidu District (68.90 per 100,000), followed by Puyang Hualong District (63.41 per 100,000), and Nanyang Wancheng District (58.64 per 100,000). The ASR China mortality rate of female breast cancer was the highest in Luohe City (12.89 per 100,000), followed by Puyang Hualong District (12.57 per 100,000), and Nanyang Wolong District (10.67 per 100,000). (Figure 5-12b)

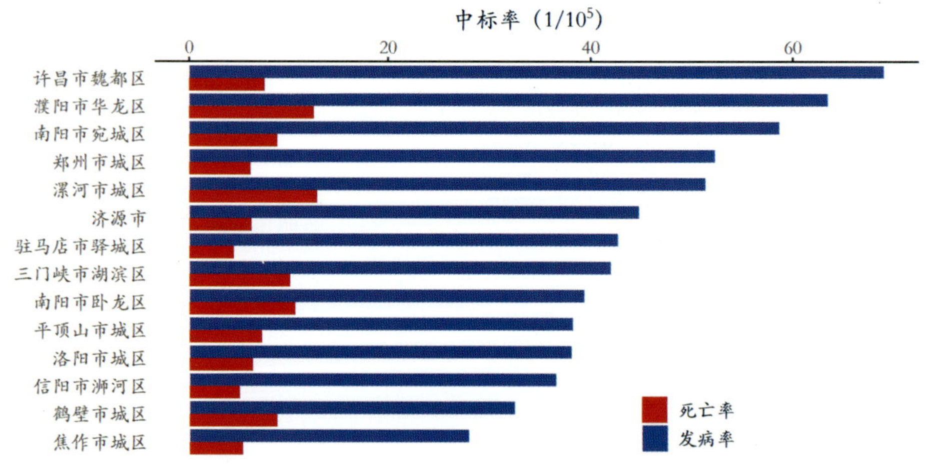

图 5-12b 2020 年河南省城市肿瘤登记地区女性乳腺癌发病率和死亡率

在 41 个农村肿瘤登记地区中，女性乳腺癌标化发病率最高的是虞城县（66.64/10 万），其次是郸城县（54.29/10 万）和濮阳县（47.57/10 万）；标化死亡率最高的是虞城县（22.33/10 万），其次是郸城县（13.03/10 万）和桐柏县（10.67/10 万）。（图 5-12c）

Among the 41 rural cancer registries, the ASR China incidence rate of female breast cancer was the highest in Yucheng County (66.64 per 100,000), followed by Dancheng County (54.29 per 100,000), and Puyang County (47.57 per 100,000). The ASR China mortality rate of female breast cancer was the highest in Yucheng County (22.33 per 100,000), followed by Dancheng County (13.03 per 100,000), and Tongbai County (10.67 per 100,000). (Figure 5-12c)

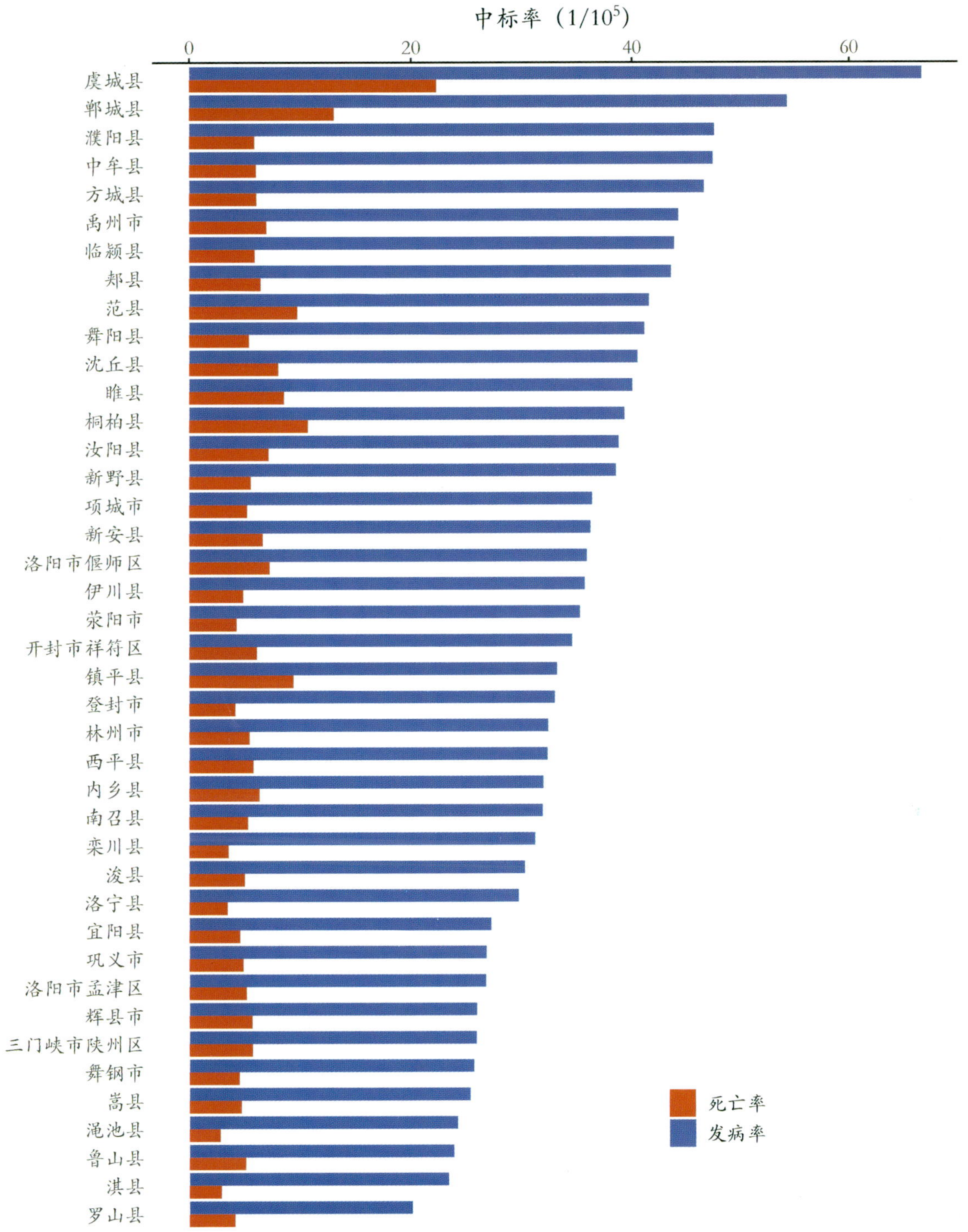

图 5-12c　2020 年河南省农村肿瘤登记地区女性乳腺癌发病率和死亡率

2020 年，河南省肿瘤登记地区女性乳腺癌发病病例中有确切解剖学亚部位信息的占 38.45%，亚部位未特指的占 61.55%。在有亚部位信息的女性乳腺病例中，乳头和乳晕占 13.4%，乳房中央占 10.44%，上内象限占 17.61%，下内象限占 7.71%，上外象限占 27.63%，下外象限占 6.18%，乳房腋尾占 0.57%，交搭跨越占 16.46%。（图 5-12d）

About 38.45% of the female breast cancer had specific subsite. Among those cases, nipple and areola accounted for 13.4%, central portion accounted for 10.44%, upper inner accounted for 17.61%, lower inner accounted for 7.71%, upper outer accounted for 27.63%, lower outer accounted for 6.18%, axillary tail accounted for 0.57%, and overlapping accounted for 16.46%. (Figure 5-12d)

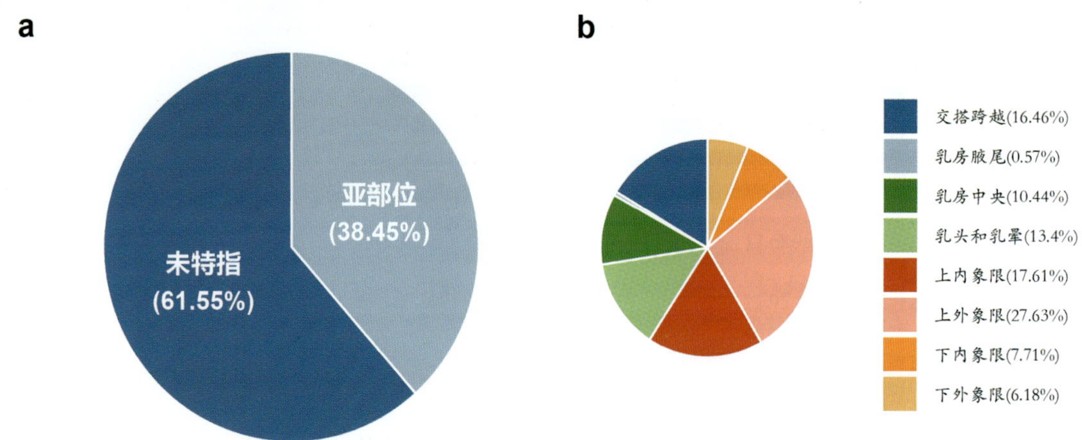

图 5-12d　2020 年河南省肿瘤登记地区女性乳腺癌发病病例亚部位构成

2020 年，河南省肿瘤登记地区女性乳腺癌发病病例中有明确组织病理学分型的占 73.18%，组织学类型未特指的占 26.82%。在有组织病理学分型的女性乳腺病例中，导管癌占 47.55%，小叶癌占 3.04%，髓样癌占 0.13%，Paget’s 病占 0.39%，其他占 48.89%。（图 5-12e）

About 73.18% of the female breast cancer had morphological verification. Among those cases, Intraductal accounted for 47.55%, Lobular accounted for 3.04%, Medullary accounted for 0.13%, Paget’s accounted for 0.39%, and Others accounted for 48.89%. (Figure 5-12e)

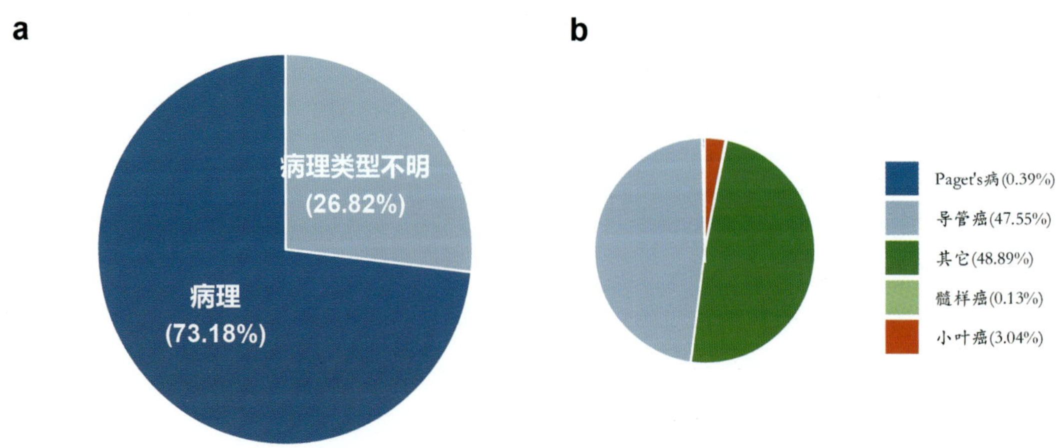

图 5-12e　2020 年河南省肿瘤登记地区女性乳腺癌发病病例形态学构成

十三、子宫颈

2020 年，河南省肿瘤登记地区子宫颈癌的发病率为 21.01/10 万，中标率为 16.38/10 万，世标率为 15.25/10 万，发病例数占全部癌症新发病例数的 3.67%；其中，城市地区和农村地区发病率分别为 19.91/10 万和 21.46/10 万；中标发病率呈现农村地区高于城市地区的特点，农村地区中标发病率是城市地区的 1.13 倍。同期，子宫颈癌的死亡率为 5.99/10 万，中标率为 4.08/10 万，世标率为 3.97/10 万，死亡病例数占全部癌症死亡病例数的 1.80%；其中，城市地区和农村地区死亡率分别为 5.70/10 万和 6.11/10 万；中标死亡率呈现农村地区高于城市地区的特点，农村地区中标死亡率是城市地区的 1.11 倍。（表 5–13）

13. Cervix

In 2020, there were 4,435 new cases diagnosed as cervix cancer in registration areas of Henan Province, China (1,226 in urban areas and 3,209 in rural areas), accounting for 3.67% of new cases of all cancers. The crude incidence rate was 21.01 per 100,000, with the ASR China 16.38 per 100,000 and the ASR World 15.25 per 100,000, respectively. Subgroup analysis showed that the incidence of ASR China was 1.13 times in rural areas as that in urban areas. The cumulative incidence rate for subjects aged 0 to 74 years was 1.66%. (Table 5–13)

A total of 1,265 cases died of cervix cancer in 2020 (351 in urban areas and 914 in rural areas), accounting for 1.80% of all cancer deaths. The crude mortality rate was 5.99 per 100,000, with the ASR China 4.08 per 100,000 and the ASR World 3.97 per 100,000, respectively. Subgroup analysis showed that the mortality of ASR China was 1.11 times in rural areas as that in urban areas. The cumulative mortality rate for subjects aged 0 to 74 years was 0.47%. (Table 5–13)

表 5–13　2020 年河南省肿瘤登记地区子宫颈癌发病与死亡情况

地区	病例数	粗率 ($1/10^5$)	构成 (%)	中标率 ($1/10^5$)	世标率 ($1/10^5$)	累积率 0 ~ 74 (%)
发病						
全省	4 435	21.01	3.67	16.38	15.25	1.66
城市地区	1 226	19.91	3.34	14.98	14.02	1.56
农村地区	3 209	21.46	3.82	16.99	15.78	1.70
死亡						
全省	1 265	5.99	1.80	4.08	3.97	0.47
城市地区	351	5.70	1.78	3.78	3.69	0.44
农村地区	914	6.11	1.80	4.20	4.10	0.49

子宫颈癌年龄别发病率在 0~19 岁年龄段处于较低水平，20 岁以后快速上升，在 50 岁达到峰值；年龄别死亡率在 0~39 岁年龄段处于较低水平，40 岁以后快速上升，在 85 岁达到峰值；城市地区和农村地区年龄别率虽然有一定差异，但是总体趋势类同。（图 5–13a）

The age specific incidence of cervix cancer was low at age group of 0~19, and it started increasing sharply at age group of 20, it reached the peak at age of 50. The age specific mortality was low at age group of 0~39, and it started increasing sharply at age group of 40, it reached the peak at age of 85. The change pattern of age specific incidence and mortality were similar in urban areas and rural areas. (Figure 5–13a)

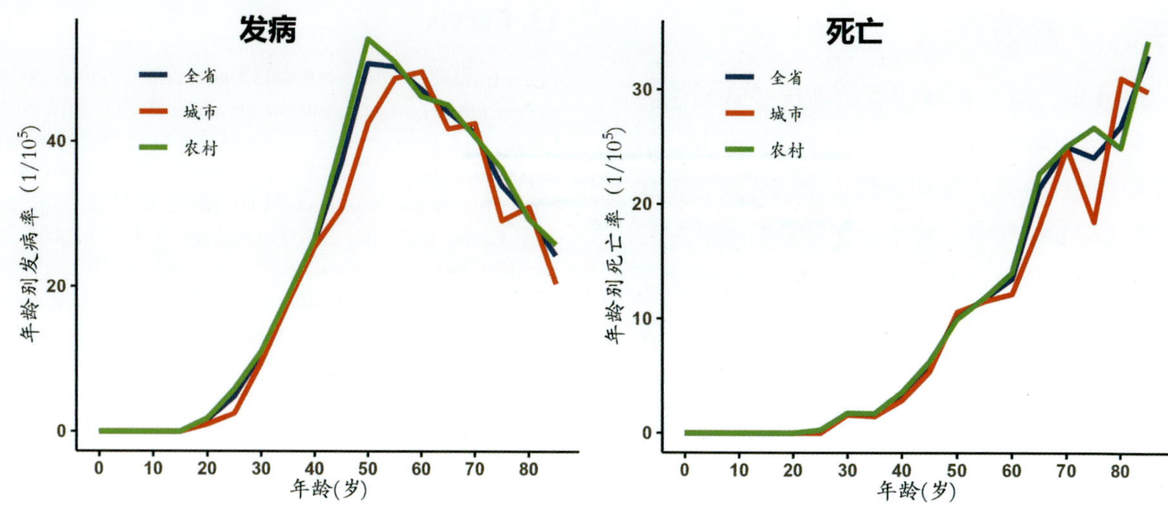

图 5-13a　2020 年河南省肿瘤登记地区子宫颈癌年龄别发病率和死亡率

在 14 个城市肿瘤登记地区中，子宫颈癌标化发病率最高的是济源市（46.18/10 万），其次是濮阳市华龙区（20.37/10 万）和漯河市城区（19.80/10 万）；标化死亡率最高的是三门峡市湖滨区（6.96/10 万），其次是濮阳市华龙区（6.79/10 万）和南阳市宛城区（5.70/10 万）。（图 5-13b）

Among the 14 urban cancer registries, the ASR China incidence rate of cervix was the highest in Jiyuan City (46.18 per 100,000), followed by Puyang Hualong District (20.37 per 100,000), and Luohe City (19.80 per 100,000). The ASR China mortality rate of cervix cancer was the highest in Sanmenxia Hubin District (6.96 per 100,000), followed by Puyang Hualong District (6.79 per 100,000), and Nanyang Wancheng District (5.70 per 100,000). (Figure 5-13b)

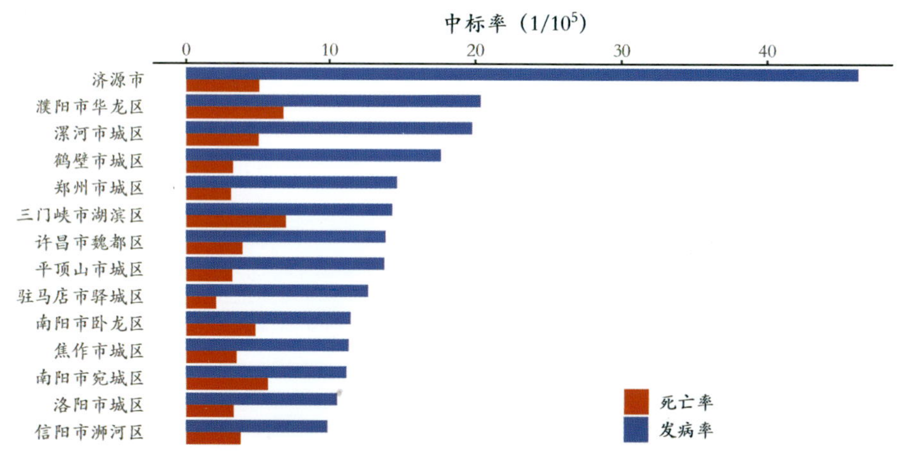

图 5-13b　2020 年河南省城市肿瘤登记地区子宫颈癌发病率和死亡率

在 41 个农村肿瘤登记地区中，子宫颈癌标化发病率最高的是舞阳县（38.18/10 万），其次是虞城县（26.8/10 万）和方城县（25.88/10 万）；标化死亡率最高的是虞城县（9.04/10 万），其次是栾川县（7.72/10 万）和睢县（7.43/10 万）。（图 5-13c）

Among the 41 rural cancer registries, the ASR China incidence rate of cervix cancer was the highest in Wuyang County (38.18 per 100,000), followed by Yucheng County (26.8 per 100,000), and Fangcheng County (25.88 per 100,000). The ASR China mortality rate of cervix cancer was the highest in Yucheng County (9.04 per 100,000), followed by Luanchuan County (7.72 per 100,000), and Sui County (7.43 per 100,000). (Figure 5-13c)

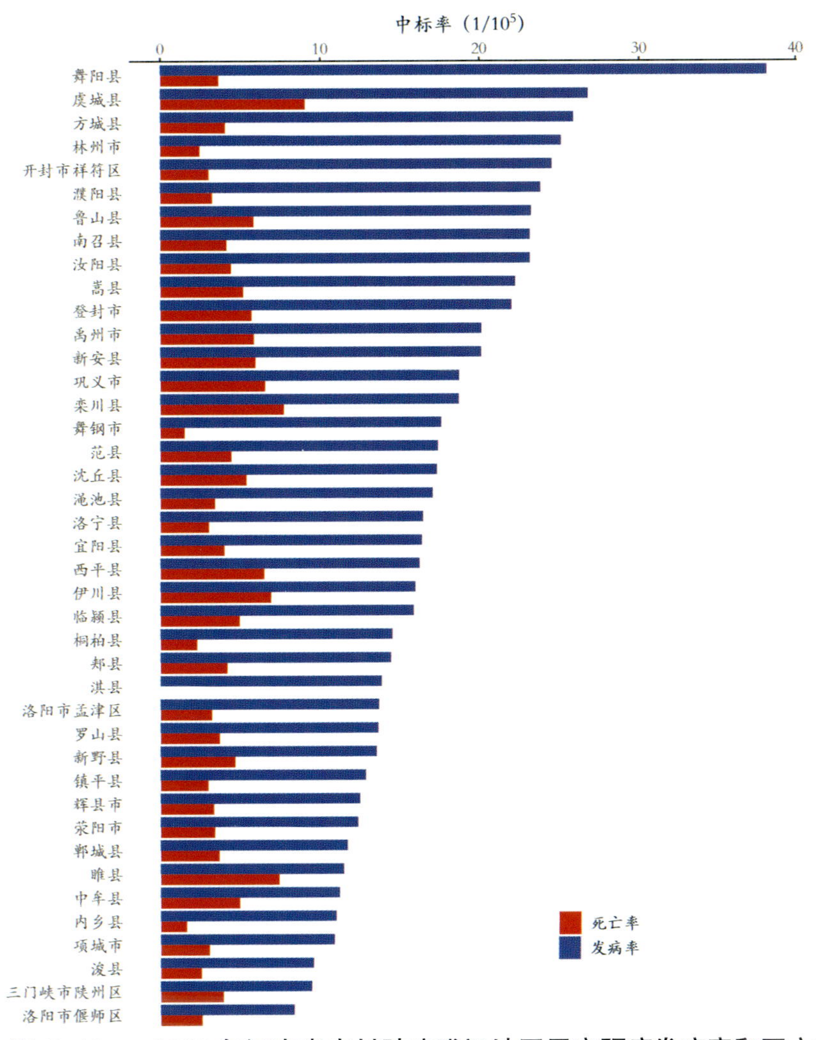

图 5-13c　2020 年河南省农村肿瘤登记地区子宫颈癌发病率和死亡率

2020 年，河南省肿瘤登记地区子宫颈癌发病病例中有确切解剖学亚部位信息的占 20.45%，亚部位未特指的占 79.55%。在有亚部位信息的子宫颈病例中，宫颈内膜占 70.67%，外宫颈占 24.73%，交搭跨越占 4.60%。（图 5-13d）

About 20.45% of the cervix cancer had specific subsite. Among those cases, endocervix accounted for 70.67%, exocervix accounted for 24.73%, and overlapping accounted for 4.60%. (Figure 5-13d)

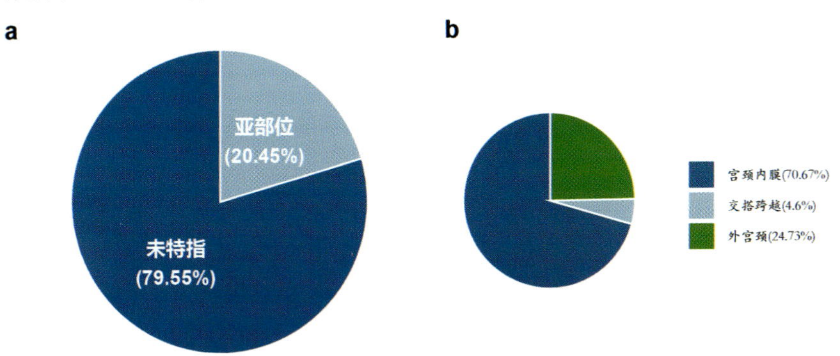

图 5-13d　2020 年河南省肿瘤登记地区子宫颈癌发病病例亚部位构成

十四、子宫体

2020 年，河南省肿瘤登记地区子宫体癌的发病率为 10.86/10 万，中标率为 7.96/10 万，世标率为 7.74/10 万，发病例数占全部癌症新发病例数的 1.90%；其中，城市地区和农村地区发病率分别为 11.27/10 万和 10.69/10 万；中标发病率呈现城市地区高于农村地区的特点，城市地区中标发病率是农村地区的 1.01 倍。同期，子宫体癌的死亡率为 2.01/10 万，中标率为 1.28/10 万，世标率为 1.27/10 万，死亡病例数占全部癌症死亡病例数的 0.60%；其中，城市地区和农村地区死亡率分别为 2.03/10 万和 2.00/10 万；中标死亡率呈现农村地区高于城市地区的特点，农村地区中标死亡率是城市地区的 1.02 倍。（表 5-14）

14. Uterus

In 2020, there were 2,292 new cases diagnosed as uterus cancer in registration areas of Henan Province, China (694 in urban areas and 1,598 in rural areas), accounting for 1.9% of new cases of all cancers. The crude incidence rate was 10.86 per 100,000, with the ASR China 7.96 per 100,000 and the ASR World 7.74 per 100,000, respectively. Subgroup analysis showed that the incidence of ASR China was 1.01 times in urban areas as that in rural areas. The cumulative incidence rate for subjects aged 0 to 74 years was 0.89%. (Table 5-14)

A total of 424 cases died of uterus cancer in 2020 (125 in urban areas and 299 in rural areas), accounting for 0.6% of all cancer deaths. The crude mortality rate was 2.01 per 100,000, with the ASR China 1.28 per 100,000 and the ASR World 1.27 per 100,000, respectively. Subgroup analysis showed that the mortality of ASR China was 1.02 times in rural areas as that in urban areas. The cumulative mortality rate for subjects aged 0 to 74 years was 0.14%. (Table 5-14)

表 5-14　2020 年河南省肿瘤登记地区子宫体癌发病与死亡情况

地区	病例数	粗率（$1/10^5$）	构成（%）	中标率（$1/10^5$）	世标率（$1/10^5$）	累积率 0～74（%）
发病						
全省	2 292	10.86	1.90	7.96	7.74	0.89
城市地区	694	11.27	1.89	8.04	7.84	0.91
农村地区	1 598	10.69	1.90	7.94	7.71	0.89
死亡						
全省	424	2.01	0.60	1.28	1.27	0.14
城市地区	125	2.03	0.63	1.26	1.26	0.15
农村地区	299	2.00	0.59	1.28	1.28	0.14

子宫体癌年龄别发病率在 0~29 岁年龄段处于较低水平，30 岁以后快速上升，在 55 岁达到峰值；年龄别死亡率在 0~39 岁年龄段处于较低水平，40 岁以后快速上升，在 85 岁达到峰值；城市地区和农村地区年龄别率虽然有一定差异，但是总体趋势类同。（图 5-14a）

The age specific incidence of uterus cancer was low at age group of 0~29, and it started increasing sharply at age group of 30, it reached the peak at age of 55. The age specific mortality was low at age group of 0~39, and it started increasing sharply at age group of 40, it reached the peak at age of 85. The change pattern of age specific incidence and mortality were similar in urban areas and rural areas. (Figure 5-14a)

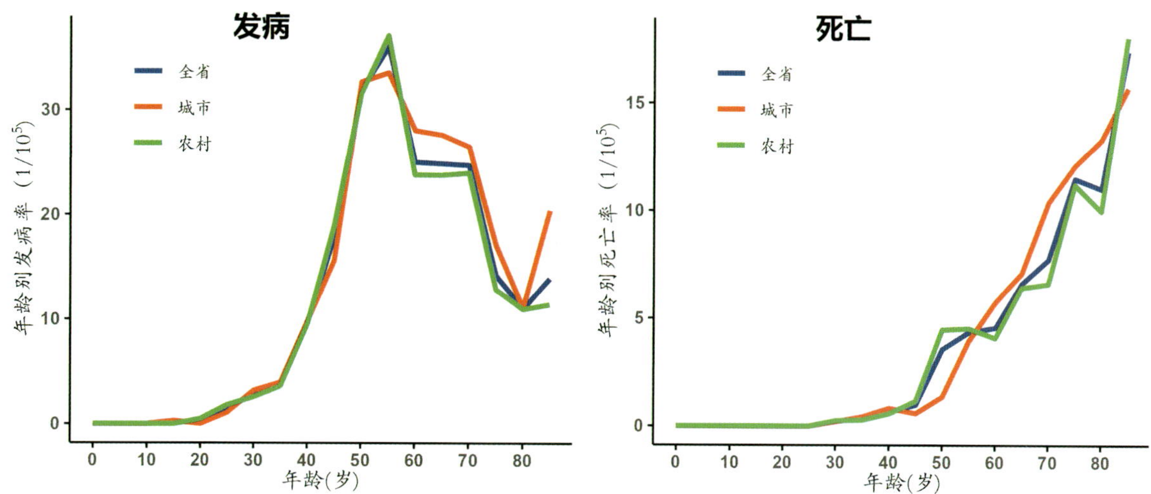

图 5-14a 2020 年河南省肿瘤登记地区子宫体癌年龄别发病率和死亡率

在 14 个城市肿瘤登记地区中，子宫体癌标化发病率最高的是南阳市宛城区（18.50/10 万），其次是南阳市卧龙区（11.52/10 万）和郑州市城区（10.23/10 万）；标化死亡率最高的是济源市（2.55/10 万），其次是濮阳市华龙区（2.22/10 万）和南阳市卧龙区（2.02/10 万）。（图 5-14b）

Among the 14 urban cancer registries, the ASR China incidence rate of uterus was the highest in Nanyang Wancheng District (18.50 per 100,000), followed by Nanyang Wolong District (11.52 per 100,000), and Zhengzhou City (10.23 per 100,000). The ASR China mortality rate of uterus cancer was the highest in Jiyuan City (2.55 per 100,000), followed by Puyang Hualong District (2.22 per 100,000), and Nanyang Wolong District (2.02 per 100,000). (Figure 5-14b)

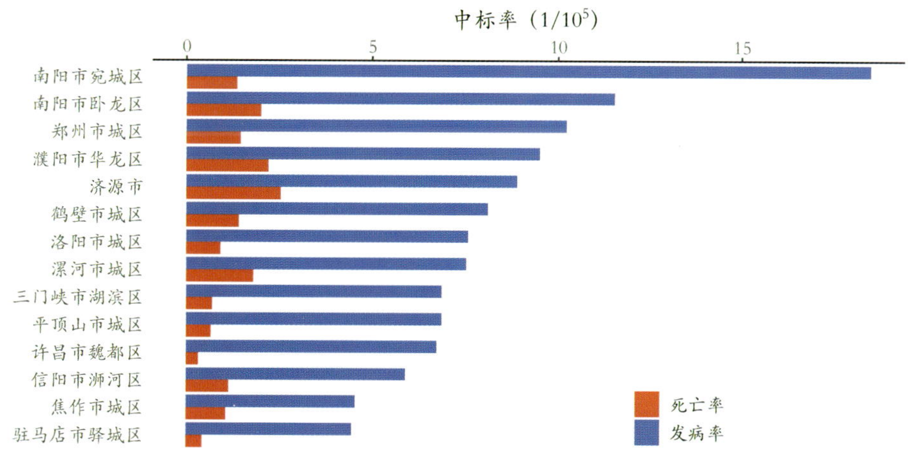

图 5-14b 2020 年河南省城市肿瘤登记地区子宫体癌发病率和死亡率

在 41 个农村肿瘤登记地区中，子宫体癌标化发病率最高的是虞城县（18.38/10 万），其次是方城县（13.56/10 万）和范县（13.33/10 万）；标化死亡率最高的是虞城县（6.35/10 万），其次是禹州市（3.48/10 万）和方城县（2.81/10 万）。（图 5-14c）

Among the 41 rural cancer registries, the ASR China incidence rate of uterus cancer was the highest in Yucheng County (18.38 per 100,000), followed by Fangcheng County (13.56 per 100,000), and Fan County (13.33 per 100,000). The ASR China mortality rate of uterus cancer was the highest in Yucheng County (6.35 per 100,000), followed by Yuzhou City (3.48 per 100,000), and Fangcheng County (2.81 per 100,000). (Figure 5-14c)

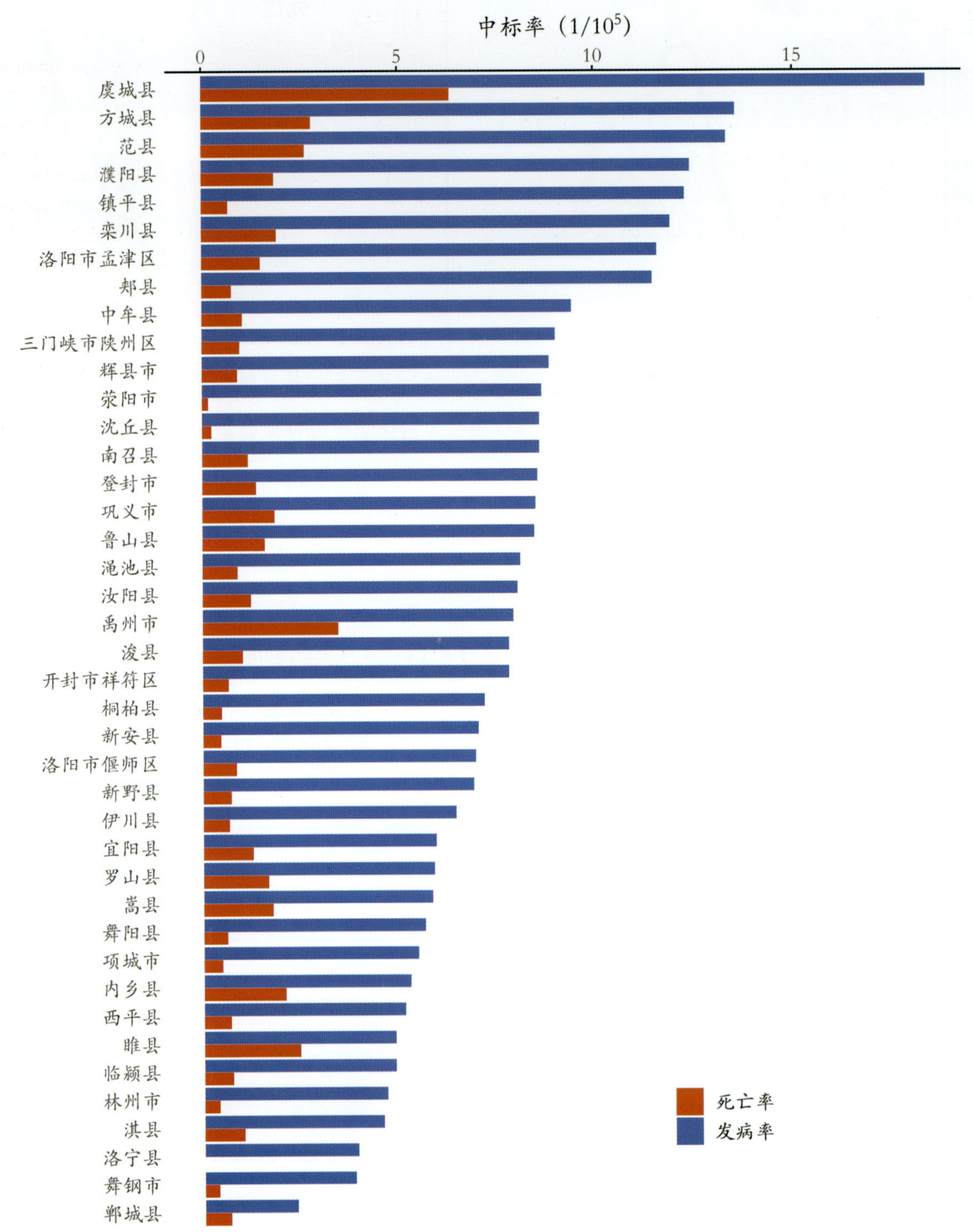

图 5-14c　2020 年河南省农村肿瘤登记地区子宫体癌发病率和死亡率

十五、卵巢

2020 年，河南省肿瘤登记地区卵巢癌的发病率为 8.06/10 万，中标率为 6.39/10 万，世标率为 6.03/10 万，发病例数占全部癌症新发病例数的 1.41%；其中，城市地区和农村地区发病率分别为 8.13/10 万和 8.03/10 万；中标发病率呈现农村地区高于城市地区的特点，农村地区中标发病率是城市地区的 1.07 倍。同期，卵巢癌的死亡率为 3.31/10 万，中标率为 2.20/10 万，世标率为 2.16/10 万，死亡病例数占全部癌症死亡病例数的 0.99%；其中，城市地区和农村地区死亡率分别为 4.12/10 万和 2.97/10 万；中标死亡率呈现城市地区高于农村地区的特点，城市地区中标死亡率是农村地区的 1.26 倍。（表 5–15）

15. Ovary

In 2020, there were 1,701 new cases diagnosed as ovary cancer in registration areas of Henan Province, China (501 in urban areas and 1,200 in rural areas), accounting for 1.41% of new cases of all cancers. The crude incidence rate was 8.06 per 100,000, with the ASR China 6.39 per 100,000 and the ASR World 6.03 per 100,000, respectively. Subgroup analysis showed that the incidence of ASR China was 1.07 times in rural areas as that in urban areas. The cumulative incidence rate for subjects aged 0 to 74 years was 0.64%. (Table 5–15)

A total of 698 cases died of ovary cancer in 2020 (254 in urban areas and 444 in rural areas), accounting for 0.99% of all cancer deaths. The crude mortality rate was 3.31 per 100,000, with the ASR China 2.20 per 100,000 and the ASR World 2.16 per 100,000, respectively. Subgroup analysis showed that the mortality of ASR China was 1.26 times in urban areas as that in rural areas. The cumulative mortality rate for subjects aged 0 to 74 years was 0.26%. (Table 5–15)

表 5–15　2020 年河南省肿瘤登记地区卵巢癌发病与死亡情况

地区	病例数	粗率（1/10^5）	构成（%）	中标率（1/10^5）	世标率（1/10^5）	累积率 0～74（%）
发病						
全省	1 701	8.06	1.41	6.39	6.03	0.64
城市地区	501	8.13	1.37	6.08	5.78	0.62
农村地区	1 200	8.03	1.43	6.52	6.12	0.65
死亡						
全省	698	3.31	0.99	2.20	2.16	0.26
城市地区	254	4.12	1.29	2.58	2.60	0.30
农村地区	444	2.97	0.88	2.04	1.98	0.24

卵巢癌年龄别发病率在 0~29 岁年龄段处于较低水平，30 岁以后快速上升，在 65 岁达到峰值；年龄别死亡率在 0~39 岁年龄段处于较低水平，40 岁以后快速上升，在 80 岁达到峰值；城市地区和农村地区年龄别率虽然有一定差异，但是总体趋势类同。（图 5–15a）

The age specific incidence of ovary cancer was low at age group of 0~29, and it started increasing sharply at age group of 30, it reached the peak at age of 65. The age specific mortality was low at age group of 0~39, and it started increasing sharply at age group of 40, it reached the peak at age of 80. The change pattern of age specific incidence and mortality were similar in urban areas and rural areas. (Figure 5–15a)

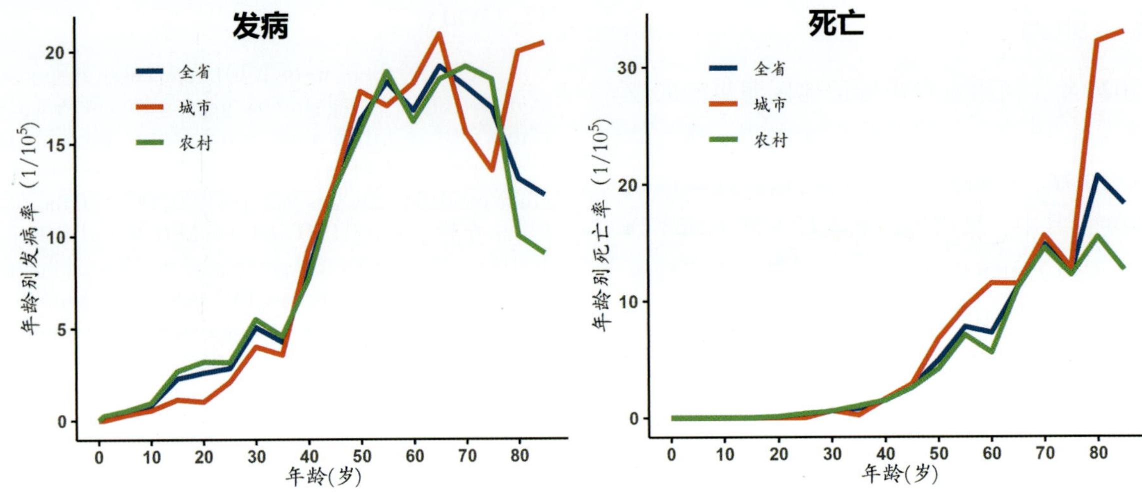

图 5-15a　2020 年河南省肿瘤登记地区卵巢癌年龄别发病率和死亡率

在 14 个城市肿瘤登记地区中，卵巢癌标化发病率最高的是濮阳市华龙区（11.38/10 万），其次是济源市（8.64/10 万）和驻马店市驿城区（7.83/10 万）；标化死亡率最高的是三门峡市湖滨区（4.97/10 万），其次是许昌市魏都区（4.22/10 万）和漯河市城区（3.96/10 万）。（图 5-15b）

Among the 14 urban cancer registries, the ASR China incidence rate of ovary was the highest in Puyang Hualong District (11.38 per 100,000), followed by Jiyuan City (8.64 per 100,000), and Zhumadian Yicheng District (7.83 per 100,000). The ASR China mortality rate of ovary cancer was the highest in Sanmenxia Hubin District (4.97 per 100,000), followed by Xuchang Weidu District (4.22 per 100,000), and Luohe City (3.96 per 100,000). (Figure 5-15b)

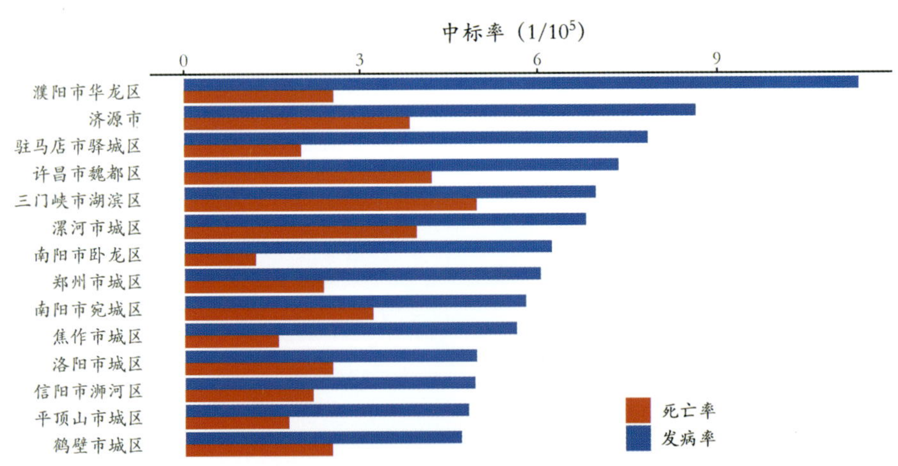

图 5-15b　2020 年河南省城市肿瘤登记地区卵巢癌发病率和死亡率

在 41 个农村肿瘤登记地区中，卵巢癌标化发病率最高的是中牟县（24.13/10 万），其次是虞城县（12.82/10 万）和方城县（10.95/10 万）；标化死亡率最高的是栾川县（4.58/10 万），其次是三门峡市陕州区（4.04/10 万）和登封市（3.69/10 万）。（图 5-15c）

Among the 41 rural cancer registries, the ASR China incidence rate of ovary cancer was the highest in Zhongmu County (24.13 per 100,000), followed by Yucheng County (12.82 per 100,000), and Fangcheng County (10.95 per 100,000). The ASR China mortality rate of ovary cancer was the highest in Luanchuan County (4.58 per 100,000), followed by Sanmenxia Shanzhou District (4.04 per 100,000), and Dengfeng City (3.69 per 100,000). (Figure 5-15c)

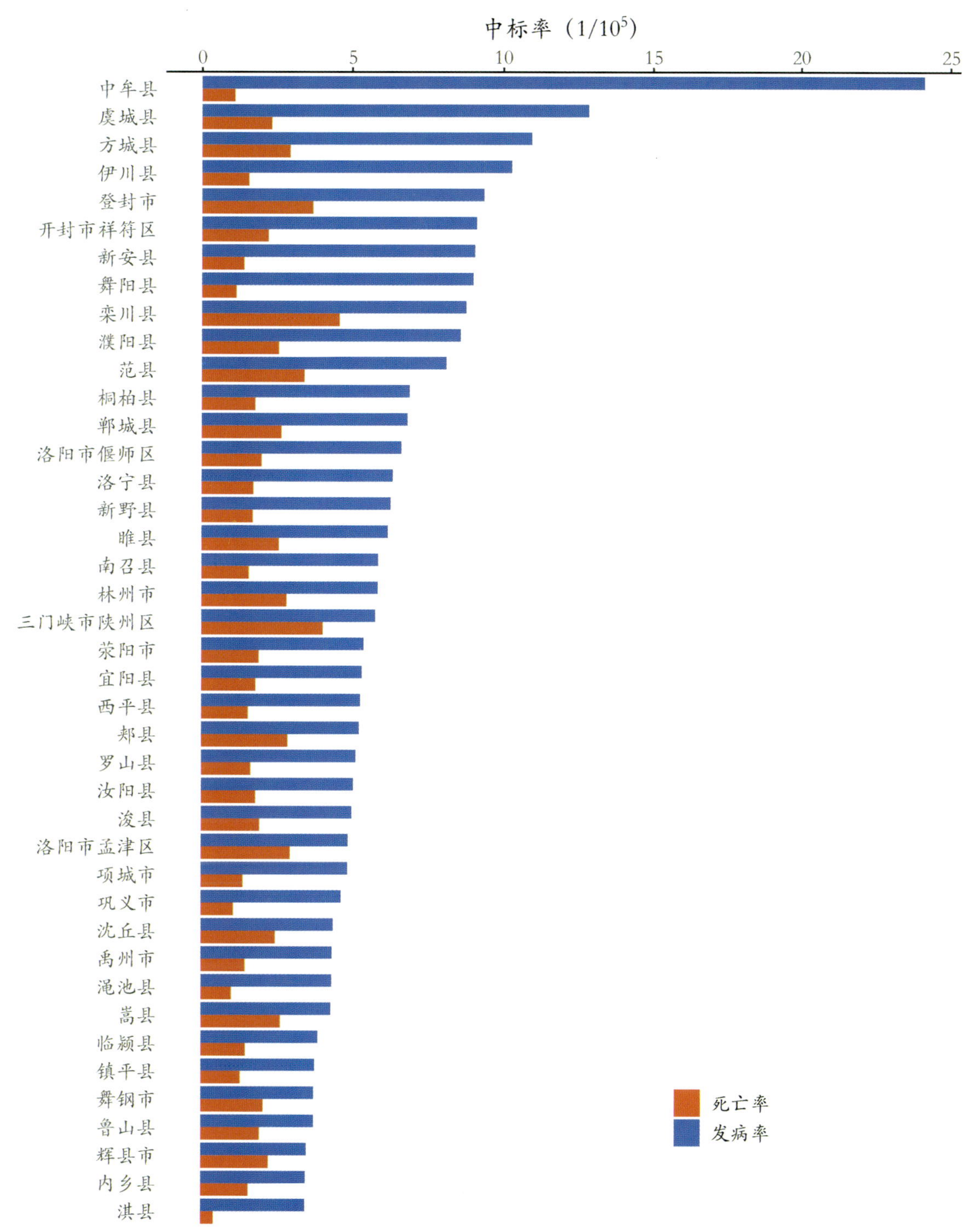

图 5-15c 2020 年河南省农村肿瘤登记地区卵巢癌发病率和死亡率

十六、前列腺

2020 年，河南省肿瘤登记地区前列腺癌的发病率为 8.09/10 万，中标率为 5.50/10 万，世标率为 5.45/10 万，发病例数占全部癌症新发病例数的 1.48%；其中，城市地区和农村地区发病率分别为 12.34/10 万和 6.45/10 万；中标发病率呈现城市地区高于农村地区的特点，城市地区中标发病率是农村地区的 1.69 倍。同期，前列腺癌的死亡率为 3.58/10 万，中标率为 2.30/10 万，世标率为 2.33/10 万，死亡病例数占全部癌症死亡病例数的 1.12%；其中，城市地区和农村地区死亡率分别为 5.53/10 万和 2.83/10 万；中标死亡率呈现城市地区高于农村地区的特点，城市地区中标死亡率是农村地区的 1.60 倍。（表 5–16）

16. Prostate

In 2020, there were 1,782 new cases diagnosed as prostate cancer in registration areas of Henan Province, China (757 in urban areas and 1,025 in rural areas), accounting for 1.48% of new cases of all cancers. The crude incidence rate was 8.09 per 100,000, with the ASR China 5.50 per 100,000 and the ASR World 5.45 per 100,000, respectively. Subgroup analysis showed that the incidence of ASR China was 1.69 times in urban areas as that in rural areas. The cumulative incidence rate for subjects aged 0 to 74 years was 0.61%. (Table 5–16)

A total of 789 cases died of prostate cancer in 2020 (339 in urban areas and 450 in rural areas), accounting for 1.12% of all cancer deaths. The crude mortality rate was 3.58 per 100,000, with the ASR China 2.30 per 100,000 and the ASR World 2.33 per 100,000, respectively. Subgroup analysis showed that the mortality of ASR China was 1.60 times in urban areas as that in rural areas. The cumulative mortality rate for subjects aged 0 to 74 years was 0.17%. (Table 5–16)

表 5–16　2020 年河南省肿瘤登记地区前列腺癌发病与死亡情况

地区	病例数	粗率（$1/10^5$）	构成（%）	中标率（$1/10^5$）	世标率（$1/10^5$）	累积率 0 ~ 74（%）
发病						
全省	1 782	8.09	1.48	5.50	5.45	0.61
城市地区	757	12.34	2.06	7.69	7.71	0.87
农村地区	1 025	6.45	1.22	4.56	4.48	0.51
死亡						
全省	789	3.58	1.12	2.30	2.33	0.17
城市地区	339	5.53	1.72	3.10	3.21	0.18
农村地区	450	2.83	0.89	1.94	1.93	0.17

前列腺癌年龄别发病率在 0~59 岁年龄段处于较低水平，60 岁以后快速上升，在 85 岁达到峰值；年龄别死亡率在 0~64 岁年龄段处于较低水平，65 岁以后快速上升，在 85 岁达到峰值；城市地区和农村地区年龄别率虽然有一定差异，但是总体趋势类同。（图 5–16a）

The age specific incidence of prostate cancer was low at age group of 0~59, and it started increasing sharply at age group of 60, it reached the peak at age of 85. The age specific mortality was low at age group of 0~64, and it started increasing sharply at age group of 65, it reached the peak at age of 85. The change pattern of age specific incidence and mortality were similar in urban areas and rural areas. (Figure 5–16a)

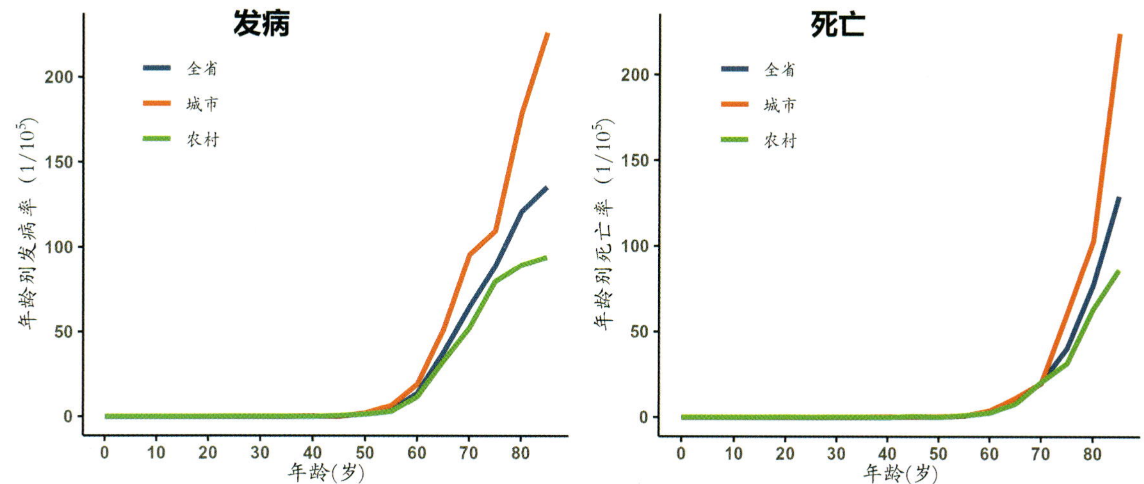

图 5-16a　2020 年河南省肿瘤登记地区前列腺癌年龄别发病率和死亡率

在 14 个城市肿瘤登记地区中，前列腺癌标化发病率最高的是三门峡市湖滨区（11.17/10 万），其次是郑州市城区（10.79/10 万）和漯河市城区（10.17/10 万）；标化死亡率最高的是三门峡市湖滨区（9.31/10 万），其次是南阳市卧龙区（6.56/10 万）和济源市（5.71/10 万）。（图 5-16b）

Among the 14 urban cancer registries, the ASR China incidence rate of prostate was the highest in Sanmenxia Hubin District (11.17 per 100,000), followed by Zhengzhou City (10.79 per 100,000), and Luohe City (10.17 per 100,000). The ASR China mortality rate of prostate cancer was the highest in Sanmenxia Hubin District (9.31 per 100,000), followed by Nanyang Wolong District (6.56 per 100,000), and Jiyuan City (5.71 per 100,000). (Figure 5-16b)

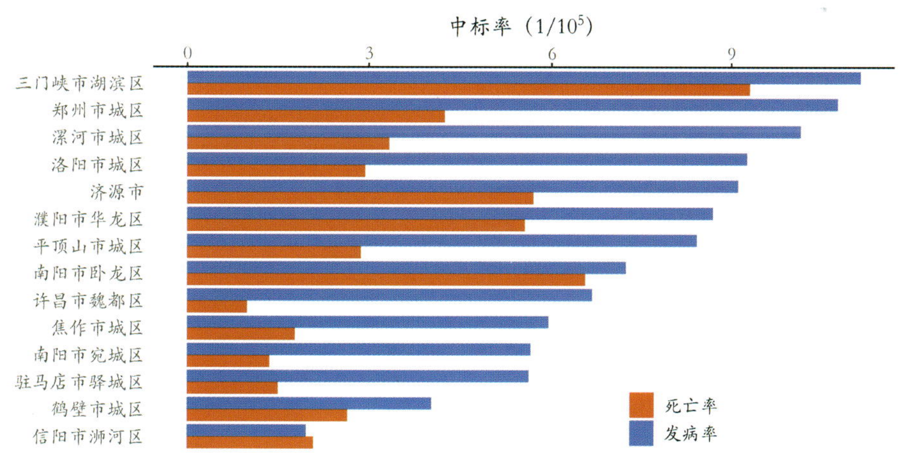

图 5-16b　2020 年河南省城市肿瘤登记地区前列腺癌发病率和死亡率

在 41 个农村肿瘤登记地区中，前列腺癌标化发病率最高的是桐柏县（10.56/10 万），其次是禹州市（9.35/10 万）和洛阳市孟津区（8.35/10 万）；标化死亡率最高的是中牟县（3.92/10 万），其次是虞城县（3.87/10 万）和禹州市（3.74/10 万）。（图 5-16c）

Among the 41 rural cancer registries, the ASR China incidence rate of prostate cancer was the highest in Tongbai County (10.56 per 100,000), followed by Yuzhou City (9.35 per 100,000), and Luoyang Mengjin District (8.35 per 100,000). The ASR China mortality rate of prostate cancer was the highest in Zhongmu County (3.92 per 100,000), followed by Yucheng County (3.87 per 100,000), and Yuzhou City (3.74 per 100,000). (Figure 5-16c)

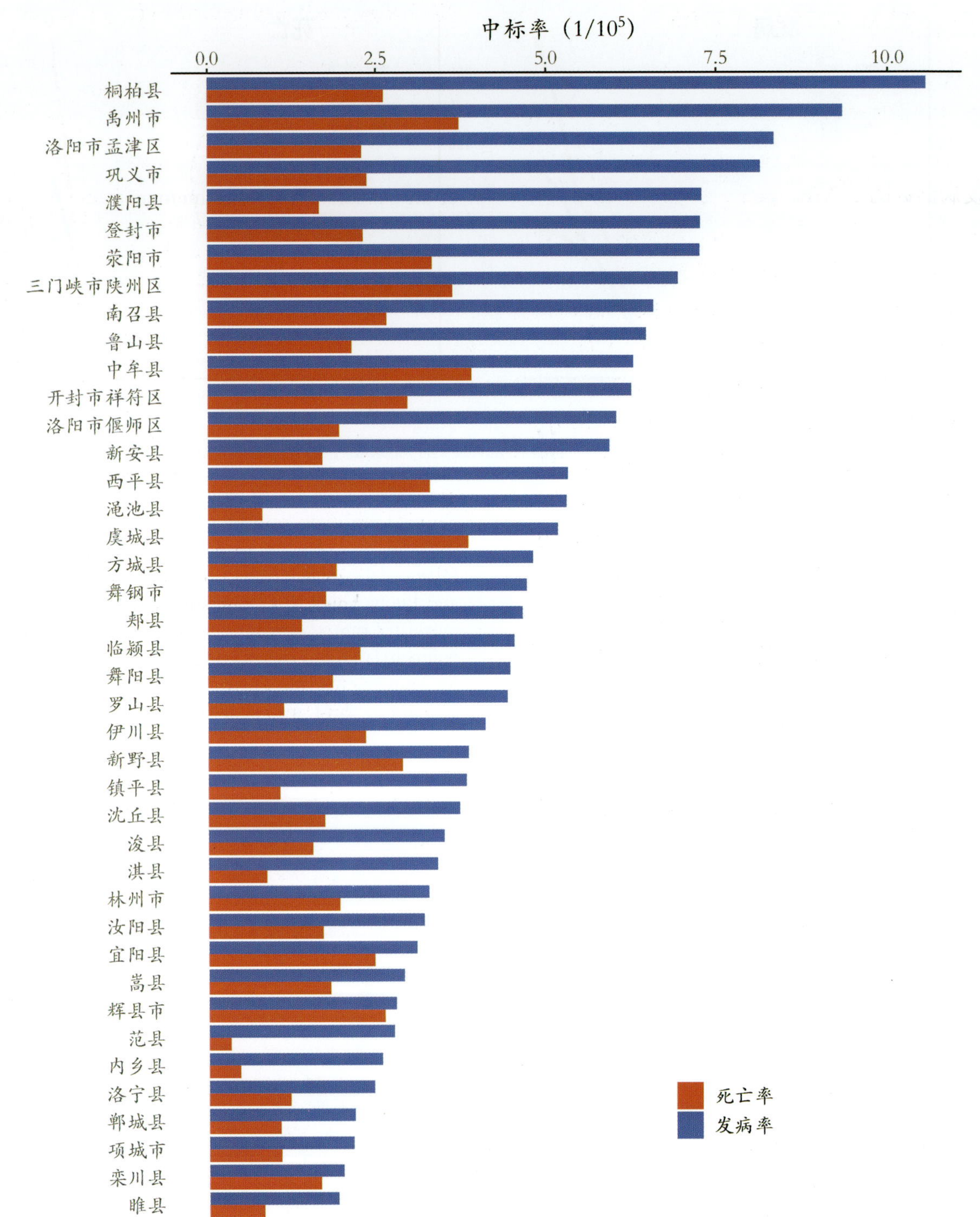

图 5-16c　2020 年河南省农村肿瘤登记地区前列腺癌发病率和死亡率

十七、肾及泌尿系统不明

2020 年，河南省肿瘤登记地区肾及泌尿系统不明癌的发病率为 4.45/10 万，中标率为 3.23/10 万，世标率为 3.17/10 万，发病例数占全部癌症新发病例数的 1.59%；其中，男性和女性发病率分别为 5.43/10 万和 3.44/10 万，城市地区和农村地区发病率分别为 5.75/10 万和 3.94/10 万；中标发病率呈现男性高于女性、城市地区高于农村地区的特点，男性中标发病率是女性的 1.71 倍，城市地区中标发病率是农村地区的 1.35 倍。同期，肾及泌尿系统不明癌的死亡率为 1.92/10 万，中标率为 1.26/10 万，世标率为 1.25/10 万，死亡病例数占全部癌症死亡病例数的 1.18%；其中，男性和女性死亡率分别为 2.44/10 万和 1.38/10 万，城市地区和农村地区死亡率分别为 2.42/10 万和 1.72/10 万；中标死亡率呈现男性高于女性、城市地区高于农村地区的特点，男性中标死亡率是女性的 2.08 倍，城市地区中标死亡率是农村地区的 1.26 倍。（表 5–17）

17. Kidney & unspecified urinary organs

In 2020, there were 1,922 new cases diagnosed as kidney & unspecified urinary organs cancer in registration areas of Henan Province, China (1,196 males and 726 females, 707 in urban areas and 1,215 in rural areas), accounting for 1.59% of new cases of all cancers. The crude incidence rate was 4.45 per 100,000, with the ASR China 3.23 per 100,000 and the ASR World 3.17 per 100,000, respectively. Subgroup analysis showed that the incidence of ASR China was 1.71 times in males as that in females, and it was 1.35 times in urban areas as that in rural areas. The cumulative incidence rate for subjects aged 0 to 74 years was 0.38%. (Table 5–17)

A total of 828 cases died of kidney & unspecified urinary organs cancer in 2,020 (537 males and 291 females, 298 in urban areas and 530 in rural areas), accounting for 1.18% of all cancer deaths. The crude mortality rate was 1.92 per 100,000, with the ASR China of 1.26 per 100,000 and the ASR World of 1.25 per 100,000, respectively. Subgroup analysis showed that the mortality of ASR China was 2.08 times in males as that in females, and it was 1.26 times in urban areas as that in rural areas. The cumulative mortality rate for subjects aged 0 to 74 years was 0.14%. (Table 5–17)

表 5–17　2020 年河南省肿瘤登记地区肾及泌尿系统不明癌发病与死亡情况

地区	性别	病例数	粗率（1/10^5）	构成（%）	中标率（1/10^5）	世标率（1/10^5）	累积率 0～74（%）
发病							
全省	合计	1 922	4.45	1.59	3.23	3.17	0.38
	男性	1 196	5.43	1.93	4.08	4.00	0.49
	女性	726	3.44	1.23	2.39	2.35	0.27
城市地区	合计	707	5.75	1.93	3.95	3.91	0.48
	男性	448	7.30	2.45	5.20	5.13	0.65
	女性	259	4.21	1.41	2.77	2.76	0.31
农村地区	合计	1 215	3.94	1.45	2.93	2.86	0.33
	男性	748	4.70	1.72	3.63	3.54	0.42
	女性	467	3.12	1.15	2.23	2.18	0.25

续表

地区	性别	病例数	粗率（1/10^5）	构成（%）	中标率（1/10^5）	世标率（1/10^5）	累积率 0～74（%）
死亡							
全省	合计	828	1.92	1.18	1.26	1.25	0.14
	男性	537	2.44	1.24	1.73	1.73	0.20
	女性	291	1.38	1.08	0.83	0.81	0.08
城市地区	合计	298	2.42	1.51	1.48	1.48	0.16
	男性	197	3.21	1.63	2.10	2.12	0.24
	女性	101	1.64	1.33	0.91	0.90	0.08
农村地区	合计	530	1.72	1.05	1.17	1.16	0.13
	男性	340	2.14	1.09	1.57	1.56	0.19
	女性	190	1.27	0.98	0.79	0.77	0.08

肾及泌尿系统不明癌年龄别发病率在0~39岁年龄段处于较低水平，40岁以后快速上升，在60岁达到峰值；年龄别死亡率在0~49岁年龄段处于较低水平，50岁以后快速上升，在85岁达到峰值；年龄别发病率和死亡率均呈现男性高于女性的特点；城市地区和农村地区年龄别率虽然有一定差异，但是总体趋势类同。（图5–17a）

在14个城市肿瘤登记地区中，男性肾及泌尿系统不明癌标化发病率最高的是郑州市城区（8.52/10万），其次是济源市（6.01/10万）和洛阳市城区（5.98/10万）；女性标化发病率最高的是三门峡市湖滨区（4.17/10万），其次是郑州市城区（3.87/10万）和洛阳市城区（3.52/10万）。男性标化死亡率最高的是漯河市城区（2.74/10万），其次是濮阳市华龙区（2.73/10万）和济源市（2.70/10万）；女性标化死亡率最高的是南阳市宛城区（2.19/10万），其次是济源市（2.08/10万）和三门峡市湖滨区（2.00/10万）。（图5–17b）

The age specific incidence of kidney & unspecified urinary organs cancer was low at age group of 0~39, and it started increasing sharply at age group of 40, it reached the peak at age of 60. The age specific mortality was low at age group of 0~49, and it started increasing sharply at age group of 50, it reached the peak at age of 85. Age specific incidence and mortality were all higher in males than in females, The change pattern of age specific incidence and mortality were similar in urban areas and rural areas. (Figure 5–17a)

Among the 14 urban cancer registries, the ASR China incidence rate of kidney & unspecified urinary organs cancer in males was the highest in Zhengzhou City (8.52 per 100,000) followed by Jiyuan City (6.01 per 100,000), and Luoyang City (5.98 per 100,000). For females, it was the highest in Sanmenxia Hubin District (4.17 per 100,000), followed by Zhengzhou City (3.87 per 100,000), and Luoyang City (3.52 per 100,000). The ASR China mortality rate of kidney & unspecified urinary organs cancer in males was the highest in Luohe City (2.74 per 100,000) followed by Puyang Hualong District (2.73 per 100,000), and Jiyuan City (2.70 per 100,000). For females, it was the highest in Nanyang Wancheng District (2.19 per 100,000), followed by Jiyuan City (2.08 per 100,000), and Sanmenxia Hubin District (2.00 per 100,000). (Figure 5–17b)

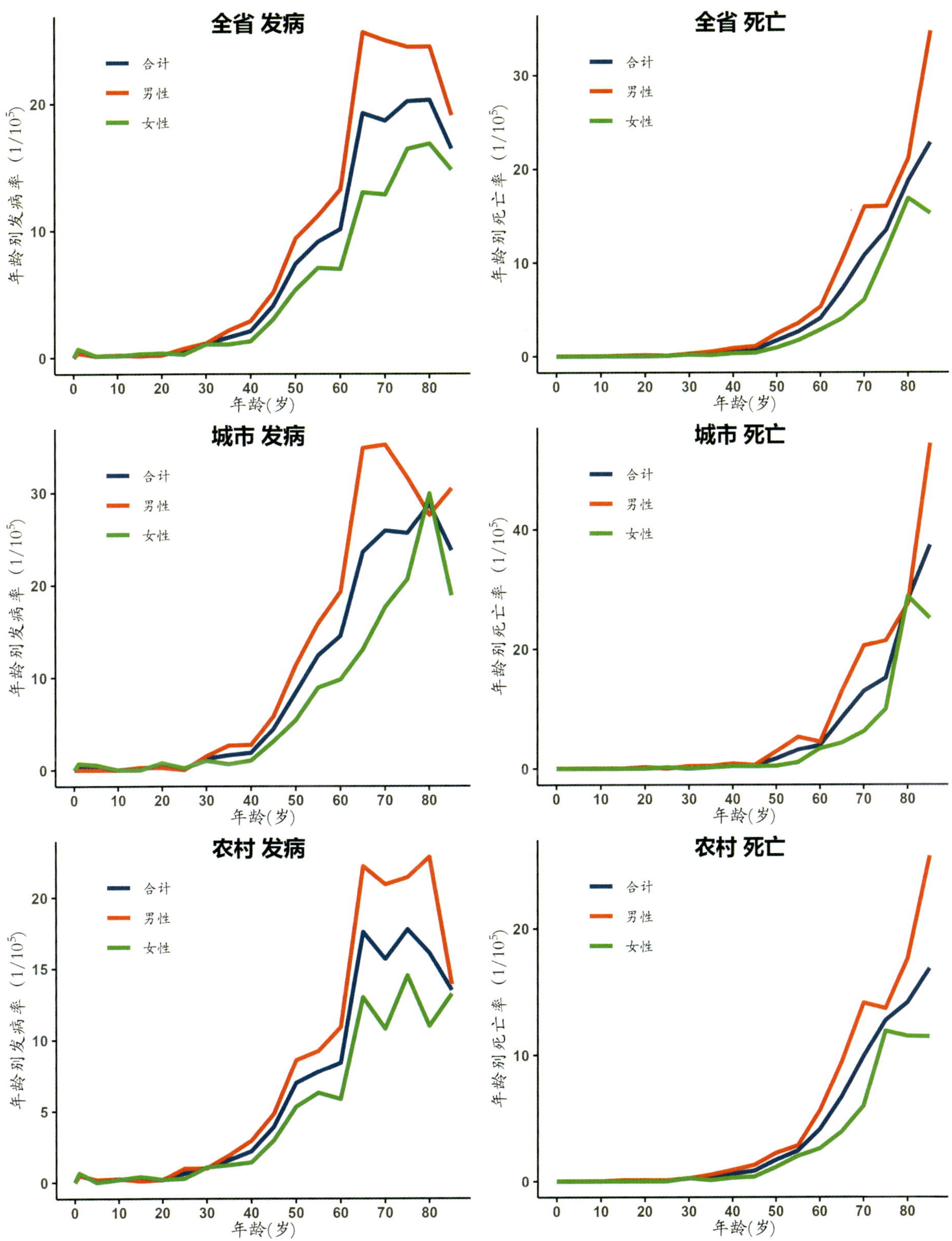

图 5–17a　2020 年河南省肿瘤登记地区肾及泌尿系统不明癌年龄别发病率和死亡率

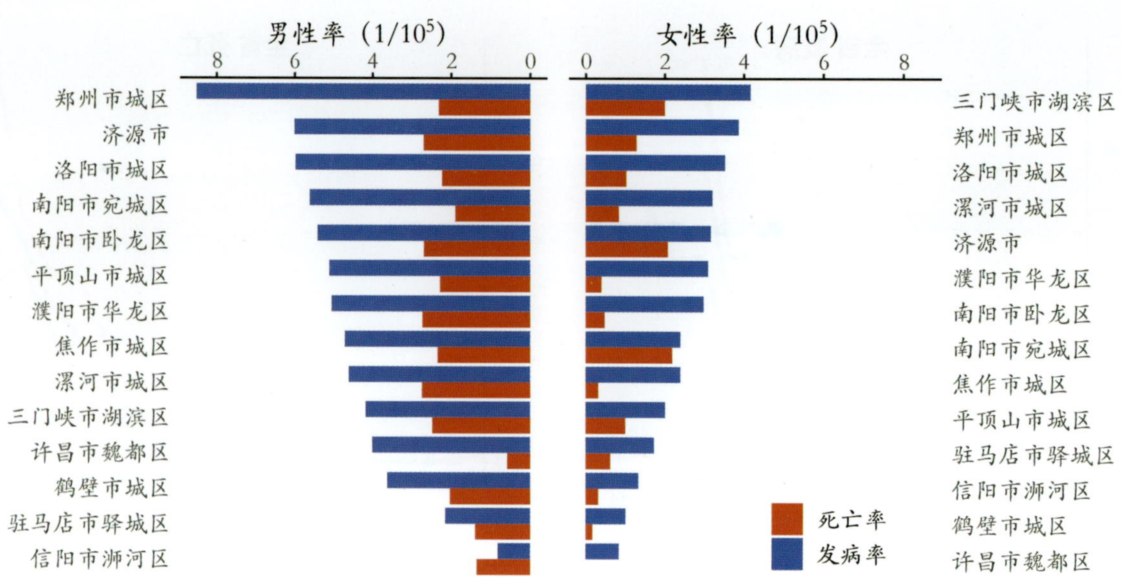

图 5-17b　2020 年河南省城市肿瘤登记地区肾及泌尿系统不明癌发病率和死亡率

在 41 个农村肿瘤登记地区中，男性肾及泌尿系统不明癌标化发病率最高的是中牟县（8.80/10 万），其次是睢县（7.57/10 万）和洛宁县（5.60/10 万）；女性标化发病率最高的是桐柏县（4.51/10 万），其次是淇县（4.34/10 万）和范县（4.28/10 万）。男性标化死亡率最高的是睢县（4.93/10 万），其次是虞城县（3.16/10 万）和范县（3.12/10 万）；女性标化死亡率最高的是开封市祥符区（2.08/10 万），其次是中牟县（2.06/10 万）和范县（1.95/10 万）。（图 5-17c）

Among the 41 rural cancer registries, the ASR China incidence rate of kidney & unspecified urinary organs cancer in males was the highest in Zhongmu County (8.80 per 100,000) followed by Sui County (7.57 per 100,000), and Luoning County (5.60 per 100,000). For females, it was the highest in Tongbai County (4.51 per 100,000), followed by Qi County (4.34 per 100,000), and Fan County (4.28 per 100,000). The ASR China mortality rate of kidney & unspecified urinary organs cancer in males was the highest in Sui County (4.93 per 100,000) followed by Yucheng County (3.16 per 100,000), and Fan County (3.12 per 100,000). For females, it was the highest in Kaifeng Xiangfu District (2.08 per 100,000), followed by Zhongmu County (2.06 per 100,000), and Fan County (1.95 per 100,000). (Figure 5-17c)

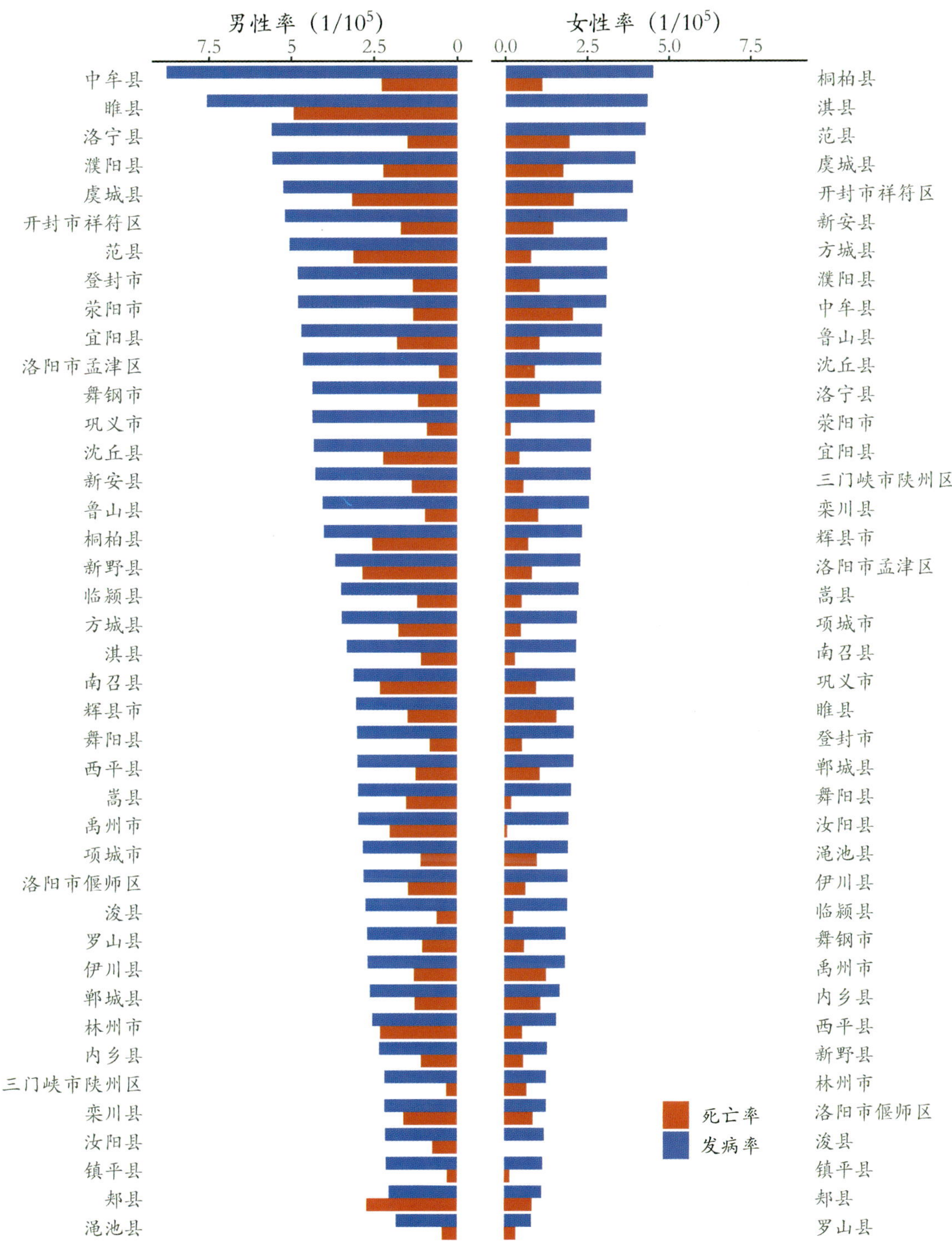

图 5-17c 2020 年河南省农村肿瘤登记地区肾及泌尿系统不明癌发病率和死亡率

十八、膀胱

2020 年，河南省肿瘤登记地区膀胱癌的发病率为 4.43/10 万，中标率为 2.95/10 万，世标率为 2.94/10 万，发病例数占全部癌症新发病例数的 1.58%；其中，男性和女性发病率分别为 6.76/10 万和 2.00/10 万，城市地区和农村地区发病率分别为 5.73/10 万和 3.92/10 万；中标发病率呈现男性高于女性、城市地区高于农村地区的特点，男性中标发病率是女性的 3.67 倍，城市地区中标发病率是农村地区的 1.34 倍。同期，膀胱癌的死亡率为 1.73/10 万，中标率为 1.02/10 万，世标率为 1.04/10 万，死亡病例数占全部癌症死亡病例数的 1.06%；其中，男性和女性死亡率分别为 2.64/10 万和 0.79/10 万，城市地区和农村地区死亡率分别为 1.99/10 万和 1.63/10 万；中标死亡率呈现男性高于女性、城市地区高于农村地区的特点，男性中标死亡率是女性的 4.10 倍，城市地区中标死亡率是农村地区的 1.02 倍。（表 5-18）

18. Bladder

In 2020, there were 1,912 new cases diagnosed as bladder cancer in registration areas of Henan Province, China (1,490 males and 422 females, 704 in urban areas and 1,208 in rural areas), accounting for 1.58% of new cases of all cancers. The crude incidence rate was 4.43 per 100,000, with the ASR China 2.95 per 100,000 and the ASR World 2.94 per 100,000, respectively. Subgroup analysis showed that the incidence of ASR China was 3.67 times in males as that in females, and it was 1.34 times in urban areas as that in rural areas. The cumulative incidence rate for subjects aged 0 to 74 years was 0.34%. (Table 5–18)

A total of 748 cases died of bladder cancer in 2020 (581 males and 167 females, 244 in urban areas and 504 in rural areas), accounting for 1.06% of all cancer deaths. The crude mortality rate was 1.73 per 100,000, with the ASR China of 1.02 per 100,000 and the ASR World of 1.04 per 100,000, respectively. Subgroup analysis showed that the mortality of ASR China was 4.10 times in males as that in females, and it was 1.02 times in urban areas as that in rural areas. The cumulative mortality rate for subjects aged 0 to 74 years was 0.08%. (Table 5–18)

表 5–18　2020 年河南省肿瘤登记地区膀胱癌发病与死亡情况

地区	性别	病例数	粗率（$1/10^5$）	构成（%）	中标率（$1/10^5$）	世标率（$1/10^5$）	累积率 0～74（%）
发病							
全省	合计	1 912	4.43	1.58	2.95	2.94	0.34
	男性	1 490	6.76	2.41	4.74	4.77	0.56
	女性	422	2.00	0.72	1.29	1.26	0.14
城市地区	合计	704	5.73	1.92	3.59	3.63	0.42
	男性	562	9.16	3.07	5.99	6.17	0.72
	女性	142	2.31	0.77	1.40	1.33	0.14
农村地区	合计	1 208	3.92	1.44	2.68	2.65	0.31
	男性	928	5.84	2.13	4.22	4.19	0.49
	女性	280	1.87	0.69	1.24	1.22	0.14

续表

地区	性别	病例数	粗率（1/10⁵）	构成（%）	中标率（1/10⁵）	世标率（1/10⁵）	累积率 0～74（%）
死亡							
全省	合计	748	1.73	1.06	1.02	1.04	0.08
	男性	581	2.64	1.34	1.72	1.76	0.13
	女性	167	0.79	0.62	0.42	0.43	0.04
城市地区	合计	244	1.99	1.24	1.03	1.09	0.07
	男性	195	3.18	1.61	1.78	1.89	0.11
	女性	49	0.80	0.64	0.39	0.42	0.03
农村地区	合计	504	1.63	1.00	1.01	1.02	0.09
	男性	386	2.43	1.24	1.67	1.69	0.14
	女性	118	0.79	0.61	0.44	0.44	0.04

膀胱癌年龄别发病率在0~44岁年龄段处于较低水平，45岁以后快速上升，在85岁达到峰值；年龄别死亡率在0~54岁年龄段处于较低水平，55岁以后快速上升，在85岁达到峰值；年龄别发病率和死亡率均呈现男性高于女性的特点；城市地区和农村地区年龄别率虽然有一定差异，但是总体趋势类同。（图5-18a）

在14个城市肿瘤登记地区中，男性膀胱癌标化发病率最高的是济源市（11.32/10万），其次是南阳市卧龙区（9.79/10万）和郑州市城区（7.75/10万）；女性标化发病率最高的是南阳市卧龙区（3.02/10万），其次是许昌市魏都区（1.90/10万）和郑州市城区（1.87/10万）。男性标化死亡率最高的是济源市（4.08/10万），其次是濮阳市华龙区（3.61/10万）和南阳市卧龙区（2.70/10万）；女性标化死亡率最高的是濮阳市华龙区（1.16/10万），其次是济源市（0.69/10万）和郑州市城区（0.57/10万）。（图5-18b）

The age specific incidence of bladder cancer was low at age group of 0~44, and it started increasing sharply at age group of 45, it reached the peak at age of 85. The age specific mortality was low at age group of 0~54, and it started increasing sharply at age group of 55, it reached the peak at age of 85. Age specific incidence and mortality were all higher in males than in females, The change pattern of age specific incidence and mortality were similar in urban areas and rural areas. (Figure 5-18a)

Among the 14 urban cancer registries, the ASR China incidence rate of bladder cancer in males was the highest in Jiyuan City (11.32 per 100,000) followed by Nanyang Wolong District (9.79 per 100,000), and Zhengzhou City (7.75 per 100,000). For females, it was the highest in Nanyang Wolong District (3.02 per 100,000), followed by Xuchang Weidu District (1.90 per 100,000), and Zhengzhou City (1.87 per 100,000). The ASR China mortality rate of bladder cancer in males was the highest in Jiyuan City (4.08 per 100,000) followed by Puyang Hualong District (3.61 per 100,000), and Nanyang Wolong District (2.70 per 100,000). For females, it was the highest in Puyang Hualong District (1.16 per 100,000), followed by Jiyuan City (0.69 per 100,000), and Zhengzhou City (0.57 per 100,000). (Figure 5-18b)

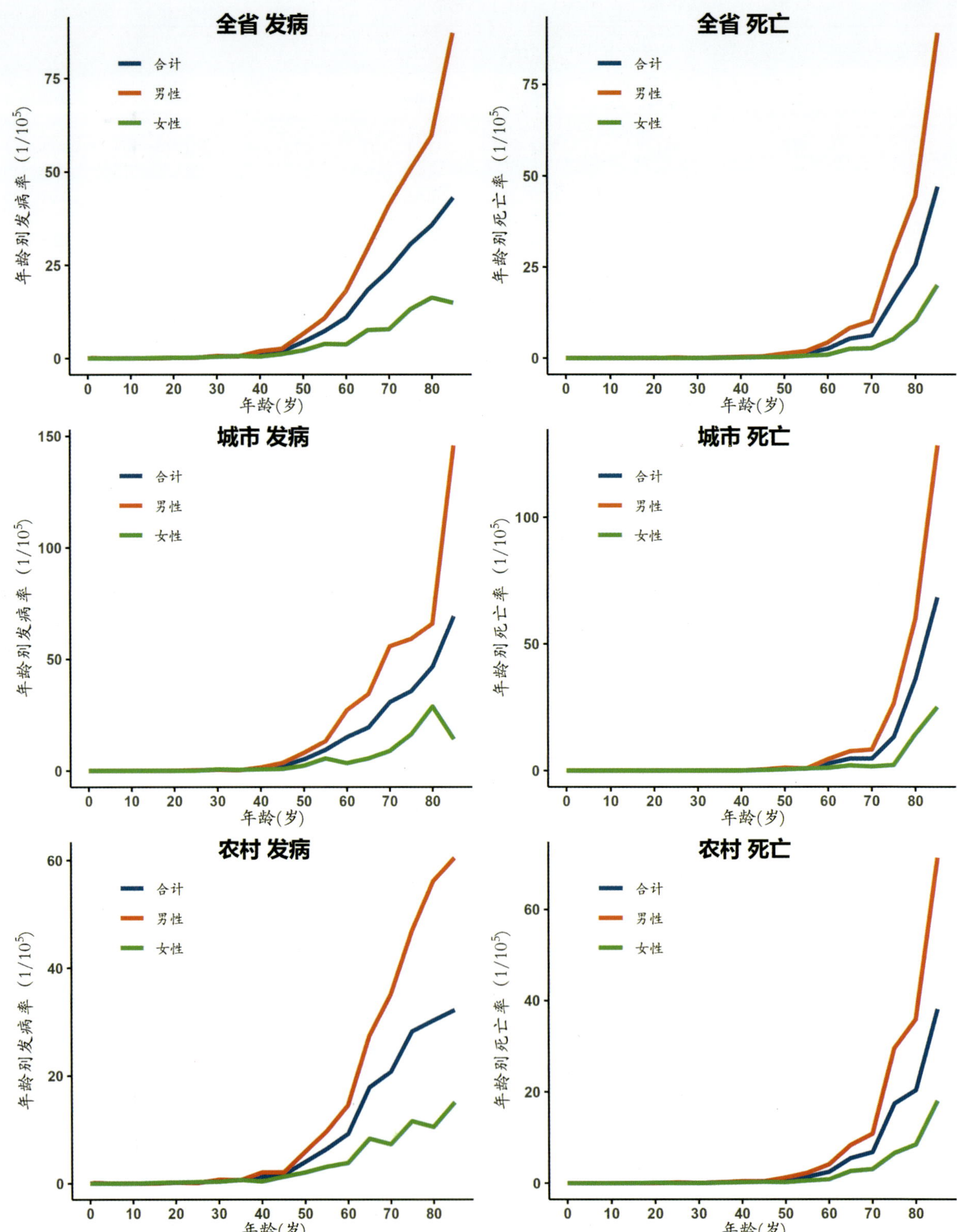

图 5-18a　2020 年河南省肿瘤登记地区膀胱癌年龄别发病率和死亡率

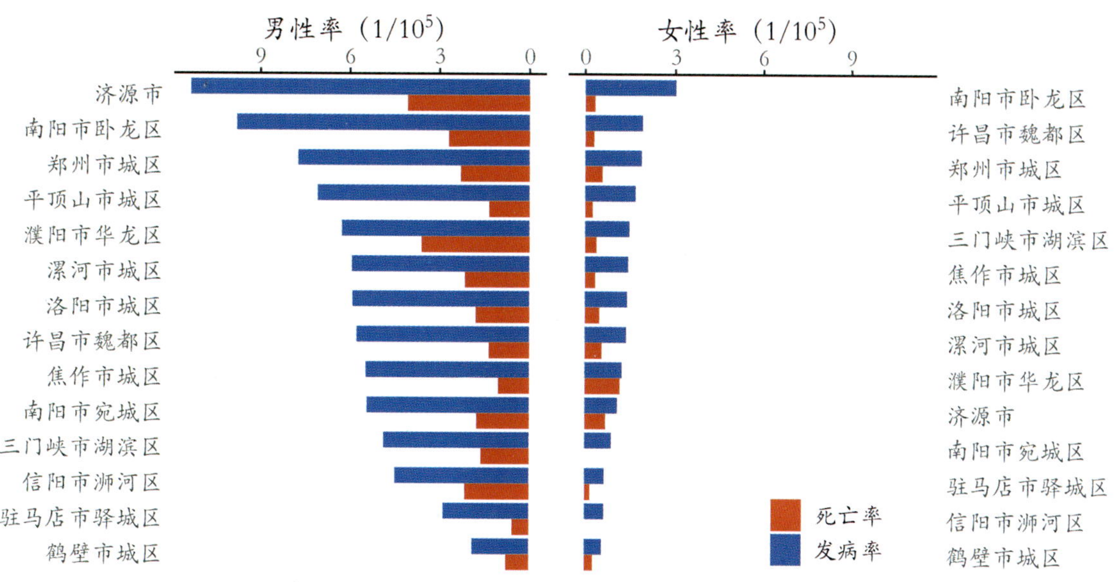

图 5-18b　2020 年河南省城市肿瘤登记地区膀胱癌发病率和死亡率

在 41 个农村肿瘤登记地区中，男性膀胱癌标化发病率最高的是禹州市（10.19/10 万），其次是桐柏县（8.80/10 万）和中牟县（6.70/10 万）；女性标化发病率最高的是桐柏县（2.51/10 万），其次是登封市（2.28/10 万）和虞城县（2.13/10 万）。男性标化死亡率最高的是禹州市（4.96/10 万），其次是鲁山县（4.17/10 万）和桐柏县（3.75/10 万）；女性标化死亡率最高的是郏县（1.31/10 万），其次是登封市（1.27/10 万）和郸城县（1.05/10 万）。（图 5-18c）

Among the 41 rural cancer registries, the ASR China incidence rate of bladder cancer in males was the highest in Yuzhou City (10.19 per 100,000) followed by Tongbai County (8.80 per 100,000), and Zhongmu County (6.70 per 100,000). For females, it was the highest in Tongbai County (2.51 per 100,000), followed by Dengfeng City (2.28 per 100,000), and Yucheng County (2.13 per 100,000). The ASR China mortality rate of bladder cancer in males was the highest in Yuzhou City (4.96 per 100,000) followed by Lushan County (4.17 per 100,000), and Tongbai County (3.75 per 100,000). For females, it was the highest in Jia County (1.31 per 100,000), followed by Dengfeng City (1.27 per 100,000), and Dancheng County (1.05 per 100,000). (Figure 5-18c)

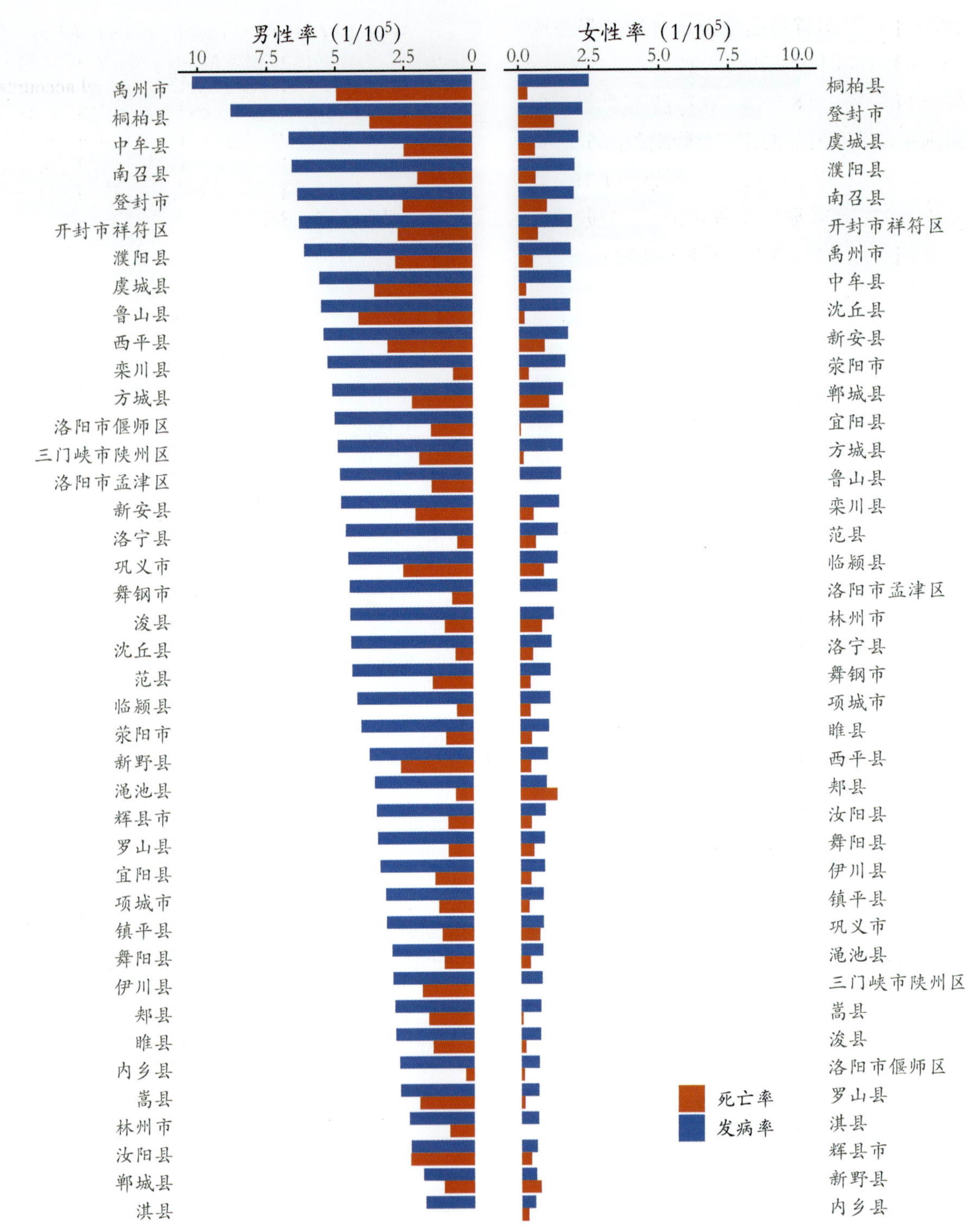

图 5-18c　2020 年河南省农村肿瘤登记地区膀胱癌发病率和死亡率

2020年，河南省肿瘤登记地区膀胱癌发病病例中有确切解剖学亚部位信息的占31.24%，亚部位未特指的占68.76%。在有亚部位信息的膀胱病例中，三角区占32.10%，膀胱顶占6.53%，侧壁占25.19%，前壁占7.01%，后壁占6.16%，膀胱颈占4.07%，输尿管口占8.90%，脐尿管占1.42%，交搭跨越占8.62%。（图5-18d）

About 31.24% of the bladder cancer had specific subsite. Among those cases, trigone accounted for 32.10%, dome accounted for 6.53%, lateral accounted for 25.19%, anterior accounted for 7.01%, posterior accounted for 6.16%, bladder neck accounted for 4.07%, ureteric orifice accounted for 8.90%, urachus accounted for 1.42%, and overlapping accounted for 8.62%. (Figure 5-18d)

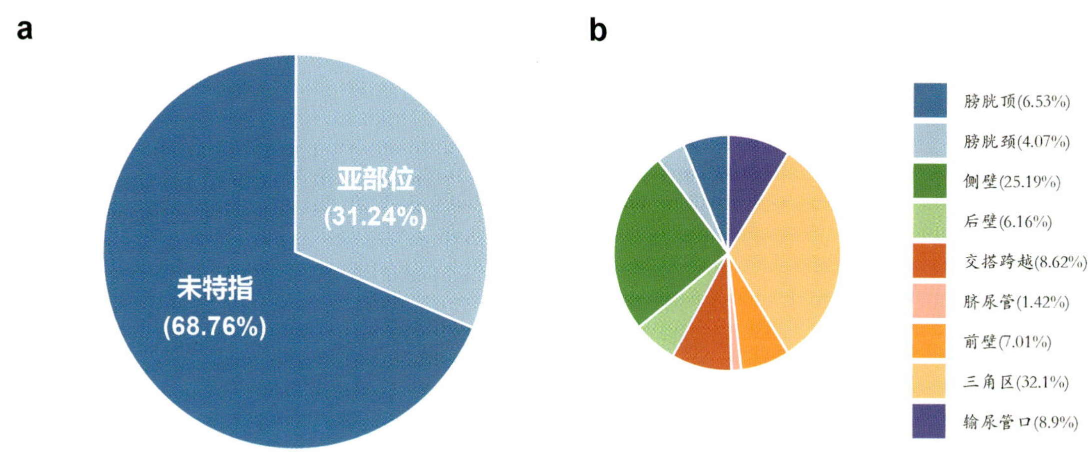

图5-18d 2020年河南省肿瘤登记地区膀胱癌发病病例亚部位构成

2020年，河南省肿瘤登记地区膀胱癌发病病例中有明确组织病理学分型的占62.75%，组织学类型未特指的占37.25%。在有组织病理学分型的膀胱病例中，鳞状细胞癌占7.96%，腺癌占5.50%，移行细胞癌占33.61%，其他占52.93%。（图5-18e）

About 62.75% of the bladder cancer had morphological verification. Among those cases, Squamous cell accounted for 7.96%, Adenocarcinoma accounted for 5.50%, Transitional cell accounted for 33.61%, and Others accounted for 52.93%. (Figure 5-18e)

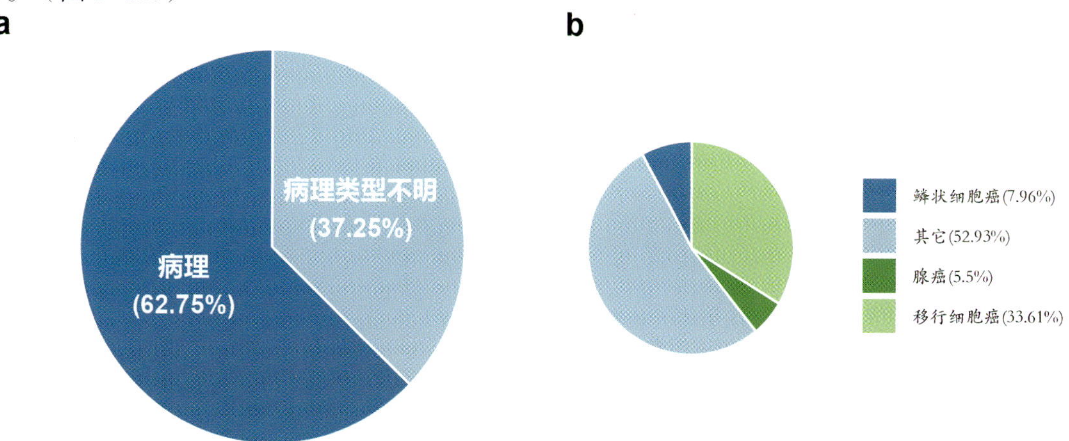

图5-18e 2020年河南省肿瘤登记地区膀胱癌发病病例形态学构成

十九、脑

2020 年，河南省肿瘤登记地区脑癌的发病率为 6.61/10 万，中标率为 5.16/10 万，世标率为 5.08/10 万，发病例数占全部癌症新发病例数的 2.36%；其中，男性和女性发病率分别为 6.39/10 万和 6.84/10 万，城市地区和农村地区发病率分别为 5.87/10 万和 6.91/10 万；中标发病率呈现男性高于女性、农村地区高于城市地区的特点，男性中标发病率是女性的 1.03 倍，农村地区中标发病率是城市地区的 1.23 倍。同期，脑癌的死亡率为 4.27/10 万，中标率为 3.15/10 万，世标率为 3.11/10 万，死亡病例数占全部癌症死亡病例数的 2.62%；其中，男性和女性死亡率分别为 4.61/10 万和 3.93/10 万，城市地区和农村地区死亡率分别为 3.95/10 万和 4.40/10 万；中标死亡率呈现男性高于女性、农村地区高于城市地区的特点，男性中标死亡率是女性的 1.33 倍，农村地区中标死亡率是城市地区的 1.17 倍。（表 5–19）

19. Brain

In 2020, there were 2,854 new cases diagnosed as brain cancer in registration areas of Henan Province, China (1,409 males and 1445 females, 722 in urban areas and 2,132 in rural areas), accounting for 2.36% of new cases of all cancers. The crude incidence rate was 6.61 per 100,000, with the ASR China 5.16 per 100,000 and the ASR World 5.08 per 100,000, respectively. Subgroup analysis showed that the incidence of ASR China was 1.03 times in males as that in females, and it was 1.23 times in rural areas as that in urban areas. The cumulative incidence rate for subjects aged 0 to 74 years was 0.54%. (Table 5–19)

A total of 1,844 cases died of brain cancer in 2020 (1,015 males and 829 females, 485 in urban areas and 1,359 in rural areas), accounting for 2.62% of all cancer deaths. The crude mortality rate was 4.27 per 100,000, with the ASR China of 3.15 per 100,000 and the ASR World of 3.11 per 100,000, respectively. Subgroup analysis showed that the mortality of ASR China was 1.33 times in males as that in females, and it was 1.17 times in rural areas as that in urban areas. The cumulative mortality rate for subjects aged 0 to 74 years was 0.35%. (Table 5–19)

表 5–19　2020 年河南省肿瘤登记地区脑癌发病与死亡情况

地区	性别	病例数	粗率（1/10^5）	构成（%）	中标率（1/10^5）	世标率（1/10^5）	累积率 0 ~ 74（%）
发病							
全省	合计	2 854	6.61	2.36	5.16	5.08	0.54
	男性	1 409	6.39	2.28	5.23	5.11	0.54
	女性	1 445	6.84	2.45	5.09	5.04	0.53
城市地区	合计	722	5.87	1.97	4.43	4.42	0.46
	男性	359	5.85	1.96	4.57	4.60	0.47
	女性	363	5.89	1.97	4.28	4.22	0.45
农村地区	合计	2 132	6.91	2.54	5.45	5.34	0.57
	男性	1 050	6.60	2.41	5.48	5.31	0.57
	女性	1 082	7.24	2.67	5.42	5.37	0.57

续表

地区	性别	病例数	粗率（1/10⁵）	构成（%）	中标率（1/10⁵）	世标率（1/10⁵）	累积率 0～74（%）
死亡							
全省	合计	1 844	4.27	2.62	3.15	3.11	0.35
	男性	1 015	4.61	2.35	3.60	3.52	0.39
	女性	829	3.93	3.06	2.70	2.70	0.30
城市地区	合计	485	3.95	2.46	2.81	2.84	0.32
	男性	279	4.55	2.31	3.37	3.39	0.38
	女性	206	3.34	2.71	2.28	2.32	0.26
农村地区	合计	1 359	4.40	2.68	3.30	3.23	0.36
	男性	736	4.63	2.36	3.69	3.58	0.40
	女性	623	4.17	3.20	2.88	2.87	0.32

脑癌年龄别发病率在0~34岁年龄段处于较低水平，35岁以后快速上升，在75岁达到峰值；年龄别死亡率在0~39岁年龄段处于较低水平，40岁以后快速上升，在85岁达到峰值；年龄别发病率和死亡率均呈现男性高于女性的特点；城市地区和农村地区年龄别率虽然有一定差异，但是总体趋势类同。（图5-19a）

在14个城市肿瘤登记地区中，男性脑癌标化发病率最高的是济源市（9.57/10万），其次是南阳市卧龙区（8.21/10万）和漯河市城区（6.39/10万）；女性标化发病率最高的是南阳市宛城区（7.79/10万），其次是漯河市城区（5.98/10万）和南阳市卧龙区（5.92/10万）。男性标化死亡率最高的是济源市（9.17/10万），其次是南阳市卧龙区（5.60/10万）和濮阳市华龙区（5.47/10万）；女性标化死亡率最高的是三门峡市湖滨区（3.67/10万），其次是南阳市卧龙区（3.47/10万）和漯河市城区（3.39/10万）。（图5-19b）

The age specific incidence of brain cancer was low at age group of 0~34, and it started increasing sharply at age group of 35, it reached the peak at age of 75. The age specific mortality was low at age group of 0~39, and it started increasing sharply at age group of 40, it reached the peak at age of 85. Age specific incidence and mortality were all higher in males than in females, The change pattern of age specific incidence and mortality were similar in urban areas and rural areas. (Figure 5-19a)

Among the 14 urban cancer registries, the ASR China incidence rate of brain cancer in males was the highest in Jiyuan City (9.57 per 100,000) followed by Nanyang Wolong District (8.21 per 100,000), and Luohe City (6.39 per 100,000). For females, it was the highest in Nanyang Wancheng District (7.79 per 100,000), followed by Luohe City (5.98 per 100,000), and Nanyang Wolong District (5.92 per 100,000). The ASR China mortality rate of brain cancer in males was the highest in Jiyuan City (9.17 per 100,000) followed by Nanyang Wolong District (5.60 per 100,000), and Puyang Hualong District (5.47 per 100,000). For females, it was the highest in Sanmenxia Hubin District (3.67 per 100,000), followed by Nanyang Wolong District (3.47 per 100,000), and Luohe City (3.39 per 100,000). (Figure 5-19b)

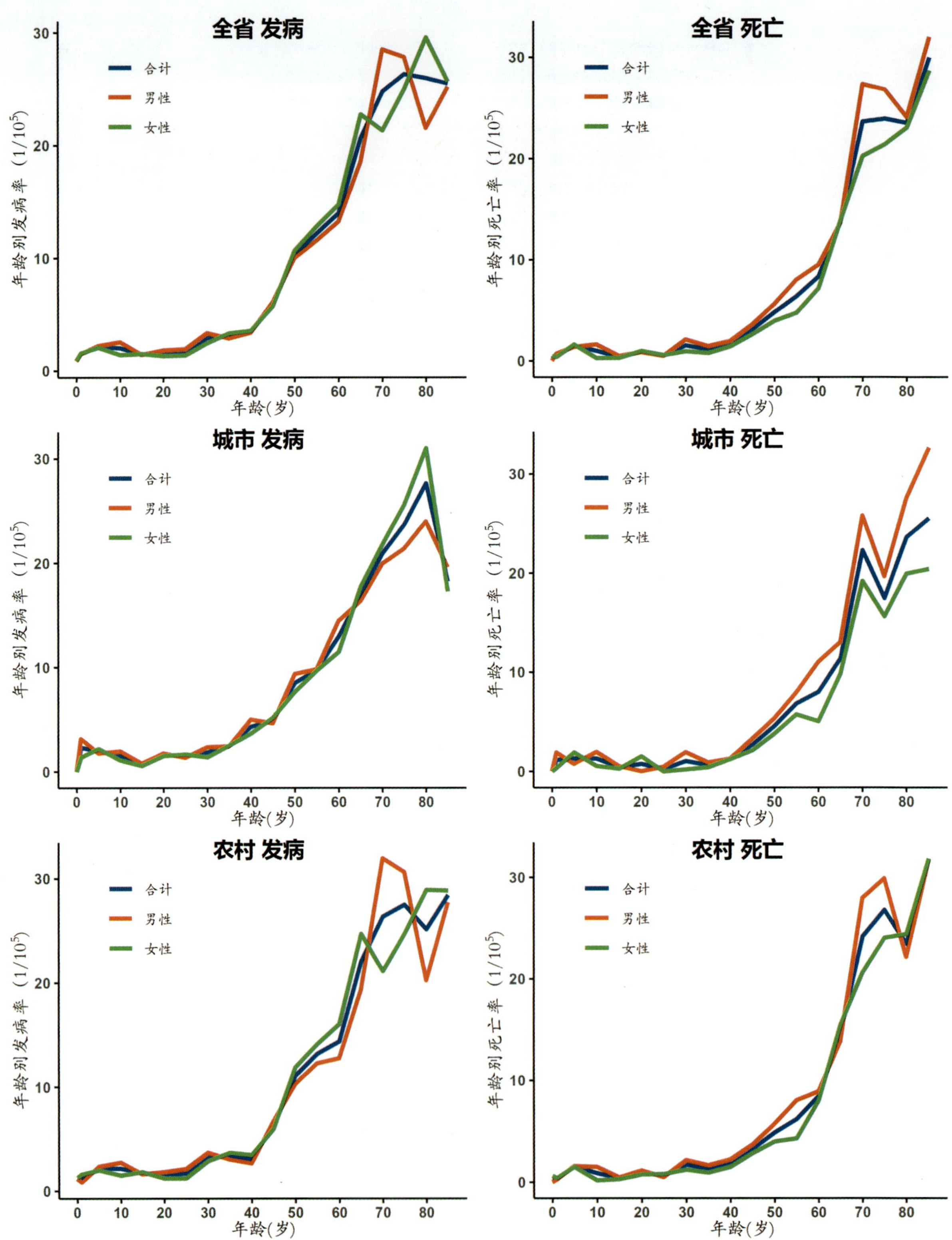

图 5-19a　2020 年河南省肿瘤登记地区脑癌年龄别发病率和死亡率

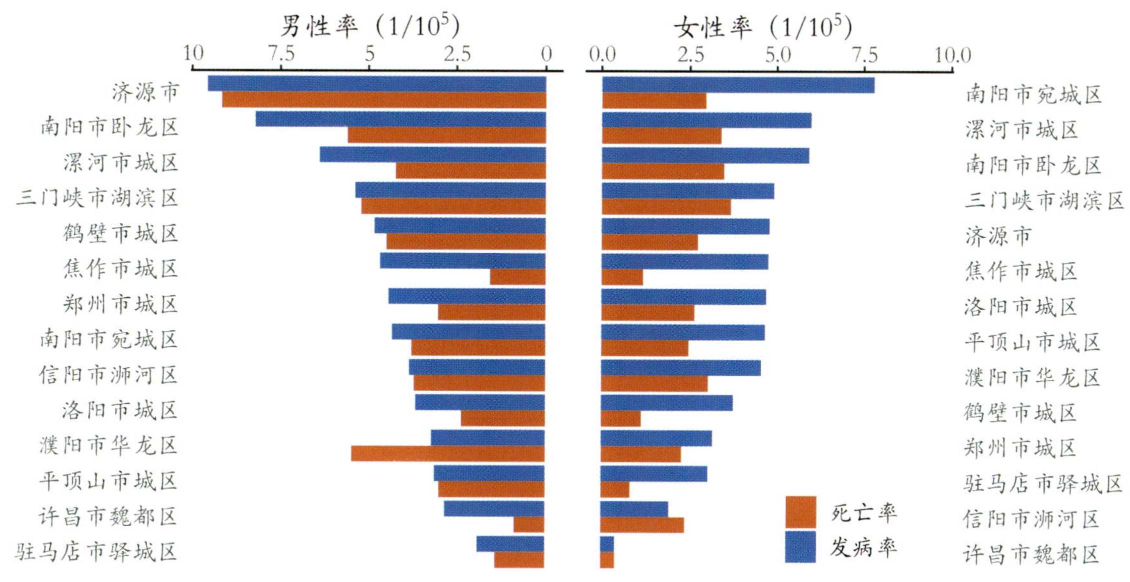

图 5-19b 2020 年河南省城市肿瘤登记地区脑癌发病率和死亡率

在 41 个农村肿瘤登记地区中，男性脑癌标化发病率最高的是范县（9.86/10 万），其次是桐柏县（9.49/10 万）和方城县（9.23/10 万）；女性标化发病率最高的是桐柏县（11.57/10 万），其次是林州市（8.56/10 万）和新野县（7.90/10 万）。男性标化死亡率最高的是范县（7.81/10 万），其次是桐柏县（7.32/10 万）和郏县（5.44/10 万）；女性标化死亡率最高的是淇县（5.66/10 万），其次是桐柏县（5.30/10 万）和栾川县（5.02/10 万）。（图 5-19c）

Among the 41 rural cancer registries, the ASR China incidence rate of brain cancer in males was the highest in Fan County (9.86 per 100,000) followed by Tongbai County (9.49 per 100,000), and Fangcheng County (9.23 per 100,000). For females, it was the highest in Tongbai County (11.57 per 100,000), followed by Linzhou City (8.56 per 100,000), and Xinye County (7.90 per 100,000). The ASR China mortality rate of brain cancer in males was the highest in Fan County (7.81 per 100,000) followed by Tongbai County (7.32 per 100,000), and Jia County (5.44 per 100,000). For females, it was the highest in Qi County (5.66 per 100,000), followed by Tongbai County (5.30 per 100,000), and Luanchuan County (5.02 per 100,000). (Figure 5-19c)

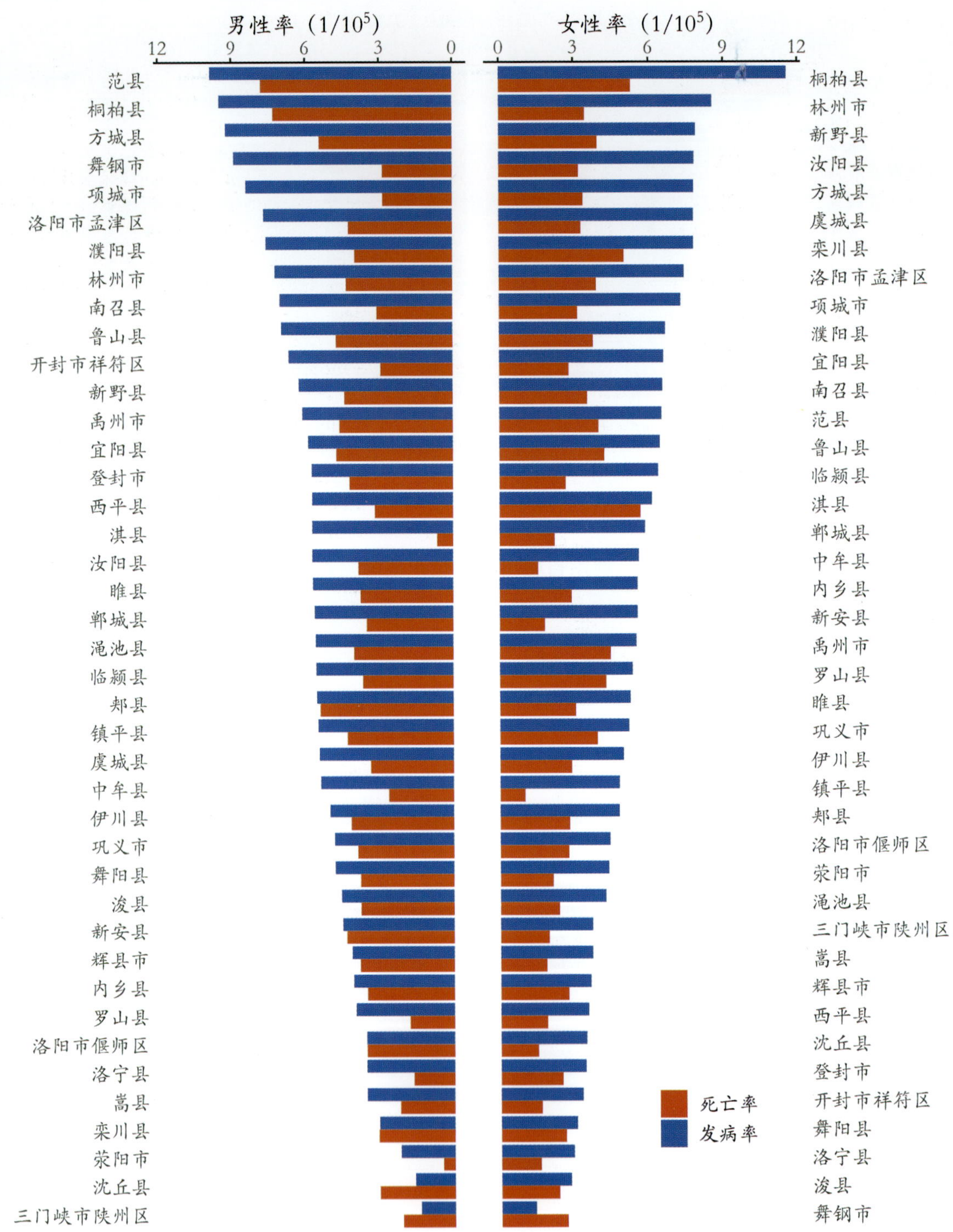

图 5-19c 2020 年河南省农村肿瘤登记地区脑癌发病率和死亡率

二十、甲状腺

2020 年，河南省肿瘤登记地区甲状腺癌的发病率为 17.69/10 万，中标率为 15.76/10 万，世标率为 13.76/10 万，发病例数占全部癌症新发病例数的 6.32%；其中，男性和女性发病率分别为 8.16/10 万和 27.64/10 万，城市地区和农村地区发病率分别为 29.40/10 万和 13.03/10 万；中标发病率呈现女性高于男性、城市地区高于农村地区的特点，女性中标发病率是男性的 3.23 倍，城市地区中标发病率是农村地区的 2.23 倍。同期，甲状腺癌的死亡率为 0.79/10 万，中标率为 0.54/10 万，世标率为 0.52/10 万，死亡病例数占全部癌症死亡病例数的 0.48%；其中，男性和女性死亡率分别为 0.51/10 万和 1.08/10 万，城市地区和农村地区死亡率分别为 0.78/10 万和 0.79/10 万；中标死亡率呈现女性高于男性、农村地区高于城市地区的特点，女性中标死亡率是男性的 2.00 倍，农村地区中标死亡率是城市地区的 1.19 倍。（表 5–20）

20. Thyroid

In 2020, there were 7,633 new cases diagnosed as thyroid cancer in registration areas of Henan Province, China (1,797 males and 5,836 females, 3,614 in urban areas and 4,019 in rural areas), accounting for 6.32% of new cases of all cancers. The crude incidence rate was 17.69 per 100,000, with the ASR China 15.76 per 100,000 and the ASR World 13.76 per 100,000, respectively. Subgroup analysis showed that the incidence of ASR China was 3.23 times in females as that in males, and it was 2.23 times in urban areas as that in rural areas. The cumulative incidence rate for subjects aged 0 to 74 years was 1.34%. (Table 5–20)

A total of 341 cases died of thyroid cancer in 2020 (112 males and 229 females, 96 in urban areas and 245 in rural areas), accounting for 0.48% of all cancer deaths. The crude mortality rate was 0.79 per 100,000, with the ASR China of 0.54 per 100,000 and the ASR World of 0.52 per 100,000, respectively. Subgroup analysis showed that the mortality of ASR China was 2.00 times in females as that in males, and it was 1.19 times in rural areas as that in urban areas. The cumulative mortality rate for subjects aged 0 to 74 years was 0.06%. (Table 5–20)

表 5–20　2020 年河南省肿瘤登记地区甲状腺癌发病与死亡情况

地区	性别	病例数	粗率（1/10^5）	构成（%）	中标率（1/10^5）	世标率（1/10^5）	累积率 0～74（%）
发病							
全省	合计	7 633	17.69	6.32	15.76	13.76	1.34
	男性	1 797	8.16	2.91	7.51	6.51	0.63
	女性	5 836	27.64	9.91	24.23	21.18	2.07
城市地区	合计	3 614	29.40	9.85	25.81	22.20	2.16
	男性	913	14.89	4.99	13.69	11.60	1.11
	女性	2 701	43.86	14.68	37.58	32.53	3.18
农村地区	合计	4 019	13.03	4.78	11.57	10.23	1.01
	男性	884	5.56	2.03	5.07	4.49	0.44
	女性	3 135	20.97	7.75	18.40	16.24	1.59

续表

地区	性别	病例数	粗率（1/10^5）	构成（%）	中标率（1/10^5）	世标率（1/10^5）	累积率 0～74（%）
死亡							
全省	合计	341	0.79	0.48	0.54	0.52	0.06
	男性	112	0.51	0.26	0.36	0.35	0.04
	女性	229	1.08	0.85	0.72	0.68	0.08
城市地区	合计	96	0.78	0.49	0.48	0.47	0.05
	男性	33	0.54	0.27	0.34	0.34	0.04
	女性	63	1.02	0.83	0.61	0.60	0.06
农村地区	合计	245	0.79	0.48	0.57	0.54	0.06
	男性	79	0.50	0.25	0.37	0.35	0.04
	女性	166	1.11	0.85	0.76	0.72	0.08

甲状腺癌年龄别发病率在0~19岁年龄段处于较低水平，20岁以后快速上升，在55岁达到峰值；年龄别死亡率在0~39岁年龄段处于较低水平，40岁以后快速上升，在80岁达到峰值；年龄别发病率和死亡率均呈现女性高于男性的特点；城市地区和农村地区年龄别率虽然有一定差异，但是总体趋势类同。（图5-20a）

在14个城市肿瘤登记地区中，男性甲状腺癌标化发病率最高的是郑州市城区（31.47/10万），其次是许昌市魏都区（22.02/10万）和平顶山市城区（16.17/10万）；女性标化发病率最高的是郑州市城区（71.63/10万），其次是许昌市魏都区（55.72/10万）和濮阳市华龙区（49.80/10万）。男性标化死亡率最高的是鹤壁市城区（1.22/10万），其次是济源市（0.55/10万）和漯河市城区（0.54/10万）；女性标化死亡率最高的是三门峡市湖滨区（1.59/10万），其次是漯河市城区（1.42/10万）和濮阳市华龙区（1.31/10万）。（图5-20b）

The age specific incidence of thyroid cancer was low at age group of 0~19, and it started increasing sharply at age group of 20, it reached the peak at age of 55. The age specific mortality was low at age group of 0~39, and it started increasing sharply at age group of 40, it reached the peak at age of 80. Age specific incidence and mortality were all higher in females than in males, The change pattern of age specific incidence and mortality were similar in urban areas and rural areas. (Figure 5-20a)

Among the 14 urban cancer registries, the ASR China incidence rate of thyroid cancer in males was the highest in Zhengzhou City (31.47 per 100,000) followed by Xuchang Weidu District (22.02 per 100,000), and Pingdingshan City (16.17 per 100,000). For females, it was the highest in Zhengzhou City (71.63 per 100,000), followed by Xuchang Weidu District (55.72 per 100,000), and Puyang Hualong District (49.80 per 100,000). The ASR China mortality rate of thyroid cancer in males was the highest in Hebi City (1.22 per 100,000) followed by Jiyuan City (0.55 per 100,000), and Luohe City (0.54 per 100,000). For females, it was the highest in Sanmenxia Hubin District (1.59 per 100,000), followed by Luohe City (1.42 per 100,000), and Puyang Hualong District (1.31 per 100,000). (Figure 5-20b)

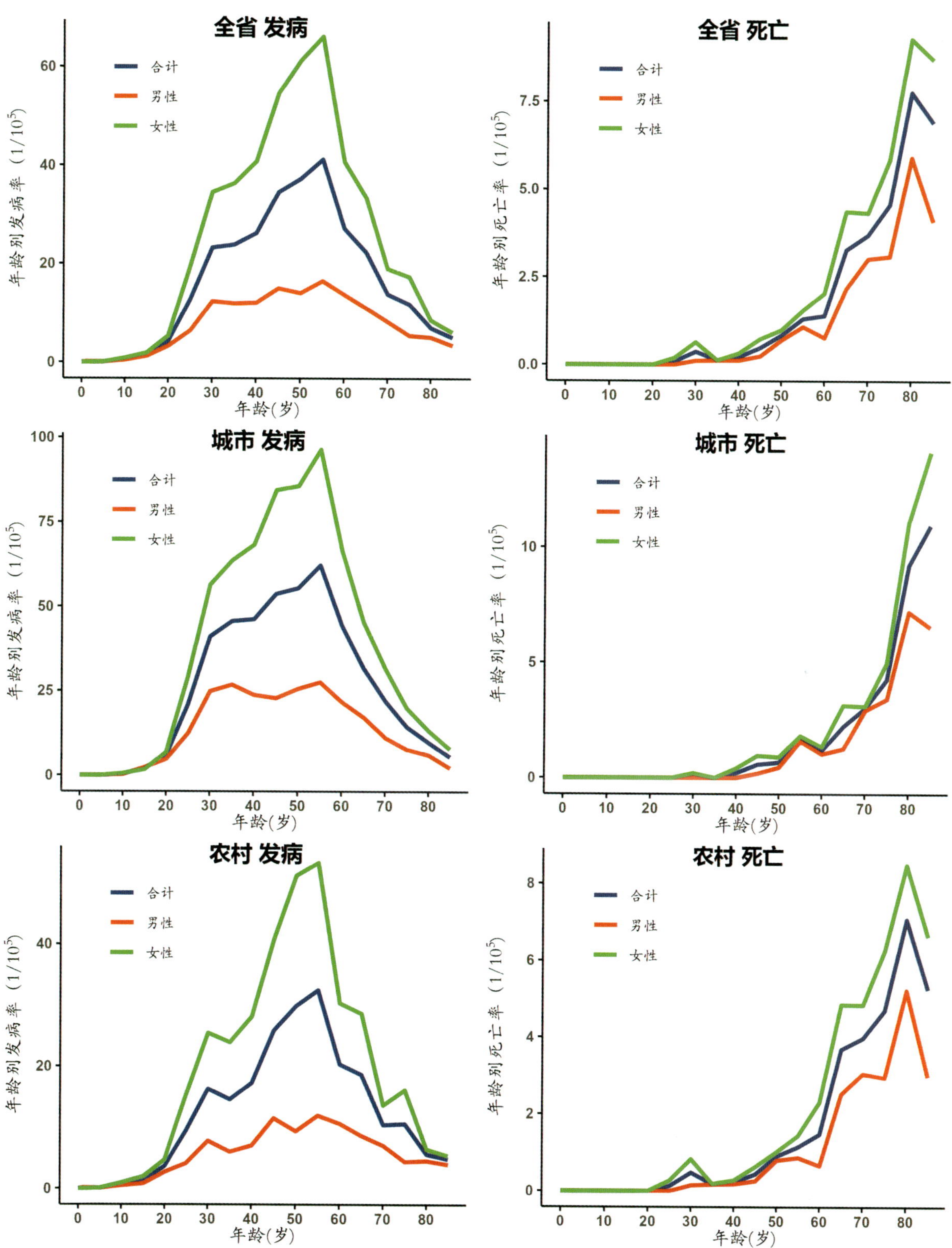

图 5-20a　2020 年河南省肿瘤登记地区甲状腺癌年龄别发病率和死亡率

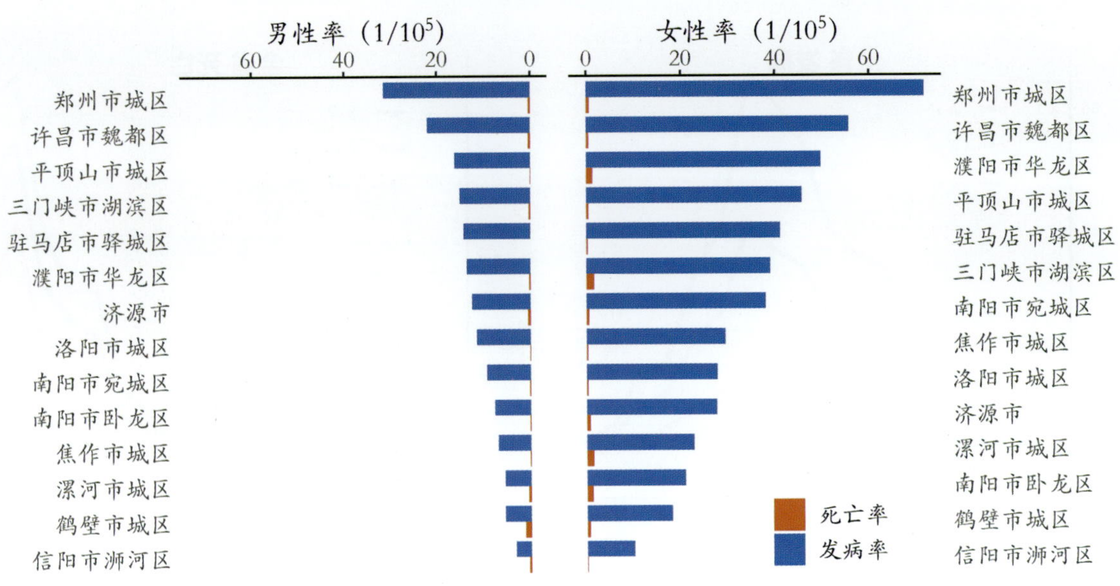

图 5-20b　2020 年河南省城市肿瘤登记地区甲状腺癌发病率和死亡率

在 41 个农村肿瘤登记地区中，男性甲状腺癌标化发病率最高的是中牟县（21.92/10 万），其次是荥阳市（11.44/10 万）和开封市祥符区（10.74/10 万）；女性标化发病率最高的是中牟县（54.15/10 万），其次是开封市祥符区（43.56/10 万）和登封市（38.47/10 万）。男性标化死亡率最高的是三门峡市陕州区（1.17/10 万），其次是郸城县（1.17/10 万）和开封市祥符区（1.07/10 万）；女性标化死亡率最高的是范县（6.90/10 万），其次是虞城县（3.61/10 万）和开封市祥符区（1.85/10 万）。（图 5-20c）

Among the 41 rural cancer registries, the ASR China incidence rate of thyroid cancer in males was the highest in Zhongmu County (21.92 per 100,000) followed by Xingyang City (11.44 per 100,000), and Kaifeng Xiangfu District (10.74 per 100,000). For females, it was the highest in Zhongmu County (54.15 per 100,000), followed by Kaifeng Xiangfu District (43.56 per 100,000), and Dengfeng City (38.47 per 100,000). The ASR China mortality rate of thyroid cancer in males was the highest in Sanmenxia Shanzhou District (1.17 per 100,000) followed by Dancheng County (1.17 per 100,000), and Kaifeng Xiangfu District (1.07 per 100,000). For females, it was the highest in Fan County (6.90 per 100,000), followed by Yucheng County (3.61 per 100,000), and Kaifeng Xiangfu District (1.85 per 100,000). (Figure 5-20c)

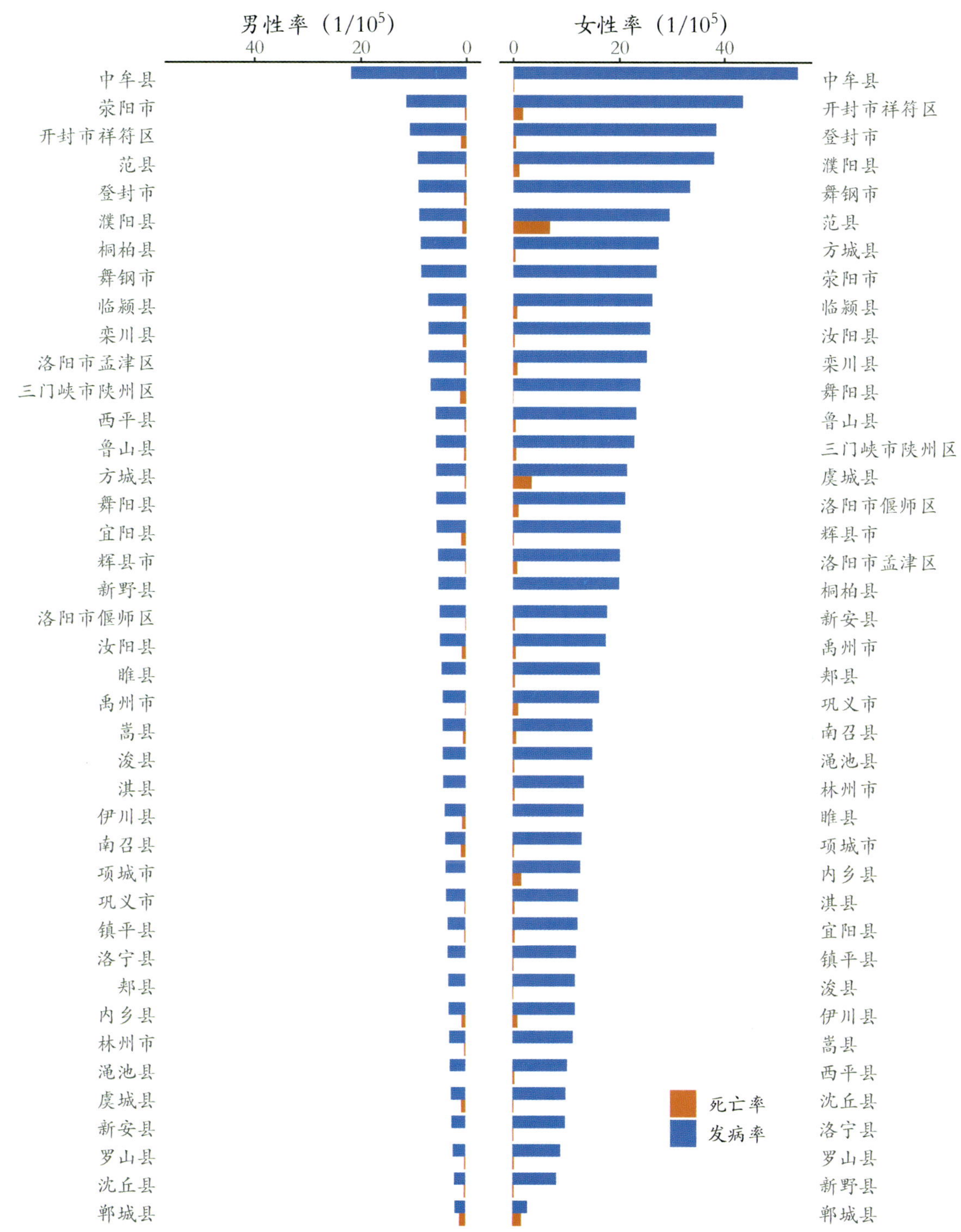

图 5-20c　2020 年河南省农村肿瘤登记地区甲状腺癌发病率和死亡率

二十一、淋巴

2020 年，河南省肿瘤登记地区淋巴瘤的发病率为 4.83/10 万，中标率为 3.59/10 万，世标率为 3.56/10 万，发病例数占全部癌症新发病例数的 1.73%；其中，男性和女性发病率分别为 5.29/10 万和 4.35/10 万，城市地区和农村地区发病率分别为 6.52/10 万和 4.16/10 万；中标发病率呈现男性高于女性、城市地区高于农村地区的特点，男性中标发病率是女性的 1.31 倍，城市地区中标发病率是农村地区的 1.45 倍。同期，淋巴瘤的死亡率为 2.61/10 万，中标率为 1.81/10 万，世标率为 1.79/10 万，死亡病例数占全部癌症死亡病例数的 1.60%；其中，男性和女性死亡率分别为 2.98/10 万和 2.23/10 万，城市地区和农村地区死亡率分别为 3.18/10 万和 2.38/10 万；中标死亡率呈现男性高于女性、城市地区高于农村地区的特点，男性中标死亡率是女性的 1.53 倍，城市地区中标死亡率是农村地区的 1.20 倍。（表 5–21）

21. Lymphoma

In 2020, there were 2,085 new cases diagnosed as lymphoma cancer in registration areas of Henan Province, China (1,166 males and 919 females, 801 in urban areas and 1,284 in rural areas), accounting for 1.73% of new cases of all cancers. The crude incidence rate was 4.83 per 100,000, with the ASR China 3.59 per 100,000 and the ASR World 3.56 per 100,000, respectively. Subgroup analysis showed that the incidence of ASR China was 1.31 times in males as that in females, and it was 1.45 times in urban areas as that in rural areas. The cumulative incidence rate for subjects aged 0 to 74 years was 0.42%. (Table 5–21)

A total of 1,126 cases died of lymphoma cancer in 2020 (656 males and 470 females, 391 in urban areas and 735 in rural areas), accounting for 1.60% of all cancer deaths. The crude mortality rate was 2.61 per 100,000, with the ASR China of 1.81 per 100,000 and the ASR World of 1.79 per 100,000, respectively. Subgroup analysis showed that the mortality of ASR China was 1.53 times in males as that in females, and it was 1.20 times in urban areas as that in rural areas. The cumulative mortality rate for subjects aged 0 to 74 years was 0.22%. (Table 5–21)

表 5–21　2020 年河南省肿瘤登记地区淋巴瘤发病与死亡情况

地区	性别	病例数	粗率（$1/10^5$）	构成（%）	中标率（$1/10^5$）	世标率（$1/10^5$）	累积率 0～74（%）
发病							
全省	合计	2 085	4.83	1.73	3.59	3.56	0.42
	男性	1 166	5.29	1.89	4.08	4.05	0.48
	女性	919	4.35	1.56	3.11	3.08	0.36
城市地区	合计	801	6.52	2.18	4.59	4.56	0.54
	男性	446	7.27	2.44	5.30	5.31	0.66
	女性	355	5.76	1.93	3.91	3.85	0.43
农村地区	合计	1 284	4.16	1.53	3.17	3.14	0.36
	男性	720	4.53	1.65	3.59	3.55	0.41
	女性	564	3.77	1.39	2.77	2.75	0.32

续表

地区	性别	病例数	粗率（1/10^5）	构成（%）	中标率（1/10^5）	世标率（1/10^5）	累积率 0~74（%）
死亡							
全省	合计	1 126	2.61	1.60	1.81	1.79	0.22
	男性	656	2.98	1.52	2.20	2.16	0.27
	女性	470	2.23	1.74	1.44	1.43	0.17
城市地区	合计	391	3.18	1.99	2.05	2.04	0.24
	男性	219	3.57	1.81	2.43	2.40	0.29
	女性	172	2.79	2.26	1.69	1.70	0.19
农村地区	合计	735	2.38	1.45	1.71	1.68	0.21
	男性	437	2.75	1.40	2.09	2.05	0.26
	女性	298	1.99	1.53	1.33	1.31	0.17

淋巴瘤年龄别发病率在0~39岁年龄段处于较低水平，40岁以后快速上升，在70岁达到峰值；年龄别死亡率在0~39岁年龄段处于较低水平，40岁以后快速上升，在85岁达到峰值；年龄别发病率和死亡率均呈现男性高于女性的特点；城市地区和农村地区年龄别率虽然有一定差异，但是总体趋势类同。（图5-21a）

在14个城市肿瘤登记地区中，男性淋巴瘤标化发病率最高的是三门峡市湖滨区（9.36/10万），其次是南阳市卧龙区（8.46/10万）和漯河市城区（7.80/10万）；女性标化发病率最高的是郑州市城区（6.47/10万），其次是南阳市卧龙区（5.27/10万）和漯河市城区（4.85/10万）。男性标化死亡率最高的是南阳市卧龙区（3.75/10万），其次是郑州市城区（3.39/10万）和漯河市城区（3.20/10万）；女性标化死亡率最高的是洛阳市城区（2.51/10万），其次是郑州市城区（2.39/10万）和济源市（2.37/10万）。（图5-21b）

The age specific incidence of lymphoma cancer was low at age group of 0~39, and it started increasing sharply at age group of 40, it reached the peak at age of 70. The age specific mortality was low at age group of 0~39, and it started increasing sharply at age group of 40, it reached the peak at age of 85. Age specific incidence and mortality were all higher in males than in females. The change pattern of age specific incidence and mortality were similar in urban areas and rural areas. (Figure 5–21a)

Among the 14 urban cancer registries, the ASR China incidence rate of lymphoma cancer in males was the highest in Sanmenxia Hubin District (9.36 per 100,000) followed by Nanyang Wolong District (8.46 per 100,000), and Luohe City (7.80 per 100,000). For females, it was the highest in Zhengzhou City (6.47 per 100,000), followed by Nanyang Wolong District (5.27 per 100,000), and Luohe City (4.85 per 100,000). The ASR China mortality rate of lymphoma cancer in males was the highest in Nanyang Wolong District (3.75 per 100,000) followed by Zhengzhou City (3.39 per 100,000), and Luohe City (3.20 per 100,000). For females, it was the highest in Luoyang City (2.51 per 100,000), followed by Zhengzhou City (2.39 per 100,000), and Jiyuan City (2.37 per 100,000). (Figure 5–21b)

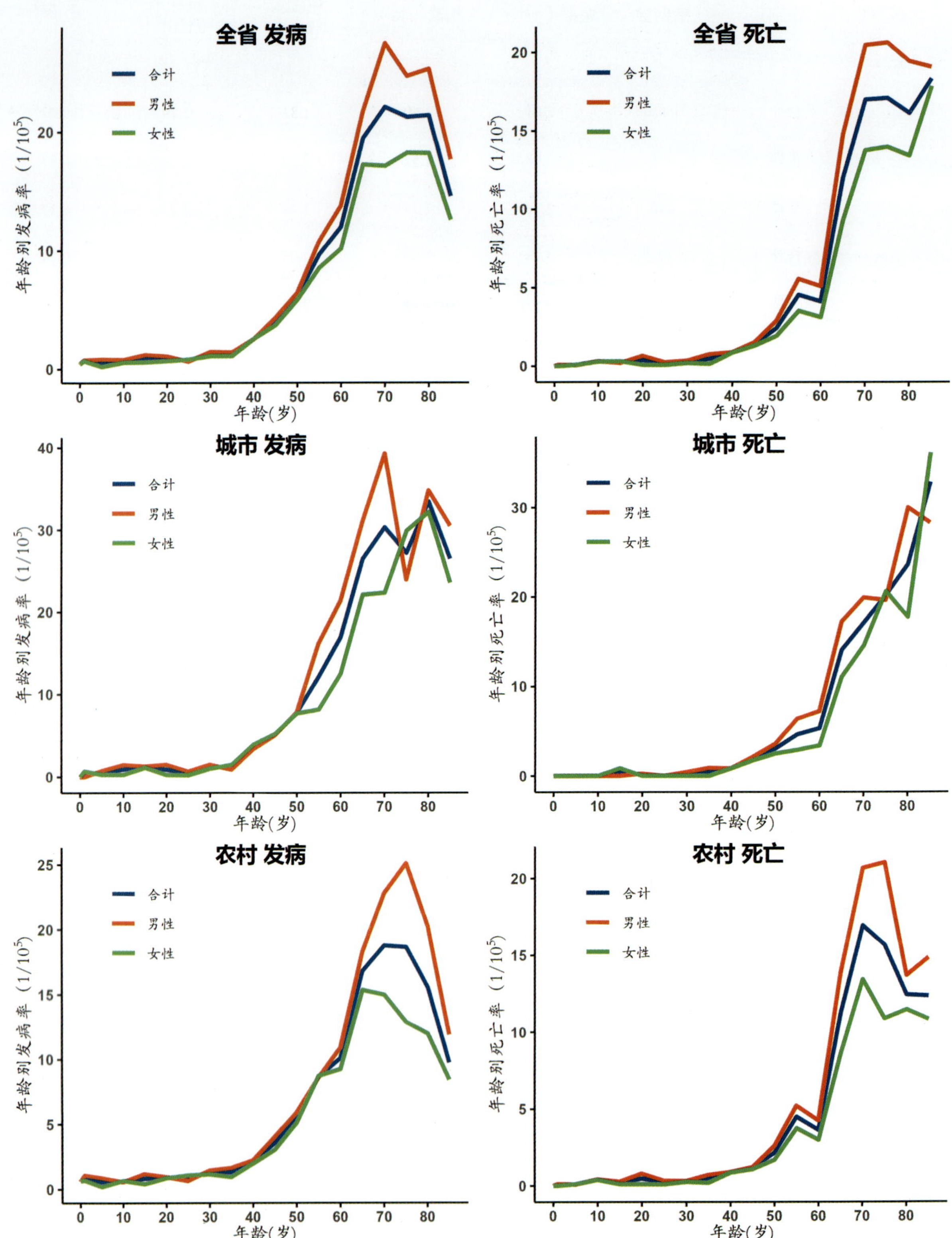

图 5-21a　2020 年河南省肿瘤登记地区淋巴瘤年龄别发病率和死亡率

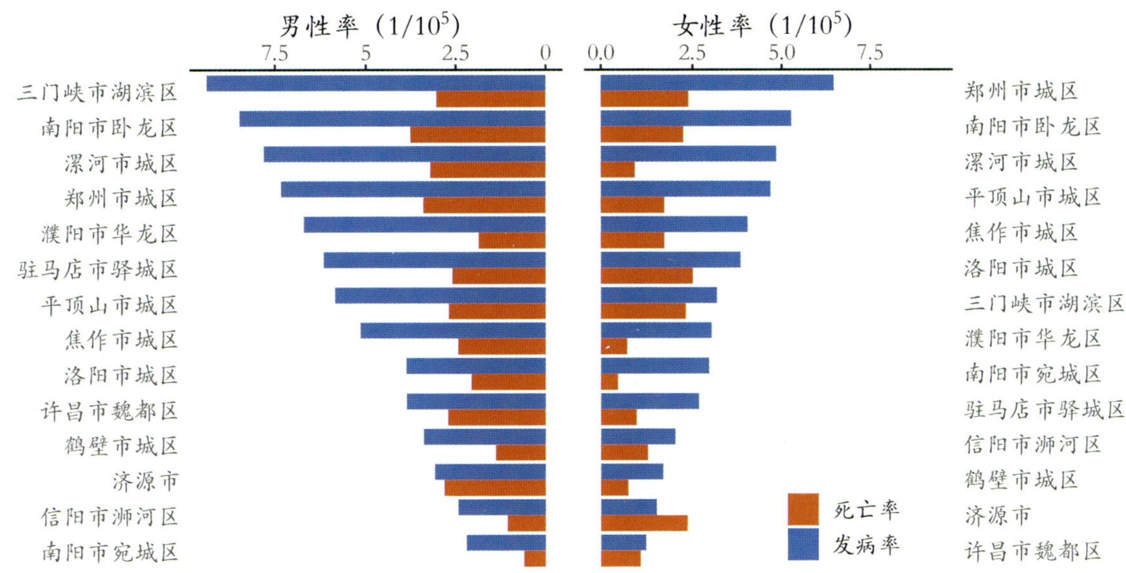

图 5-21b　2020 年河南省城市肿瘤登记地区淋巴瘤发病率和死亡率

在 41 个农村肿瘤登记地区中，男性淋巴瘤标化发病率最高的是洛阳市偃师区（8.42/10 万），其次是开封市祥符区（7.28/10 万）和洛阳市孟津区（6.98/10 万）；女性标化发病率最高的是开封市祥符区（7.31/10 万），其次是西平县（6.61/10 万）和中牟县（5.8/10 万）。男性标化死亡率最高的是开封市祥符区（8.35/10 万），其次是西平县（5.01/10 万）和新野县（3.97/10 万）；女性标化死亡率最高的是开封市祥符区（4.72/10 万），其次是西平县（4.04/10 万）和内乡县（3.11/10 万）。（图 5-21c）

Among the 41 rural cancer registries, the ASR China incidence rate of lymphoma cancer in males was the highest in Luoyang Yanshi District (8.42 per 100,000) followed by Kaifeng Xiangfu District (7.28 per 100,000), and Luoyang Mengjin District (6.98 per 100,000). For females, it was the highest in Kaifeng Xiangfu District (7.31 per 100,000), followed by Xiping County (6.61 per 100,000), and Zhongmu County (5.80 per 100,000). The ASR China mortality rate of lymphoma cancer in males was the highest in Kaifeng Xiangfu District (8.35 per 100,000) followed by Xiping County (5.01 per 100,000), and Xinye County (3.97 per 100,000). For females, it was the highest in Kaifeng Xiangfu District (4.72 per 100,000), followed by Xiping County (4.04 per 100,000), and Neixiang County (3.11 per 100,000). (Figure 5-21c)

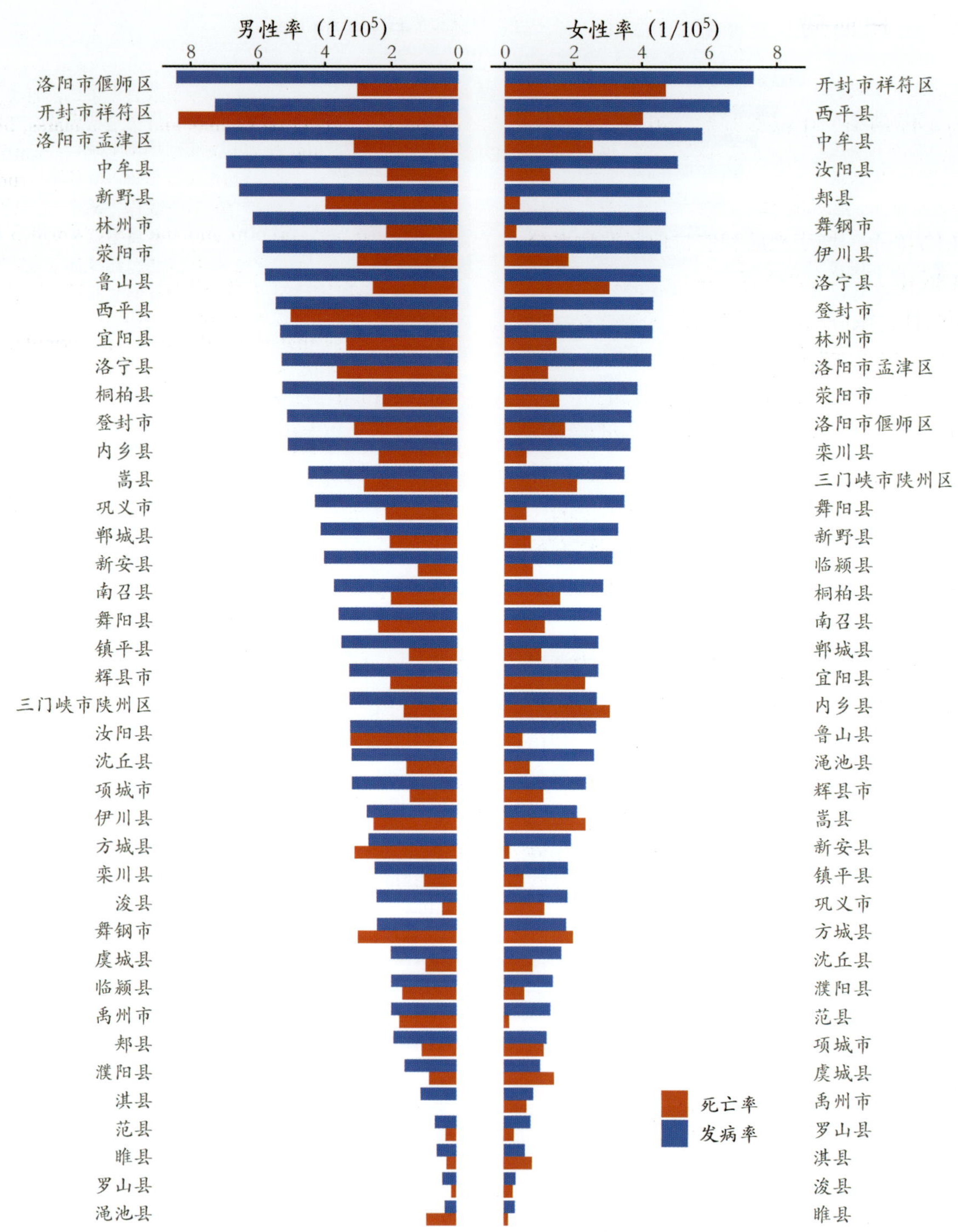

图 5-21c　2020 年河南省农村肿瘤登记地区淋巴瘤发病率和死亡率

二十二、白血病

2020 年，河南省肿瘤登记地区白血病的发病率为 4.45/10 万，中标率为 3.70/10 万，世标率为 3.85/10 万，发病例数占全部癌症新发病例数的 1.59%；其中，男性和女性发病率分别为 4.76/10 万和 4.13/10 万，城市地区和农村地区发病率分别为 4.86/10 万和 4.29/10 万；中标发病率呈现男性高于女性、城市地区高于农村地区的特点，男性中标发病率是女性的 1.18 倍，城市地区中标发病率是农村地区的 1.05 倍。同期，白血病的死亡率为 2.61/10 万，中标率为 2.00/10 万，世标率为 2.02/10 万，死亡病例数占全部癌症死亡病例数的 1.60%；其中，男性和女性死亡率分别为 2.92/10 万和 2.29/10 万，城市地区和农村地区死亡率分别为 3.11/10 万和 2.41/10 万；中标死亡率呈现男性高于女性、城市地区高于农村地区的特点，男性中标死亡率是女性的 1.34 倍，城市地区中标死亡率是农村地区的 1.16 倍。（表 5-22）

22. Leukemia

In 2020, there were 1,921 new cases diagnosed as leukemia cancer in registration areas of Henan Province, China (1,049 males and 872 females, 597 in urban areas and 1,324 in rural areas), accounting for 1.59% of new cases of all cancers. The crude incidence rate was 4.45 per 100,000, with the ASR China 3.70 per 100,000 and the ASR World 3.85 per 100,000, respectively. Subgroup analysis showed that the incidence of ASR China was 1.18 times in males as that in females, and it was 1.05 times in urban areas as that in rural areas. The cumulative incidence rate for subjects aged 0 to 74 years was 0.36%. (Table 5-22)

A total of 1,127 cases died of leukemia cancer in 2020 (643 males and 484 females, 382 in urban areas and 745 in rural areas), accounting for 1.60% of all cancer deaths. The crude mortality rate was 2.61 per 100,000, with the ASR China of 2.00 per 100,000 and the ASR World of 2.02 per 100,000, respectively. Subgroup analysis showed that the mortality of ASR China was 1.34 times in males as that in females, and it was 1.16 times in urban areas as that in rural areas. The cumulative mortality rate for subjects aged 0 to 74 years was 0.20%. (Table 5-22)

表 5-22 2020 年河南省肿瘤登记地区白血病发病与死亡情况

地区	性别	病例数	粗率（$1/10^5$）	构成（%）	中标率（$1/10^5$）	世标率（$1/10^5$）	累积率 0～74（%）
发病							
全省	合计	1 921	4.45	1.59	3.70	3.85	0.36
	男性	1 049	4.76	1.70	4.01	4.21	0.40
	女性	872	4.13	1.48	3.39	3.50	0.32
城市地区	合计	597	4.86	1.63	3.84	4.11	0.37
	男性	332	5.41	1.82	4.26	4.68	0.42
	女性	265	4.30	1.44	3.46	3.57	0.33
农村地区	合计	1 324	4.29	1.58	3.64	3.75	0.36
	男性	717	4.51	1.65	3.89	4.02	0.40
	女性	607	4.06	1.50	3.38	3.48	0.32

续表

地区	性别	病例数	粗率（1/10^5）	构成（%）	中标率（1/10^5）	世标率（1/10^5）	累积率 0～74（%）
死亡							
全省	合计	1 127	2.61	1.60	2.00	2.02	0.20
	男性	643	2.92	1.49	2.31	2.30	0.23
	女性	484	2.29	1.79	1.72	1.77	0.17
城市地区	合计	382	3.11	1.94	2.22	2.26	0.23
	男性	232	3.78	1.92	2.77	2.78	0.28
	女性	150	2.44	1.97	1.72	1.79	0.18
农村地区	合计	745	2.41	1.47	1.91	1.92	0.19
	男性	411	2.58	1.32	2.11	2.10	0.21
	女性	334	2.23	1.72	1.72	1.75	0.17

白血病年龄别发病率在0~34岁年龄段处于较低水平，35岁以后快速上升，在80岁达到峰值；年龄别死亡率在0~39岁年龄段处于较低水平，40岁以后快速上升，在85岁达到峰值；年龄别发病率和死亡率均呈现男性高于女性的特点；城市地区和农村地区年龄别率虽然有一定差异，但是总体趋势类同。（图5–22a）

在14个城市肿瘤登记地区中，男性白血病标化发病率最高的是鹤壁市城区（8.05/10万），其次是三门峡市湖滨区（6.76/10万）和漯河市城区（5.48/10万）；女性标化发病率最高的是焦作市城区（5.05/10万），其次是漯河市城区（5.03/10万）和鹤壁市城区（4.94/10万）。男性标化死亡率最高的是鹤壁市城区（5.43/10万），其次是漯河市城区（5.10/10万）和三门峡市湖滨区（4.46/10万）；女性标化死亡率最高的是漯河市城区（3.45/10万），其次是鹤壁市城区（3.28/10万）和郑州市城区（1.89/10万）。（图5–22b）

The age specific incidence of leukemia cancer was low at age group of 0~34, and it started increasing sharply at age group of 35, it reached the peak at age of 80. The age specific mortality was low at age group of 0~39, and it started increasing sharply at age group of 40, it reached the peak at age of 85. Age specific incidence and mortality were all higher in males than in females. The change pattern of age specific incidence and mortality were similar in urban areas and rural areas. (Figure 5–22a)

Among the 14 urban cancer registries, the ASR China incidence rate of leukemia cancer in males was the highest in Hebi City (8.05 per 100,000) followed by Sanmenxia Hubin District (6.76 per 100,000), and Luohe City (5.48 per 100,000). For females, it was the highest in Jiaozuo City (5.05 per 100,000), followed by Luohe City (5.03 per 100,000), and Hebi City (4.94 per 100,000). The ASR China mortality rate of leukemia cancer in males was the highest in Hebi City (5.43 per 100,000) followed by Luohe City (5.10 per 100,000), and Sanmenxia Hubin District (4.46 per 100,000). For females, it was the highest in Luohe City (3.45 per 100,000), followed by Hebi City (3.28 per 100,000), and Zhengzhou City (1.89 per 100,000). (Figure 5–22b)

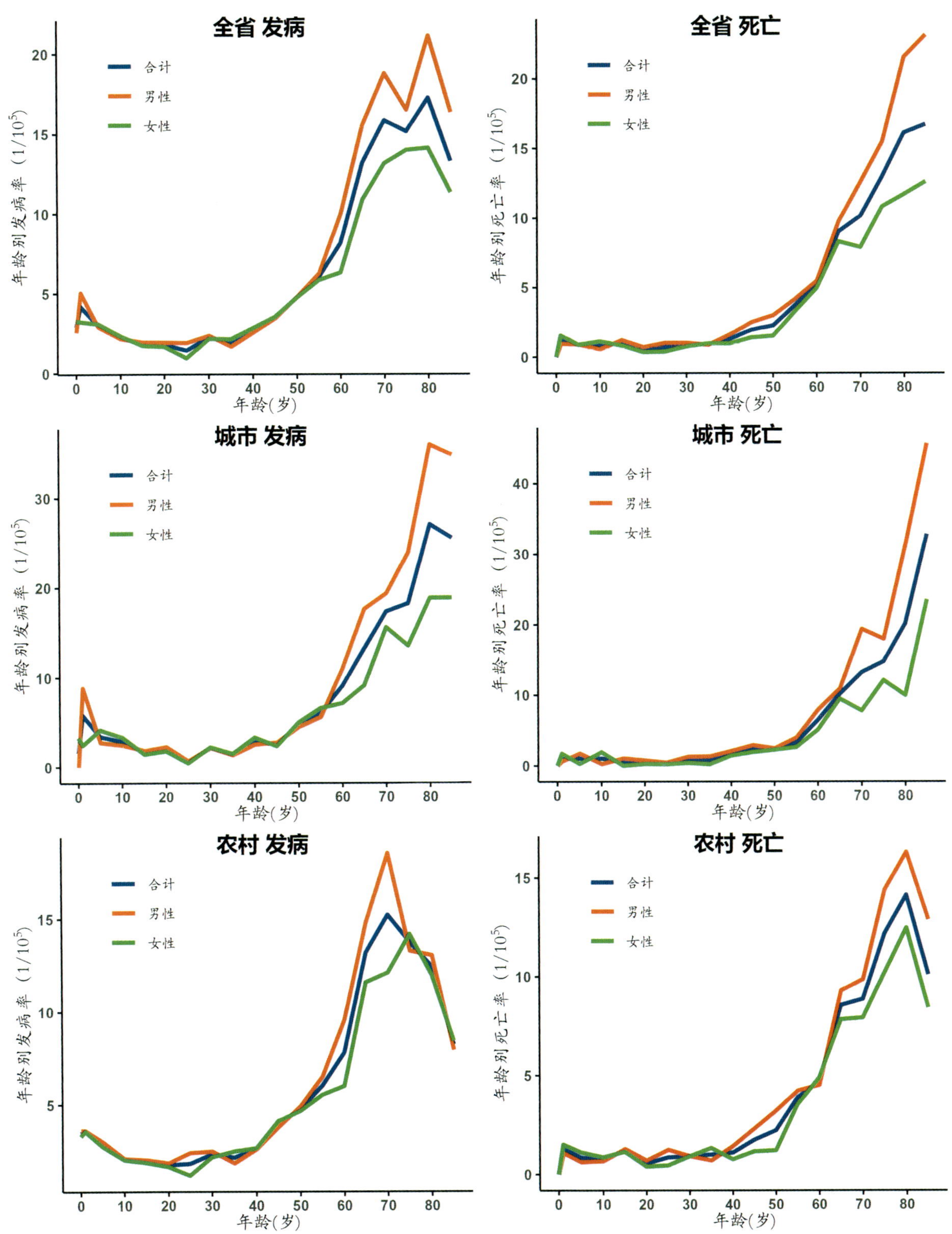

图 5-22a 2020 年河南省肿瘤登记地区白血病年龄别发病率和死亡率

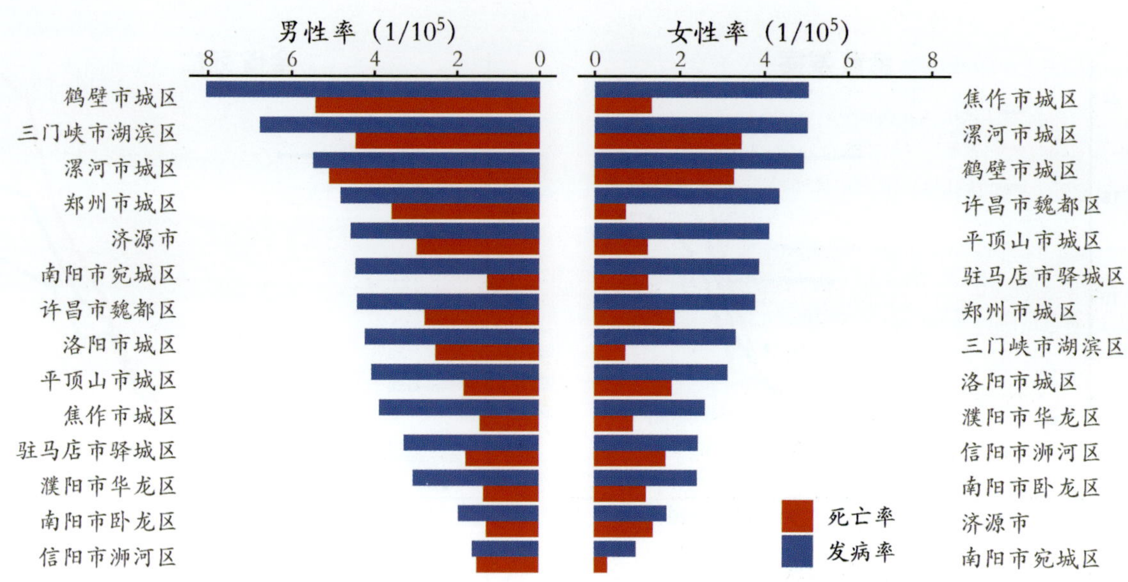

图 5-22b　2020 年河南省城市肿瘤登记地区白血病发病率和死亡率

在 41 个农村肿瘤登记地区中，男性白血病标化发病率最高的是郸城县（9.01/10 万），其次是沈丘县（8.59/10 万）和洛阳市偃师区（6.86/10 万）；女性标化发病率最高的是沈丘县（7.9/10 万），其次是郸城县（7.53/10 万）和宜阳县（7.40/10 万）。男性标化死亡率最高的是开封市祥符区（4.66/10 万），其次是罗山县（4.35/10 万）和洛阳市偃师区（4.28/10 万）；女性标化死亡率最高的是开封市祥符区（4.36/10 万），其次是临颍县（4.16/10 万）和西平县（4.14/10 万）。（图 5-22c）

Among the 41 rural cancer registries, the ASR China incidence rate of leukemia cancer in males was the highest in Dancheng County (9.01 per 100,000) followed by Shenqiu County (8.59 per 100,000), and Luoyang Yanshi District (6.86 per 100,000). For females, it was the highest in Shenqiu County (7.9 per 100,000), followed by Dancheng County (7.53 per 100,000), and Yiyang County (7.40 per 100,000). The ASR China mortality rate of leukemia cancer in males was the highest in Kaifeng Xiangfu District (4.66 per 100,000) followed by Luoshan County (4.35 per 100,000), and Luoyang Yanshi District (4.28 per 100,000). For females, it was the highest in Kaifeng Xiangfu District (4.36 per 100,000), followed by Linying County (4.16 per 100,000), and Xiping County (4.14 per 100,000). (Figure 5-22c)

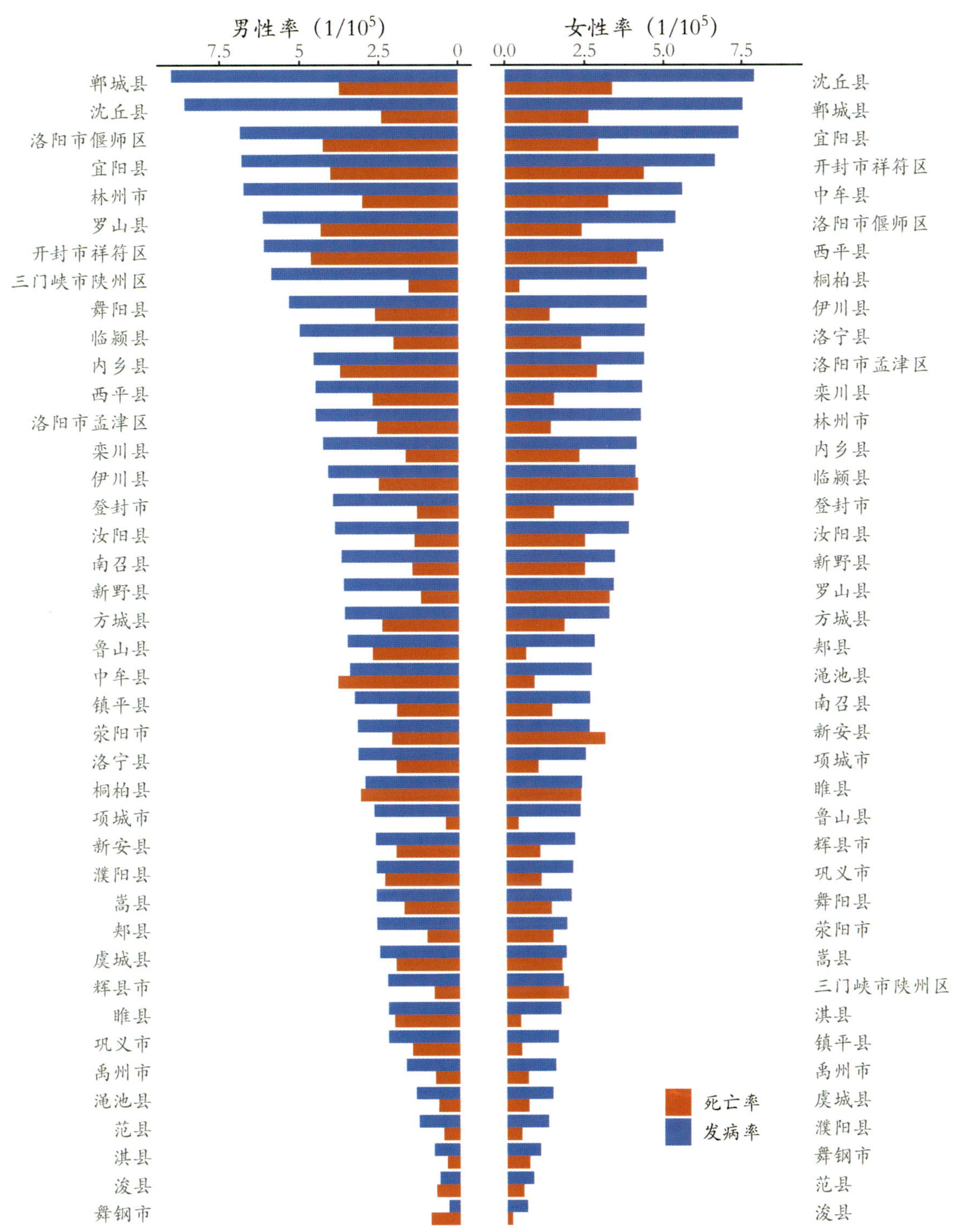

图 5-22c　2020 年河南省农村肿瘤登记地区白血病发病率和死亡率

第六章　附　录

Chapter 6　Appendix

一、河南省肿瘤登记地区合计发病和死亡情况

1. Overall incidence and mortality in Henan cancer registries

表 6-1　河南省肿瘤登记地区

部位	ICD-10	病例数	构成(%)	年龄组 0~	1~	5~	10~	15~	20~	25~
唇	C00	97	0.08	0.00	0.05	0.00	0.00	0.04	0.03	0.03
舌	C01–C02	253	0.21	0.00	0.05	0.07	0.00	0.00	0.00	0.15
口	C03–C06	405	0.34	0.00	0.00	0.07	0.03	0.00	0.13	0.06
唾液腺	C07–C08	277	0.23	0.00	0.05	0.03	0.03	0.14	0.17	0.15
扁桃体	C09	49	0.04	0.00	0.05	0.03	0.03	0.07	0.00	0.00
其他的口咽	C10	88	0.07	0.00	0.00	0.00	0.00	0.04	0.07	0.00
鼻咽	C11	418	0.35	0.00	0.05	0.07	0.13	0.18	0.10	0.09
喉咽	C12–C13	145	0.12	0.00	0.05	0.03	0.00	0.00	0.00	0.00
咽，部位不明	C14	115	0.10	0.00	0.00	0.03	0.03	0.00	0.07	0.06
食管	C15	11 678	9.68	0.00	0.05	0.03	0.00	0.00	0.20	0.40
胃	C16	13 094	10.85	0.00	0.05	0.07	0.20	0.21	0.50	0.74
小肠	C17	553	0.46	0.00	0.00	0.00	0.00	0.00	0.03	0.09
结肠	C18	4 189	3.47	0.00	0.00	0.00	0.03	0.14	0.27	0.83
直肠	C19–C20	4 737	3.92	0.00	0.00	0.03	0.00	0.04	0.20	0.68
肛门	C21	165	0.14	0.00	0.00	0.00	0.00	0.00	0.00	0.03
肝脏	C22	10 545	8.74	0.45	0.18	0.07	0.20	0.29	0.34	1.20
胆囊及其他	C23–C24	1 898	1.57	0.00	0.09	0.00	0.00	0.00	0.03	0.15
胰腺	C25	2 093	1.73	0.00	0.00	0.07	0.07	0.11	0.03	0.18
鼻、鼻窦及其他	C30–C31	204	0.17	0.00	0.09	0.07	0.10	0.14	0.07	0.03
喉	C32	609	0.50	0.00	0.05	0.07	0.03	0.00	0.00	0.06
气管、支气管、肺	C33–C34	23 397	19.39	0.22	0.00	0.07	0.03	0.07	0.57	0.98
其他的胸腔器官	C37–C38	389	0.32	0.00	0.23	0.00	0.00	0.29	0.17	0.12
骨	C40–C41	893	0.74	0.00	0.60	0.90	1.55	1.25	0.34	0.46
皮肤的黑色素瘤	C43	141	0.12	0.00	0.00	0.07	0.03	0.00	0.00	0.03
其他的皮肤	C44	869	0.72	0.00	0.14	0.28	0.03	0.25	0.07	0.15
间皮瘤	C45	43	0.04	0.00	0.00	0.00	0.00	0.07	0.00	0.00
卡波西肉瘤	C46	3	0.00	0.00	0.00	0.00	0.00	0.00	0.00	0.03
周围神经、其他结缔组织、软组织	C47;C49	329	0.27	0.22	0.28	0.24	0.20	0.32	0.07	0.18
乳房	C50	10 265	8.50	0.00	0.00	0.00	0.14	0.91	5.94	9.69
外阴	C51	86	0.07	0.00	0.00	0.00	0.00	0.08	0.00	0.06
阴道	C52	77	0.06	0.00	0.10	0.07	0.00	0.00	0.21	0.00
子宫颈	C53	4 435	3.67	0.00	0.00	0.00	0.00	0.00	1.61	4.85
子宫体	C54	2 292	1.90	0.00	0.00	0.00	0.00	0.08	0.35	1.57
子宫，部位不明	C55	351	0.29	0.00	0.00	0.00	0.07	0.00	0.07	0.13
卵巢	C56	1 701	1.41	0.00	0.20	0.44	0.85	2.27	2.58	2.83
女性其他的生殖器	C57	113	0.09	0.00	0.00	0.07	0.14	0.15	0.14	0.19
胎盘	C58	11	0.01	0.00	0.00	0.00	0.00	0.00	0.21	0.06
阴茎	C60	148	0.12	0.00	0.00	0.00	0.00	0.00	0.00	0.00
前列腺	C61	1 782	1.48	0.00	0.00	0.00	0.00	0.00	0.00	0.06
睾丸	C62	76	0.06	0.43	0.35	0.00	0.00	0.07	0.13	0.24
男性其他的生殖器	C63	24	0.02	0.00	0.00	0.00	0.00	0.07	0.00	0.00
肾	C64	1 563	1.30	0.00	0.51	0.14	0.17	0.21	0.24	0.49
肾盂	C65	132	0.11	0.00	0.00	0.00	0.00	0.00	0.00	0.00
输尿管	C66	195	0.16	0.00	0.00	0.00	0.00	0.00	0.03	0.00
膀胱	C67	1 912	1.58	0.00	0.05	0.00	0.00	0.04	0.13	0.15
其他的泌尿器官	C68	32	0.03	0.00	0.00	0.00	0.00	0.00	0.00	0.00
眼	C69	78	0.06	0.45	0.60	0.24	0.00	0.00	0.00	0.03
脑、神经系统	C70–C72	2 854	2.36	0.89	1.52	2.14	2.02	1.46	1.58	1.66
甲状腺	C73	7 633	6.32	0.00	0.05	0.07	0.63	1.53	4.23	12.76
肾上腺	C74	124	0.10	0.00	0.23	0.00	0.03	0.00	0.00	0.09
其他的内分泌腺	C75	82	0.07	0.00	0.05	0.03	0.03	0.07	0.07	0.03
霍奇金病	C81	137	0.11	0.00	0.00	0.03	0.13	0.04	0.10	0.31
非霍奇金淋巴瘤	C82–C85;C96	1 517	1.26	0.45	0.64	0.55	0.69	0.89	0.87	0.71
免疫增生性疾病	C88	11	0.01	0.00	0.09	0.00	0.00	0.00	0.00	0.03
多发性骨髓瘤	C90	557	0.46	0.00	0.00	0.00	0.00	0.04	0.03	0.00
淋巴样白血病	C91	282	0.23	0.00	1.43	1.24	0.60	0.14	0.20	0.09
髓样白血病	C92–C94	770	0.64	0.00	0.51	0.66	0.69	0.68	0.84	0.43
白血病，未特指	C95	869	0.72	2.90	2.26	1.11	0.96	1.03	0.77	0.92
其他的或未指明部位	O&U	2 647	2.19	2.23	1.52	1.38	0.60	1.36	0.91	1.32
骨髓增殖性疾病	MPD	101	0.08	0.22	0.00	0.00	0.03	0.11	0.07	0.09
骨髓增生异常综合征	MDS	23	0.02	0.00	0.09	0.00	0.03	0.00	0.00	0.03
合计	ALL	120 694	100.00	8.27	11.88	10.16	9.92	12.95	18.96	35.71
C44 以外的部位	ALL but C44	119 825	99.28	8.27	11.74	9.88	9.89	12.70	18.89	35.56

2020 年合计发病主要指标

												粗率	世标率	累积率 (%)	
30~	35~	40~	45~	50~	55~	60~	65~	70~	75~	80~	85+	($1/10^5$)	($1/10^5$)	0~64	0~74
0.12	0.03	0.03	0.03	0.26	0.19	0.43	1.08	1.37	0.72	2.65	2.12	0.22	0.15	0.01	0.02
0.43	0.13	0.57	0.75	0.91	0.97	1.59	1.53	2.65	1.32	3.41	2.12	0.59	0.42	0.03	0.05
0.17	0.19	0.38	0.78	0.94	2.09	1.78	2.89	5.63	5.41	7.20	5.84	0.94	0.64	0.03	0.08
0.43	0.41	0.73	0.63	1.00	1.24	1.49	2.15	2.41	1.20	1.52	2.12	0.64	0.48	0.03	0.06
0.00	0.03	0.10	0.06	0.13	0.35	0.29	0.23	0.56	0.60	0.38	0.53	0.11	0.09	0.01	0.01
0.00	0.16	0.13	0.24	0.39	0.31	0.34	0.68	0.64	1.44	1.33	0.53	0.20	0.14	0.01	0.01
0.40	0.45	0.76	1.14	1.85	2.90	2.07	3.17	3.22	2.40	1.71	2.65	0.97	0.72	0.05	0.08
0.06	0.10	0.13	0.15	0.36	0.70	0.82	1.30	1.77	1.92	2.65	2.12	0.34	0.23	0.01	0.03
0.03	0.06	0.13	0.18	0.39	0.46	0.63	1.25	1.21	1.44	0.95	1.33	0.27	0.19	0.01	0.02
0.29	0.89	1.65	5.69	17.31	35.19	68.84	139.49	185.93	204.94	219.92	229.52	27.07	17.79	0.65	2.28
1.90	3.44	5.46	12.89	29.20	46.21	81.76	146.34	184.08	195.68	216.32	220.50	30.35	20.36	0.91	2.57
0.17	0.19	0.38	1.38	1.88	2.13	3.42	5.83	6.43	5.65	7.96	6.10	1.28	0.88	0.05	0.11
1.67	2.26	3.68	7.17	12.74	17.13	24.78	40.20	47.61	53.85	66.35	57.31	9.71	6.62	0.35	0.79
1.21	1.79	3.40	7.74	13.87	20.61	29.36	48.01	57.98	60.82	70.53	60.50	10.98	7.48	0.39	0.92
0.09	0.13	0.13	0.30	0.52	0.62	0.82	1.36	2.73	1.68	2.46	2.39	0.38	0.26	0.01	0.03
3.08	5.04	11.46	23.48	37.66	51.27	66.48	95.11	112.75	107.34	123.80	152.04	24.44	16.94	1.00	2.04
0.17	0.26	0.73	1.51	3.79	5.95	10.41	20.61	24.77	31.97	40.19	44.05	4.40	2.88	0.12	0.34
0.55	0.70	1.24	2.68	5.19	7.54	11.71	21.91	25.33	29.09	40.19	41.39	4.85	3.24	0.15	0.39
0.12	0.32	0.16	0.33	0.75	1.01	1.35	1.64	1.37	2.28	1.90	2.12	0.47	0.35	0.02	0.04
0.09	0.16	0.35	0.63	2.04	3.67	3.81	6.62	7.64	8.53	3.79	6.10	1.41	0.98	0.05	0.13
3.51	5.13	10.95	27.58	57.88	97.02	146.31	242.02	310.75	339.08	383.34	394.30	54.23	36.36	1.75	4.51
0.49	0.26	0.70	0.96	1.49	1.89	1.88	3.40	2.57	3.13	4.93	2.65	0.90	0.66	0.04	0.07
0.66	0.92	1.14	1.42	2.27	3.36	4.29	6.45	7.56	7.93	10.81	9.29	2.07	1.66	0.10	0.17
0.12	0.10	0.22	0.18	0.32	0.58	0.72	1.53	1.61	1.68	2.09	1.33	0.33	0.23	0.01	0.03
0.32	0.29	0.67	0.87	1.85	2.24	2.84	7.47	9.17	13.94	21.04	33.43	2.01	1.33	0.05	0.13
0.03	0.00	0.00	0.06	0.19	0.23	0.29	0.51	0.32	0.36	0.76	0.00	0.10	0.07	0.00	0.01
0.00	0.00	0.00	0.00	0.00	0.00	0.05	0.06	0.00	0.00	0.00	0.00	0.01	0.01	0.00	0.00
0.72	0.26	0.63	0.84	1.23	1.20	1.83	1.75	2.09	2.52	3.22	2.39	0.76	0.60	0.04	0.06
23.48	40.97	64.05	101.14	121.60	108.06	96.00	110.37	82.22	68.03	61.23	47.84	48.62	35.55	2.86	3.82
0.12	0.20	0.19	0.43	0.46	0.70	0.68	1.57	2.32	1.80	1.72	1.74	0.41	0.27	0.01	0.03
0.06	0.13	0.32	0.55	0.26	0.85	0.87	1.01	1.55	1.13	1.38	1.30	0.36	0.27	0.02	0.03
10.60	18.33	26.21	37.03	50.75	50.34	47.22	44.15	41.26	34.02	29.92	24.35	21.01	15.25	1.23	1.66
2.75	3.72	9.62	17.87	31.90	36.05	25.02	24.88	24.73	14.19	11.01	13.92	10.86	7.74	0.64	0.89
0.70	0.85	1.81	2.50	4.55	4.27	3.88	4.71	2.78	2.48	3.10	3.91	1.66	1.18	0.09	0.13
5.04	4.24	8.13	12.63	16.28	18.33	16.78	19.16	18.08	16.90	13.07	12.18	8.06	6.03	0.45	0.64
0.06	0.33	0.32	0.92	1.12	0.78	1.84	1.46	0.77	1.35	1.03	1.74	0.54	0.40	0.03	0.04
0.12	0.13	0.06	0.00	0.13	0.00	0.00	0.00	0.00	0.00	0.00	0.00	0.05	0.05	0.00	0.00
0.06	0.06	0.19	0.71	1.08	1.08	1.53	2.86	4.19	3.35	5.49	5.44	0.67	0.48	0.02	0.06
0.06	0.06	0.12	0.42	1.59	4.08	14.00	37.88	64.72	88.65	120.81	135.44	8.09	5.45	0.10	0.61
0.68	0.44	0.50	0.59	0.26	0.15	0.48	0.80	0.67	0.77	0.42	0.68	0.34	0.30	0.02	0.03
0.00	0.00	0.00	0.06	0.19	0.23	0.48	0.46	0.17	0.26	1.27	1.36	0.11	0.08	0.01	0.01
0.92	1.43	1.84	3.52	6.51	7.97	8.20	14.72	15.20	15.14	12.13	12.21	3.62	2.61	0.16	0.31
0.12	0.06	0.10	0.21	0.29	0.50	0.67	1.53	1.13	2.40	2.09	2.12	0.31	0.20	0.01	0.02
0.03	0.03	0.13	0.27	0.42	0.54	1.16	2.49	2.09	2.52	5.50	2.12	0.45	0.30	0.01	0.04
0.52	0.54	1.17	1.81	4.34	7.27	10.89	18.29	23.64	30.53	35.64	42.99	4.43	2.94	0.13	0.34
0.03	0.06	0.03	0.06	0.16	0.12	0.10	0.51	0.24	0.12	0.57	0.00	0.07	0.05	0.00	0.01
0.03	0.03	0.10	0.12	0.26	0.35	0.19	0.40	0.97	0.48	0.00	0.53	0.18	0.19	0.01	0.02
2.91	3.09	3.46	5.90	10.34	12.18	13.98	20.66	24.77	26.32	25.97	25.47	6.61	5.08	0.31	0.54
23.24	23.84	26.19	34.56	37.27	41.18	27.14	22.31	13.83	11.78	7.01	5.04	17.69	13.76	1.16	1.34
0.14	0.10	0.29	0.21	0.49	0.54	0.48	0.74	1.29	1.44	1.14	1.33	0.29	0.22	0.01	0.02
0.14	0.13	0.13	0.15	0.36	0.46	0.48	0.23	0.40	1.32	0.38	0.27	0.19	0.15	0.01	0.01
0.29	0.22	0.29	0.30	0.39	0.39	0.63	0.74	1.69	0.96	0.38	0.80	0.32	0.25	0.02	0.03
1.18	1.05	2.22	3.10	4.28	6.77	8.29	12.34	15.52	15.87	15.74	10.08	3.52	2.64	0.16	0.30
0.00	0.00	0.03	0.00	0.00	0.04	0.14	0.11	0.00	0.12	0.00	0.00	0.03	0.03	0.00	0.00
0.12	0.22	0.32	0.93	1.88	2.86	3.57	7.02	6.59	5.29	5.69	4.51	1.29	0.90	0.05	0.12
0.14	0.06	0.29	0.48	0.26	1.04	1.01	1.36	2.98	2.40	0.76	2.92	0.65	0.65	0.03	0.06
0.98	0.96	1.40	1.75	2.59	2.51	3.52	6.17	6.27	6.01	4.93	3.71	1.78	1.43	0.09	0.15
1.15	0.89	1.02	1.26	1.91	2.47	3.62	5.66	6.59	6.73	11.56	6.63	2.01	1.77	0.10	0.16
2.16	2.07	3.17	4.79	7.58	10.13	13.40	19.93	25.82	31.37	40.19	31.58	6.14	4.53	0.25	0.48
0.09	0.06	0.13	0.18	0.32	0.54	0.67	0.79	0.40	0.96	1.14	1.33	0.23	0.18	0.01	0.02
0.06	0.00	0.00	0.03	0.13	0.08	0.05	0.17	0.00	0.12	0.38	0.80	0.05	0.04	0.00	0.00
72.58	92.64	143.19	246.07	389.97	517.77	673.10	1 067.55	1 284.65	1 367.97	1 539.63	1 561.27	279.74	196.11	11.17	22.93
72.26	92.35	142.52	245.20	388.13	515.53	670.26	1 060.08	1 275.48	1 354.03	1 518.58	1 527.84	277.72	194.78	11.12	22.80

表 6-2 河南省肿瘤登记地区

部位	ICD-10	病例数	构成(%)	年龄组						
				0~	1~	5~	10~	15~	20~	25~
唇	C00	58	0.09	0.00	0.09	0.00	0.00	0.07	0.06	0.06
舌	C01–C02	151	0.24	0.00	0.09	0.06	0.00	0.00	0.00	0.24
口	C03–C06	235	0.38	0.00	0.00	0.00	0.06	0.00	0.13	0.06
唾液腺	C07–C08	154	0.25	0.00	0.09	0.00	0.06	0.14	0.19	0.00
扁桃体	C09	30	0.05	0.00	0.00	0.00	0.06	0.07	0.00	0.00
其他的口咽	C10	66	0.11	0.00	0.00	0.00	0.00	0.00	0.06	0.00
鼻咽	C11	285	0.46	0.00	0.09	0.13	0.19	0.34	0.06	0.06
喉咽	C12–C13	121	0.20	0.00	0.09	0.06	0.00	0.00	0.00	0.00
咽，部位不明	C14	78	0.13	0.00	0.00	0.00	0.00	0.00	0.06	0.06
食管	C15	7 239	11.71	0.00	0.09	0.06	0.00	0.00	0.13	0.36
胃	C16	9 147	14.80	0.00	0.09	0.06	0.19	0.20	0.52	0.36
小肠	C17	327	0.53	0.00	0.00	0.00	0.00	0.00	0.00	0.06
结肠	C18	2 252	3.64	0.00	0.00	0.00	0.06	0.27	0.32	0.96
直肠	C19–C20	2 650	4.29	0.00	0.00	0.06	0.00	0.07	0.13	0.72
肛门	C21	88	0.14	0.00	0.00	0.00	0.00	0.00	0.00	0.06
肝脏	C22	7 242	11.71	0.86	0.26	0.13	0.19	0.41	0.45	1.44
胆囊及其他	C23–C24	862	1.39	0.00	0.09	0.00	0.00	0.00	0.00	0.18
胰腺	C25	1 106	1.79	0.00	0.00	0.00	0.12	0.14	0.00	0.24
鼻、鼻窦及其他	C30–C31	119	0.19	0.00	0.09	0.13	0.12	0.20	0.13	0.00
喉	C32	539	0.87	0.00	0.09	0.13	0.00	0.00	0.00	0.12
气管、支气管、肺	C33–C34	15 678	25.36	0.00	0.00	0.06	0.06	0.07	0.65	0.96
其他的胸腔器官	C37–C38	220	0.36	0.00	0.17	0.00	0.00	0.34	0.32	0.12
骨	C40–C41	491	0.79	0.00	0.96	0.97	1.67	1.42	0.19	0.72
皮肤的黑色素瘤	C43	62	0.10	0.00	0.00	0.06	0.06	0.00	0.00	0.00
其他的皮肤	C44	435	0.70	0.00	0.09	0.32	0.00	0.27	0.00	0.18
间皮瘤	C45	26	0.04	0.00	0.00	0.00	0.00	0.14	0.00	0.00
卡波西肉瘤	C46	2	0.00	0.00	0.00	0.00	0.00	0.00	0.00	0.06
周围神经、其他结缔组织、软组织	C47;C49	163	0.26	0.00	0.17	0.06	0.19	0.20	0.13	0.24
乳房	C50	135	0.22	0.00	0.00	0.00	0.00	0.00	0.00	0.06
外阴	C51	0	0.00	0.00	0.00	0.00	0.00	0.00	0.00	0.00
阴道	C52	0	0.00	0.00	0.00	0.00	0.00	0.00	0.00	0.00
子宫颈	C53	1	0.00	0.00	0.00	0.00	0.00	0.00	0.00	0.00
子宫体	C54	0	0.00	0.00	0.00	0.00	0.00	0.00	0.00	0.00
子宫，部位不明	C55	0	0.00	0.00	0.00	0.00	0.00	0.00	0.00	0.00
卵巢	C56	0	0.00	0.00	0.00	0.00	0.00	0.00	0.00	0.00
女性其他的生殖器	C57	0	0.00	0.00	0.00	0.00	0.00	0.00	0.00	0.00
胎盘	C58	0	0.00	0.00	0.00	0.00	0.00	0.00	0.00	0.00
阴茎	C60	148	0.24	0.00	0.00	0.00	0.00	0.00	0.00	0.00
前列腺	C61	1 782	2.88	0.00	0.00	0.00	0.00	0.00	0.00	0.06
睾丸	C62	76	0.12	0.43	0.35	0.00	0.00	0.07	0.13	0.24
男性其他的生殖器	C63	24	0.04	0.00	0.00	0.00	0.00	0.07	0.00	0.00
肾	C64	986	1.59	0.00	0.35	0.13	0.19	0.14	0.13	0.72
肾盂	C65	80	0.13	0.00	0.00	0.00	0.00	0.00	0.00	0.00
输尿管	C66	113	0.18	0.00	0.00	0.00	0.00	0.00	0.06	0.00
膀胱	C67	1 490	2.41	0.00	0.09	0.00	0.00	0.00	0.13	0.12
其他的泌尿器官	C68	17	0.03	0.00	0.00	0.00	0.00	0.00	0.00	0.00
眼	C69	41	0.07	0.86	0.43	0.39	0.00	0.00	0.00	0.00
脑、神经系统	C70–C72	1 409	2.28	0.86	1.48	2.21	2.54	1.42	1.81	1.92
甲状腺	C73	1 797	2.91	0.00	0.09	0.06	0.43	1.22	3.24	6.37
肾上腺	C74	80	0.13	0.00	0.35	0.00	0.06	0.00	0.00	0.06
其他的内分泌腺	C75	45	0.07	0.00	0.09	0.00	0.00	0.07	0.13	0.06
霍奇金病	C81	80	0.13	0.00	0.00	0.06	0.25	0.07	0.13	0.30
非霍奇金淋巴瘤	C82–C85;C96	853	1.38	0.43	0.70	0.84	0.81	1.15	1.10	0.60
免疫增生性疾病	C88	5	0.01	0.00	0.09	0.00	0.00	0.00	0.00	0.06
多发性骨髓瘤	C90	308	0.50	0.00	0.00	0.00	0.00	0.07	0.00	0.00
淋巴样白血病	C91	155	0.25	0.00	1.91	1.10	0.50	0.14	0.19	0.06
髓样白血病	C92–C94	431	0.70	0.00	0.70	0.65	0.74	0.68	0.84	0.42
白血病，未特指	C95	463	0.75	2.57	2.43	1.17	0.93	1.15	0.91	1.44
其他的或未指明部位	O&U	1 400	2.26	1.71	1.65	1.23	0.56	1.76	0.97	1.56
骨髓增殖性疾病	MPD	61	0.10	0.00	0.00	0.00	0.06	0.20	0.06	0.18
骨髓增生异常综合征	MDS	14	0.02	0.00	0.09	0.00	0.06	0.00	0.00	0.06
合计	ALL	61 820	100.00	7.71	13.29	10.19	10.17	12.51	13.41	21.56
C44 以外的部位	ALL but C44	61 385	99.30	7.71	13.21	9.87	10.17	12.24	13.41	21.38

2020 年男性发病主要指标

30~	35~	40~	45~	50~	55~	60~	65~	70~	75~	80~	85+	粗率 (1/10^5)	世标率 (1/10^5)	累积率 (%) 0~64	累积率 (%) 0~74
0.06	0.06	0.06	0.00	0.32	0.23	0.29	1.60	1.84	0.52	3.80	2.72	0.26	0.20	0.01	0.02
0.68	0.12	0.37	1.07	1.15	1.23	1.92	1.60	3.19	0.77	4.65	4.08	0.69	0.52	0.03	0.06
0.23	0.25	0.19	1.07	1.28	2.85	2.01	3.89	7.04	6.18	7.60	4.08	1.07	0.76	0.04	0.10
0.40	0.12	1.00	0.65	1.08	1.31	2.20	2.40	2.18	2.58	2.53	2.72	0.70	0.53	0.04	0.06
0.00	0.00	0.19	0.12	0.13	0.54	0.38	0.23	0.67	0.52	0.42	0.68	0.14	0.10	0.01	0.01
0.00	0.19	0.19	0.30	0.64	0.54	0.38	1.14	1.17	2.58	1.69	1.36	0.30	0.21	0.01	0.02
0.62	0.50	1.19	1.78	2.36	4.54	2.68	3.78	4.19	2.32	2.11	5.44	1.29	0.99	0.07	0.11
0.11	0.00	0.12	0.30	0.70	1.15	1.44	2.17	3.19	3.61	4.22	4.76	0.55	0.40	0.02	0.05
0.06	0.00	0.19	0.30	0.45	0.92	0.96	1.95	2.01	1.80	0.84	0.00	0.35	0.26	0.01	0.03
0.34	0.94	2.06	7.79	23.78	47.04	92.98	182.74	239.94	255.90	277.52	280.42	32.85	23.14	0.88	2.99
1.64	3.30	6.56	15.81	39.41	66.21	122.70	217.64	288.74	288.88	306.24	302.19	41.51	29.52	1.29	3.82
0.23	0.31	0.56	1.55	2.30	2.93	4.31	7.44	7.38	6.70	7.60	6.81	1.48	1.08	0.06	0.14
1.98	2.99	4.25	8.03	14.16	16.63	27.13	41.65	58.02	61.59	71.81	68.06	10.22	7.35	0.38	0.88
1.30	2.12	3.93	8.14	15.49	23.48	33.74	53.32	71.43	75.76	82.37	65.34	12.03	8.60	0.45	1.07
0.17	0.19	0.19	0.30	0.51	0.62	0.96	1.72	2.68	2.58	2.11	0.68	0.40	0.29	0.01	0.04
4.75	7.79	18.48	37.04	57.83	78.38	96.63	127.93	147.72	138.90	137.70	183.77	32.87	24.03	1.52	2.90
0.11	0.37	1.00	1.49	3.25	5.39	10.83	18.99	24.31	32.21	34.64	38.80	3.91	2.76	0.11	0.33
0.51	0.94	1.69	2.91	5.93	8.08	12.65	24.37	30.85	27.83	40.55	45.60	5.02	3.59	0.17	0.44
0.11	0.31	0.19	0.36	1.02	1.15	1.82	1.72	1.68	3.09	2.11	0.68	0.54	0.42	0.03	0.05
0.17	0.25	0.56	1.13	3.44	6.54	7.29	11.44	14.59	16.24	7.60	10.89	2.45	1.77	0.10	0.23
3.51	5.11	10.99	30.85	65.93	128.27	208.69	344.42	469.66	503.29	563.91	567.64	71.15	50.37	2.28	6.35
0.45	0.25	0.94	1.07	1.53	2.23	2.11	4.69	2.52	4.38	4.22	2.04	1.00	0.76	0.05	0.08
0.51	0.62	1.37	1.72	2.23	3.70	5.56	6.52	8.72	10.31	10.98	10.89	2.23	1.86	0.11	0.18
0.11	0.12	0.06	0.24	0.38	0.69	0.58	1.37	0.84	1.55	1.69	2.04	0.28	0.21	0.01	0.02
0.17	0.25	0.87	0.95	1.91	2.39	3.16	7.32	8.38	18.55	22.81	34.71	1.97	1.39	0.05	0.13
0.00	0.00	0.00	0.06	0.19	0.46	0.19	0.57	0.50	0.26	1.27	0.00	0.12	0.09	0.01	0.01
0.00	0.00	0.00	0.00	0.00	0.00	0.00	0.11	0.00	0.00	0.00	0.00	0.01	0.01	0.00	0.00
0.73	0.31	0.44	0.77	1.08	1.39	1.63	1.83	2.68	3.09	3.80	3.40	0.74	0.57	0.04	0.06
0.11	0.25	0.31	0.77	1.08	1.54	1.25	2.52	2.52	2.06	4.65	2.72	0.61	0.44	0.03	0.05
0.00	0.00	0.00	0.00	0.00	0.00	0.00	0.00	0.00	0.00	0.00	0.00	0.00	0.00	0.00	0.00
0.00	0.00	0.00	0.00	0.00	0.00	0.00	0.00	0.00	0.00	0.00	0.00	0.00	0.00	0.00	0.00
0.00	0.00	0.00	0.00	0.00	0.00	0.00	0.11	0.00	0.00	0.00	0.00	0.00	0.00	0.00	0.00
0.00	0.00	0.00	0.00	0.00	0.00	0.00	0.00	0.00	0.00	0.00	0.00	0.00	0.00	0.00	0.00
0.00	0.00	0.00	0.00	0.00	0.00	0.00	0.00	0.00	0.00	0.00	0.00	0.00	0.00	0.00	0.00
0.00	0.00	0.00	0.00	0.00	0.00	0.00	0.00	0.00	0.00	0.00	0.00	0.00	0.00	0.00	0.00
0.00	0.00	0.00	0.00	0.00	0.00	0.00	0.00	0.00	0.00	0.00	0.00	0.00	0.00	0.00	0.00
0.00	0.00	0.00	0.00	0.00	0.00	0.00	0.00	0.00	0.00	0.00	0.00	0.00	0.00	0.00	0.00
0.06	0.06	0.19	0.71	1.08	1.08	1.53	2.86	4.19	3.35	5.49	5.44	0.67	0.48	0.02	0.06
0.06	0.06	0.12	0.42	1.59	4.08	14.00	37.88	64.72	88.65	120.81	135.44	8.09	5.45	0.10	0.61
0.68	0.44	0.50	0.59	0.26	0.15	0.48	0.80	0.67	0.77	0.42	0.68	0.34	0.30	0.02	0.03
0.00	0.00	0.00	0.06	0.19	0.23	0.48	0.46	0.17	0.26	1.27	1.36	0.11	0.08	0.01	0.01
1.07	1.93	2.44	4.34	8.10	9.47	10.83	20.60	21.63	18.55	14.78	13.61	4.47	3.33	0.20	0.41
0.06	0.12	0.19	0.36	0.45	0.77	0.67	1.83	1.01	2.83	2.53	3.40	0.36	0.26	0.01	0.03
0.00	0.00	0.19	0.36	0.57	0.85	1.63	2.86	1.84	3.09	6.34	2.04	0.51	0.36	0.02	0.04
0.62	0.50	1.87	2.50	6.50	10.70	18.02	29.29	40.91	50.51	59.56	87.12	6.76	4.77	0.21	0.56
0.00	0.06	0.06	0.06	0.26	0.08	0.10	0.34	0.50	0.00	0.84	0.00	0.08	0.06	0.00	0.01
0.06	0.06	0.06	0.12	0.26	0.08	0.19	0.57	1.34	0.26	0.00	1.36	0.19	0.19	0.01	0.02
3.34	2.87	3.37	6.06	10.01	11.55	13.23	18.54	28.50	27.83	21.54	25.18	6.39	5.11	0.31	0.54
12.32	11.91	12.05	14.98	14.03	16.48	13.71	10.98	8.22	5.41	5.07	3.40	8.16	6.51	0.53	0.63
0.06	0.06	0.44	0.24	0.77	0.46	0.58	0.92	2.35	2.06	1.69	2.04	0.36	0.29	0.02	0.03
0.11	0.12	0.06	0.06	0.32	0.46	0.58	0.23	0.67	2.58	0.42	0.00	0.20	0.16	0.01	0.01
0.17	0.25	0.25	0.48	0.51	0.31	0.96	0.92	2.01	1.03	0.42	0.68	0.36	0.30	0.02	0.03
1.30	1.25	2.25	3.51	4.21	8.08	10.26	12.47	19.12	19.07	19.43	10.21	3.87	3.01	0.18	0.34
0.00	0.00	0.06	0.00	0.00	0.00	0.00	0.11	0.00	0.26	0.00	0.00	0.02	0.02	0.00	0.00
0.17	0.19	0.25	0.83	2.23	2.69	3.55	9.15	8.38	5.41	5.91	7.49	1.40	1.02	0.05	0.14
0.11	0.06	0.31	0.36	0.38	1.08	1.25	2.06	3.52	2.32	1.27	2.72	0.70	0.72	0.04	0.06
0.96	0.81	1.19	1.66	2.61	2.62	4.12	8.01	8.38	7.99	7.18	5.44	1.96	1.59	0.09	0.17
1.30	0.81	1.06	1.43	1.79	2.54	4.60	5.49	6.87	6.18	12.67	8.17	2.10	1.91	0.11	0.17
1.75	2.74	3.31	4.64	7.78	9.93	13.71	23.46	30.18	32.73	46.89	40.16	6.35	4.88	0.26	0.53
0.17	0.12	0.25	0.12	0.45	0.62	0.67	0.80	0.67	1.29	1.27	0.68	0.28	0.22	0.01	0.02
0.06	0.00	0.00	0.00	0.19	0.08	0.10	0.23	0.00	0.00	0.84	0.68	0.06	0.05	0.00	0.00
43.48	52.11	88.42	170.44	314.10	494.83	761.71	1 268.07	1 664.52	1 756.50	1 948.14	2 009.87	280.56	203.26	10.03	24.69
43.31	51.86	87.54	169.49	312.18	492.44	758.54	1 260.75	1 656.14	1 737.94	1 925.33	1 975.16	278.58	201.87	9.97	24.56

表 6-3 河南省肿瘤登记地区

部位	ICD-10	病例数	构成(%)	年龄组						
				0~	1~	5~	10~	15~	20~	25~
唇	C00	39	0.07	0.00	0.00	0.00	0.00	0.00	0.00	0.00
舌	C01–C02	102	0.17	0.00	0.00	0.07	0.00	0.00	0.00	0.06
口	C03–C06	170	0.29	0.00	0.00	0.15	0.00	0.00	0.14	0.06
唾液腺	C07–C08	123	0.21	0.00	0.00	0.07	0.00	0.15	0.14	0.31
扁桃体	C09	19	0.03	0.00	0.10	0.00	0.00	0.08	0.00	0.00
其他的口咽	C10	22	0.04	0.00	0.00	0.00	0.00	0.08	0.07	0.00
鼻咽	C11	133	0.23	0.00	0.00	0.00	0.07	0.00	0.14	0.13
喉咽	C12–C13	24	0.04	0.00	0.00	0.00	0.00	0.00	0.00	0.00
咽，部位不明	C14	37	0.06	0.00	0.00	0.07	0.07	0.00	0.07	0.06
食管	C15	4 439	7.54	0.00	0.00	0.00	0.00	0.00	0.28	0.44
胃	C16	3 947	6.70	0.00	0.00	0.07	0.21	0.23	0.49	1.13
小肠	C17	226	0.38	0.00	0.00	0.00	0.00	0.00	0.07	0.13
结肠	C18	1 937	3.29	0.00	0.00	0.00	0.00	0.00	0.21	0.69
直肠	C19–C20	2 087	3.54	0.00	0.00	0.00	0.00	0.00	0.28	0.63
肛门	C21	77	0.13	0.00	0.00	0.00	0.00	0.00	0.00	0.00
肝脏	C22	3 303	5.61	0.00	0.10	0.00	0.21	0.15	0.21	0.94
胆囊及其他	C23–C24	1 036	1.76	0.00	0.10	0.00	0.00	0.00	0.07	0.13
胰腺	C25	987	1.68	0.00	0.00	0.15	0.00	0.08	0.07	0.13
鼻、鼻窦及其他	C30–C31	85	0.14	0.00	0.10	0.00	0.07	0.08	0.00	0.06
喉	C32	70	0.12	0.00	0.00	0.00	0.07	0.00	0.00	0.00
气管、支气管、肺	C33–C34	7 719	13.11	0.47	0.00	0.07	0.00	0.08	0.49	1.01
其他的胸腔器官	C37–C38	169	0.29	0.00	0.29	0.00	0.00	0.23	0.00	0.13
骨	C40–C41	402	0.68	0.00	0.20	0.81	1.42	1.06	0.49	0.19
皮肤的黑色素瘤	C43	79	0.13	0.00	0.00	0.07	0.00	0.00	0.00	0.06
其他的皮肤	C44	434	0.74	0.00	0.20	0.22	0.07	0.23	0.14	0.13
间皮瘤	C45	17	0.03	0.00	0.00	0.00	0.00	0.00	0.00	0.00
卡波西肉瘤	C46	1	0.00	0.00	0.00	0.00	0.00	0.00	0.00	0.00
周围神经、其他结缔组织、软组织	C47;C49	166	0.28	0.47	0.39	0.44	0.21	0.45	0.00	0.13
乳房	C50	10 265	17.44	0.00	0.00	0.00	0.14	0.91	5.94	9.69
外阴	C51	86	0.15	0.00	0.00	0.00	0.00	0.08	0.00	0.06
阴道	C52	77	0.13	0.00	0.10	0.07	0.00	0.00	0.21	0.00
子宫颈	C53	4 435	7.53	0.00	0.00	0.00	0.00	0.00	1.61	4.85
子宫体	C54	2 292	3.89	0.00	0.00	0.00	0.00	0.08	0.35	1.57
子宫，部位不明	C55	351	0.60	0.00	0.00	0.00	0.07	0.00	0.07	0.13
卵巢	C56	1 701	2.89	0.00	0.20	0.44	0.85	2.27	2.58	2.83
女性其他的生殖器	C57	113	0.19	0.00	0.00	0.07	0.14	0.15	0.14	0.19
胎盘	C58	11	0.02	0.00	0.00	0.00	0.00	0.00	0.21	0.06
阴茎	C60	0	0.00	0.00	0.00	0.00	0.00	0.00	0.00	0.00
前列腺	C61	1	0.00	0.00	0.00	0.00	0.00	0.00	0.00	0.00
睾丸	C62	1	0.00	0.00	0.00	0.00	0.00	0.00	0.00	0.00
男性其他的生殖器	C63	0	0.00	0.00	0.00	0.00	0.00	0.00	0.00	0.00
肾	C64	577	0.98	0.00	0.69	0.15	0.14	0.30	0.35	0.25
肾盂	C65	52	0.09	0.00	0.00	0.00	0.00	0.00	0.00	0.00
输尿管	C66	82	0.14	0.00	0.00	0.00	0.00	0.00	0.00	0.00
膀胱	C67	422	0.72	0.00	0.00	0.00	0.00	0.08	0.14	0.19
其他的泌尿器官	C68	15	0.03	0.00	0.00	0.00	0.00	0.00	0.00	0.00
眼	C69	37	0.06	0.00	0.78	0.07	0.00	0.00	0.00	0.06
脑、神经系统	C70–C72	1 445	2.45	0.93	1.57	2.07	1.42	1.51	1.33	1.38
甲状腺	C73	5 836	9.91	0.00	0.00	0.07	0.85	1.89	5.31	19.45
肾上腺	C74	44	0.07	0.00	0.10	0.00	0.00	0.00	0.00	0.13
其他的内分泌腺	C75	37	0.06	0.00	0.00	0.07	0.07	0.08	0.00	0.00
霍奇金病	C81	57	0.10	0.00	0.00	0.00	0.00	0.00	0.07	0.31
非霍奇金淋巴瘤	C82–C85;C96	664	1.13	0.47	0.59	0.22	0.57	0.60	0.63	0.82
免疫增生性疾病	C88	6	0.01	0.00	0.10	0.00	0.00	0.00	0.00	0.00
多发性骨髓瘤	C90	249	0.42	0.00	0.00	0.00	0.00	0.00	0.07	0.00
淋巴样白血病	C91	127	0.22	0.00	0.88	1.40	0.71	0.15	0.21	0.13
髓样白血病	C92–C94	339	0.58	0.00	0.29	0.66	0.64	0.68	0.84	0.44
白血病，未特指	C95	406	0.69	3.27	2.06	1.03	0.99	0.91	0.63	0.38
其他的或未指明部位	O&U	1 247	2.12	2.80	1.37	1.55	0.64	0.91	0.84	1.07
骨髓增殖性疾病	MPD	40	0.07	0.47	0.00	0.00	0.00	0.00	0.07	0.00
骨髓增生异常综合征	MDS	9	0.02	0.00	0.10	0.00	0.00	0.00	0.00	0.00
合计	ALL	58 874	100.00	8.87	10.29	10.12	9.64	13.46	24.94	50.54
C44 以外的部位	ALL but C44	58 440	99.26	8.87	10.09	9.90	9.57	13.23	24.80	50.42

2020 年女性发病主要指标

30~	35~	40~	45~	50~	55~	60~	65~	70~	75~	80~	85+	粗率 (1/10⁵)	世标率 (1/10⁵)	累积率 (%) 0~64	0~74
0.18	0.00	0.00	0.06	0.20	0.16	0.58	0.56	0.93	0.90	1.72	1.74	0.18	0.12	0.01	0.01
0.18	0.13	0.77	0.43	0.66	0.70	1.26	1.46	2.16	1.80	2.41	0.87	0.48	0.34	0.02	0.04
0.12	0.13	0.58	0.49	0.59	1.32	1.55	1.90	4.33	4.73	6.88	6.96	0.81	0.51	0.03	0.06
0.47	0.72	0.45	0.61	0.92	1.17	0.78	1.90	2.63	0.00	0.69	1.74	0.58	0.44	0.03	0.05
0.00	0.07	0.00	0.00	0.13	0.16	0.19	0.22	0.46	0.68	0.34	0.43	0.09	0.07	0.00	0.01
0.00	0.13	0.06	0.18	0.13	0.08	0.29	0.22	0.15	0.45	1.03	0.00	0.10	0.08	0.01	0.01
0.18	0.39	0.32	0.49	1.32	1.24	1.45	2.58	2.32	2.48	1.38	0.87	0.63	0.44	0.03	0.05
0.00	0.20	0.13	0.00	0.00	0.23	0.19	0.45	0.46	0.45	1.38	0.43	0.11	0.07	0.00	0.01
0.00	0.13	0.06	0.06	0.33	0.00	0.29	0.56	0.46	1.13	1.03	2.17	0.18	0.12	0.01	0.01
0.23	0.85	1.23	3.54	10.61	23.23	44.41	97.15	136.15	160.39	173.01	197.00	21.03	12.74	0.42	1.59
2.17	3.59	4.33	9.88	18.65	26.02	40.34	76.53	87.63	114.21	143.09	168.30	18.70	11.71	0.54	1.36
0.12	0.07	0.19	1.22	1.45	1.32	2.52	4.26	5.56	4.73	8.26	5.65	1.07	0.69	0.04	0.08
1.35	1.50	3.10	6.28	11.27	17.63	22.40	38.77	38.02	47.08	61.91	50.45	9.18	5.93	0.32	0.71
1.11	1.44	2.84	7.32	12.19	17.71	24.92	42.80	45.59	47.76	60.88	57.40	9.89	6.42	0.34	0.78
0.00	0.07	0.06	0.31	0.53	0.62	0.68	1.01	2.78	0.90	2.75	3.48	0.36	0.23	0.01	0.03
1.35	2.15	4.20	9.58	16.81	23.93	35.98	62.97	80.52	79.74	112.48	131.77	15.65	9.93	0.48	1.20
0.23	0.13	0.45	1.53	4.35	6.53	9.99	22.19	25.19	31.76	44.72	47.40	4.91	2.99	0.12	0.35
0.59	0.46	0.77	2.44	4.42	6.99	10.76	19.50	20.25	30.19	39.90	38.70	4.68	2.91	0.13	0.33
0.12	0.33	0.13	0.31	0.46	0.85	0.87	1.57	1.08	1.58	1.72	3.04	0.40	0.28	0.02	0.03
0.00	0.07	0.13	0.12	0.59	0.78	0.29	1.90	1.24	1.80	0.69	3.04	0.33	0.22	0.01	0.03
3.51	5.15	10.91	24.22	49.56	65.49	83.20	141.74	164.28	195.53	236.30	283.54	36.56	23.29	1.22	2.75
0.53	0.26	0.45	0.85	1.45	1.55	1.65	2.13	2.63	2.03	5.50	3.04	0.80	0.57	0.04	0.06
0.82	1.24	0.90	1.10	2.31	3.03	3.01	6.39	6.49	5.86	10.66	8.26	1.90	1.45	0.08	0.15
0.12	0.07	0.39	0.12	0.26	0.47	0.87	1.68	2.32	1.80	2.41	0.87	0.37	0.25	0.01	0.03
0.47	0.33	0.45	0.79	1.78	2.10	2.52	7.62	9.89	9.91	19.61	32.62	2.06	1.27	0.05	0.13
0.06	0.00	0.00	0.06	0.20	0.00	0.39	0.45	0.15	0.45	0.34	0.00	0.08	0.06	0.00	0.01
0.00	0.00	0.00	0.00	0.00	0.00	0.10	0.00	0.00	0.00	0.00	0.00	0.00	0.00	0.00	0.00
0.70	0.20	0.84	0.92	1.38	1.01	2.04	1.68	1.55	2.03	2.75	1.74	0.79	0.64	0.04	0.06
23.48	40.97	64.05	101.14	121.60	108.06	96.00	110.37	82.22	68.03	61.23	47.84	48.62	35.55	2.86	3.82
0.12	0.20	0.19	0.43	0.46	0.70	0.68	1.57	2.32	1.80	1.72	1.74	0.41	0.27	0.01	0.03
0.06	0.13	0.32	0.55	0.26	0.85	0.87	1.01	1.55	1.13	1.38	1.30	0.36	0.27	0.02	0.03
10.60	18.33	26.21	37.03	50.75	50.34	47.22	44.15	41.26	34.02	29.92	24.35	21.01	15.25	1.23	1.66
2.75	3.72	9.62	17.87	31.90	36.05	25.02	24.88	24.73	14.19	11.01	13.92	10.86	7.74	0.64	0.89
0.70	0.85	1.81	2.50	4.55	4.27	3.88	4.71	2.78	2.48	3.10	3.91	1.66	1.18	0.09	0.13
5.04	4.24	8.13	12.63	16.28	18.33	16.78	19.16	18.08	16.90	13.07	12.18	8.06	6.03	0.45	0.64
0.06	0.33	0.32	0.92	1.12	0.78	1.84	1.46	0.77	1.35	1.03	1.74	0.54	0.40	0.03	0.04
0.12	0.13	0.06	0.00	0.13	0.00	0.00	0.00	0.00	0.00	0.00	0.00	0.05	0.05	0.00	0.00
0.00	0.00	0.00	0.00	0.00	0.00	0.00	0.00	0.00	0.00	0.00	0.00	0.00	0.00	0.00	0.00
0.00	0.00	0.00	0.06	0.00	0.00	0.00	0.00	0.00	0.00	0.00	0.00	0.00	0.00	0.00	0.00
0.00	0.00	0.00	0.00	0.00	0.00	0.00	0.00	0.00	0.23	0.00	0.00	0.00	0.00	0.00	0.00
0.00	0.00	0.00	0.00	0.00	0.00	0.00	0.00	0.00	0.00	0.00	0.00	0.00	0.00	0.00	0.00
0.76	0.91	1.23	2.68	4.88	6.45	5.53	8.96	9.27	12.16	9.97	11.31	2.73	1.91	0.12	0.21
0.18	0.00	0.00	0.06	0.13	0.23	0.68	1.23	1.24	2.03	1.72	1.30	0.25	0.15	0.01	0.02
0.06	0.07	0.06	0.18	0.26	0.23	0.68	2.13	2.32	2.03	4.82	2.17	0.39	0.24	0.01	0.03
0.41	0.59	0.45	1.10	2.11	3.81	3.68	7.51	7.73	13.07	16.17	14.79	2.00	1.26	0.06	0.14
0.06	0.07	0.00	0.06	0.07	0.16	0.10	0.67	0.00	0.23	0.34	0.00	0.07	0.05	0.00	0.01
0.00	0.00	0.13	0.12	0.26	0.62	0.19	0.22	0.62	0.68	0.00	0.00	0.18	0.18	0.01	0.01
2.46	3.33	3.55	5.73	10.68	12.82	14.74	22.75	21.33	25.00	29.58	25.66	6.84	5.04	0.31	0.53
34.55	36.34	40.80	54.66	61.29	66.11	40.73	33.39	19.01	17.35	8.60	6.09	27.64	21.18	1.81	2.07
0.23	0.13	0.13	0.18	0.20	0.62	0.39	0.56	0.31	0.90	0.69	0.87	0.21	0.15	0.01	0.01
0.18	0.13	0.19	0.24	0.40	0.47	0.39	0.22	0.15	0.23	0.34	0.43	0.18	0.14	0.01	0.01
0.41	0.20	0.32	0.12	0.26	0.47	0.29	0.56	1.39	0.90	0.34	0.87	0.27	0.20	0.01	0.02
1.05	0.85	2.20	2.68	4.35	5.44	6.30	12.21	12.21	13.07	12.73	10.00	3.15	2.26	0.13	0.25
0.00	0.00	0.00	0.00	0.00	0.08	0.29	0.11	0.00	0.00	0.00	0.00	0.03	0.03	0.00	0.00
0.06	0.26	0.39	1.04	1.52	3.03	3.59	4.93	4.95	5.18	5.50	2.61	1.18	0.79	0.05	0.10
0.18	0.07	0.26	0.61	0.13	1.01	0.78	0.67	2.47	2.48	0.34	3.04	0.60	0.59	0.03	0.05
1.00	1.11	1.61	1.83	2.57	2.41	2.91	4.37	4.33	4.28	3.10	2.61	1.61	1.28	0.08	0.13
1.00	0.98	0.97	1.10	2.04	2.41	2.62	5.83	6.34	7.21	10.66	5.65	1.92	1.63	0.09	0.15
2.58	1.37	3.03	4.94	7.38	10.33	13.09	16.47	21.79	30.19	34.74	26.09	5.91	4.20	0.25	0.44
0.00	0.00	0.00	0.24	0.20	0.47	0.68	0.78	0.15	0.68	1.03	1.74	0.19	0.13	0.01	0.01
0.06	0.00	0.00	0.06	0.07	0.08	0.00	0.11	0.00	0.23	0.00	0.87	0.04	0.03	0.00	0.00
102.72	135.05	199.82	323.67	468.40	540.91	583.48	871.19	934.53	1 028.35	1 206.97	1 274.64	278.88	191.92	12.36	21.39
102.25	134.72	199.37	322.88	466.62	538.82	580.95	863.57	924.64	1 018.44	1 187.37	1 242.03	276.82	190.65	12.32	21.26

表 6-4 河南省城市肿瘤登记地区

部位	ICD-10	病例数	构成 (%)	年龄组						
				0~	1~	5~	10~	15~	20~	25~
唇	C00	35	0.10	0.00	0.00	0.00	0.00	0.00	0.13	0.00
舌	C01–C02	97	0.26	0.00	0.16	0.13	0.00	0.00	0.00	0.11
口	C03–C06	142	0.39	0.00	0.00	0.00	0.13	0.00	0.25	0.00
唾液腺	C07–C08	69	0.19	0.00	0.00	0.00	0.00	0.00	0.13	0.22
扁桃体	C09	17	0.05	0.00	0.00	0.00	0.00	0.00	0.00	0.00
其他的口咽	C10	30	0.08	0.00	0.00	0.00	0.00	0.14	0.00	0.00
鼻咽	C11	107	0.29	0.00	0.00	0.00	0.00	0.14	0.13	0.00
喉咽	C12–C13	71	0.19	0.00	0.16	0.00	0.00	0.00	0.00	0.00
咽，部位不明	C14	28	0.08	0.00	0.00	0.00	0.13	0.00	0.00	0.00
食管	C15	2 211	6.03	0.00	0.16	0.00	0.00	0.00	0.13	0.22
胃	C16	3 126	8.52	0.00	0.00	0.00	0.26	0.00	0.25	0.32
小肠	C17	174	0.47	0.00	0.00	0.00	0.00	0.00	0.00	0.00
结肠	C18	1 652	4.50	0.00	0.00	0.00	0.00	0.27	0.38	0.32
直肠	C19–C20	1 534	4.18	0.00	0.00	0.00	0.00	0.00	0.00	0.43
肛门	C21	30	0.08	0.00	0.00	0.00	0.00	0.00	0.00	0.00
肝脏	C22	2 723	7.42	0.00	0.33	0.00	0.13	0.14	0.00	0.75
胆囊及其他	C23–C24	627	1.71	0.00	0.00	0.00	0.00	0.00	0.00	0.11
胰腺	C25	757	2.06	0.00	0.00	0.13	0.00	0.00	0.00	0.32
鼻、鼻窦及其他	C30–C31	57	0.16	0.00	0.33	0.00	0.00	0.14	0.13	0.00
喉	C32	208	0.57	0.00	0.00	0.00	0.00	0.00	0.00	0.00
气管、支气管、肺	C33–C34	6 861	18.70	0.78	0.00	0.00	0.00	0.00	0.13	1.08
其他的胸腔器官	C37–C38	113	0.31	0.00	0.33	0.00	0.00	0.41	0.13	0.00
骨	C40–C41	208	0.57	0.00	0.49	1.17	1.42	0.95	0.38	0.22
皮肤的黑色素瘤	C43	61	0.17	0.00	0.00	0.13	0.13	0.00	0.00	0.00
其他的皮肤	C44	280	0.76	0.00	0.16	0.13	0.00	0.00	0.00	0.11
间皮瘤	C45	10	0.03	0.00	0.00	0.00	0.00	0.14	0.00	0.00
卡波西肉瘤	C46	0	0.00	0.00	0.00	0.00	0.00	0.00	0.00	0.00
周围神经、其他结缔组织、软组织	C47;C49	122	0.33	0.78	0.33	0.39	0.39	0.00	0.00	0.11
乳房	C50	3 572	9.74	0.00	0.00	0.00	0.27	0.57	2.03	7.54
外阴	C51	32	0.09	0.00	0.00	0.00	0.00	0.28	0.00	0.00
阴道	C52	22	0.06	0.00	0.00	0.27	0.00	0.00	0.00	0.00
子宫颈	C53	1 226	3.34	0.00	0.00	0.00	0.00	0.00	1.01	2.51
子宫体	C54	694	1.89	0.00	0.00	0.00	0.00	0.28	0.00	1.05
子宫，部位不明	C55	86	0.23	0.00	0.00	0.00	0.00	0.00	0.00	0.00
卵巢	C56	501	1.37	0.00	0.00	0.27	0.55	1.13	1.01	2.09
女性其他的生殖器	C57	34	0.09	0.00	0.00	0.00	0.27	0.00	0.25	0.00
胎盘	C58	4	0.01	0.00	0.00	0.00	0.00	0.00	0.00	0.21
阴茎	C60	39	0.11	0.00	0.00	0.00	0.00	0.00	0.00	0.00
前列腺	C61	757	2.06	0.00	0.00	0.00	0.00	0.00	0.00	0.00
睾丸	C62	17	0.05	0.00	0.00	0.00	0.00	0.26	0.25	0.66
男性其他的生殖器	C63	13	0.04	0.00	0.00	0.00	0.00	0.26	0.00	0.00
肾	C64	571	1.56	0.00	0.33	0.26	0.00	0.14	0.38	0.11
肾盂	C65	47	0.13	0.00	0.00	0.00	0.00	0.00	0.00	0.00
输尿管	C66	78	0.21	0.00	0.00	0.00	0.00	0.00	0.13	0.00
膀胱	C67	704	1.92	0.00	0.00	0.00	0.00	0.00	0.00	0.11
其他的泌尿器官	C68	11	0.03	0.00	0.00	0.00	0.00	0.00	0.00	0.00
眼	C69	22	0.06	1.56	0.49	0.39	0.00	0.00	0.00	0.00
脑、神经系统	C70–C72	722	1.97	0.00	2.31	1.95	1.55	0.68	1.63	1.51
甲状腺	C73	3 614	9.85	0.00	0.00	0.00	0.39	2.03	5.77	20.98
肾上腺	C74	45	0.12	0.00	0.66	0.00	0.00	0.00	0.00	0.11
其他的内分泌腺	C75	31	0.08	0.00	0.00	0.00	0.13	0.00	0.00	0.11
霍奇金病	C81	53	0.14	0.00	0.00	0.00	0.26	0.00	0.25	0.22
非霍奇金淋巴瘤	C82–C85;C96	583	1.59	0.00	0.33	0.52	0.90	1.22	0.88	0.32
免疫增生性疾病	C88	1	0.00	0.00	0.00	0.00	0.00	0.00	0.00	0.11
多发性骨髓瘤	C90	217	0.59	0.00	0.00	0.00	0.00	0.00	0.00	0.00
淋巴样白血病	C91	109	0.30	0.00	2.14	1.82	0.64	0.27	0.38	0.11
髓样白血病	C92–C94	262	0.71	0.00	0.99	0.26	0.77	0.68	1.26	0.22
白血病，未特指	C95	226	0.62	1.56	2.63	1.30	1.42	0.68	0.38	0.22
其他的或未指明部位	O&U	961	2.62	6.26	0.82	1.56	0.26	1.49	0.38	1.29
骨髓增殖性疾病	MPD	48	0.13	0.00	0.00	0.00	0.13	0.27	0.13	0.11
骨髓增生异常综合征	MDS	3	0.01	0.00	0.00	0.00	0.00	0.00	0.00	0.00
合计	ALL	36 690	100.00	10.95	13.17	10.42	9.54	11.11	15.94	37.01
C44 以外的部位	ALL but C44	36 410	99.24	10.95	13.01	10.29	9.54	11.11	15.94	36.90

2020 年合计发病主要指标

30~	35~	40~	45~	50~	55~	60~	65~	70~	75~	80~	85+	粗率 $(1/10^5)$	世标率 $(1/10^5)$	累积率 (%)	
														0~64	0~74
0.10	0.00	0.10	0.00	0.22	0.00	1.02	1.02	1.38	1.16	3.46	4.56	0.28	0.18	0.01	0.02
0.41	0.21	0.72	0.96	0.90	1.71	2.39	2.24	2.48	1.55	4.61	3.65	0.79	0.56	0.04	0.06
0.21	0.00	0.41	0.68	0.90	2.11	3.07	3.05	7.16	6.21	7.49	12.77	1.16	0.76	0.04	0.09
0.51	0.21	0.83	0.29	1.12	0.92	1.02	1.22	2.75	0.78	2.88	1.82	0.56	0.39	0.03	0.05
0.00	0.00	0.00	0.19	0.22	0.66	0.68	0.20	0.55	0.00	0.00	0.91	0.14	0.10	0.01	0.01
0.00	0.00	0.21	0.29	0.56	0.53	0.17	0.61	1.38	1.55	1.15	0.00	0.24	0.16	0.01	0.02
0.31	0.32	0.83	1.06	2.02	2.63	2.05	3.05	2.48	1.55	0.58	0.91	0.87	0.63	0.05	0.07
0.00	0.32	0.21	0.29	0.56	1.84	1.70	1.83	2.48	1.94	3.46	3.65	0.58	0.39	0.03	0.05
0.00	0.00	0.10	0.19	0.22	0.40	0.51	1.63	0.55	1.16	1.15	0.91	0.23	0.16	0.01	0.02
0.21	0.11	1.34	3.38	10.86	24.89	45.35	88.83	118.37	118.79	157.24	144.12	17.99	11.43	0.43	1.47
1.95	2.99	4.33	9.94	22.73	36.61	72.97	119.53	155.26	145.96	166.46	183.34	25.43	16.64	0.76	2.14
0.10	0.00	0.41	1.74	1.90	2.11	3.58	4.88	7.71	6.60	9.79	10.03	1.42	0.92	0.05	0.11
1.64	2.57	3.51	8.78	12.65	23.04	33.25	55.50	62.77	71.43	111.74	106.72	13.44	8.68	0.43	1.02
0.92	1.82	4.33	8.30	13.77	23.83	36.66	51.63	60.01	59.00	89.85	70.23	12.48	8.20	0.45	1.01
0.10	0.11	0.00	0.19	0.34	0.40	0.51	0.00	1.93	1.16	2.88	1.82	0.24	0.15	0.01	0.02
2.47	4.17	10.63	18.43	31.69	50.83	59.67	81.92	94.15	93.16	107.71	149.59	22.15	14.82	0.90	1.78
0.10	0.11	1.03	1.45	3.14	6.32	11.59	20.94	26.43	35.32	54.14	64.76	5.10	3.15	0.12	0.36
0.31	0.64	1.44	2.60	5.15	10.27	15.17	23.38	30.83	32.22	62.78	64.76	6.16	3.89	0.18	0.45
0.21	0.21	0.00	0.19	0.56	0.79	0.68	2.03	1.93	2.72	2.88	2.74	0.46	0.33	0.02	0.04
0.10	0.00	0.52	0.68	2.69	4.61	5.97	6.30	7.71	8.93	6.34	7.30	1.69	1.14	0.07	0.14
4.32	6.63	11.45	28.07	58.34	103.89	160.94	236.62	286.58	301.23	378.99	410.46	55.82	36.44	1.87	4.49
0.21	0.11	1.13	0.77	1.68	1.84	1.53	3.66	3.03	3.88	3.46	1.82	0.92	0.67	0.04	0.07
0.21	0.53	1.03	1.25	1.34	2.11	4.09	3.86	6.88	6.99	9.22	11.86	1.69	1.35	0.08	0.13
0.21	0.21	0.41	0.19	0.45	0.79	0.85	2.03	2.75	1.94	4.03	1.82	0.50	0.34	0.02	0.04
0.41	0.43	1.03	0.87	1.34	2.37	3.92	7.32	11.01	13.59	26.49	36.49	2.28	1.41	0.05	0.15
0.10	0.00	0.00	0.00	0.11	0.13	0.17	0.41	0.00	0.00	1.73	0.00	0.08	0.06	0.00	0.01
0.00	0.00	0.00	0.00	0.00	0.00	0.00	0.00	0.00	0.00	0.00	0.00	0.00	0.00	0.00	0.00
0.92	0.32	0.72	0.96	1.01	1.45	3.07	3.05	1.93	4.66	5.18	1.82	0.99	0.75	0.05	0.07
26.10	42.71	71.27	115.64	135.23	130.47	133.05	124.22	97.05	83.21	104.18	53.40	58.00	40.77	3.32	4.43
0.00	0.21	0.41	0.38	0.45	0.79	1.01	1.18	3.63	2.13	2.22	4.71	0.52	0.34	0.02	0.04
0.00	0.00	0.00	0.58	0.23	0.79	1.01	1.58	2.08	1.42	1.11	0.00	0.36	0.25	0.01	0.03
9.56	17.71	25.53	30.79	42.60	48.73	49.64	41.80	42.55	29.16	31.03	20.42	19.91	14.02	1.14	1.56
3.19	3.96	9.80	15.59	32.68	33.54	28.03	27.60	26.47	17.07	11.08	20.42	11.27	7.84	0.64	0.91
0.40	0.21	2.04	0.77	3.83	4.45	4.05	5.52	1.56	0.71	2.22	4.71	1.40	0.98	0.08	0.11
3.98	3.54	9.19	12.89	17.81	17.03	18.24	20.90	15.57	13.51	19.95	20.42	8.13	5.78	0.44	0.62
0.00	0.42	0.20	0.58	1.35	0.52	2.03	1.58	1.04	1.42	2.22	3.14	0.55	0.40	0.03	0.04
0.00	0.42	0.00	0.00	0.23	0.00	0.00	0.00	0.00	0.00	0.00	0.00	0.06	0.05	0.00	0.00
0.21	0.22	0.00	0.58	0.67	0.53	1.03	2.52	5.86	1.71	6.00	6.53	0.64	0.43	0.02	0.06
0.00	0.00	0.21	0.00	2.00	6.62	19.28	51.19	95.57	109.39	178.68	226.29	12.34	7.71	0.14	0.87
0.64	0.44	0.42	0.19	0.00	0.00	0.34	0.84	0.00	0.00	0.00	2.18	0.28	0.25	0.02	0.02
0.00	0.00	0.00	0.19	0.45	0.79	0.69	0.00	0.00	0.85	2.40	2.18	0.21	0.15	0.01	0.01
1.03	1.39	1.55	4.24	7.50	11.19	11.42	18.30	21.20	18.63	15.55	17.33	4.65	3.21	0.20	0.39
0.21	0.11	0.10	0.10	0.22	0.53	1.36	2.03	1.10	3.11	2.30	1.82	0.38	0.25	0.01	0.03
0.00	0.11	0.10	0.10	0.45	0.53	1.53	2.64	3.58	3.49	9.79	4.56	0.63	0.39	0.01	0.05
0.51	0.32	1.03	2.12	5.15	9.35	15.17	19.51	30.83	35.71	46.65	69.32	5.73	3.63	0.17	0.42
0.00	0.00	0.10	0.00	0.22	0.13	0.17	0.61	0.00	0.39	1.15	0.00	0.09	0.06	0.00	0.01
0.00	0.11	0.00	0.00	0.11	0.53	0.17	0.41	0.83	0.78	0.00	0.00	0.18	0.20	0.01	0.02
1.85	2.46	4.33	4.92	8.51	9.74	12.96	17.08	20.92	23.68	27.65	18.24	5.87	4.42	0.27	0.46
41.11	45.64	46.21	53.74	55.43	62.15	44.33	31.71	22.02	14.36	9.79	5.47	29.40	22.20	1.89	2.16
0.21	0.11	0.31	0.39	0.56	0.79	0.17	0.81	0.83	1.55	1.73	3.65	0.37	0.28	0.02	0.02
0.10	0.11	0.00	0.39	0.34	0.66	0.68	0.20	0.55	3.11	0.00	0.00	0.25	0.17	0.01	0.02
0.41	0.43	0.52	0.19	0.67	0.53	0.34	1.02	2.20	0.78	1.15	2.74	0.43	0.32	0.02	0.04
1.13	1.07	3.30	3.67	5.49	8.56	12.79	17.89	21.47	19.41	22.46	14.59	4.74	3.40	0.20	0.40
0.00	0.00	0.00	0.00	0.00	0.00	0.00	0.00	0.00	0.00	0.00	0.00	0.01	0.01	0.00	0.00
0.10	0.11	0.31	1.45	2.24	3.56	4.09	8.54	8.81	7.76	10.94	11.86	1.77	1.16	0.06	0.15
0.21	0.11	0.10	0.68	0.34	1.19	1.19	2.24	2.75	4.27	1.15	6.38	0.89	0.90	0.04	0.07
1.03	0.64	2.06	1.06	2.69	3.03	4.43	7.32	8.81	6.60	10.37	7.30	2.13	1.64	0.09	0.18
0.92	0.64	0.72	0.77	1.68	1.84	3.41	3.66	5.78	7.38	15.55	11.86	1.84	1.57	0.08	0.13
2.26	1.82	4.54	4.44	8.96	12.77	17.73	25.00	34.96	41.54	53.57	43.78	7.82	5.46	0.30	0.60
0.00	0.11	0.31	0.29	0.78	0.40	0.68	1.42	1.10	1.94	1.73	2.74	0.39	0.29	0.02	0.03
0.00	0.00	0.00	0.00	0.11	0.00	0.17	0.00	0.00	0.00	0.58	0.00	0.02	0.02	0.00	0.00
89.82	113.19	172.68	259.90	396.31	557.92	736.52	1 030.43	1 237.43	1 251.13	1 639.23	1 695.64	298.49	203.25	12.12	23.46
89.41	112.76	171.65	259.03	394.97	555.55	732.60	1 023.11	1 226.42	1 237.54	1 612.74	1 659.16	296.21	201.84	12.06	23.31

表 6-5 河南省城市肿瘤登记地区

部位	ICD-10	病例数	构成 (%)	年龄组						
				0~	1~	5~	10~	15~	20~	25~
唇	C00	22	0.12	0	0.00	0.00	0.00	0.00	0.25	0.00
舌	C01–C02	61	0.33	0	0.31	0.00	0.00	0.00	0.00	0.22
口	C03–C06	81	0.44	0	0.00	0.00	0.24	0.00	0.25	0.00
唾液腺	C07–C08	38	0.21	0	0.00	0.00	0.00	0.00	0.00	0.00
扁桃体	C09	14	0.08	0	0.00	0.00	0.00	0.00	0.00	0.00
其他的口咽	C10	24	0.13	0	0.00	0.00	0.00	0.00	0.00	0.00
鼻咽	C11	79	0.43	0	0.00	0.00	0.00	0.26	0.25	0.00
喉咽	C12–C13	60	0.33	0	0.31	0.00	0.00	0.00	0.00	0.00
咽，部位不明	C14	22	0.12	0	0.00	0.00	0.00	0.00	0.00	0.00
食管	C15	1 436	7.85	0	0.31	0.00	0.00	0.00	0.25	0.22
胃	C16	2 240	12.25	0	0.00	0.00	0.49	0.00	0.25	0.00
小肠	C17	99	0.54	0	0.00	0.00	0.00	0.00	0.00	0.00
结肠	C18	892	4.88	0	0.00	0.00	0.00	0.52	0.50	0.22
直肠	C19–C20	886	4.85	0	0.00	0.00	0.00	0.00	0.00	0.00
肛门	C21	10	0.05	0	0.00	0.00	0.00	0.00	0.00	0.00
肝脏	C22	1 936	10.59	0	0.31	0.00	0.24	0.00	0.00	1.11
胆囊及其他	C23–C24	301	1.65	0	0.00	0.00	0.00	0.00	0.00	0.22
胰腺	C25	399	2.18	0	0.00	0.00	0.00	0.00	0.00	0.22
鼻、鼻窦及其他	C30–C31	31	0.17	0	0.31	0.00	0.00	0.26	0.25	0.00
喉	C32	192	1.05	0	0.00	0.00	0.00	0.00	0.00	0.00
气管、支气管、肺	C33–C34	4 479	24.50	0	0.00	0.00	0.00	0.00	0.00	0.44
其他的胸腔器官	C37–C38	70	0.38	0	0.31	0.00	0.00	0.26	0.25	0.00
骨	C40–C41	124	0.68	0	0.63	0.99	1.21	1.04	0.00	0.44
皮肤的黑色素瘤	C43	25	0.14	0	0.00	0.25	0.24	0.00	0.00	0.00
其他的皮肤	C44	131	0.72	0	0.31	0.00	0.00	0.00	0.00	0.00
间皮瘤	C45	8	0.04	0	0.00	0.00	0.00	0.26	0.00	0.00
卡波西肉瘤	C46	0	0.00	0	0.00	0.00	0.00	0.00	0.00	0.00
周围神经、其他结缔组织、软组织	C47;C49	57	0.31	0	0.31	0.00	0.49	0.00	0.00	0.22
乳房	C50	35	0.19	0	0.00	0.00	0.00	0.00	0.00	0.00
外阴	C51	0	0.00	0	0.00	0.00	0.00	0.00	0.00	0.00
阴道	C52	0	0.00	0	0.00	0.00	0.00	0.00	0.00	0.00
子宫颈	C53	0	0.00	0	0.00	0.00	0.00	0.00	0.00	0.00
子宫体	C54	0	0.00	0	0.00	0.00	0.00	0.00	0.00	0.00
子宫，部位不明	C55	0	0.00	0	0.00	0.00	0.00	0.00	0.00	0.00
卵巢	C56	0	0.00	0	0.00	0.00	0.00	0.00	0.00	0.00
女性其他的生殖器	C57	0	0.00	0	0.00	0.00	0.00	0.00	0.00	0.00
胎盘	C58	0	0.00	0	0.00	0.00	0.00	0.00	0.00	0.00
阴茎	C60	39	0.21	0	0.00	0.00	0.00	0.00	0.00	0.00
前列腺	C61	757	4.14	0	0.00	0.00	0.00	0.00	0.00	0.00
睾丸	C62	17	0.09	0	0.00	0.00	0.00	0.26	0.25	0.66
男性其他的生殖器	C63	13	0.07	0	0.00	0.00	0.00	0.26	0.00	0.00
肾	C64	371	2.03	0	0.00	0.00	0.00	0.26	0.00	0.00
肾盂	C65	30	0.16	0	0.00	0.00	0.00	0.00	0.00	0.00
输尿管	C66	41	0.22	0	0.00	0.00	0.00	0.00	0.25	0.00
膀胱	C67	562	3.07	0	0.00	0.00	0.00	0.00	0.00	0.22
其他的泌尿器官	C68	6	0.03	0	0.00	0.00	0.00	0.00	0.00	0.00
眼	C69	13	0.07	3	0.31	0.74	0.00	0.00	0.00	0.00
脑、神经系统	C70–C72	359	1.96	0	3.15	1.74	1.94	0.78	1.74	1.33
甲状腺	C73	913	4.99	0	0.00	0.00	0.24	2.34	4.73	12.40
肾上腺	C74	30	0.16	0	0.94	0.00	0.00	0.00	0.00	0.22
其他的内分泌腺	C75	20	0.11	0	0.00	0.00	0.00	0.00	0.00	0.22
霍奇金病	C81	33	0.18	0	0.00	0.00	0.49	0.00	0.25	0.22
非霍奇金淋巴瘤	C82–C85;C96	324	1.77	0	0.00	0.74	1.46	1.30	1.49	0.44
免疫增生性疾病	C88	1	0.01	0	0.00	0.00	0.00	0.00	0.00	0.22
多发性骨髓瘤	C90	121	0.66	0	0.00	0.00	0.00	0.00	0.00	0.00
淋巴样白血病	C91	59	0.32	0	3.15	1.49	0.24	0.00	0.25	0.22
髓样白血病	C92–C94	151	0.83	0	1.26	0.00	0.49	0.78	1.49	0.00
白血病，未特指	C95	122	0.67	0	4.40	1.24	1.70	1.04	0.50	0.44
其他的或未指明部位	O&U	518	2.83	3	1.26	0.99	0.24	1.82	0.75	1.33
骨髓增殖性疾病	MPD	30	0.16	0	0.00	0.00	0.24	0.52	0.00	0.22
骨髓增生异常综合征	MDS	3	0.02	0	0.00	0.00	0.00	0.00	0.00	0.00
合计	ALL	18 285	100.00	6	17.62	8.18	9.96	11.98	13.94	21.48
C44 以外的部位	ALL but C44	18 154	99.28	6	17.30	8.18	9.96	11.98	13.94	21.48

2020 年男性发病主要指标

30~	35~	40~	45~	50~	55~	60~	65~	70~	75~	80~	85+	粗率 (1/10^5)	世标率 (1/10^5)	累积率 (%) 0~64	累积率 (%) 0~74
0.00	0.00	0.21	0.00	0.45	0.00	1.03	1.68	1.17	1.71	4.80	6.53	0.36	0.24	0.01	0.02
0.64	0.22	0.21	1.16	1.56	2.38	3.79	2.10	3.52	0.85	7.20	6.53	0.99	0.72	0.05	0.08
0.21	0.00	0.21	0.77	1.34	3.18	4.48	4.20	7.04	7.69	6.00	13.06	1.32	0.93	0.05	0.11
0.64	0.00	1.04	0.19	1.11	1.06	2.07	1.26	2.35	1.71	4.80	2.18	0.62	0.43	0.03	0.05
0.00	0.00	0.00	0.39	0.22	1.32	1.03	0.42	1.17	0.00	0.00	0.00	0.23	0.16	0.01	0.02
0.00	0.00	0.42	0.39	0.89	0.79	0.34	1.26	2.35	2.56	2.40	0.00	0.39	0.26	0.01	0.03
0.42	0.22	1.25	1.74	2.67	5.29	3.10	3.36	3.52	1.71	1.20	2.18	1.29	0.94	0.08	0.11
0.00	0.00	0.21	0.58	1.11	3.18	2.75	3.78	4.69	4.27	4.80	8.70	0.98	0.69	0.04	0.08
0.00	0.00	0.21	0.19	0.45	0.79	1.03	2.94	1.17	1.71	1.20	0.00	0.36	0.25	0.01	0.03
0.42	0.22	2.29	5.80	19.36	38.65	65.43	124.19	149.51	151.27	184.67	182.77	23.41	15.79	0.66	2.03
2.34	3.73	4.59	12.38	31.60	56.12	109.16	189.64	256.21	217.93	233.84	245.87	36.52	25.03	1.10	3.33
0.21	0.00	0.63	1.93	2.67	3.44	4.48	5.87	6.45	8.55	8.39	10.88	1.61	1.10	0.07	0.13
2.34	3.51	4.38	9.87	15.36	24.09	35.47	57.06	79.15	82.05	119.92	126.20	14.54	9.81	0.48	1.16
0.42	1.98	5.21	9.29	16.25	30.97	40.98	64.19	77.39	75.21	98.33	82.68	14.45	9.83	0.53	1.23
0.21	0.00	0.00	0.19	0.00	0.26	0.69	0.00	1.17	1.71	1.20	0.00	0.16	0.11	0.01	0.01
4.03	6.80	18.55	32.31	50.30	81.27	91.94	111.18	128.99	122.21	127.11	193.65	31.57	22.03	1.43	2.63
0.00	0.22	1.04	1.55	4.01	6.09	14.46	22.24	25.80	35.04	39.57	69.63	4.91	3.29	0.14	0.38
0.21	0.88	1.88	2.90	8.46	12.44	16.87	28.11	35.18	23.93	58.76	67.45	6.51	4.38	0.22	0.54
0.21	0.22	0.00	0.19	0.89	1.06	0.69	2.10	1.17	3.42	3.60	2.18	0.51	0.38	0.02	0.04
0.21	0.00	0.63	1.35	4.90	8.74	12.05	11.75	14.66	18.80	11.99	13.06	3.13	2.17	0.14	0.27
2.97	7.02	8.55	28.63	55.86	137.66	230.02	338.58	447.94	439.29	526.44	607.06	73.03	49.54	2.36	6.29
0.21	0.22	1.88	0.77	1.78	2.65	2.07	5.87	2.35	6.84	2.40	0.00	1.14	0.84	0.05	0.09
0.42	0.44	1.04	1.55	2.23	2.38	5.51	5.03	9.38	8.55	11.99	15.23	2.02	1.59	0.09	0.16
0.00	0.22	0.00	0.39	0.67	1.06	1.03	1.68	0.59	0.85	3.60	2.18	0.41	0.30	0.02	0.03
0.42	0.44	1.25	0.58	1.11	2.65	3.44	7.13	9.38	17.09	28.78	32.64	2.14	1.37	0.05	0.13
0.00	0.00	0.00	0.00	0.00	0.26	0.34	0.84	0.00	0.00	3.60	0.00	0.13	0.09	0.00	0.01
0.00	0.00	0.00	0.00	0.00	0.00	0.00	0.00	0.00	0.00	0.00	0.00	0.00	0.00	0.00	0.00
1.06	0.44	0.42	0.97	0.67	1.85	2.41	2.52	3.52	4.27	3.60	4.35	0.93	0.70	0.04	0.07
0.00	0.22	0.42	0.58	0.67	1.32	1.72	2.52	1.76	2.56	2.40	4.35	0.57	0.40	0.02	0.05
0.00	0.00	0.00	0.00	0.00	0.00	0.00	0.00	0.00	0.00	0.00	0.00	0.00	0.00	0.00	0.00
0.00	0.00	0.00	0.00	0.00	0.00	0.00	0.00	0.00	0.00	0.00	0.00	0.00	0.00	0.00	0.00
0.00	0.00	0.00	0.00	0.00	0.00	0.00	0.00	0.00	0.00	0.00	0.00	0.00	0.00	0.00	0.00
0.00	0.00	0.00	0.00	0.00	0.00	0.00	0.00	0.00	0.00	0.00	0.00	0.00	0.00	0.00	0.00
0.00	0.00	0.00	0.00	0.00	0.00	0.00	0.00	0.00	0.00	0.00	0.00	0.00	0.00	0.00	0.00
0.00	0.00	0.00	0.00	0.00	0.00	0.00	0.00	0.00	0.00	0.00	0.00	0.00	0.00	0.00	0.00
0.00	0.00	0.00	0.00	0.00	0.00	0.00	0.00	0.00	0.00	0.00	0.00	0.00	0.00	0.00	0.00
0.00	0.00	0.00	0.00	0.00	0.00	0.00	0.00	0.00	0.00	0.00	0.00	0.00	0.00	0.00	0.00
0.21	0.22	0.00	0.58	0.67	0.53	1.03	2.52	5.86	1.71	6.00	6.53	0.64	0.43	0.02	0.06
0.00	0.00	0.21	0.00	2.00	6.62	19.28	51.19	95.57	109.39	178.68	226.29	12.34	7.71	0.14	0.87
0.64	0.44	0.42	0.19	0.00	0.00	0.34	0.84	0.00	0.00	0.00	2.18	0.28	0.25	0.02	0.02
0.00	0.00	0.00	0.19	0.45	0.79	0.69	0.00	0.00	0.85	2.40	2.18	0.21	0.15	0.01	0.01
1.27	2.41	2.29	5.42	10.02	14.30	15.84	27.27	31.07	23.08	16.79	21.76	6.05	4.28	0.26	0.55
0.21	0.22	0.21	0.19	0.45	0.79	1.03	3.78	0.59	4.27	1.20	4.35	0.49	0.34	0.02	0.04
0.00	0.00	0.00	0.19	0.45	0.79	2.41	2.94	3.52	4.27	8.39	4.35	0.67	0.45	0.02	0.05
0.42	0.22	1.46	3.48	8.01	13.24	27.20	34.40	55.70	58.97	65.96	145.78	9.16	6.17	0.27	0.72
0.00	0.00	0.21	0.00	0.45	0.00	0.00	0.84	0.00	0.00	1.20	0.00	0.10	0.07	0.00	0.01
0.00	0.22	0.00	0.00	0.22	0.00	0.34	0.84	1.17	0.00	0.00	0.00	0.21	0.25	0.01	0.02
2.34	2.41	5.00	4.64	9.35	9.80	14.46	16.36	19.93	21.37	23.98	19.58	5.85	4.60	0.29	0.47
24.84	26.77	23.76	22.83	25.59	27.53	21.69	17.20	11.14	7.69	6.00	2.18	14.89	11.60	0.96	1.11
0.21	0.00	0.42	0.39	0.89	1.06	0.34	0.84	1.76	3.42	1.20	4.35	0.49	0.40	0.02	0.03
0.21	0.22	0.00	0.00	0.45	0.79	0.69	0.42	1.17	5.98	0.00	0.00	0.33	0.22	0.01	0.02
0.42	0.66	0.63	0.39	0.89	0.53	0.69	1.26	2.93	0.85	1.20	2.18	0.54	0.42	0.03	0.05
1.27	0.88	3.34	3.68	5.56	11.38	16.87	18.04	27.56	18.80	26.38	13.06	5.28	3.91	0.24	0.47
0.00	0.00	0.00	0.00	0.00	0.00	0.00	0.00	0.00	0.00	0.00	0.00	0.02	0.02	0.00	0.00
0.21	0.00	0.00	1.35	2.23	4.77	4.48	13.01	11.73	5.13	8.39	17.41	1.97	1.38	0.07	0.19
0.42	0.00	0.00	0.58	0.45	1.06	1.03	4.62	1.76	6.84	1.20	6.53	0.96	0.97	0.04	0.07
0.85	0.66	1.88	1.16	2.67	3.18	4.82	10.49	11.14	11.11	16.79	10.88	2.46	1.87	0.10	0.20
0.85	0.66	0.63	0.97	1.34	1.32	5.17	2.52	6.45	5.98	17.99	17.41	1.99	1.84	0.10	0.14
2.12	2.63	4.79	3.87	8.46	13.77	19.97	33.56	44.56	42.73	56.36	54.40	8.45	6.10	0.31	0.70
0.00	0.22	0.63	0.19	0.89	0.26	1.03	1.68	1.76	3.42	2.40	0.00	0.49	0.38	0.02	0.04
0.00	0.00	0.00	0.00	0.22	0.00	0.34	0.00	0.00	0.00	1.20	0.00	0.05	0.03	0.00	0.00
54.13	65.84	102.35	166.97	308.25	543.50	818.16	1 246.07	1 612.92	1 577.67	1 946.28	2 260.71	298.14	207.19	10.70	25.00
53.71	65.40	101.10	166.39	307.14	540.86	814.72	1 238.93	1 603.54	1 560.58	1 917.50	2 228.07	296.01	205.81	10.65	24.86

表 6-6 河南省城市肿瘤登记地区

部位	ICD-10	病例数	构成(%)	年龄组 0~	1~	5~	10~	15~	20~	25~
唇	C00	13	0.07	0.00	0.00	0.00	0.00	0.00	0.00	0.00
舌	C01–C02	36	0.20	0.00	0.00	0.27	0.00	0.00	0.00	0.00
口	C03–C06	61	0.33	0.00	0.00	0.00	0.00	0.00	0.25	0.00
唾液腺	C07–C08	31	0.17	0.00	0.00	0.00	0.00	0.00	0.25	0.42
扁桃体	C09	3	0.02	0.00	0.00	0.00	0.00	0.00	0.00	0.00
其他的口咽	C10	6	0.03	0.00	0.00	0.00	0.00	0.28	0.00	0.00
鼻咽	C11	28	0.15	0.00	0.00	0.00	0.00	0.00	0.00	0.00
喉咽	C12–C13	11	0.06	0.00	0.00	0.00	0.00	0.00	0.00	0.00
咽，部位不明	C14	6	0.03	0.00	0.00	0.00	0.27	0.00	0.00	0.00
食管	C15	775	4.21	0.00	0.00	0.00	0.00	0.00	0.00	0.21
胃	C16	886	4.81	0.00	0.00	0.00	0.00	0.00	0.25	0.63
小肠	C17	75	0.41	0.00	0.00	0.00	0.00	0.00	0.00	0.00
结肠	C18	760	4.13	0.00	0.00	0.00	0.00	0.00	0.25	0.42
直肠	C19–C20	648	3.52	0.00	0.00	0.00	0.00	0.00	0.00	0.84
肛门	C21	20	0.11	0.00	0.00	0.00	0.00	0.00	0.00	0.00
肝脏	C22	787	4.28	0.00	0.35	0.00	0.00	0.28	0.00	0.42
胆囊及其他	C23–C24	326	1.77	0.00	0.00	0.00	0.00	0.00	0.00	0.00
胰腺	C25	358	1.95	0.00	0.00	0.27	0.00	0.00	0.00	0.42
鼻、鼻窦及其他	C30–C31	26	0.14	0.00	0.35	0.00	0.00	0.00	0.00	0.00
喉	C32	16	0.09	0.00	0.00	0.00	0.00	0.00	0.00	0.00
气管、支气管、肺	C33–C34	2 382	12.94	1.64	0.00	0.00	0.00	0.00	0.25	1.67
其他的胸腔器官	C37–C38	43	0.23	0.00	0.35	0.00	0.00	0.57	0.00	0.00
骨	C40–C41	84	0.46	0.00	0.35	1.37	1.65	0.85	0.76	0.00
皮肤的黑色素瘤	C43	36	0.20	0.00	0.00	0.00	0.00	0.00	0.00	0.00
其他的皮肤	C44	149	0.81	0.00	0.00	0.27	0.00	0.00	0.00	0.21
间皮瘤	C45	2	0.01	0.00	0.00	0.00	0.00	0.00	0.00	0.00
卡波西肉瘤	C46	0	0.00	0.00	0.00	0.00	0.00	0.00	0.00	0.00
周围神经、其他结缔组织、软组织	C47;C49	65	0.35	1.64	0.35	0.82	0.27	0.00	0.00	0.00
乳房	C50	3 572	19.41	0.00	0.00	0.00	0.27	0.57	2.03	7.54
外阴	C51	32	0.17	0.00	0.00	0.00	0.00	0.28	0.00	0.00
阴道	C52	22	0.12	0.00	0.00	0.27	0.00	0.00	0.00	0.00
子宫颈	C53	1 226	6.66	0.00	0.00	0.00	0.00	0.00	1.01	2.51
子宫体	C54	694	3.77	0.00	0.00	0.00	0.00	0.28	0.00	1.05
子宫，部位不明	C55	86	0.47	0.00	0.00	0.00	0.00	0.00	0.00	0.00
卵巢	C56	501	2.72	0.00	0.00	0.27	0.55	1.13	1.01	2.09
女性其他的生殖器	C57	34	0.18	0.00	0.00	0.00	0.27	0.00	0.25	0.00
胎盘	C58	4	0.02	0.00	0.00	0.00	0.00	0.00	0.00	0.21
阴茎	C60	0	0.00	0.00	0.00	0.00	0.00	0.00	0.00	0.00
前列腺	C61	0	0.00	0.00	0.00	0.00	0.00	0.00	0.00	0.00
睾丸	C62	0	0.00	0.00	0.00	0.00	0.00	0.00	0.00	0.00
男性其他的生殖器	C63	0	0.00	0.00	0.00	0.00	0.00	0.00	0.00	0.00
肾	C64	200	1.09	0.00	0.69	0.55	0.00	0.00	0.76	0.21
肾盂	C65	17	0.09	0.00	0.00	0.00	0.00	0.00	0.00	0.00
输尿管	C66	37	0.20	0.00	0.00	0.00	0.00	0.00	0.00	0.00
膀胱	C67	142	0.77	0.00	0.00	0.00	0.00	0.00	0.00	0.00
其他的泌尿器官	C68	5	0.03	0.00	0.00	0.00	0.00	0.00	0.00	0.00
眼	C69	9	0.05	0.00	0.69	0.00	0.00	0.00	0.00	0.00
脑、神经系统	C70–C72	363	1.97	0.00	1.38	2.20	1.10	0.57	1.52	1.67
甲状腺	C73	2 701	14.68	0.00	0.00	0.00	0.55	1.70	6.84	29.09
肾上腺	C74	15	0.08	0.00	0.35	0.00	0.00	0.00	0.00	0.00
其他的内分泌腺	C75	11	0.06	0.00	0.00	0.00	0.27	0.00	0.00	0.00
霍奇金病	C81	20	0.11	0.00	0.00	0.00	0.00	0.00	0.25	0.21
非霍奇金淋巴瘤	C82–C85;C96	259	1.41	0.00	0.69	0.27	0.27	1.13	0.25	0.21
免疫增生性疾病	C88	0	0.00	0.00	0.00	0.00	0.00	0.00	0.00	0.00
多发性骨髓瘤	C90	96	0.52	0.00	0.00	0.00	0.00	0.00	0.00	0.00
淋巴样白血病	C91	50	0.27	0.00	1.04	2.20	1.10	0.57	0.51	0.00
髓样白血病	C92–C94	111	0.60	0.00	0.69	0.55	1.10	0.57	1.01	0.42
白血病，未特指	C95	104	0.57	3.27	0.69	1.37	1.10	0.28	0.25	0.00
其他的或未指明部位	O&U	443	2.41	9.81	0.35	2.20	0.27	1.13	0.00	1.26
骨髓增殖性疾病	MPD	18	0.10	0.00	0.00	0.00	0.00	0.00	0.25	0.00
骨髓增生异常综合征	MDS	0	0.00	0.00	0.00	0.00	0.00	0.00	0.00	0.00
合计	ALL	18 405	100.00	16.36	8.29	12.91	9.06	10.17	17.98	51.70
C44 以外的部位	ALL but C44	18 256	99.19	16.36	8.29	12.63	9.06	10.17	17.98	51.49

2020 年女性发病主要指标

30~	35~	40~	45~	50~	55~	60~	65~	70~	75~	80~	85+	粗率 (1/10^5)	世标率 (1/10^5)	累积率 (%) 0~64	累积率 (%) 0~74
0.20	0.00	0.00	0.00	0.00	0.00	1.01	0.39	1.56	0.71	2.22	3.14	0.21	0.13	0.01	0.02
0.20	0.21	1.23	0.77	0.23	1.05	1.01	2.37	1.56	2.13	2.22	1.57	0.58	0.41	0.02	0.04
0.20	0.00	0.61	0.58	0.45	1.05	1.69	1.97	7.27	4.98	8.87	12.56	0.99	0.60	0.02	0.07
0.40	0.42	0.61	0.38	1.13	0.79	0.00	1.18	3.11	0.00	1.11	1.57	0.50	0.36	0.02	0.04
0.00	0.00	0.00	0.00	0.23	0.00	0.34	0.00	0.00	0.00	0.00	1.57	0.05	0.03	0.00	0.00
0.00	0.00	0.00	0.19	0.23	0.26	0.00	0.00	0.52	0.71	0.00	0.00	0.10	0.08	0.00	0.01
0.20	0.42	0.41	0.38	1.35	0.00	1.01	2.76	1.56	1.42	0.00	0.00	0.45	0.32	0.02	0.04
0.00	0.63	0.20	0.00	0.00	0.52	0.68	0.00	0.52	0.00	2.22	0.00	0.18	0.12	0.01	0.01
0.00	0.00	0.00	0.19	0.00	0.00	0.00	0.39	0.00	0.71	1.11	1.57	0.10	0.07	0.00	0.00
0.00	0.00	0.41	0.96	2.25	11.27	25.66	55.60	90.82	91.75	131.89	116.22	12.58	7.33	0.20	0.94
1.59	2.29	4.08	7.50	13.75	17.29	37.48	53.63	65.91	86.06	104.18	138.20	14.39	8.88	0.42	1.02
0.00	0.00	0.20	1.54	1.13	0.79	2.70	3.94	8.82	4.98	11.08	9.42	1.22	0.75	0.03	0.10
1.00	1.67	2.65	7.70	9.92	22.01	31.07	54.03	48.26	62.59	104.18	92.66	12.34	7.65	0.38	0.89
1.39	1.67	3.47	7.31	11.27	16.77	32.42	39.83	44.63	45.52	82.01	61.25	10.52	6.69	0.38	0.80
0.00	0.21	0.00	0.19	0.68	0.52	0.34	0.00	2.59	0.71	4.43	3.14	0.32	0.19	0.01	0.02
1.00	1.67	2.86	4.62	12.85	20.70	28.03	54.42	63.31	68.99	89.77	117.79	12.78	7.92	0.36	0.95
0.20	0.00	1.02	1.35	2.25	6.55	8.78	19.72	26.99	35.56	67.61	61.25	5.29	3.01	0.10	0.33
0.40	0.42	1.02	2.31	1.80	8.12	13.51	18.93	26.99	39.12	66.50	62.82	5.81	3.41	0.14	0.37
0.20	0.21	0.00	0.19	0.23	0.52	0.68	1.97	2.59	2.13	2.22	3.14	0.42	0.29	0.01	0.03
0.00	0.00	0.41	0.00	0.45	0.52	0.00	1.18	1.56	0.71	1.11	3.14	0.26	0.16	0.01	0.02
5.58	6.25	14.30	27.52	60.85	70.48	93.20	140.78	143.75	186.34	242.72	268.55	38.68	24.52	1.40	2.82
0.20	0.00	0.41	0.77	1.58	1.05	1.01	1.58	3.63	1.42	4.43	3.14	0.70	0.50	0.03	0.06
0.00	0.63	1.02	0.96	0.45	1.83	2.70	2.76	4.67	5.69	6.65	9.42	1.36	1.13	0.06	0.10
0.40	0.21	0.82	0.00	0.23	0.52	0.68	2.37	4.67	2.84	4.43	1.57	0.58	0.37	0.01	0.05
0.40	0.42	0.82	1.15	1.58	2.10	4.39	7.49	12.46	10.67	24.38	39.26	2.42	1.45	0.06	0.16
0.20	0.00	0.00	0.00	0.23	0.00	0.00	0.00	0.00	0.00	0.00	0.00	0.03	0.02	0.00	0.00
0.00	0.00	0.00	0.00	0.00	0.00	0.00	0.00	0.00	0.00	0.00	0.00	0.00	0.00	0.00	0.00
0.80	0.21	1.02	0.96	1.35	1.05	3.71	3.55	0.52	4.98	6.65	0.00	1.06	0.81	0.05	0.07
26.10	42.71	71.27	115.64	135.23	130.47	133.05	124.22	97.05	83.21	104.18	53.40	58.00	40.77	3.32	4.43
0.00	0.21	0.41	0.38	0.45	0.79	1.01	1.18	3.63	2.13	2.22	4.71	0.52	0.34	0.02	0.04
0.00	0.00	0.00	0.58	0.23	0.79	1.01	1.58	2.08	1.42	1.11	0.00	0.36	0.25	0.01	0.03
9.56	17.71	25.53	30.79	42.60	48.73	49.64	41.80	42.55	29.16	31.03	20.42	19.91	14.02	1.14	1.56
3.19	3.96	9.80	15.59	32.68	33.54	28.03	27.60	26.47	17.07	11.08	20.42	11.27	7.84	0.64	0.91
0.40	0.21	2.04	0.77	3.83	4.45	4.05	5.52	1.56	0.71	2.22	4.71	1.40	0.98	0.08	0.11
3.98	3.54	9.19	12.89	17.81	17.03	18.24	20.90	15.57	13.51	19.95	20.42	8.13	5.78	0.44	0.62
0.00	0.42	0.20	0.58	1.35	0.52	2.03	1.58	1.04	1.42	2.22	3.14	0.55	0.40	0.03	0.04
0.00	0.42	0.00	0.00	0.23	0.00	0.00	0.00	0.00	0.00	0.00	0.00	0.06	0.05	0.00	0.00
0.00	0.00	0.00	0.00	0.00	0.00	0.00	0.00	0.00	0.00	0.00	0.00	0.00	0.00	0.00	0.00
0.00	0.00	0.00	0.00	0.00	0.00	0.00	0.00	0.00	0.00	0.00	0.00	0.00	0.00	0.00	0.00
0.00	0.00	0.00	0.00	0.00	0.00	0.00	0.00	0.00	0.00	0.00	0.00	0.00	0.00	0.00	0.00
0.00	0.00	0.00	0.00	0.00	0.00	0.00	0.00	0.00	0.00	0.00	0.00	0.00	0.00	0.00	0.00
0.80	0.42	0.82	3.08	4.96	8.12	7.09	9.86	12.46	14.94	14.41	14.13	3.25	2.20	0.14	0.25
0.20	0.00	0.00	0.00	0.00	0.26	1.69	0.39	1.56	2.13	3.32	0.00	0.28	0.17	0.01	0.02
0.00	0.21	0.20	0.00	0.45	0.26	0.68	2.37	3.63	2.84	11.08	4.71	0.60	0.34	0.01	0.04
0.60	0.42	0.61	0.77	2.25	5.50	3.38	5.52	8.82	16.36	28.82	14.13	2.31	1.33	0.07	0.14
0.00	0.00	0.00	0.00	0.00	0.26	0.34	0.39	0.00	0.71	1.11	0.00	0.08	0.05	0.00	0.00
0.00	0.00	0.00	0.00	0.00	1.05	0.00	0.00	0.52	1.42	0.00	0.00	0.15	0.13	0.01	0.01
1.39	2.50	3.68	5.20	7.66	9.69	11.48	17.75	21.80	25.60	31.03	17.28	5.89	4.22	0.25	0.45
56.38	63.55	68.21	84.47	85.65	96.41	66.52	45.35	31.66	19.91	13.30	7.85	43.86	32.53	2.80	3.18
0.20	0.21	0.20	0.38	0.23	0.52	0.00	0.79	0.00	0.00	2.22	3.14	0.24	0.18	0.01	0.01
0.00	0.00	0.00	0.77	0.23	0.52	0.68	0.00	0.00	0.71	0.00	0.00	0.18	0.14	0.01	0.01
0.40	0.21	0.41	0.00	0.45	0.52	0.00	0.79	1.56	0.71	1.11	3.14	0.32	0.22	0.01	0.02
1.00	1.25	3.27	3.66	5.41	5.76	8.78	17.75	16.09	19.91	18.84	15.70	4.21	2.89	0.16	0.33
0.00	0.00	0.00	0.00	0.00	0.00	0.00	0.00	0.00	0.00	0.00	0.00	0.00	0.00	0.00	0.00
0.00	0.21	0.61	1.54	2.25	2.36	3.71	4.34	6.23	9.96	13.30	7.85	1.56	0.96	0.05	0.11
0.00	0.21	0.20	0.77	0.23	1.31	1.35	0.00	3.63	2.13	1.11	6.28	0.81	0.83	0.05	0.06
1.20	0.63	2.25	0.96	2.70	2.88	4.05	4.34	6.75	2.84	4.43	4.71	1.80	1.44	0.09	0.15
1.00	0.63	0.82	0.58	2.03	2.36	1.69	4.73	5.19	8.53	13.30	7.85	1.69	1.30	0.07	0.12
2.39	1.04	4.29	5.00	9.47	11.79	15.53	16.96	26.47	40.54	50.98	36.12	7.19	4.89	0.28	0.50
0.00	0.00	0.00	0.38	0.68	0.52	0.34	1.18	0.52	0.71	1.11	4.71	0.29	0.19	0.01	0.02
0.00	0.00	0.00	0.00	0.00	0.00	0.00	0.00	0.00	0.00	0.00	0.00	0.00	0.00	0.00	0.00
123.31	158.14	241.60	352.32	485.49	572.19	656.46	827.75	905.07	979.37	1 355.46	1 287.79	298.84	201.65	13.51	22.17
122.91	157.72	240.78	351.17	483.91	570.10	652.07	820.25	892.61	968.71	1 331.07	1 248.53	296.42	200.20	13.45	22.01

表 6-7 河南省农村肿瘤登记地区

部位	ICD-10	病例数	构成 (%)	年龄组						
				0~	1~	5~	10~	15~	20~	25~
唇	C00	62	0.07	0.00	0.06	0.00	0.00	0.05	0.00	0.04
舌	C01–C02	156	0.19	0.00	0.00	0.05	0.00	0.00	0.00	0.17
口	C03–C06	263	0.31	0.00	0.00	0.09	0.00	0.00	0.09	0.09
唾液腺	C07–C08	208	0.25	0.00	0.06	0.05	0.04	0.19	0.18	0.13
扁桃体	C09	32	0.04	0.00	0.06	0.00	0.04	0.10	0.00	0.00
其他的口咽	C10	58	0.07	0.00	0.00	0.00	0.00	0.00	0.09	0.00
鼻咽	C11	311	0.37	0.00	0.06	0.09	0.18	0.19	0.09	0.13
喉咽	C12–C13	74	0.09	0.00	0.00	0.05	0.00	0.00	0.00	0.00
咽，部位不明	C14	87	0.10	0.00	0.00	0.05	0.00	0.00	0.09	0.09
食管	C15	9 467	11.27	0.00	0.00	0.05	0.00	0.00	0.23	0.47
胃	C16	9 968	11.87	0.00	0.06	0.09	0.18	0.29	0.60	0.90
小肠	C17	379	0.45	0.00	0.00	0.00	0.00	0.00	0.05	0.13
结肠	C18	2 537	3.02	0.00	0.00	0.00	0.04	0.10	0.23	1.03
直肠	C19–C20	3 203	3.81	0.00	0.00	0.05	0.00	0.05	0.28	0.77
肛门	C21	135	0.16	0.00	0.00	0.00	0.00	0.00	0.00	0.04
肝脏	C22	7 822	9.31	0.63	0.13	0.09	0.22	0.34	0.46	1.38
胆囊及其他	C23–C24	1 271	1.51	0.00	0.13	0.00	0.00	0.00	0.05	0.17
胰腺	C25	1 336	1.59	0.00	0.00	0.05	0.09	0.15	0.05	0.13
鼻、鼻窦及其他	C30–C31	147	0.17	0.00	0.00	0.09	0.13	0.15	0.05	0.04
喉	C32	401	0.48	0.00	0.06	0.09	0.04	0.00	0.00	0.09
气管、支气管、肺	C33–C34	16 536	19.68	0.00	0.00	0.09	0.04	0.10	0.73	0.95
其他的胸腔器官	C37–C38	276	0.33	0.00	0.19	0.00	0.00	0.24	0.18	0.17
骨	C40–C41	685	0.82	0.00	0.64	0.80	1.60	1.36	0.32	0.56
皮肤的黑色素瘤	C43	80	0.10	0.00	0.00	0.05	0.00	0.00	0.00	0.04
其他的皮肤	C44	589	0.70	0.00	0.13	0.33	0.04	0.34	0.09	0.17
间皮瘤	C45	33	0.04	0.00	0.00	0.00	0.00	0.05	0.00	0.00
卡波西肉瘤	C46	3	0.00	0.00	0.00	0.00	0.00	0.00	0.00	0.04
周围神经、其他结缔组织、软组织	C47;C49	207	0.25	0.00	0.26	0.19	0.13	0.44	0.09	0.22
乳房	C50	6 693	7.97	0.00	0.00	0.00	0.10	1.03	7.43	10.62
外阴	C51	54	0.06	0.00	0.00	0.00	0.00	0.00	0.00	0.09
阴道	C52	55	0.07	0.00	0.14	0.00	0.00	0.00	0.29	0.00
子宫颈	C53	3 209	3.82	0.00	0.00	0.00	0.00	0.00	1.83	5.85
子宫体	C54	1 598	1.90	0.00	0.00	0.00	0.00	0.00	0.48	1.80
子宫，部位不明	C55	265	0.32	0.00	0.00	0.00	0.10	0.00	0.10	0.18
卵巢	C56	1 200	1.43	0.00	0.27	0.51	0.96	2.68	3.18	3.15
女性其他的生殖器	C57	79	0.09	0.00	0.00	0.10	0.10	0.21	0.10	0.27
胎盘	C58	7	0.01	0.00	0.00	0.00	0.00	0.00	0.29	0.00
阴茎	C60	109	0.13	0.00	0.00	0.00	0.00	0.00	0.00	0.00
前列腺	C61	1 025	1.22	0.00	0.00	0.00	0.00	0.00	0.00	0.08
睾丸	C62	59	0.07	0.60	0.48	0.00	0.00	0.00	0.09	0.08
男性其他的生殖器	C63	11	0.01	0.00	0.00	0.00	0.00	0.00	0.00	0.00
肾	C64	992	1.18	0.00	0.58	0.09	0.22	0.24	0.18	0.65
肾盂	C65	85	0.10	0.00	0.00	0.00	0.00	0.00	0.00	0.00
输尿管	C66	117	0.14	0.00	0.00	0.00	0.00	0.00	0.00	0.00
膀胱	C67	1 208	1.44	0.00	0.06	0.00	0.00	0.05	0.18	0.17
其他的泌尿器官	C68	21	0.02	0.00	0.00	0.00	0.00	0.00	0.00	0.00
眼	C69	56	0.07	0.00	0.64	0.19	0.00	0.00	0.00	0.04
脑、神经系统	C70–C72	2 132	2.54	1.25	1.21	2.21	2.18	1.74	1.56	1.72
甲状腺	C73	4 019	4.78	0.00	0.06	0.09	0.71	1.36	3.67	9.47
肾上腺	C74	79	0.09	0.00	0.06	0.00	0.04	0.00	0.00	0.09
其他的内分泌腺	C75	51	0.06	0.00	0.06	0.05	0.00	0.10	0.09	0.00
霍奇金病	C81	84	0.10	0.00	0.00	0.05	0.09	0.05	0.05	0.34
非霍奇金淋巴瘤	C82–C85;C96	934	1.11	0.63	0.77	0.56	0.62	0.78	0.87	0.86
免疫增生性疾病	C88	10	0.01	0.00	0.13	0.00	0.00	0.00	0.00	0.00
多发性骨髓瘤	C90	340	0.40	0.00	0.00	0.00	0.00	0.05	0.05	0.00
淋巴样白血病	C91	173	0.21	0.00	1.15	1.03	0.58	0.10	0.14	0.09
髓样白血病	C92–C94	508	0.60	0.00	0.32	0.80	0.67	0.68	0.69	0.52
白血病，未特指	C95	643	0.77	3.44	2.11	1.03	0.80	1.16	0.92	1.20
其他的或未指明部位	O&U	1 686	2.01	0.63	1.79	1.32	0.71	1.31	1.10	1.33
骨髓增殖性疾病	MPD	53	0.06	0.31	0.00	0.00	0.00	0.05	0.05	0.09
骨髓增生异常综合征	MDS	20	0.02	0.00	0.13	0.00	0.04	0.00	0.00	0.04
合计	ALL	84 004	100.00	7.19	11.38	10.06	10.05	13.61	20.06	35.20
C44 以外的部位	ALL but C44	83 415	99.30	7.19	11.25	9.73	10.01	13.27	19.97	35.02

2020 年合计发病主要指标

30~	35~	40~	45~	50~	55~	60~	65~	70~	75~	80~	85+	粗率 ($1/10^5$)	世标率 ($1/10^5$)	累积率 (%) 0~64	累积率 (%) 0~74
0.12	0.05	0.00	0.04	0.27	0.27	0.20	1.10	1.36	0.52	2.26	1.12	0.20	0.14	0.01	0.02
0.44	0.09	0.50	0.66	0.91	0.66	1.28	1.26	2.73	1.22	2.83	1.50	0.51	0.37	0.02	0.04
0.16	0.27	0.37	0.83	0.96	2.08	1.28	2.82	5.00	5.05	7.07	2.99	0.85	0.59	0.03	0.07
0.40	0.50	0.69	0.79	0.96	1.37	1.68	2.51	2.27	1.39	0.85	2.25	0.67	0.52	0.04	0.06
0.00	0.05	0.14	0.00	0.09	0.22	0.13	0.24	0.57	0.87	0.57	0.37	0.10	0.08	0.00	0.01
0.00	0.23	0.09	0.22	0.32	0.22	0.40	0.71	0.34	1.39	1.41	0.75	0.19	0.13	0.01	0.01
0.44	0.50	0.73	1.18	1.78	3.01	2.08	3.22	3.52	2.79	2.26	3.37	1.01	0.75	0.05	0.09
0.08	0.00	0.09	0.09	0.27	0.22	0.47	1.10	1.48	1.92	2.26	1.50	0.24	0.16	0.01	0.02
0.04	0.09	0.14	0.18	0.46	0.49	0.67	1.10	1.48	1.57	0.85	1.50	0.28	0.20	0.01	0.02
0.32	1.23	1.79	6.74	19.93	39.47	78.10	159.05	213.82	243.58	250.67	264.56	30.68	20.42	0.74	2.61
1.88	3.63	5.96	14.22	31.83	50.20	85.22	156.69	195.98	217.98	240.78	235.74	32.31	21.91	0.98	2.74
0.20	0.27	0.37	1.23	1.87	2.14	3.36	6.20	5.91	5.22	7.07	4.49	1.23	0.87	0.05	0.11
1.68	2.14	3.76	6.43	12.77	14.67	21.44	34.29	41.35	45.96	44.09	37.05	8.22	5.76	0.32	0.70
1.32	1.77	2.98	7.48	13.91	19.27	26.48	46.61	57.15	61.63	61.04	56.50	10.38	7.18	0.37	0.89
0.08	0.14	0.18	0.35	0.59	0.71	0.94	1.88	3.07	1.92	2.26	2.62	0.44	0.31	0.02	0.04
3.32	5.41	11.83	25.78	40.09	51.46	69.16	100.20	120.43	113.69	131.69	153.05	25.35	17.82	1.05	2.15
0.20	0.32	0.60	1.53	4.06	5.80	9.95	20.48	24.09	30.47	33.35	35.55	4.12	2.77	0.11	0.34
0.64	0.73	1.15	2.71	5.20	6.41	10.35	21.34	23.06	27.68	29.11	31.81	4.33	2.97	0.14	0.36
0.08	0.36	0.23	0.39	0.82	1.09	1.61	1.49	1.14	2.09	1.41	1.87	0.48	0.36	0.03	0.04
0.08	0.23	0.28	0.61	1.78	3.28	2.96	6.75	7.61	8.36	2.54	5.61	1.30	0.92	0.05	0.12
3.20	4.50	10.73	27.35	57.69	94.16	140.54	244.10	320.72	356.05	385.48	387.67	53.59	36.34	1.70	4.52
0.60	0.32	0.50	1.05	1.41	1.92	2.02	3.30	2.39	2.79	5.65	2.99	0.89	0.66	0.04	0.07
0.84	1.09	1.19	1.49	2.65	3.89	4.37	7.45	7.84	8.36	11.59	8.23	2.22	1.78	0.10	0.18
0.08	0.05	0.14	0.18	0.27	0.49	0.67	1.33	1.14	1.57	1.13	1.12	0.26	0.18	0.01	0.02
0.28	0.23	0.50	0.88	2.05	2.19	2.42	7.53	8.41	14.10	18.37	32.18	1.91	1.29	0.05	0.13
0.00	0.00	0.00	0.09	0.23	0.27	0.34	0.55	0.45	0.52	0.28	0.00	0.11	0.08	0.00	0.01
0.00	0.00	0.00	0.00	0.00	0.00	0.07	0.08	0.00	0.00	0.00	0.00	0.01	0.01	0.00	0.00
0.64	0.23	0.60	0.79	1.32	1.09	1.34	1.26	2.16	1.57	2.26	2.62	0.67	0.54	0.04	0.05
22.40	40.18	60.70	94.41	115.96	98.61	81.08	104.87	75.93	60.99	41.90	45.71	44.76	33.30	2.66	3.57
0.17	0.19	0.09	0.45	0.47	0.66	0.54	1.72	1.76	1.65	1.50	0.60	0.36	0.25	0.01	0.03
0.08	0.19	0.47	0.54	0.28	0.88	0.82	0.78	1.32	0.99	1.50	1.80	0.37	0.27	0.02	0.03
11.03	18.62	26.53	39.92	54.12	51.02	46.25	45.08	40.72	36.27	29.43	25.86	21.46	15.78	1.28	1.70
2.57	3.61	9.54	18.94	31.58	37.10	23.81	23.79	23.99	12.86	10.97	11.43	10.69	7.71	0.65	0.89
0.83	1.14	1.70	3.30	4.84	4.20	3.81	4.38	3.30	3.30	3.49	3.61	1.77	1.28	0.10	0.14
5.47	4.56	7.65	12.50	15.65	18.88	16.19	18.47	19.15	18.46	9.98	9.02	8.03	6.12	0.46	0.65
0.08	0.28	0.38	1.07	1.02	0.88	1.77	1.41	0.66	1.32	0.50	1.20	0.53	0.41	0.03	0.04
0.17	0.00	0.09	0.00	0.09	0.00	0.00	0.00	0.00	0.00	0.00	0.00	0.05	0.04	0.00	0.00
0.00	0.00	0.27	0.77	1.25	1.30	1.73	2.99	3.52	4.06	5.22	4.95	0.69	0.50	0.03	0.06
0.08	0.09	0.09	0.60	1.43	3.04	11.96	32.88	52.37	79.69	89.34	94.09	6.45	4.48	0.09	0.51
0.69	0.44	0.53	0.77	0.36	0.22	0.53	0.79	0.94	1.11	0.65	0.00	0.37	0.32	0.02	0.03
0.00	0.00	0.00	0.00	0.09	0.00	0.40	0.63	0.23	0.00	0.65	0.99	0.07	0.05	0.00	0.01
0.88	1.45	1.97	3.19	6.11	6.62	6.92	13.34	12.72	13.58	10.46	10.10	3.22	2.37	0.15	0.28
0.08	0.05	0.09	0.26	0.32	0.49	0.40	1.33	1.14	2.09	1.98	2.25	0.28	0.19	0.01	0.02
0.04	0.00	0.14	0.35	0.41	0.55	1.01	2.43	1.48	2.09	3.39	1.12	0.38	0.26	0.01	0.03
0.52	0.64	1.24	1.66	4.01	6.41	9.21	17.81	20.68	28.21	30.24	32.18	3.92	2.65	0.12	0.31
0.04	0.09	0.00	0.09	0.14	0.11	0.07	0.47	0.34	0.00	0.28	0.00	0.07	0.05	0.00	0.01
0.04	0.00	0.14	0.18	0.32	0.27	0.20	0.39	1.02	0.35	0.00	0.75	0.18	0.18	0.01	0.02
3.32	3.36	3.07	6.35	11.08	13.19	14.38	22.05	26.36	27.51	25.15	28.44	6.91	5.34	0.33	0.57
16.30	14.58	17.29	25.87	29.87	32.46	20.36	18.67	10.45	10.62	5.65	4.86	13.03	10.23	0.86	1.01
0.12	0.09	0.28	0.13	0.46	0.44	0.60	0.71	1.48	1.39	0.85	0.37	0.26	0.19	0.01	0.02
0.16	0.14	0.18	0.04	0.36	0.38	0.40	0.24	0.34	0.52	0.57	0.37	0.17	0.13	0.01	0.01
0.24	0.14	0.18	0.35	0.27	0.33	0.74	0.63	1.48	1.04	0.00	0.00	0.27	0.22	0.01	0.02
1.20	1.04	1.74	2.84	3.79	6.02	6.52	10.20	13.07	14.28	12.43	8.23	3.03	2.32	0.14	0.25
0.00	0.00	0.05	0.00	0.00	0.05	0.20	0.16	0.00	0.17	0.00	0.00	0.03	0.03	0.00	0.00
0.12	0.27	0.32	0.70	1.73	2.57	3.36	6.43	5.68	4.18	3.11	1.50	1.10	0.79	0.05	0.11
0.12	0.05	0.37	0.39	0.23	0.99	0.94	1.02	3.07	1.57	0.57	1.50	0.56	0.56	0.03	0.05
0.96	1.09	1.10	2.06	2.55	2.30	3.16	5.73	5.23	5.75	2.26	2.25	1.65	1.34	0.08	0.14
1.24	1.00	1.15	1.49	2.01	2.74	3.70	6.43	6.93	6.44	9.61	4.49	2.08	1.85	0.10	0.17
2.12	2.18	2.57	4.95	7.02	9.03	11.69	17.97	22.04	26.81	33.63	26.57	5.46	4.14	0.23	0.43
0.12	0.05	0.05	0.13	0.14	0.60	0.67	0.55	0.11	0.52	0.85	0.75	0.17	0.13	0.01	0.01
0.08	0.00	0.00	0.04	0.14	0.11	0.00	0.24	0.00	0.17	0.28	1.12	0.06	0.05	0.00	0.00
65.87	83.90	130.08	239.79	387.39	501.08	648.10	1 081.88	1 304.14	1 420.38	1 490.75	1 506.15	272.26	193.08	10.78	22.71
65.59	83.68	129.57	238.92	385.34	498.89	645.68	1 074.34	1 295.73	1 406.28	1 472.38	1 473.97	270.36	191.79	10.73	22.58

表 6-8 河南省农村肿瘤登记地区

部位	ICD-10	病例数	构成(%)	年龄组						
				0~	1~	5~	10~	15~	20~	25~
唇	C00	36	0.08	0.0	0.12	0.00	0.00	0.09	0.00	0.08
舌	C01–C02	90	0.21	0.0	0.00	0.09	0.00	0.00	0.00	0.25
口	C03–C06	154	0.35	0.0	0.00	0.00	0.00	0.00	0.09	0.08
唾液腺	C07–C08	116	0.27	0.0	0.12	0.00	0.08	0.18	0.26	0.00
扁桃体	C09	16	0.04	0.0	0.00	0.00	0.08	0.09	0.00	0.00
其他的口咽	C10	42	0.10	0.0	0.00	0.00	0.00	0.00	0.09	0.00
鼻咽	C11	206	0.47	0.0	0.12	0.18	0.25	0.37	0.00	0.08
喉咽	C12–C13	61	0.14	0.0	0.00	0.09	0.00	0.00	0.00	0.00
咽，部位不明	C14	56	0.13	0.0	0.00	0.00	0.00	0.00	0.09	0.08
食管	C15	5 803	13.33	0.0	0.00	0.09	0.00	0.00	0.09	0.41
胃	C16	6 907	15.87	0.0	0.12	0.09	0.08	0.27	0.61	0.49
小肠	C17	228	0.52	0.0	0.00	0.00	0.00	0.00	0.00	0.08
结肠	C18	1 360	3.12	0.0	0.00	0.00	0.08	0.18	0.26	1.24
直肠	C19–C20	1 764	4.05	0.0	0.00	0.09	0.00	0.09	0.18	0.99
肛门	C21	78	0.18	0.0	0.00	0.00	0.00	0.00	0.00	0.08
肝脏	C22	5 306	12.19	1.2	0.24	0.18	0.17	0.55	0.61	1.57
胆囊及其他	C23–C24	561	1.29	0.0	0.12	0.00	0.00	0.00	0.00	0.16
胰腺	C25	707	1.62	0.0	0.00	0.00	0.17	0.18	0.00	0.25
鼻、鼻窦及其他	C30–C31	88	0.20	0.0	0.00	0.18	0.17	0.18	0.09	0.00
喉	C32	347	0.80	0.0	0.12	0.18	0.00	0.00	0.00	0.16
气管、支气管、肺	C33–C34	11 199	25.72	0.0	0.00	0.09	0.08	0.09	0.88	1.15
其他的胸腔器官	C37–C38	150	0.34	0.0	0.12	0.00	0.00	0.37	0.35	0.16
骨	C40–C41	367	0.84	0.0	1.08	0.97	1.83	1.55	0.26	0.82
皮肤的黑色素瘤	C43	37	0.08	0.0	0.00	0.00	0.00	0.00	0.00	0.00
其他的皮肤	C44	304	0.70	0.0	0.00	0.44	0.00	0.37	0.00	0.25
间皮瘤	C45	18	0.04	0.0	0.00	0.00	0.00	0.09	0.00	0.00
卡波西肉瘤	C46	2	0.00	0.0	0.00	0.00	0.00	0.00	0.00	0.08
周围神经、其他结缔组织、软组织	C47;C49	106	0.24	0.0	0.12	0.09	0.08	0.27	0.18	0.25
乳房	C50	100	0.23	0.0	0.00	0.00	0.00	0.00	0.00	0.08
外阴	C51	0	0.00	0.0	0.00	0.00	0.00	0.00	0.00	0.00
阴道	C52	0	0.00	0.0	0.00	0.00	0.00	0.00	0.00	0.00
子宫颈	C53	1	0.00	0.0	0.00	0.00	0.00	0.00	0.00	0.00
子宫体	C54	0	0.00	0.0	0.00	0.00	0.00	0.00	0.00	0.00
子宫，部位不明	C55	0	0.00	0.0	0.00	0.00	0.00	0.00	0.00	0.00
卵巢	C56	0	0.00	0.0	0.00	0.00	0.00	0.00	0.00	0.00
女性其他的生殖器	C57	0	0.00	0.0	0.00	0.00	0.00	0.00	0.00	0.00
胎盘	C58	0	0.00	0.0	0.00	0.00	0.00	0.00	0.00	0.00
阴茎	C60	109	0.25	0.0	0.00	0.00	0.00	0.00	0.00	0.00
前列腺	C61	1 025	2.35	0.0	0.00	0.00	0.00	0.00	0.00	0.08
睾丸	C62	59	0.14	0.6	0.48	0.00	0.00	0.00	0.09	0.08
男性其他的生殖器	C63	11	0.03	0.0	0.00	0.00	0.00	0.00	0.00	0.00
肾	C64	615	1.41	0.0	0.48	0.18	0.25	0.09	0.18	0.99
肾盂	C65	50	0.11	0.0	0.00	0.00	0.00	0.00	0.00	0.00
输尿管	C66	72	0.17	0.0	0.00	0.00	0.00	0.00	0.00	0.00
膀胱	C67	928	2.13	0.0	0.12	0.00	0.00	0.00	0.18	0.08
其他的泌尿器官	C68	11	0.03	0.0	0.00	0.00	0.00	0.00	0.00	0.00
眼	C69	28	0.06	0.0	0.48	0.26	0.00	0.00	0.00	0.00
脑、神经系统	C70–C72	1 050	2.41	1.2	0.84	2.37	2.75	1.64	1.84	2.14
甲状腺	C73	884	2.03	0.0	0.12	0.09	0.50	0.82	2.71	4.12
肾上腺	C74	50	0.11	0.0	0.12	0.00	0.08	0.00	0.00	0.00
其他的内分泌腺	C75	25	0.06	0.0	0.12	0.00	0.00	0.09	0.18	0.00
霍奇金病	C81	47	0.11	0.0	0.00	0.09	0.17	0.09	0.09	0.33
非霍奇金淋巴瘤	C82–C85;C96	529	1.22	0.6	0.96	0.88	0.58	1.10	0.96	0.66
免疫增生性疾病	C88	4	0.01	0.0	0.12	0.00	0.00	0.00	0.00	0.00
多发性骨髓瘤	C90	187	0.43	0.0	0.00	0.00	0.00	0.09	0.00	0.00
淋巴样白血病	C91	96	0.22	0.0	1.44	0.97	0.58	0.18	0.18	0.00
髓样白血病	C92–C94	280	0.64	0.0	0.48	0.88	0.83	0.64	0.61	0.58
白血病，未特指	C95	341	0.78	3.6	1.68	1.14	0.67	1.19	1.05	1.81
其他的或未指明部位	O&U	882	2.03	1.2	1.80	1.32	0.67	1.73	1.05	1.65
骨髓增殖性疾病	MPD	31	0.07	0.0	0.00	0.00	0.00	0.09	0.09	0.16
骨髓增生异常综合征	MDS	11	0.03	0.0	0.12	0.00	0.08	0.00	0.00	0.08
合计	ALL	43 535	100.00	8.4	11.64	10.90	10.24	12.69	13.22	21.60
C44 以外的部位	ALL but C44	43 231	99.30	8.4	11.64	10.46	10.24	12.33	13.22	21.35

2020 年男性发病主要指标

30~	35~	40~	45~	50~	55~	60~	65~	70~	75~	80~	85+	粗率 (1/10[5])	世标率 (1/10[5])	累积率 (%)	
														0~64	0~74
0.08	0.09	0.00	0.00	0.27	0.33	0.00	1.57	2.11	0.00	3.26	0.99	0.23	0.17	0.01	0.02
0.69	0.09	0.45	1.03	0.98	0.76	1.20	1.42	3.05	0.74	3.26	2.97	0.57	0.43	0.03	0.05
0.23	0.35	0.18	1.20	1.25	2.71	1.06	3.78	7.05	5.53	8.48	0.00	0.97	0.70	0.04	0.09
0.31	0.17	0.98	0.86	1.07	1.41	2.26	2.83	2.11	2.95	1.30	2.97	0.73	0.57	0.04	0.06
0.00	0.00	0.27	0.00	0.09	0.22	0.13	0.16	0.47	0.74	0.65	0.99	0.10	0.08	0.00	0.01
0.00	0.26	0.09	0.26	0.54	0.43	0.40	1.10	0.70	2.58	1.30	1.98	0.26	0.19	0.01	0.02
0.69	0.61	1.16	1.80	2.23	4.23	2.52	3.93	4.46	2.58	2.61	6.93	1.30	1.01	0.07	0.11
0.15	0.00	0.09	0.17	0.54	0.33	0.93	1.57	2.58	3.32	3.91	2.97	0.38	0.28	0.01	0.03
0.08	0.00	0.18	0.34	0.45	0.98	0.93	1.57	2.35	1.84	0.65	0.00	0.35	0.26	0.02	0.04
0.31	1.22	1.96	8.67	25.56	50.48	103.62	204.70	276.17	301.07	328.01	324.86	36.49	26.16	0.96	3.37
1.39	3.13	7.40	17.34	42.54	70.35	127.93	228.14	301.77	319.51	345.62	327.83	43.44	31.40	1.36	4.01
0.23	0.44	0.53	1.37	2.14	2.71	4.25	8.02	7.75	5.90	7.17	4.95	1.43	1.06	0.06	0.14
1.85	2.79	4.19	7.21	13.67	13.57	23.91	35.87	49.55	52.76	45.65	41.60	8.55	6.32	0.34	0.77
1.62	2.18	3.39	7.64	15.19	20.41	30.95	49.25	69.04	76.00	73.69	57.45	11.09	8.09	0.41	1.01
0.15	0.26	0.27	0.34	0.71	0.76	1.06	2.36	3.29	2.95	2.61	0.99	0.49	0.36	0.02	0.05
5.01	8.18	18.45	39.13	60.86	77.19	98.44	134.21	155.23	146.11	143.46	179.27	33.37	24.82	1.55	3.00
0.15	0.44	0.98	1.46	2.95	5.10	9.43	17.78	23.72	30.99	31.95	24.76	3.53	2.54	0.10	0.31
0.62	0.96	1.60	2.92	4.92	6.30	11.03	22.97	29.12	29.52	30.65	35.66	4.45	3.25	0.14	0.41
0.08	0.35	0.27	0.43	1.07	1.19	2.26	1.57	1.88	2.95	1.30	0.00	0.55	0.44	0.03	0.05
0.15	0.35	0.53	1.03	2.86	5.65	5.45	11.33	14.56	15.13	5.22	9.90	2.18	1.61	0.08	0.21
3.70	4.35	12.03	31.84	69.97	124.42	200.46	346.62	478.36	530.92	584.29	549.69	70.43	50.74	2.25	6.37
0.54	0.26	0.53	1.20	1.43	2.06	2.13	4.25	2.58	3.32	5.22	2.97	0.94	0.73	0.05	0.08
0.54	0.70	1.52	1.80	2.23	4.23	5.58	7.08	8.45	11.07	10.43	8.91	2.31	1.96	0.11	0.19
0.15	0.09	0.09	0.17	0.27	0.54	0.40	1.26	0.94	1.84	0.65	1.98	0.23	0.17	0.01	0.02
0.08	0.17	0.71	1.12	2.23	2.28	3.06	7.39	7.98	19.19	19.56	35.66	1.91	1.40	0.05	0.13
0.00	0.00	0.00	0.09	0.27	0.54	0.13	0.47	0.70	0.37	0.00	0.00	0.11	0.09	0.01	0.01
0.00	0.00	0.00	0.00	0.00	0.00	0.00	0.16	0.00	0.00	0.00	0.00	0.01	0.01	0.00	0.00
0.62	0.26	0.45	0.69	1.25	1.19	1.33	1.57	2.35	2.58	3.91	2.97	0.67	0.53	0.03	0.05
0.15	0.26	0.27	0.86	1.25	1.63	1.06	2.52	2.82	1.84	5.87	1.98	0.63	0.46	0.03	0.05
0.00	0.00	0.00	0.00	0.00	0.00	0.00	0.00	0.00	0.00	0.00	0.00	0.00	0.00	0.00	0.00
0.00	0.00	0.00	0.00	0.00	0.00	0.00	0.00	0.00	0.00	0.00	0.00	0.00	0.00	0.00	0.00
0.00	0.00	0.00	0.00	0.00	0.00	0.00	0.16	0.00	0.00	0.00	0.00	0.01	0.00	0.00	0.00
0.00	0.00	0.00	0.00	0.00	0.00	0.00	0.00	0.00	0.00	0.00	0.00	0.00	0.00	0.00	0.00
0.00	0.00	0.00	0.00	0.00	0.00	0.00	0.00	0.00	0.00	0.00	0.00	0.00	0.00	0.00	0.00
0.00	0.00	0.00	0.00	0.00	0.00	0.00	0.00	0.00	0.00	0.00	0.00	0.00	0.00	0.00	0.00
0.00	0.00	0.00	0.00	0.00	0.00	0.00	0.00	0.00	0.00	0.00	0.00	0.00	0.00	0.00	0.00
0.00	0.00	0.00	0.00	0.00	0.00	0.00	0.00	0.00	0.00	0.00	0.00	0.00	0.00	0.00	0.00
0.00	0.00	0.27	0.77	1.25	1.30	1.73	2.99	3.52	4.06	5.22	4.95	0.69	0.50	0.03	0.06
0.08	0.09	0.09	0.60	1.43	3.04	11.96	32.88	52.37	79.69	89.34	94.09	6.45	4.48	0.09	0.51
0.69	0.44	0.53	0.77	0.36	0.22	0.53	0.79	0.94	1.11	0.65	0.00	0.37	0.32	0.02	0.03
0.00	0.00	0.00	0.00	0.09	0.00	0.40	0.63	0.23	0.00	0.65	0.99	0.07	0.05	0.00	0.01
1.00	1.74	2.50	3.86	7.33	7.49	8.90	18.09	17.85	16.60	13.69	9.90	3.87	2.94	0.17	0.35
0.00	0.09	0.18	0.43	0.45	0.76	0.53	1.10	1.17	2.21	3.26	2.97	0.31	0.23	0.01	0.02
0.00	0.00	0.27	0.43	0.63	0.87	1.33	2.83	1.17	2.58	5.22	0.99	0.45	0.33	0.02	0.04
0.69	0.61	2.05	2.06	5.90	9.66	14.48	27.38	34.99	46.86	56.08	60.42	5.84	4.19	0.18	0.49
0.00	0.09	0.00	0.09	0.18	0.11	0.13	0.16	0.70	0.00	0.65	0.00	0.07	0.05	0.00	0.01
0.08	0.00	0.09	0.17	0.27	0.11	0.13	0.47	1.41	0.37	0.00	1.98	0.18	0.17	0.01	0.02
3.70	3.05	2.67	6.69	10.28	12.27	12.75	19.35	31.94	30.62	20.22	27.73	6.60	5.31	0.32	0.57
7.78	6.01	7.04	11.50	9.38	11.94	10.63	8.65	7.05	4.43	4.56	3.96	5.56	4.49	0.36	0.44
0.00	0.09	0.45	0.17	0.71	0.22	0.66	0.94	2.58	1.48	1.96	0.99	0.31	0.24	0.01	0.03
0.08	0.09	0.09	0.09	0.27	0.33	0.53	0.16	0.47	1.11	0.65	0.00	0.16	0.13	0.01	0.01
0.08	0.09	0.09	0.51	0.36	0.22	1.06	0.79	1.64	1.11	0.00	0.00	0.30	0.25	0.02	0.03
1.31	1.39	1.78	3.43	3.66	6.73	7.70	10.38	15.73	19.19	15.65	8.91	3.33	2.65	0.16	0.29
0.00	0.00	0.09	0.00	0.00	0.00	0.00	0.16	0.00	0.37	0.00	0.00	0.03	0.03	0.00	0.00
0.15	0.26	0.36	0.60	2.23	1.85	3.19	7.71	7.05	5.53	4.56	2.97	1.18	0.87	0.04	0.12
0.00	0.09	0.45	0.26	0.36	1.09	1.33	1.10	4.23	0.37	1.30	0.99	0.60	0.62	0.03	0.06
1.00	0.87	0.89	1.89	2.59	2.39	3.85	7.08	7.28	6.64	1.96	2.97	1.76	1.47	0.09	0.16
1.46	0.87	1.25	1.63	1.97	3.04	4.38	6.61	7.05	6.27	9.78	3.96	2.14	1.93	0.11	0.18
1.62	2.79	2.67	4.98	7.51	8.36	11.29	19.67	24.42	28.41	41.73	33.67	5.55	4.39	0.24	0.46
0.23	0.09	0.09	0.09	0.27	0.76	0.53	0.47	0.23	0.37	0.65	0.99	0.19	0.15	0.01	0.02
0.08	0.00	0.00	0.00	0.18	0.11	0.00	0.31	0.00	0.00	0.65	0.99	0.07	0.06	0.00	0.00
39.61	46.67	82.46	171.98	316.44	474.87	739.93	1 276.33	1 685.19	1 833.70	1 949.15	1 895.69	273.77	201.68	9.76	24.57
39.53	46.49	81.75	170.86	314.21	472.59	736.87	1 268.93	1 677.21	1 814.51	1 929.59	1 860.03	271.86	200.29	9.71	24.44

表 6-9 河南省农村肿瘤登记地区

部位	ICD-10	病例数	构成 (%)	年龄组						
				0~	1~	5~	10~	15~	20~	25~
唇	C00	26	0.06	0.00	0.00	0.00	0.00	0.00	0.00	0.00
舌	C01–C02	66	0.16	0.00	0.00	0.00	0.00	0.00	0.00	0.09
口	C03–C06	109	0.27	0.00	0.00	0.20	0.00	0.00	0.10	0.09
唾液腺	C07–C08	92	0.23	0.00	0.00	0.10	0.00	0.21	0.10	0.27
扁桃体	C09	16	0.04	0.00	0.14	0.00	0.00	0.10	0.00	0.00
其他的口咽	C10	16	0.04	0.00	0.00	0.00	0.00	0.00	0.10	0.00
鼻咽	C11	105	0.26	0.00	0.00	0.00	0.10	0.00	0.19	0.18
喉咽	C12–C13	13	0.03	0.00	0.00	0.00	0.00	0.00	0.00	0.00
咽，部位不明	C14	31	0.08	0.00	0.00	0.10	0.00	0.00	0.10	0.09
食管	C15	3 664	9.05	0.00	0.00	0.00	0.00	0.00	0.39	0.54
胃	C16	3 061	7.56	0.00	0.00	0.10	0.29	0.31	0.58	1.35
小肠	C17	151	0.37	0.00	0.00	0.00	0.00	0.00	0.10	0.18
结肠	C18	1 177	2.91	0.00	0.00	0.00	0.00	0.00	0.19	0.81
直肠	C19–C20	1 439	3.56	0.00	0.00	0.00	0.00	0.00	0.39	0.54
肛门	C21	57	0.14	0.00	0.00	0.00	0.00	0.00	0.00	0.00
肝脏	C22	2 516	6.22	0.00	0.00	0.00	0.29	0.10	0.29	1.17
胆囊及其他	C23–C24	710	1.75	0.00	0.14	0.00	0.00	0.00	0.10	0.18
胰腺	C25	629	1.55	0.00	0.00	0.10	0.00	0.10	0.10	0.00
鼻、鼻窦及其他	C30–C31	59	0.15	0.00	0.00	0.00	0.10	0.10	0.00	0.09
喉	C32	54	0.13	0.00	0.00	0.00	0.10	0.00	0.00	0.00
气管、支气管、肺	C33–C34	5 337	13.19	0.00	0.00	0.10	0.00	0.10	0.58	0.72
其他的胸腔器官	C37–C38	126	0.31	0.00	0.27	0.00	0.00	0.10	0.00	0.18
骨	C40–C41	318	0.79	0.00	0.14	0.61	1.34	1.14	0.39	0.27
皮肤的黑色素瘤	C43	43	0.11	0.00	0.00	0.10	0.00	0.00	0.00	0.09
其他的皮肤	C44	285	0.70	0.00	0.27	0.20	0.10	0.31	0.19	0.09
间皮瘤	C45	15	0.04	0.00	0.00	0.00	0.00	0.00	0.00	0.00
卡波西肉瘤	C46	1	0.00	0.00	0.00	0.00	0.00	0.00	0.00	0.00
周围神经、其他结缔组织、软组织	C47;C49	101	0.25	0.00	0.41	0.30	0.19	0.62	0.00	0.18
乳房	C50	6 693	16.54	0.00	0.00	0.00	0.10	1.03	7.43	10.62
外阴	C51	54	0.13	0.00	0.00	0.00	0.00	0.00	0.00	0.09
阴道	C52	55	0.14	0.00	0.14	0.00	0.00	0.00	0.29	0.00
子宫颈	C53	3 209	7.93	0.00	0.00	0.00	0.00	0.00	1.83	5.85
子宫体	C54	1 598	3.95	0.00	0.00	0.00	0.00	0.00	0.48	1.80
子宫，部位不明	C55	265	0.65	0.00	0.00	0.00	0.10	0.00	0.10	0.18
卵巢	C56	1 200	2.97	0.00	0.27	0.51	0.96	2.68	3.18	3.15
女性其他的生殖器	C57	79	0.20	0.00	0.00	0.10	0.10	0.21	0.10	0.27
胎盘	C58	7	0.02	0.00	0.00	0.00	0.00	0.00	0.29	0.00
阴茎	C60	0	0.00	0.00	0.00	0.00	0.00	0.00	0.00	0.00
前列腺	C61	1	0.00	0.00	0.00	0.00	0.00	0.00	0.00	0.00
睾丸	C62	1	0.00	0.00	0.00	0.00	0.00	0.00	0.00	0.00
男性其他的生殖器	C63	0	0.00	0.00	0.00	0.00	0.00	0.00	0.00	0.00
肾	C64	377	0.93	0.00	0.68	0.00	0.19	0.41	0.19	0.27
肾盂	C65	35	0.09	0.00	0.00	0.00	0.00	0.00	0.00	0.00
输尿管	C66	45	0.11	0.00	0.00	0.00	0.00	0.00	0.00	0.00
膀胱	C67	280	0.69	0.00	0.00	0.00	0.00	0.10	0.19	0.27
其他的泌尿器官	C68	10	0.02	0.00	0.00	0.00	0.00	0.00	0.00	0.00
眼	C69	28	0.07	0.00	0.82	0.10	0.00	0.00	0.00	0.09
脑、神经系统	C70–C72	1 082	2.67	1.31	1.64	2.02	1.53	1.86	1.25	1.26
甲状腺	C73	3 135	7.75	0.00	0.00	0.10	0.96	1.96	4.73	15.30
肾上腺	C74	29	0.07	0.00	0.00	0.00	0.00	0.00	0.00	0.18
其他的内分泌腺	C75	26	0.06	0.00	0.00	0.10	0.00	0.10	0.00	0.00
霍奇金病	C81	37	0.09	0.00	0.00	0.00	0.00	0.00	0.00	0.36
非霍奇金淋巴瘤	C82–C85;C96	405	1.00	0.65	0.55	0.20	0.67	0.41	0.77	1.08
免疫增生性疾病	C88	6	0.01	0.00	0.14	0.00	0.00	0.00	0.00	0.00
多发性骨髓瘤	C90	153	0.38	0.00	0.00	0.00	0.00	0.00	0.10	0.00
淋巴样白血病	C91	77	0.19	0.00	0.82	1.11	0.57	0.00	0.10	0.18
髓样白血病	C92–C94	228	0.56	0.00	0.14	0.71	0.48	0.72	0.77	0.45
白血病，未特指	C95	302	0.75	3.27	2.60	0.91	0.96	1.14	0.77	0.54
其他的或未指明部位	O&U	804	1.99	0.00	1.78	1.31	0.76	0.83	1.16	0.99
骨髓增殖性疾病	MPD	22	0.05	0.65	0.00	0.00	0.00	0.00	0.00	0.00
骨髓增生异常综合征	MDS	9	0.02	0.00	0.14	0.00	0.00	0.00	0.00	0.00
合计	ALL	40 469	100.00	5.88	11.07	9.09	9.84	14.65	27.59	50.05
C44 以外的部位	ALL but C44	40 184	99.30	5.88	10.80	8.89	9.75	14.35	27.39	49.96

2020 年女性发病主要指标

30~	35~	40~	45~	50~	55~	60~	65~	70~	75~	80~	85+	粗率 (1/10^5)	世标率 (1/10^5)	累积率 (%) 0~64	累积率 (%) 0~74
0.17	0.00	0.00	0.09	0.28	0.22	0.41	0.63	0.66	0.99	1.50	1.20	0.17	0.11	0.01	0.01
0.17	0.09	0.57	0.27	0.84	0.55	1.36	1.10	2.42	1.65	2.49	0.60	0.44	0.30	0.02	0.04
0.08	0.19	0.57	0.45	0.65	1.44	1.50	1.88	3.08	4.62	5.99	4.81	0.73	0.48	0.03	0.05
0.50	0.85	0.38	0.71	0.84	1.33	1.09	2.19	2.42	0.00	0.50	1.80	0.62	0.47	0.03	0.05
0.00	0.09	0.00	0.00	0.09	0.22	0.14	0.31	0.66	0.99	0.50	0.00	0.11	0.08	0.00	0.01
0.00	0.19	0.09	0.18	0.09	0.00	0.41	0.31	0.00	0.33	1.50	0.00	0.11	0.08	0.01	0.01
0.17	0.38	0.28	0.54	1.30	1.77	1.63	2.50	2.64	2.97	2.00	1.20	0.70	0.50	0.03	0.06
0.00	0.00	0.09	0.00	0.00	0.11	0.00	0.63	0.44	0.66	1.00	0.60	0.09	0.05	0.00	0.01
0.00	0.19	0.09	0.00	0.47	0.00	0.41	0.63	0.66	1.32	1.00	2.41	0.21	0.14	0.01	0.01
0.33	1.23	1.60	4.73	14.06	28.27	51.97	113.64	155.38	192.21	191.52	227.94	24.51	15.00	0.52	1.86
2.41	4.18	4.44	10.99	20.68	29.70	41.49	85.62	96.84	127.26	160.60	179.83	20.47	12.90	0.58	1.49
0.17	0.09	0.19	1.07	1.58	1.55	2.45	4.38	4.18	4.62	6.98	4.21	1.01	0.67	0.04	0.08
1.49	1.42	3.30	5.63	11.83	15.79	18.91	32.71	33.67	39.89	42.89	34.28	7.87	5.21	0.30	0.63
1.00	1.33	2.55	7.32	12.57	18.11	21.90	43.98	46.00	48.79	51.37	55.93	9.62	6.30	0.33	0.78
0.00	0.00	0.09	0.36	0.47	0.66	0.82	1.41	2.86	0.99	2.00	3.61	0.38	0.25	0.01	0.03
1.49	2.37	4.81	11.88	18.44	25.29	39.18	66.37	87.81	84.73	122.69	137.12	16.83	10.78	0.53	1.30
0.25	0.19	0.19	1.61	5.22	6.52	10.47	23.17	24.43	30.00	34.41	42.10	4.75	2.98	0.12	0.36
0.66	0.47	0.66	2.50	5.50	6.52	9.66	19.72	17.39	26.05	27.93	29.47	4.21	2.69	0.13	0.32
0.08	0.38	0.19	0.36	0.56	0.99	0.95	1.41	0.44	1.32	1.50	3.01	0.39	0.28	0.02	0.03
0.00	0.09	0.00	0.18	0.65	0.88	0.41	2.19	1.10	2.31	0.50	3.01	0.36	0.24	0.01	0.03
2.65	4.65	9.35	22.69	44.90	63.38	79.17	142.12	172.99	199.79	233.42	289.29	35.69	22.77	1.14	2.72
0.66	0.38	0.47	0.89	1.40	1.77	1.90	2.35	2.20	2.31	5.99	3.01	0.84	0.59	0.04	0.06
1.16	1.52	0.85	1.16	3.07	3.53	3.13	7.83	7.26	5.93	12.47	7.82	2.13	1.59	0.09	0.17
0.00	0.00	0.19	0.18	0.28	0.44	0.95	1.41	1.32	1.32	1.50	0.60	0.29	0.20	0.01	0.02
0.50	0.28	0.28	0.63	1.86	2.10	1.77	7.67	8.80	9.56	17.46	30.07	1.91	1.20	0.04	0.13
0.00	0.00	0.00	0.09	0.19	0.00	0.54	0.63	0.22	0.66	0.50	0.00	0.10	0.07	0.00	0.01
0.00	0.00	0.00	0.00	0.00	0.00	0.14	0.00	0.00	0.00	0.00	0.00	0.01	0.01	0.00	0.00
0.66	0.19	0.76	0.89	1.40	0.99	1.36	0.94	1.98	0.66	1.00	2.41	0.68	0.56	0.04	0.05
22.40	40.18	60.70	94.41	115.96	98.61	81.08	104.87	75.93	60.99	41.90	45.71	44.76	33.30	2.66	3.57
0.17	0.19	0.09	0.45	0.47	0.66	0.54	1.72	1.76	1.65	1.50	0.60	0.36	0.25	0.01	0.03
0.08	0.19	0.47	0.54	0.28	0.88	0.82	0.78	1.32	0.99	1.50	1.80	0.37	0.27	0.02	0.03
11.03	18.62	26.53	39.92	54.12	51.02	46.25	45.08	40.72	36.27	29.43	25.86	21.46	15.78	1.28	1.70
2.57	3.61	9.54	18.94	31.58	37.10	23.81	23.79	23.99	12.86	10.97	11.43	10.69	7.71	0.65	0.89
0.83	1.14	1.70	3.30	4.84	4.20	3.81	4.38	3.30	3.30	3.49	3.61	1.77	1.28	0.10	0.14
5.47	4.56	7.65	12.50	15.65	18.88	16.19	18.47	19.15	18.46	9.98	9.02	8.03	6.12	0.46	0.65
0.08	0.28	0.38	1.07	1.02	0.88	1.77	1.41	0.66	1.32	0.50	1.20	0.53	0.41	0.03	0.04
0.17	0.00	0.09	0.00	0.09	0.00	0.00	0.00	0.00	0.00	0.00	0.00	0.05	0.04	0.00	0.00
0.00	0.00	0.00	0.00	0.00	0.00	0.00	0.00	0.00	0.00	0.00	0.00	0.00	0.00	0.00	0.00
0.00	0.00	0.00	0.09	0.00	0.00	0.00	0.00	0.00	0.00	0.00	0.00	0.01	0.01	0.00	0.00
0.00	0.00	0.00	0.00	0.00	0.00	0.00	0.00	0.00	0.33	0.00	0.00	0.01	0.00	0.00	0.00
0.00	0.00	0.00	0.00	0.00	0.00	0.00	0.00	0.00	0.00	0.00	0.00	0.00	0.00	0.00	0.00
0.75	1.14	1.42	2.50	4.84	5.74	4.90	8.61	7.92	10.88	7.98	10.22	2.52	1.79	0.11	0.20
0.17	0.00	0.00	0.09	0.19	0.22	0.27	1.57	1.10	1.98	1.00	1.80	0.23	0.15	0.00	0.02
0.08	0.00	0.00	0.27	0.19	0.22	0.68	2.03	1.76	1.65	2.00	1.20	0.30	0.20	0.01	0.03
0.33	0.66	0.38	1.25	2.05	3.09	3.81	8.30	7.26	11.54	10.47	15.04	1.87	1.22	0.06	0.14
0.08	0.09	0.00	0.09	0.09	0.11	0.00	0.78	0.00	0.00	0.00	0.00	0.07	0.05	0.00	0.01
0.00	0.00	0.19	0.18	0.37	0.44	0.27	0.31	0.66	0.33	0.00	0.00	0.19	0.19	0.01	0.02
2.90	3.70	3.49	5.98	11.92	14.13	16.05	24.73	21.13	24.73	28.93	28.87	7.24	5.37	0.34	0.57
25.46	23.94	28.13	40.82	51.23	53.34	30.34	28.64	13.65	16.15	6.48	5.41	20.97	16.24	1.38	1.59
0.25	0.09	0.09	0.09	0.19	0.66	0.54	0.47	0.44	1.32	0.00	0.00	0.19	0.14	0.01	0.02
0.25	0.19	0.28	0.00	0.47	0.44	0.27	0.31	0.22	0.00	0.50	0.60	0.17	0.13	0.01	0.01
0.41	0.19	0.28	0.18	0.19	0.44	0.41	0.47	1.32	0.99	0.00	0.00	0.25	0.19	0.01	0.02
1.08	0.66	1.70	2.23	3.91	5.30	5.31	10.02	10.56	9.89	9.98	7.82	2.71	1.99	0.12	0.22
0.00	0.00	0.00	0.00	0.00	0.11	0.41	0.16	0.00	0.00	0.00	0.00	0.04	0.04	0.00	0.00
0.08	0.28	0.28	0.80	1.21	3.31	3.54	5.17	4.40	2.97	2.00	0.60	1.02	0.72	0.05	0.10
0.25	0.00	0.28	0.54	0.09	0.88	0.54	0.94	1.98	2.64	0.00	1.80	0.51	0.50	0.03	0.04
0.91	1.33	1.32	2.23	2.51	2.21	2.45	4.38	3.30	4.95	2.49	1.80	1.52	1.22	0.08	0.12
1.00	1.14	1.04	1.34	2.05	2.43	2.99	6.26	6.82	6.59	9.48	4.81	2.02	1.76	0.10	0.16
2.65	1.52	2.45	4.91	6.52	9.72	12.11	16.28	19.81	25.39	27.43	22.25	5.38	3.90	0.23	0.41
0.00	0.00	0.00	0.18	0.00	0.44	0.82	0.63	0.00	0.66	1.00	0.60	0.15	0.11	0.01	0.01
0.08	0.00	0.00	0.09	0.09	0.11	0.00	0.16	0.00	0.33	0.00	1.20	0.06	0.05	0.00	0.00
94.14	124.52	180.51	310.38	461.34	527.73	554.07	888.43	947.02	1 051.05	1 140.16	1 269.61	270.66	187.61	11.87	21.05
93.65	124.24	180.22	309.75	459.48	525.63	552.30	880.76	938.22	1 041.49	1 122.70	1 239.54	268.75	186.42	11.83	20.92

表 6-10 河南省肿瘤登记地区

部位	ICD-10	病例数	构成(%)	年龄组						
				0~	1~	5~	10~	15~	20~	25~
唇	C00	44	0.06	0.00	0.00	0.00	0.00	0.00	0.00	0.03
舌	C01–C02	112	0.16	0.00	0.05	0.00	0.00	0.00	0.00	0.00
口	C03–C06	165	0.23	0.00	0.00	0.00	0.00	0.00	0.00	0.00
唾液腺	C07–C08	83	0.12	0.00	0.00	0.00	0.00	0.00	0.00	0.00
扁桃体	C09	23	0.03	0.00	0.00	0.00	0.00	0.00	0.00	0.00
其他的口咽	C10	50	0.07	0.00	0.00	0.03	0.00	0.00	0.00	0.00
鼻咽	C11	223	0.32	0.00	0.00	0.00	0.00	0.00	0.00	0.00
喉咽	C12–C13	75	0.11	0.00	0.00	0.00	0.00	0.00	0.00	0.00
咽，部位不明	C14	82	0.12	0.00	0.00	0.00	0.03	0.00	0.00	0.00
食管	C15	9 122	12.97	0.00	0.05	0.00	0.00	0.00	0.03	0.15
胃	C16	10 260	14.59	0.00	0.05	0.03	0.07	0.04	0.17	0.25
小肠	C17	310	0.44	0.00	0.00	0.00	0.00	0.00	0.00	0.00
结肠	C18	1 993	2.83	0.00	0.00	0.00	0.00	0.04	0.07	0.28
直肠	C19–C20	2 180	3.10	0.00	0.00	0.03	0.00	0.00	0.00	0.09
肛门	C21	170	0.24	0.00	0.00	0.00	0.00	0.00	0.00	0.00
肝脏	C22	9 221	13.11	0.00	0.14	0.10	0.13	0.11	0.10	0.22
胆囊及其他	C23–C24	1 520	2.16	0.00	0.00	0.00	0.00	0.00	0.00	0.06
胰腺	C25	1 765	2.51	0.00	0.00	0.03	0.00	0.00	0.03	0.03
鼻、鼻窦及其他	C30–C31	107	0.15	0.00	0.00	0.00	0.00	0.00	0.03	0.03
喉	C32	313	0.44	0.00	0.00	0.00	0.00	0.00	0.00	0.00
气管、支气管、肺	C33–C34	17 574	24.99	0.00	0.00	0.00	0.07	0.04	0.20	0.49
其他的胸腔器官	C37–C38	229	0.33	0.00	0.05	0.00	0.03	0.14	0.10	0.03
骨	C40–C41	544	0.77	0.00	0.05	0.21	0.33	0.36	0.44	0.28
皮肤的黑色素瘤	C43	64	0.09	0.00	0.00	0.00	0.00	0.00	0.00	0.00
其他的皮肤	C44	349	0.50	0.00	0.00	0.00	0.00	0.00	0.03	0.00
间皮瘤	C45	36	0.05	0.00	0.00	0.00	0.00	0.00	0.00	0.00
卡波西肉瘤	C46	1	0.00	0.00	0.00	0.00	0.00	0.00	0.00	0.00
周围神经、其他结缔组织、软组织	C47;C49	118	0.17	0.22	0.09	0.07	0.17	0.04	0.00	0.03
乳房	C50	2 123	3.02	0.00	0.00	0.00	0.00	0.00	0.14	0.31
外阴	C51	33	0.05	0.00	0.00	0.00	0.00	0.00	0.00	0.00
阴道	C52	31	0.04	0.00	0.00	0.00	0.00	0.00	0.00	0.00
子宫颈	C53	1 265	1.80	0.00	0.00	0.00	0.00	0.00	0.00	0.19
子宫体	C54	424	0.60	0.00	0.00	0.00	0.00	0.00	0.00	0.00
子宫，部位不明	C55	128	0.18	0.00	0.00	0.00	0.00	0.00	0.00	0.00
卵巢	C56	698	0.99	0.00	0.00	0.00	0.00	0.00	0.07	0.25
女性其他的生殖器	C57	27	0.04	0.00	0.00	0.07	0.00	0.00	0.00	0.00
胎盘	C58	0	0.00	0.00	0.00	0.00	0.00	0.00	0.00	0.00
阴茎	C60	42	0.06	0.00	0.00	0.00	0.00	0.00	0.00	0.00
前列腺	C61	789	1.12	0.00	0.00	0.00	0.00	0.00	0.06	0.00
睾丸	C62	22	0.03	0.00	0.09	0.00	0.00	0.00	0.00	0.00
男性其他的生殖器	C63	11	0.02	0.00	0.00	0.00	0.00	0.00	0.00	0.00
肾	C64	630	0.90	0.00	0.00	0.00	0.00	0.04	0.07	0.06
肾盂	C65	74	0.11	0.00	0.00	0.00	0.00	0.00	0.00	0.00
输尿管	C66	107	0.15	0.00	0.00	0.00	0.00	0.00	0.00	0.00
膀胱	C67	748	1.06	0.00	0.00	0.00	0.00	0.00	0.03	0.06
其他的泌尿器官	C68	17	0.02	0.00	0.00	0.00	0.00	0.00	0.00	0.00
眼	C69	31	0.04	0.00	0.05	0.03	0.00	0.00	0.00	0.03
脑、神经系统	C70–C72	1 844	2.62	0.22	0.55	1.49	0.99	0.39	0.91	0.52
甲状腺	C73	341	0.48	0.00	0.00	0.00	0.00	0.00	0.00	0.09
肾上腺	C74	74	0.11	0.00	0.00	0.07	0.00	0.04	0.00	0.03
其他的内分泌腺	C75	30	0.04	0.00	0.00	0.00	0.00	0.00	0.03	0.00
霍奇金病	C81	72	0.10	0.00	0.00	0.00	0.00	0.00	0.00	0.09
非霍奇金淋巴瘤	C82–C85;C96	785	1.12	0.00	0.00	0.07	0.30	0.25	0.34	0.15
免疫增生性疾病	C88	2	0.00	0.00	0.00	0.00	0.00	0.00	0.00	0.00
多发性骨髓瘤	C90	339	0.48	0.00	0.05	0.00	0.00	0.00	0.03	0.00
淋巴样白血病	C91	162	0.23	0.00	0.23	0.31	0.10	0.21	0.13	0.03
髓样白血病	C92–C94	393	0.56	0.00	0.41	0.17	0.20	0.25	0.24	0.22
白血病，未特指	C95	572	0.81	0.00	0.60	0.41	0.53	0.57	0.17	0.46
其他的或未指明部位	O&U	1 572	2.23	0.45	0.41	0.48	0.26	0.61	0.34	0.37
骨髓增殖性疾病	MPD	32	0.05	0.00	0.00	0.00	0.00	0.00	0.07	0.00
骨髓增生异常综合征	MDS	129	0.18	0.00	0.09	0.03	0.00	0.00	0.03	0.03
合计	ALL	70 338	100.00	0.89	2.90	3.63	3.21	3.10	3.73	4.49
C44 以外的部位	ALL but C44	69 989	99.50	0.89	2.90	3.63	3.21	3.10	3.70	4.49

2020 年合计死亡主要指标

30~	35~	40~	45~	50~	55~	60~	65~	70~	75~	80~	85+	粗率 (1/10^5)	世标率 (1/10^5)	累积率 (%)	
														0~64	0~74
0.00	0.03	0.03	0.06	0.00	0.15	0.24	0.28	0.48	0.24	1.33	2.65	0.10	0.07	0.00	0.01
0.12	0.10	0.13	0.21	0.19	0.35	0.48	1.08	0.80	1.32	2.65	3.71	0.26	0.17	0.01	0.02
0.03	0.00	0.10	0.12	0.29	0.46	0.53	1.64	2.49	3.00	5.12	3.45	0.38	0.24	0.01	0.03
0.03	0.03	0.10	0.09	0.36	0.27	0.39	0.68	1.21	0.48	1.33	2.92	0.19	0.13	0.01	0.02
0.00	0.00	0.00	0.09	0.03	0.08	0.10	0.45	0.16	0.36	0.38	0.00	0.05	0.04	0.00	0.00
0.00	0.00	0.03	0.03	0.13	0.27	0.14	0.28	0.97	0.60	1.33	1.06	0.12	0.08	0.00	0.01
0.17	0.22	0.13	0.45	0.75	0.89	1.49	1.98	1.85	3.00	3.41	3.45	0.52	0.35	0.02	0.04
0.00	0.03	0.03	0.06	0.16	0.27	0.14	0.51	1.29	1.32	2.09	2.39	0.17	0.11	0.00	0.01
0.09	0.00	0.06	0.03	0.10	0.31	0.39	0.68	0.80	1.80	1.90	2.39	0.19	0.12	0.01	0.01
0.20	0.45	0.89	2.74	7.42	17.28	38.95	84.75	147.49	200.49	251.96	308.59	21.14	13.20	0.34	1.50
1.09	1.50	2.73	6.14	13.45	26.64	46.13	103.09	152.16	197.25	247.03	304.88	23.78	15.19	0.49	1.77
0.09	0.03	0.06	0.48	0.71	1.04	1.59	3.40	3.30	5.17	5.88	8.23	0.72	0.47	0.02	0.05
0.26	0.67	0.79	2.02	3.21	5.76	8.20	16.64	21.87	36.42	57.25	71.64	4.62	2.92	0.11	0.30
0.37	0.38	0.86	2.17	3.95	6.30	10.17	19.30	25.41	37.38	57.44	75.62	5.05	3.22	0.12	0.35
0.00	0.10	0.13	0.30	0.32	0.77	0.48	0.96	2.41	2.64	3.98	6.10	0.39	0.25	0.01	0.03
2.27	3.92	7.30	15.81	26.54	41.61	51.00	85.94	103.90	116.23	135.93	210.68	21.37	14.41	0.75	1.70
0.06	0.13	0.41	0.54	1.94	3.71	6.94	16.08	20.83	26.32	39.43	55.99	3.52	2.24	0.07	0.25
0.23	0.29	0.86	1.29	3.86	6.07	9.16	16.13	23.89	28.13	39.62	48.82	4.09	2.66	0.11	0.31
0.09	0.06	0.06	0.21	0.42	0.31	0.63	0.51	0.64	2.16	2.09	2.92	0.25	0.16	0.01	0.01
0.03	0.03	0.16	0.12	0.36	1.08	1.64	3.40	3.94	6.73	5.31	9.55	0.73	0.47	0.02	0.05
1.01	1.82	4.57	12.98	30.20	56.84	84.36	173.41	249.47	315.52	393.96	494.07	40.73	26.23	0.96	3.08
0.17	0.16	0.10	0.18	0.68	0.77	1.16	1.59	2.57	3.73	4.93	4.51	0.53	0.36	0.02	0.04
0.29	0.29	0.25	0.60	1.17	1.86	1.93	4.53	6.11	6.85	9.67	15.92	1.26	0.89	0.04	0.09
0.03	0.06	0.06	0.03	0.29	0.23	0.24	0.28	1.21	0.72	1.33	1.33	0.15	0.10	0.00	0.01
0.06	0.13	0.10	0.24	0.58	0.73	1.01	1.98	3.46	5.41	10.05	25.74	0.81	0.49	0.01	0.04
0.03	0.03	0.00	0.06	0.16	0.12	0.29	0.28	0.64	0.24	0.57	0.00	0.08	0.06	0.00	0.01
0.00	0.03	0.00	0.00	0.00	0.00	0.00	0.00	0.00	0.00	0.00	0.00	0.00	0.00	0.00	0.00
0.14	0.19	0.16	0.18	0.19	0.35	0.67	0.51	0.97	1.44	1.71	3.45	0.27	0.21	0.01	0.02
1.35	3.00	5.04	11.22	17.93	23.38	24.73	35.18	33.85	38.75	41.96	56.53	10.06	6.71	0.44	0.78
0.00	0.07	0.06	0.06	0.07	0.31	0.58	0.34	0.46	0.68	0.69	3.48	0.16	0.10	0.01	0.01
0.06	0.00	0.06	0.06	0.13	0.31	0.39	0.22	0.46	0.68	2.06	1.74	0.15	0.09	0.01	0.01
1.70	1.63	3.36	5.98	10.15	11.73	13.48	21.40	25.04	24.10	26.83	33.05	5.99	3.97	0.24	0.47
0.23	0.33	0.65	0.98	3.56	4.35	4.56	6.61	7.73	11.49	11.01	17.40	2.01	1.27	0.07	0.14
0.12	0.00	0.06	0.43	0.79	1.48	1.26	2.24	1.70	3.83	5.16	4.78	0.61	0.37	0.02	0.04
0.59	0.78	1.55	2.68	4.94	7.77	7.27	11.20	14.84	12.39	20.64	18.27	3.31	2.16	0.13	0.26
0.00	0.00	0.06	0.06	0.20	0.23	0.19	0.67	0.31	0.45	1.03	1.30	0.13	0.08	0.00	0.01
0.00	0.00	0.00	0.00	0.00	0.00	0.00	0.00	0.00	0.00	0.00	0.00	0.00	0.00	0.00	0.00
0.00	0.00	0.00	0.06	0.19	0.15	0.10	0.69	1.51	2.06	2.53	4.08	0.19	0.13	0.00	0.01
0.06	0.06	0.06	0.48	0.26	1.00	2.97	8.81	20.46	40.46	77.30	129.32	3.58	2.33	0.02	0.17
0.17	0.00	0.06	0.06	0.06	0.15	0.29	0.34	0.50	0.52	0.42	0.68	0.10	0.08	0.00	0.01
0.00	0.00	0.00	0.06	0.06	0.00	0.10	0.00	0.34	0.00	1.69	1.36	0.05	0.03	0.00	0.00
0.17	0.22	0.54	0.57	1.59	2.05	3.13	5.77	8.28	9.86	11.94	15.66	1.46	0.97	0.04	0.11
0.00	0.06	0.03	0.09	0.06	0.15	0.53	0.40	1.13	1.44	1.52	2.65	0.17	0.11	0.00	0.01
0.03	0.03	0.03	0.06	0.03	0.39	0.34	0.79	1.21	2.16	4.55	3.45	0.25	0.15	0.00	0.01
0.00	0.10	0.22	0.33	0.75	1.24	2.55	5.26	6.19	16.11	25.59	46.97	1.73	1.04	0.03	0.08
0.03	0.00	0.00	0.00	0.00	0.04	0.05	0.23	0.16	0.00	0.76	1.06	0.04	0.02	0.00	0.00
0.00	0.00	0.03	0.06	0.10	0.04	0.19	0.06	0.24	0.84	0.00	1.59	0.07	0.05	0.00	0.00
1.52	1.12	1.68	3.10	4.80	6.38	8.34	13.76	23.64	23.92	23.51	29.98	4.27	3.11	0.16	0.35
0.37	0.13	0.22	0.48	0.84	1.31	1.40	3.28	3.70	4.57	7.77	6.90	0.79	0.52	0.02	0.06
0.03	0.03	0.06	0.27	0.06	0.27	0.29	0.34	1.05	0.84	1.52	2.12	0.17	0.12	0.01	0.01
0.06	0.00	0.00	0.03	0.06	0.15	0.14	0.11	0.40	0.36	0.95	0.53	0.07	0.05	0.00	0.01
0.00	0.10	0.06	0.12	0.16	0.27	0.24	0.51	1.05	1.56	0.57	1.33	0.17	0.11	0.01	0.01
0.20	0.41	0.76	1.08	1.78	2.86	2.84	7.30	11.10	12.26	12.32	13.27	1.82	1.25	0.06	0.15
0.00	0.00	0.00	0.00	0.00	0.00	0.00	0.11	0.00	0.00	0.00	0.00	0.00	0.00	0.00	0.00
0.06	0.03	0.10	0.30	0.62	1.66	1.25	4.59	5.87	4.81	3.79	5.04	0.79	0.53	0.02	0.07
0.06	0.19	0.16	0.30	0.42	0.58	0.87	0.74	1.37	1.92	1.33	3.18	0.38	0.31	0.02	0.03
0.23	0.38	0.48	0.66	0.91	1.28	1.93	3.28	4.10	4.57	5.69	4.51	0.91	0.69	0.04	0.07
0.60	0.35	0.67	0.99	0.94	1.86	2.41	4.98	4.66	6.49	9.10	9.02	1.33	1.02	0.05	0.10
0.60	0.96	1.49	1.42	3.50	4.99	6.70	13.42	18.50	24.40	32.61	36.35	3.64	2.51	0.11	0.27
0.00	0.00	0.00	0.00	0.06	0.08	0.14	0.40	0.08	0.36	1.33	1.33	0.07	0.05	0.00	0.00
0.09	0.03	0.10	0.09	0.16	0.39	0.63	0.85	2.09	2.40	2.09	3.71	0.30	0.20	0.01	0.02
13.00	17.69	32.25	68.19	133.36	226.09	330.55	651.27	930.72	1 194.17	1 532.80	1 995.64	163.02	106.43	4.21	12.12
12.94	17.56	32.15	67.95	132.78	225.36	329.54	649.29	927.26	1 188.76	1 522.75	1 969.90	162.22	105.94	4.19	12.08

表 6-11 河南省肿瘤登记地区

部位	ICD-10	病例数	构成 (%)	年龄组 0~	1~	5~	10~	15~	20~	25~
唇	C00	29	0.07	0.00	0.00	0.00	0.00	0.00	0.00	0.06
舌	C01–C02	58	0.13	0.00	0.09	0.00	0.00	0.00	0.00	0.00
口	C03–C06	84	0.19	0.00	0.00	0.00	0.00	0.00	0.00	0.00
唾液腺	C07–C08	58	0.13	0.00	0.00	0.00	0.00	0.00	0.00	0.00
扁桃体	C09	12	0.03	0.00	0.00	0.00	0.00	0.00	0.00	0.00
其他的口咽	C10	36	0.08	0.00	0.00	0.00	0.00	0.00	0.00	0.00
鼻咽	C11	151	0.35	0.00	0.00	0.00	0.00	0.00	0.00	0.00
喉咽	C12–C13	68	0.16	0.00	0.00	0.00	0.00	0.00	0.00	0.00
咽，部位不明	C14	55	0.13	0.00	0.00	0.00	0.00	0.00	0.00	0.00
食管	C15	5 769	13.33	0.00	0.09	0.00	0.00	0.00	0.00	0.06
胃	C16	7 214	16.67	0.00	0.09	0.06	0.00	0.00	0.13	0.18
小肠	C17	188	0.43	0.00	0.00	0.00	0.00	0.00	0.00	0.00
结肠	C18	1 079	2.49	0.00	0.00	0.00	0.00	0.07	0.06	0.30
直肠	C19–C20	1 237	2.86	0.00	0.00	0.06	0.00	0.00	0.00	0.12
肛门	C21	99	0.23	0.00	0.00	0.00	0.00	0.00	0.00	0.00
肝脏	C22	6 341	14.65	0.00	0.17	0.13	0.06	0.07	0.13	0.36
胆囊及其他	C23–C24	669	1.55	0.00	0.00	0.00	0.00	0.00	0.00	0.00
胰腺	C25	941	2.17	0.00	0.00	0.00	0.00	0.00	0.00	0.06
鼻、鼻窦及其他	C30–C31	62	0.14	0.00	0.00	0.00	0.00	0.00	0.00	0.00
喉	C32	273	0.63	0.00	0.00	0.00	0.00	0.00	0.00	0.00
气管、支气管、肺	C33–C34	12 473	28.82	0.00	0.00	0.00	0.06	0.00	0.32	0.78
其他的胸腔器官	C37–C38	134	0.31	0.00	0.00	0.00	0.00	0.27	0.19	0.06
骨	C40–C41	333	0.77	0.00	0.09	0.32	0.43	0.47	0.52	0.12
皮肤的黑色素瘤	C43	35	0.08	0.00	0.00	0.00	0.00	0.00	0.00	0.00
其他的皮肤	C44	186	0.43	0.00	0.00	0.00	0.00	0.00	0.00	0.00
间皮瘤	C45	22	0.05	0.00	0.00	0.00	0.00	0.00	0.00	0.00
卡波西肉瘤	C46	0	0.00	0.00	0.00	0.00	0.00	0.00	0.00	0.00
周围神经、其他结缔组织、软组织	C47;C49	65	0.15	0.00	0.17	0.06	0.12	0.00	0.00	0.00
乳房	C50	55	0.13	0.00	0.00	0.00	0.00	0.00	0.00	0.00
外阴	C51	0	0.00	0.00	0.00	0.00	0.00	0.00	0.00	0.00
阴道	C52	0	0.00	0.00	0.00	0.00	0.00	0.00	0.00	0.00
子宫颈	C53	1	0.00	0.00	0.00	0.00	0.00	0.00	0.00	0.00
子宫体	C54	0	0.00	0.00	0.00	0.00	0.00	0.00	0.00	0.00
子宫，部位不明	C55	1	0.00	0.00	0.00	0.00	0.00	0.00	0.00	0.00
卵巢	C56	0	0.00	0.00	0.00	0.00	0.00	0.00	0.00	0.00
女性其他的生殖器	C57	0	0.00	0.00	0.00	0.00	0.00	0.00	0.00	0.00
胎盘	C58	0	0.00	0.00	0.00	0.00	0.00	0.00	0.00	0.00
阴茎	C60	42	0.10	0.00	0.00	0.00	0.00	0.00	0.00	0.00
前列腺	C61	789	1.82	0.00	0.00	0.00	0.00	0.00	0.06	0.00
睾丸	C62	22	0.05	0.00	0.09	0.00	0.00	0.00	0.00	0.00
男性其他的生殖器	C63	11	0.03	0.00	0.00	0.00	0.00	0.00	0.00	0.00
肾	C64	415	0.96	0.00	0.00	0.00	0.00	0.07	0.13	0.06
肾盂	C65	47	0.11	0.00	0.00	0.00	0.00	0.00	0.00	0.00
输尿管	C66	68	0.16	0.00	0.00	0.00	0.00	0.00	0.00	0.00
膀胱	C67	581	1.34	0.00	0.00	0.00	0.00	0.00	0.00	0.12
其他的泌尿器官	C68	7	0.02	0.00	0.00	0.00	0.00	0.00	0.00	0.00
眼	C69	18	0.04	0.00	0.09	0.06	0.00	0.00	0.00	0.00
脑、神经系统	C70–C72	1 015	2.35	0.00	0.70	1.36	1.61	0.47	0.84	0.48
甲状腺	C73	112	0.26	0.00	0.00	0.00	0.00	0.00	0.00	0.00
肾上腺	C74	57	0.13	0.00	0.00	0.13	0.00	0.07	0.00	0.00
其他的内分泌腺	C75	16	0.04	0.00	0.00	0.00	0.00	0.00	0.06	0.00
霍奇金病	C81	39	0.09	0.00	0.00	0.00	0.00	0.00	0.00	0.12
非霍奇金淋巴瘤	C82–C85;C96	451	1.04	0.00	0.00	0.06	0.31	0.20	0.58	0.24
免疫增生性疾病	C88	2	0.00	0.00	0.00	0.00	0.00	0.00	0.00	0.00
多发性骨髓瘤	C90	203	0.47	0.00	0.09	0.00	0.00	0.00	0.06	0.00
淋巴样白血病	C91	95	0.22	0.00	0.09	0.39	0.06	0.34	0.19	0.00
髓样白血病	C92–C94	230	0.53	0.00	0.35	0.26	0.19	0.34	0.26	0.30
白血病，未特指	C95	318	0.73	0.00	0.52	0.26	0.31	0.54	0.26	0.72
其他的或未指明部位	O&U	916	2.12	0.43	0.43	0.39	0.31	0.68	0.52	0.48
骨髓增殖性疾病	MPD	16	0.04	0.00	0.00	0.00	0.00	0.00	0.06	0.00
骨髓增生异常综合征	MDS	78	0.18	0.00	0.09	0.06	0.00	0.00	0.00	0.00
合计	ALL	43 276	100.00	0.43	3.13	3.64	3.47	3.58	4.40	4.63
C44 以外的部位	ALL but C44	43 090	99.57	0.43	3.13	3.64	3.47	3.58	4.40	4.63

2020 年男性死亡主要指标

												粗率	世标率	累积率 (%)	
30~	35~	40~	45~	50~	55~	60~	65~	70~	75~	80~	85+	(1/10^5)	(1/10^5)	0~64	0~74
0.00	0.00	0.06	0.06	0.00	0.15	0.29	0.34	1.01	0.26	1.27	5.44	0.13	0.10	0.00	0.01
0.06	0.12	0.12	0.30	0.13	0.46	0.77	1.26	0.17	1.29	2.96	4.76	0.26	0.19	0.01	0.02
0.00	0.00	0.12	0.18	0.32	0.69	0.48	1.83	2.68	3.87	3.80	2.72	0.38	0.26	0.01	0.03
0.06	0.06	0.19	0.06	0.32	0.38	0.58	1.14	1.84	1.03	1.27	5.44	0.26	0.19	0.01	0.02
0.00	0.00	0.00	0.00	0.06	0.08	0.10	0.80	0.17	0.26	0.00	0.00	0.05	0.04	0.00	0.01
0.00	0.00	0.00	0.06	0.19	0.23	0.29	0.57	1.34	0.77	2.53	2.72	0.16	0.11	0.00	0.01
0.17	0.31	0.25	0.59	0.89	1.46	2.30	2.86	2.68	3.87	3.80	4.76	0.69	0.50	0.03	0.06
0.00	0.06	0.06	0.12	0.32	0.54	0.29	0.92	2.35	2.58	3.80	5.44	0.31	0.21	0.01	0.02
0.17	0.00	0.06	0.06	0.13	0.54	0.58	1.03	1.01	2.32	2.53	3.40	0.25	0.17	0.01	0.02
0.23	0.56	0.87	4.70	10.97	22.94	52.72	118.66	201.71	265.18	329.05	403.61	26.18	17.88	0.47	2.07
1.02	1.68	3.25	8.62	18.04	38.27	69.79	156.65	242.12	303.06	356.93	424.03	32.74	22.62	0.71	2.70
0.17	0.06	0.12	0.77	0.83	1.23	2.30	4.35	4.53	6.44	5.91	8.17	0.85	0.61	0.03	0.07
0.34	0.75	0.94	2.50	3.83	6.70	8.63	18.19	26.83	38.66	62.52	97.33	4.90	3.38	0.12	0.35
0.40	0.56	0.81	2.62	4.59	7.55	12.37	23.23	31.52	42.01	76.88	85.76	5.61	3.87	0.15	0.42
0.00	0.19	0.12	0.48	0.26	0.77	0.58	1.03	3.35	4.12	5.49	5.44	0.45	0.31	0.01	0.03
3.34	6.42	12.11	24.97	41.51	66.37	73.81	121.52	140.35	153.33	167.70	256.59	28.78	20.68	1.15	2.46
0.06	0.06	0.50	0.54	1.28	3.70	6.61	16.48	20.46	25.25	32.53	49.00	3.04	2.11	0.06	0.25
0.23	0.37	1.12	1.37	4.34	7.08	10.45	18.08	28.67	28.35	43.09	53.77	4.27	2.99	0.13	0.36
0.17	0.12	0.06	0.30	0.64	0.23	0.86	0.92	0.50	2.32	2.11	2.72	0.28	0.20	0.01	0.02
0.06	0.06	0.19	0.24	0.57	2.08	2.97	5.72	7.71	12.63	11.40	17.02	1.24	0.86	0.03	0.10
1.24	2.74	5.43	15.58	40.55	80.46	126.92	261.46	387.67	494.79	601.08	744.60	56.61	39.19	1.37	4.62
0.17	0.19	0.06	0.12	0.96	0.85	1.15	2.29	3.52	5.15	6.76	1.36	0.61	0.44	0.02	0.05
0.45	0.44	0.37	0.89	1.02	2.46	2.40	5.84	8.38	10.05	10.56	19.74	1.51	1.14	0.05	0.12
0.06	0.06	0.06	0.06	0.26	0.31	0.29	0.34	1.34	0.77	1.27	2.04	0.16	0.11	0.01	0.01
0.00	0.12	0.00	0.18	0.64	0.85	1.15	2.98	4.02	7.22	12.67	27.22	0.84	0.57	0.01	0.05
0.06	0.00	0.00	0.12	0.26	0.15	0.48	0.11	0.50	0.52	0.84	0.00	0.10	0.07	0.01	0.01
0.00	0.00	0.00	0.00	0.00	0.00	0.00	0.00	0.00	0.00	0.00	0.00	0.00	0.00	0.00	0.00
0.11	0.19	0.19	0.24	0.13	0.23	1.15	0.80	1.01	1.80	1.69	4.76	0.29	0.23	0.01	0.02
0.00	0.00	0.25	0.12	0.26	0.46	0.58	0.92	1.51	1.80	2.53	2.04	0.25	0.17	0.01	0.02
0.00	0.00	0.00	0.00	0.00	0.00	0.00	0.00	0.00	0.00	0.00	0.00	0.00	0.00	0.00	0.00
0.00	0.00	0.00	0.00	0.00	0.00	0.00	0.00	0.00	0.00	0.00	0.00	0.00	0.00	0.00	0.00
0.00	0.00	0.00	0.00	0.00	0.00	0.00	0.11	0.00	0.00	0.00	0.00	0.00	0.00	0.00	0.00
0.00	0.00	0.00	0.00	0.00	0.00	0.00	0.00	0.00	0.00	0.00	0.00	0.00	0.00	0.00	0.00
0.00	0.00	0.00	0.00	0.06	0.00	0.00	0.00	0.00	0.00	0.00	0.00	0.00	0.00	0.00	0.00
0.00	0.00	0.00	0.00	0.00	0.00	0.00	0.00	0.00	0.00	0.00	0.00	0.00	0.00	0.00	0.00
0.00	0.00	0.00	0.00	0.00	0.00	0.00	0.00	0.00	0.00	0.00	0.00	0.00	0.00	0.00	0.00
0.00	0.00	0.00	0.00	0.00	0.00	0.00	0.00	0.00	0.00	0.00	0.00	0.00	0.00	0.00	0.00
0.00	0.00	0.00	0.06	0.19	0.15	0.10	0.69	1.51	2.06	2.53	4.08	0.19	0.13	0.00	0.01
0.06	0.06	0.06	0.48	0.26	1.00	2.97	8.81	20.46	40.46	77.30	129.32	3.58	2.33	0.02	0.17
0.17	0.00	0.06	0.06	0.06	0.15	0.29	0.34	0.50	0.52	0.42	0.68	0.10	0.08	0.00	0.01
0.00	0.00	0.00	0.06	0.06	0.00	0.10	0.00	0.34	0.00	1.69	1.36	0.05	0.03	0.00	0.00
0.23	0.31	0.75	0.89	2.23	2.77	4.03	8.58	12.07	11.85	13.94	24.50	1.88	1.35	0.06	0.16
0.00	0.12	0.06	0.12	0.13	0.31	0.77	0.57	1.68	1.29	1.69	2.72	0.21	0.15	0.01	0.02
0.06	0.06	0.06	0.06	0.06	0.38	0.48	1.14	2.01	2.83	4.65	6.13	0.31	0.21	0.01	0.02
0.00	0.12	0.31	0.42	1.21	1.85	4.22	8.12	10.06	28.60	44.35	89.16	2.64	1.76	0.04	0.13
0.00	0.00	0.00	0.00	0.00	0.08	0.00	0.11	0.17	0.00	0.84	1.36	0.03	0.02	0.00	0.00
0.00	0.00	0.06	0.00	0.06	0.08	0.10	0.11	0.34	1.03	0.00	3.40	0.08	0.07	0.00	0.00
2.09	1.43	1.94	3.57	5.61	8.01	9.49	13.62	27.33	26.80	24.08	31.99	4.61	3.52	0.19	0.39
0.11	0.12	0.12	0.24	0.70	1.08	0.77	2.17	3.02	3.09	5.91	4.08	0.51	0.35	0.02	0.04
0.00	0.06	0.12	0.42	0.13	0.38	0.48	0.57	1.84	1.29	1.69	4.76	0.26	0.20	0.01	0.02
0.00	0.00	0.00	0.00	0.00	0.23	0.19	0.23	0.34	0.52	1.27	0.68	0.07	0.05	0.00	0.01
0.00	0.06	0.00	0.24	0.26	0.23	0.29	0.57	1.01	1.80	0.84	1.36	0.18	0.13	0.01	0.01
0.28	0.69	0.81	1.13	2.17	3.54	3.64	8.47	13.75	13.66	15.21	12.25	2.05	1.49	0.07	0.18
0.00	0.00	0.00	0.00	0.00	0.00	0.00	0.23	0.00	0.00	0.00	0.00	0.01	0.01	0.00	0.00
0.06	0.06	0.06	0.36	0.70	2.00	1.44	6.06	6.71	6.96	4.22	6.81	0.92	0.66	0.02	0.09
0.11	0.25	0.19	0.24	0.51	0.69	0.86	1.03	2.01	2.06	1.69	4.76	0.43	0.36	0.02	0.03
0.34	0.25	0.69	0.89	1.15	1.23	1.63	3.32	5.87	6.18	8.03	7.49	1.04	0.81	0.04	0.08
0.57	0.37	0.75	1.37	1.34	2.23	2.97	5.38	4.69	7.22	11.83	10.89	1.44	1.13	0.06	0.11
0.85	1.18	1.56	1.49	4.08	6.47	7.86	17.39	23.31	27.57	39.28	46.28	4.16	3.03	0.13	0.33
0.00	0.00	0.00	0.00	0.13	0.15	0.10	0.11	0.17	0.52	2.11	0.68	0.07	0.05	0.00	0.00
0.11	0.06	0.12	0.12	0.13	0.46	0.67	1.03	2.35	3.87	2.96	6.13	0.35	0.25	0.01	0.03
13.57	20.38	35.09	78.00	154.50	280.72	424.28	859.11	1 270.48	1 609.86	2 019.52	2 640.80	196.40	137.37	5.14	15.79
13.57	20.26	35.09	77.82	153.86	279.87	423.13	856.14	1 266.46	1 602.65	2 006.85	2 613.58	195.55	136.80	5.13	15.74

表 6-12 河南省肿瘤登记地区

部位	ICD-10	病例数	构成 (%)	年龄组						
				0~	1~	5~	10~	15~	20~	25~
唇	C00	15	0.06	0.00	0.00	0.00	0.00	0.00	0.00	0.00
舌	C01–C02	54	0.20	0.00	0.00	0.00	0.00	0.00	0.00	0.00
口	C03–C06	81	0.30	0.00	0.00	0.00	0.00	0.00	0.00	0.00
唾液腺	C07–C08	25	0.09	0.00	0.00	0.00	0.00	0.00	0.00	0.00
扁桃体	C09	11	0.04	0.00	0.00	0.00	0.00	0.00	0.00	0.00
其他的口咽	C10	14	0.05	0.00	0.00	0.07	0.00	0.00	0.00	0.00
鼻咽	C11	72	0.27	0.00	0.00	0.00	0.00	0.00	0.00	0.00
喉咽	C12–C13	7	0.03	0.00	0.00	0.00	0.00	0.00	0.00	0.00
咽，部位不明	C14	27	0.10	0.00	0.00	0.00	0.07	0.00	0.00	0.00
食管	C15	3 353	12.39	0.00	0.00	0.00	0.00	0.00	0.07	0.25
胃	C16	3 046	11.26	0.00	0.00	0.00	0.14	0.08	0.21	0.31
小肠	C17	122	0.45	0.00	0.00	0.00	0.00	0.00	0.00	0.00
结肠	C18	914	3.38	0.00	0.00	0.00	0.00	0.00	0.07	0.25
直肠	C19–C20	943	3.48	0.00	0.00	0.00	0.00	0.00	0.00	0.06
肛门	C21	71	0.26	0.00	0.00	0.00	0.00	0.00	0.00	0.00
肝脏	C22	2 880	10.64	0.00	0.10	0.07	0.21	0.15	0.07	0.06
胆囊及其他	C23–C24	851	3.14	0.00	0.00	0.00	0.00	0.00	0.00	0.13
胰腺	C25	824	3.04	0.00	0.00	0.07	0.00	0.00	0.07	0.00
鼻、鼻窦及其他	C30–C31	45	0.17	0.00	0.00	0.00	0.00	0.00	0.07	0.06
喉	C32	40	0.15	0.00	0.00	0.00	0.00	0.00	0.00	0.00
气管、支气管、肺	C33–C34	5 101	18.85	0.00	0.00	0.00	0.07	0.08	0.07	0.19
其他的胸腔器官	C37–C38	95	0.35	0.00	0.10	0.00	0.07	0.00	0.00	0.00
骨	C40–C41	211	0.78	0.00	0.00	0.07	0.21	0.23	0.35	0.44
皮肤的黑色素瘤	C43	29	0.11	0.00	0.00	0.00	0.00	0.00	0.00	0.00
其他的皮肤	C44	163	0.60	0.00	0.00	0.00	0.00	0.00	0.07	0.00
间皮瘤	C45	14	0.05	0.00	0.00	0.00	0.00	0.00	0.00	0.00
卡波西肉瘤	C46	1	0.00	0.00	0.00	0.00	0.00	0.00	0.00	0.00
周围神经、其他结缔组织、软组织	C47;C49	53	0.20	0.47	0.00	0.07	0.21	0.08	0.00	0.06
乳房	C50	2 123	7.84	0.00	0.00	0.00	0.00	0.00	0.14	0.31
外阴	C51	33	0.12	0.00	0.00	0.00	0.00	0.00	0.00	0.00
阴道	C52	31	0.11	0.00	0.00	0.00	0.00	0.00	0.00	0.00
子宫颈	C53	1 265	4.67	0.00	0.00	0.00	0.00	0.00	0.00	0.19
子宫体	C54	424	1.57	0.00	0.00	0.00	0.00	0.00	0.00	0.00
子宫，部位不明	C55	128	0.47	0.00	0.00	0.00	0.00	0.00	0.00	0.00
卵巢	C56	698	2.58	0.00	0.00	0.00	0.00	0.00	0.07	0.25
女性其他的生殖器	C57	27	0.10	0.00	0.00	0.07	0.00	0.00	0.00	0.00
胎盘	C58	0	0.00	0.00	0.00	0.00	0.00	0.00	0.00	0.00
阴茎	C60	0	0.00	0.00	0.00	0.00	0.00	0.00	0.00	0.00
前列腺	C61	0	0.00	0.00	0.00	0.00	0.00	0.00	0.00	0.00
睾丸	C62	1	0.00	0.00	0.00	0.00	0.00	0.00	0.00	0.00
男性其他的生殖器	C63	0	0.00	0.00	0.00	0.00	0.00	0.00	0.00	0.00
肾	C64	215	0.79	0.00	0.00	0.00	0.00	0.00	0.00	0.06
肾盂	C65	27	0.10	0.00	0.00	0.00	0.00	0.00	0.00	0.00
输尿管	C66	39	0.14	0.00	0.00	0.00	0.00	0.00	0.00	0.00
膀胱	C67	167	0.62	0.00	0.00	0.00	0.00	0.00	0.07	0.00
其他的泌尿器官	C68	10	0.04	0.00	0.00	0.00	0.00	0.00	0.00	0.00
眼	C69	13	0.05	0.00	0.00	0.00	0.00	0.00	0.00	0.06
脑、神经系统	C70–C72	829	3.06	0.47	0.39	1.62	0.28	0.30	0.98	0.57
甲状腺	C73	229	0.85	0.00	0.00	0.00	0.00	0.00	0.00	0.19
肾上腺	C74	17	0.06	0.00	0.00	0.00	0.00	0.00	0.00	0.06
其他的内分泌腺	C75	14	0.05	0.00	0.00	0.00	0.00	0.00	0.00	0.00
霍奇金病	C81	33	0.12	0.00	0.00	0.00	0.00	0.00	0.00	0.06
非霍奇金淋巴瘤	C82–C85;C96	334	1.23	0.00	0.00	0.07	0.28	0.30	0.07	0.06
免疫增生性疾病	C88	0	0.00	0.00	0.00	0.00	0.00	0.00	0.00	0.00
多发性骨髓瘤	C90	136	0.50	0.00	0.00	0.00	0.00	0.00	0.00	0.00
淋巴样白血病	C91	67	0.25	0.00	0.39	0.22	0.14	0.08	0.07	0.06
髓样白血病	C92–C94	163	0.60	0.00	0.49	0.07	0.21	0.15	0.21	0.13
白血病，未特指	C95	254	0.94	0.00	0.69	0.59	0.78	0.60	0.07	0.19
其他的或未指明部位	O&U	656	2.42	0.47	0.39	0.59	0.21	0.53	0.14	0.25
骨髓增殖性疾病	MPD	16	0.06	0.00	0.00	0.00	0.00	0.00	0.07	0.00
骨髓增生异常综合征	MDS	51	0.19	0.00	0.10	0.00	0.00	0.00	0.07	0.06
合计	ALL	27 062	100.00	1.40	2.64	3.62	2.91	2.57	3.00	4.34
C44 以外的部位	ALL but C44	26 899	99.40	1.40	2.64	3.62	2.91	2.57	2.93	4.34

2020 年女性死亡主要指标

30~	35~	40~	45~	50~	55~	60~	65~	70~	75~	80~	85+	粗率 (1/10^5)	世标率 (1/10^5)	累积率 (%) 0~64	0~74
0.00	0.07	0.00	0.06	0.00	0.16	0.19	0.22	0.00	0.23	1.38	0.87	0.07	0.04	0.00	0.00
0.18	0.07	0.13	0.12	0.26	0.23	0.19	0.90	1.39	1.35	2.41	3.04	0.26	0.16	0.01	0.02
0.06	0.00	0.06	0.06	0.26	0.23	0.58	1.46	2.32	2.25	6.19	3.91	0.38	0.22	0.01	0.03
0.00	0.00	0.00	0.12	0.40	0.16	0.19	0.22	0.62	0.00	1.38	1.30	0.12	0.07	0.00	0.01
0.00	0.00	0.00	0.18	0.00	0.08	0.10	0.11	0.15	0.45	0.69	0.00	0.05	0.03	0.00	0.00
0.00	0.00	0.06	0.00	0.07	0.31	0.00	0.00	0.62	0.45	0.34	0.00	0.07	0.05	0.00	0.01
0.18	0.13	0.00	0.31	0.59	0.31	0.68	1.12	1.08	2.25	3.10	2.61	0.34	0.21	0.01	0.02
0.00	0.00	0.00	0.00	0.00	0.00	0.00	0.11	0.31	0.23	0.69	0.43	0.03	0.02	0.00	0.00
0.00	0.00	0.06	0.00	0.07	0.08	0.19	0.34	0.62	1.35	1.38	1.74	0.13	0.08	0.00	0.01
0.18	0.33	0.90	0.73	3.76	11.57	25.02	51.54	97.52	143.95	189.18	247.88	15.88	8.93	0.21	0.96
1.17	1.30	2.20	3.60	8.70	14.92	22.21	50.65	69.24	104.75	157.54	228.75	14.43	8.36	0.27	0.87
0.00	0.00	0.00	0.18	0.59	0.85	0.87	2.47	2.16	4.05	5.85	8.26	0.58	0.34	0.01	0.04
0.18	0.59	0.65	1.53	2.57	4.82	7.76	15.13	17.31	34.47	52.97	55.23	4.33	2.52	0.09	0.25
0.35	0.20	0.90	1.71	3.30	5.05	7.95	15.46	19.78	33.34	41.62	69.15	4.47	2.63	0.10	0.27
0.00	0.00	0.13	0.12	0.40	0.78	0.39	0.90	1.55	1.35	2.75	6.52	0.34	0.20	0.01	0.02
1.17	1.30	2.32	6.41	11.07	16.62	27.93	51.09	70.32	83.80	110.07	181.35	13.64	8.30	0.34	0.94
0.06	0.20	0.32	0.55	2.64	3.73	7.27	15.69	21.17	27.26	45.06	60.45	4.03	2.34	0.07	0.26
0.23	0.20	0.58	1.22	3.36	5.05	7.85	14.23	19.47	27.93	36.80	45.66	3.90	2.34	0.09	0.26
0.00	0.00	0.06	0.12	0.20	0.39	0.39	0.11	0.77	2.03	2.06	3.04	0.21	0.13	0.01	0.01
0.00	0.00	0.13	0.00	0.13	0.08	0.29	1.12	0.46	1.58	0.34	4.78	0.19	0.11	0.00	0.01
0.76	0.85	3.68	10.31	19.51	33.02	41.31	87.17	122.09	158.81	225.30	333.99	24.16	14.36	0.55	1.60
0.18	0.13	0.13	0.24	0.40	0.70	1.16	0.90	1.70	2.48	3.44	6.52	0.45	0.29	0.02	0.03
0.12	0.13	0.13	0.31	1.32	1.24	1.45	3.25	4.02	4.05	8.94	13.48	1.00	0.66	0.03	0.07
0.00	0.07	0.06	0.00	0.33	0.16	0.19	0.22	1.08	0.68	1.38	0.87	0.14	0.08	0.00	0.01
0.12	0.13	0.19	0.31	0.53	0.62	0.87	1.01	2.94	3.83	7.91	24.79	0.77	0.43	0.01	0.03
0.00	0.07	0.00	0.00	0.07	0.08	0.10	0.45	0.77	0.00	0.34	0.00	0.07	0.04	0.00	0.01
0.00	0.07	0.00	0.00	0.00	0.00	0.00	0.00	0.00	0.00	0.00	0.00	0.00	0.00	0.00	0.00
0.18	0.20	0.13	0.12	0.26	0.47	0.19	0.22	0.93	1.13	1.72	2.61	0.25	0.18	0.01	0.02
1.35	3.00	5.04	11.22	17.93	23.38	24.73	35.18	33.85	38.75	41.96	56.53	10.06	6.71	0.44	0.78
0.00	0.07	0.06	0.06	0.07	0.31	0.58	0.34	0.46	0.68	0.69	3.48	0.16	0.10	0.01	0.01
0.06	0.00	0.06	0.06	0.13	0.31	0.39	0.22	0.46	0.68	2.06	1.74	0.15	0.09	0.01	0.01
1.70	1.63	3.36	5.98	10.15	11.73	13.48	21.40	25.04	24.10	26.83	33.05	5.99	3.97	0.24	0.47
0.23	0.33	0.65	0.98	3.56	4.35	4.56	6.61	7.73	11.49	11.01	17.40	2.01	1.27	0.07	0.14
0.12	0.00	0.06	0.43	0.79	1.48	1.26	2.24	1.70	3.83	5.16	4.78	0.61	0.37	0.02	0.04
0.59	0.78	1.55	2.68	4.94	7.77	7.27	11.20	14.84	12.39	20.64	18.27	3.31	2.16	0.13	0.26
0.00	0.00	0.06	0.06	0.20	0.23	0.19	0.67	0.31	0.45	1.03	1.30	0.13	0.08	0.00	0.01
0.00	0.00	0.00	0.00	0.00	0.00	0.00	0.00	0.00	0.00	0.00	0.00	0.00	0.00	0.00	0.00
0.00	0.00	0.00	0.00	0.00	0.00	0.00	0.00	0.00	0.00	0.00	0.00	0.00	0.00	0.00	0.00
0.00	0.00	0.00	0.00	0.00	0.00	0.00	0.00	0.00	0.00	0.00	0.00	0.00	0.00	0.00	0.00
0.00	0.00	0.00	0.00	0.00	0.00	0.00	0.00	0.00	0.23	0.00	0.00	0.00	0.00	0.00	0.00
0.00	0.00	0.00	0.00	0.00	0.00	0.00	0.00	0.00	0.00	0.00	0.00	0.00	0.00	0.00	0.00
0.12	0.13	0.32	0.24	0.92	1.32	2.23	3.03	4.79	8.11	10.32	10.00	1.02	0.61	0.03	0.07
0.00	0.00	0.00	0.06	0.00	0.00	0.29	0.22	0.62	1.58	1.38	2.61	0.13	0.07	0.00	0.01
0.00	0.00	0.00	0.06	0.00	0.39	0.19	0.45	0.46	1.58	4.47	1.74	0.18	0.10	0.00	0.01
0.00	0.07	0.13	0.24	0.26	0.62	0.87	2.47	2.63	5.18	10.32	20.00	0.79	0.43	0.01	0.04
0.06	0.00	0.00	0.00	0.00	0.00	0.10	0.34	0.15	0.00	0.69	0.87	0.05	0.03	0.00	0.00
0.00	0.00	0.00	0.12	0.13	0.00	0.29	0.00	0.15	0.68	0.00	0.43	0.06	0.04	0.00	0.00
0.94	0.78	1.42	2.62	3.95	4.74	7.18	13.89	20.25	21.40	23.05	28.70	3.93	2.70	0.13	0.30
0.64	0.13	0.32	0.73	0.99	1.55	2.04	4.37	4.33	5.86	9.29	8.70	1.08	0.68	0.03	0.08
0.06	0.00	0.00	0.12	0.00	0.16	0.10	0.11	0.31	0.45	1.38	0.43	0.08	0.05	0.00	0.00
0.12	0.00	0.00	0.06	0.13	0.08	0.10	0.00	0.46	0.23	0.69	0.43	0.07	0.04	0.00	0.00
0.00	0.13	0.13	0.00	0.07	0.31	0.19	0.45	1.08	1.35	0.34	1.30	0.16	0.10	0.00	0.01
0.12	0.13	0.71	1.04	1.38	2.18	2.04	6.16	8.65	11.04	9.97	13.92	1.58	1.02	0.04	0.12
0.00	0.00	0.00	0.00	0.00	0.00	0.00	0.00	0.00	0.00	0.00	0.00	0.00	0.00	0.00	0.00
0.06	0.00	0.13	0.24	0.53	1.32	1.07	3.14	5.10	2.93	3.44	3.91	0.64	0.41	0.02	0.06
0.00	0.13	0.13	0.37	0.33	0.47	0.87	0.45	0.77	1.80	1.03	2.17	0.32	0.26	0.02	0.02
0.12	0.52	0.26	0.43	0.66	1.32	2.23	3.25	2.47	3.15	3.78	2.61	0.77	0.58	0.03	0.06
0.64	0.33	0.58	0.61	0.53	1.48	1.84	4.59	4.64	5.86	6.88	7.83	1.20	0.92	0.04	0.09
0.35	0.72	1.42	1.34	2.90	3.50	5.53	9.52	14.06	21.63	27.17	30.01	3.11	2.01	0.09	0.21
0.00	0.00	0.00	0.00	0.00	0.00	0.19	0.67	0.00	0.23	0.69	1.74	0.08	0.05	0.00	0.00
0.06	0.00	0.06	0.06	0.20	0.31	0.58	0.67	1.85	1.13	1.38	2.17	0.24	0.16	0.01	0.02
12.42	14.88	29.31	58.13	111.52	170.98	235.74	447.75	617.56	830.79	1 136.46	1 583.41	128.19	78.15	3.26	8.59
12.30	14.74	29.12	57.83	110.99	170.36	234.86	446.74	614.62	826.96	1 128.55	1 558.62	127.42	77.73	3.25	8.55

表 6-13 河南省城市肿瘤登记地区

部位	ICD-10	病例数	构成 (%)	年龄组						
				0~	1~	5~	10~	15~	20~	25~
唇	C00	10	0.05	0.00	0.00	0.00	0.00	0.00	0.00	0.00
舌	C01–C02	43	0.22	0.00	0.16	0.00	0.00	0.00	0.00	0.00
口	C03–C06	64	0.32	0.00	0.00	0.00	0.00	0.00	0.00	0.00
唾液腺	C07–C08	25	0.13	0.00	0.00	0.00	0.00	0.00	0.00	0.00
扁桃体	C09	9	0.05	0.00	0.00	0.00	0.00	0.00	0.00	0.00
其他的口咽	C10	14	0.07	0.00	0.00	0.13	0.00	0.00	0.00	0.00
鼻咽	C11	65	0.33	0.00	0.00	0.00	0.00	0.00	0.00	0.00
喉咽	C12–C13	28	0.14	0.00	0.00	0.00	0.00	0.00	0.00	0.00
咽，部位不明	C14	20	0.10	0.00	0.00	0.00	0.13	0.00	0.00	0.00
食管	C15	1 854	9.41	0.00	0.16	0.00	0.00	0.00	0.00	0.11
胃	C16	2 393	12.15	0.00	0.00	0.00	0.00	0.00	0.00	0.22
小肠	C17	102	0.52	0.00	0.00	0.00	0.00	0.00	0.00	0.00
结肠	C18	773	3.92	0.00	0.00	0.00	0.00	0.00	0.13	0.22
直肠	C19–C20	678	3.44	0.00	0.00	0.00	0.00	0.00	0.00	0.11
肛门	C21	16	0.08	0.00	0.00	0.00	0.00	0.00	0.00	0.00
肝脏	C22	2 452	12.45	0.00	0.16	0.00	0.13	0.14	0.13	0.11
胆囊及其他	C23–C24	500	2.54	0.00	0.00	0.00	0.00	0.00	0.00	0.11
胰腺	C25	658	3.34	0.00	0.00	0.13	0.00	0.00	0.00	0.11
鼻、鼻窦及其他	C30–C31	23	0.12	0.00	0.00	0.00	0.00	0.00	0.00	0.00
喉	C32	110	0.56	0.00	0.00	0.00	0.00	0.00	0.00	0.00
气管、支气管、肺	C33–C34	5 007	25.42	0.00	0.00	0.00	0.00	0.14	0.00	0.22
其他的胸腔器官	C37–C38	73	0.37	0.00	0.00	0.00	0.00	0.27	0.00	0.11
骨	C40–C41	123	0.62	0.00	0.00	0.13	0.26	0.14	0.00	0.11
皮肤的黑色素瘤	C43	19	0.10	0.00	0.00	0.00	0.00	0.00	0.00	0.00
其他的皮肤	C44	92	0.47	0.00	0.00	0.00	0.00	0.00	0.13	0.00
间皮瘤	C45	17	0.09	0.00	0.00	0.00	0.00	0.00	0.00	0.00
卡波西肉瘤	C46	0	0.00	0.00	0.00	0.00	0.00	0.00	0.00	0.00
周围神经、其他结缔组织、软组织	C47;C49	43	0.22	0.78	0.16	0.13	0.13	0.00	0.00	0.00
乳房	C50	709	3.60	0.00	0.00	0.00	0.00	0.00	0.00	0.63
外阴	C51	17	0.09	0.00	0.00	0.00	0.00	0.00	0.00	0.00
阴道	C52	9	0.05	0.00	0.00	0.00	0.00	0.00	0.00	0.00
子宫颈	C53	351	1.78	0.00	0.00	0.00	0.00	0.00	0.00	0.00
子宫体	C54	125	0.63	0.00	0.00	0.00	0.00	0.00	0.00	0.00
子宫，部位不明	C55	28	0.14	0.00	0.00	0.00	0.00	0.00	0.00	0.00
卵巢	C56	254	1.29	0.00	0.00	0.00	0.00	0.00	0.00	0.00
女性其他的生殖器	C57	8	0.04	0.00	0.00	0.00	0.00	0.00	0.00	0.00
胎盘	C58	0	0.00	0.00	0.00	0.00	0.00	0.00	0.00	0.00
阴茎	C60	11	0.06	0.00	0.00	0.00	0.00	0.00	0.00	0.00
前列腺	C61	339	1.72	0.00	0.00	0.00	0.00	0.00	0.00	0.00
睾丸	C62	4	0.02	0.00	0.31	0.00	0.00	0.00	0.00	0.00
男性其他的生殖器	C63	6	0.03	0.00	0.00	0.00	0.00	0.00	0.00	0.00
肾	C64	217	1.10	0.00	0.00	0.00	0.00	0.00	0.13	0.11
肾盂	C65	25	0.13	0.00	0.00	0.00	0.00	0.00	0.00	0.00
输尿管	C66	49	0.25	0.00	0.00	0.00	0.00	0.00	0.00	0.00
膀胱	C67	244	1.24	0.00	0.00	0.00	0.00	0.00	0.00	0.00
其他的泌尿器官	C68	7	0.04	0.00	0.00	0.00	0.00	0.00	0.00	0.00
眼	C69	9	0.05	0.00	0.00	0.13	0.00	0.00	0.00	0.00
脑、神经系统	C70–C72	485	2.46	0.00	1.15	1.30	1.29	0.41	0.75	0.22
甲状腺	C73	96	0.49	0.00	0.00	0.00	0.00	0.00	0.00	0.00
肾上腺	C74	18	0.09	0.00	0.00	0.00	0.00	0.14	0.00	0.00
其他的内分泌腺	C75	9	0.05	0.00	0.00	0.00	0.00	0.00	0.00	0.00
霍奇金病	C81	24	0.12	0.00	0.00	0.00	0.00	0.00	0.00	0.11
非霍奇金淋巴瘤	C82–C85;C96	278	1.41	0.00	0.00	0.00	0.00	0.41	0.13	0.00
免疫增生性疾病	C88	0	0.00	0.00	0.00	0.00	0.00	0.00	0.00	0.00
多发性骨髓瘤	C90	113	0.57	0.00	0.00	0.00	0.00	0.00	0.00	0.00
淋巴样白血病	C91	60	0.30	0.00	0.49	0.39	0.26	0.14	0.13	0.11
髓样白血病	C92–C94	143	0.73	0.00	0.16	0.26	0.26	0.14	0.25	0.00
白血病，未特指	C95	179	0.91	0.00	0.49	0.39	0.52	0.27	0.13	0.22
其他的或未指明部位	O&U	582	2.95	1.56	0.33	0.26	0.26	0.41	0.25	0.54
骨髓增殖性疾病	MPD	13	0.07	0.00	0.00	0.00	0.00	0.00	0.00	0.00
骨髓增生异常综合征	MDS	58	0.29	0.00	0.00	0.00	0.00	0.00	0.00	0.00
合计	ALL	19 697	100.00	2.35	3.46	3.26	3.22	2.58	2.13	3.01
C44 以外的部位	ALL but C44	19 605	99.53	2.35	3.46	3.26	3.22	2.58	2.01	3.01

2020 年合计死亡主要指标

												粗率	世标率	累积率 (%)	
30~	35~	40~	45~	50~	55~	60~	65~	70~	75~	80~	85+	(1/10⁵)	(1/10⁵)	0~64	0~74
0.00	0.11	0.00	0.00	0.00	0.13	0.17	0.20	0.00	0.00	0.58	4.56	0.08	0.05	0.00	0.00
0.10	0.21	0.00	0.39	0.45	0.53	0.34	1.22	0.55	0.78	2.88	9.12	0.35	0.23	0.01	0.02
0.00	0.00	0.21	0.29	0.22	0.13	0.85	1.63	3.30	1.94	9.22	9.12	0.52	0.31	0.01	0.03
0.00	0.00	0.10	0.00	0.22	0.40	0.68	0.61	1.38	0.39	1.73	2.74	0.20	0.13	0.01	0.02
0.00	0.00	0.00	0.19	0.00	0.00	0.34	0.61	0.28	0.39	0.00	0.00	0.07	0.05	0.00	0.01
0.00	0.00	0.00	0.00	0.11	0.40	0.00	0.41	0.55	1.16	1.15	0.00	0.11	0.08	0.00	0.01
0.10	0.21	0.21	0.39	0.67	0.92	1.70	2.64	1.38	3.49	2.30	1.82	0.53	0.36	0.02	0.04
0.00	0.00	0.00	0.19	0.22	0.79	0.34	0.81	1.38	0.78	1.15	2.74	0.23	0.15	0.01	0.02
0.00	0.00	0.00	0.00	0.11	0.53	0.17	0.20	0.55	1.16	2.88	1.82	0.16	0.10	0.00	0.01
0.00	0.00	0.72	1.83	5.94	11.59	29.50	56.11	98.83	123.06	175.67	232.59	15.08	9.05	0.25	1.02
0.92	1.50	2.79	5.50	9.74	18.57	35.97	79.08	118.10	145.18	206.78	268.16	19.47	11.89	0.38	1.36
0.10	0.00	0.10	0.39	1.01	1.05	1.36	2.85	3.30	5.43	9.79	12.77	0.83	0.50	0.02	0.05
0.62	0.43	1.13	2.32	3.25	6.06	10.74	21.55	24.23	41.54	87.55	122.22	6.29	3.73	0.12	0.35
0.31	0.43	0.62	2.03	4.93	7.37	11.08	19.92	23.95	34.16	58.75	93.95	5.52	3.38	0.13	0.35
0.00	0.00	0.00	0.10	0.11	0.26	0.00	0.20	0.83	0.78	0.58	4.56	0.13	0.08	0.00	0.01
1.75	3.63	6.60	13.89	24.41	41.61	49.95	73.18	89.19	98.21	116.35	202.49	19.95	13.05	0.71	1.52
0.10	0.21	0.31	0.29	2.13	4.08	7.67	15.25	21.47	26.40	48.38	82.09	4.07	2.44	0.07	0.26
0.00	0.21	0.72	1.93	4.70	7.90	12.10	17.28	28.08	32.22	58.17	75.71	5.35	3.30	0.14	0.37
0.00	0.00	0.21	0.29	0.11	0.26	0.34	0.20	0.83	1.94	1.73	0.91	0.19	0.11	0.01	0.01
0.00	0.00	0.31	0.29	0.45	1.84	2.39	2.64	5.78	6.60	5.76	10.03	0.89	0.57	0.03	0.07
0.72	1.18	4.02	11.67	25.87	54.38	87.46	161.41	221.33	273.28	440.05	550.01	40.73	25.00	0.93	2.84
0.10	0.21	0.10	0.00	0.56	0.66	1.70	2.03	2.75	4.27	5.18	5.47	0.59	0.39	0.02	0.04
0.21	0.32	0.31	0.48	0.67	1.32	1.53	3.86	4.96	3.88	6.91	19.15	1.00	0.67	0.03	0.07
0.00	0.00	0.21	0.10	0.22	0.13	0.17	0.00	1.65	0.00	1.73	2.74	0.15	0.10	0.00	0.01
0.00	0.00	0.21	0.48	0.22	0.53	1.36	1.22	3.85	4.27	6.34	25.54	0.75	0.45	0.01	0.04
0.00	0.00	0.00	0.10	0.34	0.00	0.51	0.20	1.38	0.78	1.15	0.00	0.14	0.09	0.00	0.01
0.00	0.00	0.00	0.00	0.00	0.00	0.00	0.00	0.00	0.00	0.00	0.00	0.00	0.00	0.00	0.00
0.10	0.21	0.10	0.19	0.34	0.40	1.19	0.61	1.10	1.55	2.30	4.56	0.35	0.26	0.02	0.02
1.79	2.92	6.54	12.31	20.06	23.32	24.65	32.73	35.29	42.67	70.93	95.80	11.51	7.33	0.46	0.80
0.00	0.21	0.20	0.00	0.00	0.79	1.01	0.79	0.00	1.42	2.22	4.71	0.28	0.17	0.01	0.02
0.00	0.00	0.20	0.00	0.00	0.26	0.00	0.79	0.52	0.71	1.11	3.14	0.15	0.09	0.00	0.01
1.59	1.46	2.86	5.39	10.59	11.53	12.16	18.14	24.91	18.49	31.03	29.84	5.70	3.69	0.23	0.44
0.20	0.42	0.82	0.58	1.35	3.93	5.74	7.10	10.38	12.09	13.30	15.70	2.03	1.26	0.07	0.15
0.00	0.00	0.20	0.19	0.45	1.83	2.03	0.79	0.52	0.71	2.22	7.85	0.45	0.29	0.02	0.03
0.60	0.21	1.63	2.89	6.76	9.43	11.48	11.44	15.57	12.80	32.14	32.98	4.12	2.60	0.17	0.30
0.00	0.00	0.20	0.00	0.23	0.26	0.00	0.79	0.00	0.00	2.22	1.57	0.13	0.08	0.00	0.01
0.00	0.00	0.00	0.00	0.00	0.00	0.00	0.00	0.00	0.00	0.00	0.00	0.00	0.00	0.00	0.00
0.00	0.00	0.00	0.00	0.22	0.00	0.00	0.84	1.17	0.85	3.60	4.35	0.18	0.11	0.00	0.01
0.00	0.00	0.21	0.19	0.45	0.79	3.79	11.33	19.93	60.68	103.13	224.11	5.53	3.21	0.03	0.18
0.21	0.00	0.21	0.00	0.00	0.00	0.00	0.42	0.00	0.00	0.00	0.00	0.07	0.07	0.00	0.01
0.00	0.00	0.00	0.19	0.00	0.00	0.00	0.00	0.00	0.00	4.80	2.18	0.10	0.05	0.00	0.00
0.21	0.21	0.52	0.19	1.46	2.50	3.24	6.71	9.91	10.87	16.13	25.54	1.77	1.11	0.04	0.13
0.00	0.11	0.00	0.10	0.11	0.13	0.17	0.61	1.38	1.55	2.30	3.65	0.20	0.12	0.00	0.01
0.00	0.00	0.10	0.19	0.11	0.53	0.34	0.81	1.65	2.72	8.06	7.30	0.40	0.22	0.01	0.02
0.00	0.00	0.00	0.29	0.78	0.79	2.73	4.68	4.68	13.20	36.29	68.41	1.99	1.09	0.02	0.07
0.00	0.00	0.00	0.00	0.00	0.00	0.17	0.41	0.00	0.00	1.73	0.91	0.06	0.03	0.00	0.00
0.00	0.00	0.10	0.10	0.00	0.00	0.17	0.00	0.55	0.78	0.00	0.91	0.07	0.06	0.00	0.01
1.03	0.64	1.24	2.70	4.59	6.85	8.01	11.38	22.30	17.47	23.62	25.54	3.95	2.84	0.15	0.32
0.10	0.00	0.21	0.58	0.67	1.71	1.19	2.24	3.03	4.27	9.22	10.95	0.78	0.47	0.02	0.05
0.00	0.00	0.00	0.19	0.11	0.13	0.17	0.20	0.28	0.39	2.88	3.65	0.15	0.09	0.00	0.01
0.21	0.00	0.00	0.00	0.00	0.13	0.17	0.20	0.55	0.00	1.15	0.00	0.07	0.05	0.00	0.01
0.00	0.11	0.00	0.19	0.11	0.26	0.17	0.61	1.65	0.78	1.15	2.74	0.20	0.13	0.00	0.02
0.10	0.43	0.72	1.45	2.35	3.03	3.58	9.55	12.39	15.14	16.70	20.07	2.26	1.46	0.06	0.17
0.00	0.00	0.00	0.00	0.00	0.00	0.00	0.00	0.00	0.00	0.00	0.00	0.00	0.00	0.00	0.00
0.10	0.00	0.10	0.48	0.67	1.58	1.70	4.47	4.68	5.05	6.91	12.77	0.92	0.58	0.02	0.07
0.10	0.21	0.21	0.48	0.34	0.40	0.51	1.02	1.93	2.33	1.73	8.21	0.49	0.40	0.02	0.03
0.21	0.21	0.41	0.77	1.01	1.19	2.90	4.88	6.61	5.82	7.49	7.30	1.16	0.82	0.04	0.10
0.51	0.32	1.13	1.16	1.01	1.71	3.07	4.27	4.68	6.60	10.94	17.33	1.46	1.04	0.05	0.10
0.51	0.86	1.75	1.45	3.47	6.58	10.91	16.06	21.75	35.71	41.47	47.43	4.73	3.08	0.14	0.33
0.00	0.00	0.00	0.00	0.22	0.13	0.00	0.41	0.28	0.39	2.30	1.82	0.11	0.06	0.00	0.01
0.21	0.00	0.00	0.00	0.34	0.66	1.19	1.83	2.75	3.49	2.88	7.30	0.47	0.30	0.01	0.03
10.69	14.64	32.29	64.64	124.30	216.61	331.44	579.76	819.54	1 017.44	1 582.21	2 224.67	160.24	100.12	4.06	11.06
10.69	14.64	32.08	64.15	124.08	216.08	330.07	578.54	815.68	1 013.17	1 575.87	2 199.14	159.50	99.66	4.05	11.02

表 6-14 河南省城市肿瘤登记地区

部位	ICD-10	病例数	构成(%)	年龄组						
				0~	1~	5~	10~	15~	20~	25~
唇	C00	8	0.07	0.0	0.00	0.00	0.00	0.00	0.00	0.00
舌	C01–C02	21	0.17	0.0	0.31	0.00	0.00	0.00	0.00	0.00
口	C03–C06	30	0.25	0.0	0.00	0.00	0.00	0.00	0.00	0.00
唾液腺	C07–C08	18	0.15	0.0	0.00	0.00	0.00	0.00	0.00	0.00
扁桃体	C09	6	0.05	0.0	0.00	0.00	0.00	0.00	0.00	0.00
其他的口咽	C10	10	0.08	0.0	0.00	0.00	0.00	0.00	0.00	0.00
鼻咽	C11	47	0.39	0.0	0.00	0.00	0.00	0.00	0.00	0.00
喉咽	C12–C13	28	0.23	0.0	0.00	0.00	0.00	0.00	0.00	0.00
咽，部位不明	C14	13	0.11	0.0	0.00	0.00	0.00	0.00	0.00	0.00
食管	C15	1 217	10.07	0.0	0.31	0.00	0.00	0.00	0.00	0.22
胃	C16	1 683	13.92	0.0	0.00	0.00	0.00	0.00	0.00	0.44
小肠	C17	61	0.50	0.0	0.00	0.00	0.00	0.00	0.00	0.00
结肠	C18	441	3.65	0.0	0.00	0.00	0.00	0.00	0.00	0.22
直肠	C19–C20	404	3.34	0.0	0.00	0.00	0.00	0.00	0.00	0.00
肛门	C21	6	0.05	0.0	0.00	0.00	0.00	0.00	0.00	0.00
肝脏	C22	1 696	14.03	0.0	0.00	0.00	0.24	0.00	0.00	0.22
胆囊及其他	C23–C24	229	1.89	0.0	0.00	0.00	0.00	0.00	0.00	0.00
胰腺	C25	337	2.79	0.0	0.00	0.00	0.00	0.00	0.00	0.22
鼻、鼻窦及其他	C30–C31	16	0.13	0.0	0.00	0.00	0.00	0.00	0.00	0.00
喉	C32	101	0.84	0.0	0.00	0.00	0.00	0.00	0.00	0.00
气管、支气管、肺	C33–C34	3 555	29.41	0.0	0.00	0.00	0.00	0.00	0.00	0.44
其他的胸腔器官	C37–C38	54	0.45	0.0	0.00	0.00	0.00	0.52	0.00	0.22
骨	C40–C41	72	0.60	0.0	0.00	0.00	0.24	0.26	0.00	0.22
皮肤的黑色素瘤	C43	11	0.09	0.0	0.00	0.00	0.00	0.00	0.00	0.00
其他的皮肤	C44	44	0.36	0.0	0.00	0.00	0.00	0.00	0.00	0.00
间皮瘤	C45	11	0.09	0.0	0.00	0.00	0.00	0.00	0.00	0.00
卡波西肉瘤	C46	0	0.00	0.0	0.00	0.00	0.00	0.00	0.00	0.00
周围神经、其他结缔组织、软组织	C47;C49	25	0.21	0.0	0.31	0.25	0.00	0.00	0.00	0.00
乳房	C50	16	0.13	0.0	0.00	0.00	0.00	0.00	0.00	0.00
外阴	C51	0	0.00	0.0	0.00	0.00	0.00	0.00	0.00	0.00
阴道	C52	0	0.00	0.0	0.00	0.00	0.00	0.00	0.00	0.00
子宫颈	C53	0	0.00	0.0	0.00	0.00	0.00	0.00	0.00	0.00
子宫体	C54	0	0.00	0.0	0.00	0.00	0.00	0.00	0.00	0.00
子宫，部位不明	C55	0	0.00	0.0	0.00	0.00	0.00	0.00	0.00	0.00
卵巢	C56	0	0.00	0.0	0.00	0.00	0.00	0.00	0.00	0.00
女性其他的生殖器	C57	0	0.00	0.0	0.00	0.00	0.00	0.00	0.00	0.00
胎盘	C58	0	0.00	0.0	0.00	0.00	0.00	0.00	0.00	0.00
阴茎	C60	11	0.09	0.0	0.00	0.00	0.00	0.00	0.00	0.00
前列腺	C61	339	2.80	0.0	0.00	0.00	0.00	0.00	0.00	0.00
睾丸	C62	4	0.03	0.0	0.31	0.00	0.00	0.00	0.00	0.00
男性其他的生殖器	C63	6	0.05	0.0	0.00	0.00	0.00	0.00	0.00	0.00
肾	C64	152	1.26	0.0	0.00	0.00	0.00	0.00	0.25	0.00
肾盂	C65	16	0.13	0.0	0.00	0.00	0.00	0.00	0.00	0.00
输尿管	C66	27	0.22	0.0	0.00	0.00	0.00	0.00	0.00	0.00
膀胱	C67	195	1.61	0.0	0.00	0.00	0.00	0.00	0.00	0.00
其他的泌尿器官	C68	2	0.02	0.0	0.00	0.00	0.00	0.00	0.00	0.00
眼	C69	6	0.05	0.0	0.00	0.25	0.00	0.00	0.00	0.00
脑、神经系统	C70–C72	279	2.31	0.0	1.89	0.74	1.94	0.52	0.00	0.44
甲状腺	C73	33	0.27	0.0	0.00	0.00	0.00	0.00	0.00	0.00
肾上腺	C74	12	0.10	0.0	0.00	0.00	0.00	0.26	0.00	0.00
其他的内分泌腺	C75	3	0.02	0.0	0.00	0.00	0.00	0.00	0.00	0.00
霍奇金病	C81	15	0.12	0.0	0.00	0.00	0.00	0.00	0.00	0.22
非霍奇金淋巴瘤	C82–C85;C96	153	1.27	0.0	0.00	0.00	0.00	0.00	0.25	0.00
免疫增生性疾病	C88	0	0.00	0.0	0.00	0.00	0.00	0.00	0.00	0.00
多发性骨髓瘤	C90	66	0.55	0.0	0.00	0.00	0.00	0.00	0.00	0.00
淋巴样白血病	C91	33	0.27	0.0	0.00	0.74	0.00	0.26	0.25	0.00
髓样白血病	C92–C94	91	0.75	0.0	0.00	0.50	0.00	0.26	0.25	0.00
白血病，未特指	C95	108	0.89	0.0	0.63	0.50	0.24	0.52	0.25	0.44
其他的或未指明部位	O&U	335	2.77	1.5	0.31	0.25	0.00	0.52	0.50	0.44
骨髓增殖性疾病	MPD	8	0.07	0.0	0.00	0.00	0.00	0.00	0.00	0.00
骨髓增生异常综合征	MDS	34	0.28	0.0	0.00	0.00	0.00	0.00	0.00	0.00
合计	ALL	12 088	100.00	1.5	4.09	3.22	2.67	3.13	1.74	3.76
C44 以外的部位	ALL but C44	12 044	99.64	1.5	4.09	3.22	2.67	3.13	1.74	3.76

2020 年男性死亡主要指标

30~	35~	40~	45~	50~	55~	60~	65~	70~	75~	80~	85+	粗率 (1/10⁵)	世标率 (1/10⁵)	累积率 (%) 0~64	累积率 (%) 0~74
0.00	0.00	0.00	0.00	0.00	0.26	0.00	0.42	0.00	0.00	1.20	10.88	0.13	0.08	0.00	0.00
0.00	0.44	0.00	0.58	0.22	0.79	0.34	1.68	0.00	0.00	1.20	10.88	0.34	0.26	0.01	0.02
0.00	0.00	0.21	0.39	0.22	0.26	1.03	1.26	4.10	1.71	7.20	8.70	0.49	0.32	0.01	0.04
0.00	0.00	0.21	0.00	0.45	0.53	0.69	1.26	2.35	0.85	0.00	6.53	0.29	0.21	0.01	0.03
0.00	0.00	0.00	0.00	0.00	0.00	0.34	1.26	0.59	0.85	0.00	0.00	0.10	0.07	0.00	0.01
0.00	0.00	0.00	0.00	0.22	0.53	0.00	0.84	1.17	0.85	2.40	0.00	0.16	0.10	0.00	0.01
0.00	0.22	0.42	0.39	1.11	1.85	2.75	3.78	1.76	5.98	2.40	2.18	0.77	0.53	0.03	0.06
0.00	0.00	0.00	0.39	0.45	1.59	0.69	1.68	2.93	1.71	2.40	6.53	0.46	0.31	0.02	0.04
0.00	0.00	0.00	0.00	0.22	1.06	0.00	0.42	1.17	0.85	3.60	2.18	0.21	0.13	0.01	0.01
0.00	0.00	0.83	3.29	10.91	18.53	43.04	83.91	145.40	158.96	209.86	306.80	19.84	12.90	0.39	1.53
0.85	1.76	3.34	6.38	13.13	28.33	57.85	125.03	195.83	217.08	279.41	363.37	27.44	17.93	0.56	2.16
0.21	0.00	0.21	0.58	1.34	1.06	2.41	4.62	5.28	5.98	8.39	10.88	0.99	0.67	0.03	0.08
0.85	0.88	1.25	2.52	3.56	7.41	11.36	27.69	31.66	44.44	99.53	176.24	7.19	4.56	0.14	0.44
0.21	0.88	0.42	2.32	6.01	9.53	16.18	26.43	34.01	42.73	67.15	104.44	6.59	4.32	0.18	0.48
0.00	0.00	0.00	0.00	0.00	0.26	0.00	0.42	1.17	0.85	1.20	0.00	0.10	0.06	0.00	0.01
2.97	5.93	11.05	22.83	39.62	68.04	73.69	99.85	117.85	131.61	141.50	265.45	27.65	18.96	1.12	2.21
0.00	0.22	0.42	0.39	1.34	4.24	9.30	17.62	21.69	25.64	37.17	76.15	3.73	2.46	0.08	0.28
0.00	0.22	1.46	1.93	6.23	9.53	13.77	21.40	29.32	27.35	56.36	73.98	5.49	3.63	0.17	0.42
0.00	0.00	0.21	0.58	0.22	0.26	0.69	0.42	1.17	2.56	1.20	2.18	0.26	0.18	0.01	0.02
0.00	0.00	0.42	0.58	0.67	3.71	4.48	5.45	11.73	14.53	10.79	15.23	1.65	1.09	0.05	0.14
0.64	1.76	3.96	13.35	34.05	84.45	133.95	248.79	347.09	433.30	621.18	833.35	57.97	37.67	1.36	4.34
0.21	0.44	0.21	0.00	0.89	1.06	2.07	4.20	4.10	7.69	8.39	0.00	0.88	0.61	0.03	0.07
0.21	0.22	0.42	0.77	1.11	2.12	1.72	4.62	8.21	4.27	4.80	19.58	1.17	0.84	0.04	0.10
0.00	0.00	0.21	0.19	0.22	0.00	0.34	0.00	2.35	0.00	1.20	4.35	0.18	0.12	0.00	0.02
0.00	0.00	0.00	0.39	0.00	0.53	1.72	2.10	3.52	5.13	7.20	26.11	0.72	0.46	0.01	0.04
0.00	0.00	0.00	0.19	0.45	0.00	1.03	0.00	1.17	1.71	1.20	0.00	0.18	0.12	0.01	0.01
0.00	0.00	0.00	0.00	0.00	0.00	0.00	0.00	0.00	0.00	0.00	0.00	0.00	0.00	0.00	0.00
0.00	0.22	0.21	0.19	0.22	0.26	2.07	0.84	1.17	1.71	2.40	8.70	0.41	0.32	0.02	0.03
0.00	0.00	0.42	0.19	0.00	0.53	1.38	0.00	2.93	1.71	0.00	0.00	0.26	0.19	0.01	0.03
0.00	0.00	0.00	0.00	0.00	0.00	0.00	0.00	0.00	0.00	0.00	0.00	0.00	0.00	0.00	0.00
0.00	0.00	0.00	0.00	0.00	0.00	0.00	0.00	0.00	0.00	0.00	0.00	0.00	0.00	0.00	0.00
0.00	0.00	0.00	0.00	0.00	0.00	0.00	0.00	0.00	0.00	0.00	0.00	0.00	0.00	0.00	0.00
0.00	0.00	0.00	0.00	0.00	0.00	0.00	0.00	0.00	0.00	0.00	0.00	0.00	0.00	0.00	0.00
0.00	0.00	0.00	0.00	0.00	0.00	0.00	0.00	0.00	0.00	0.00	0.00	0.00	0.00	0.00	0.00
0.00	0.00	0.00	0.00	0.00	0.00	0.00	0.00	0.00	0.00	0.00	0.00	0.00	0.00	0.00	0.00
0.00	0.00	0.00	0.00	0.00	0.00	0.00	0.00	0.00	0.00	0.00	0.00	0.00	0.00	0.00	0.00
0.00	0.00	0.00	0.00	0.00	0.00	0.00	0.00	0.00	0.00	0.00	0.00	0.00	0.00	0.00	0.00
0.00	0.00	0.00	0.00	0.22	0.00	0.00	0.84	1.17	0.85	3.60	4.35	0.18	0.11	0.00	0.01
0.00	0.00	0.21	0.19	0.45	0.79	3.79	11.33	19.93	60.68	103.13	224.11	5.53	3.21	0.03	0.18
0.21	0.00	0.21	0.00	0.00	0.00	0.00	0.42	0.00	0.00	0.00	0.00	0.07	0.07	0.00	0.01
0.00	0.00	0.00	0.19	0.00	0.00	0.00	0.00	0.00	0.00	4.80	2.18	0.10	0.05	0.00	0.00
0.42	0.22	0.63	0.19	2.45	3.97	4.13	10.91	16.42	16.24	16.79	41.34	2.48	1.66	0.06	0.20
0.00	0.22	0.00	0.19	0.22	0.26	0.00	1.26	1.76	1.71	2.40	4.35	0.26	0.17	0.00	0.02
0.00	0.00	0.21	0.19	0.22	1.06	0.34	0.84	2.35	3.42	6.00	8.70	0.44	0.27	0.01	0.03
0.00	0.00	0.00	0.39	1.11	0.79	4.48	7.55	8.21	26.49	59.96	128.38	3.18	1.89	0.03	0.11
0.00	0.00	0.00	0.00	0.00	0.00	0.00	0.00	0.00	0.00	2.40	0.00	0.03	0.01	0.00	0.00
0.00	0.00	0.21	0.00	0.00	0.00	0.34	0.00	0.59	0.85	0.00	2.18	0.10	0.08	0.00	0.01
1.91	0.88	1.25	3.29	5.34	7.94	11.02	13.01	25.80	19.66	27.58	32.64	4.55	3.39	0.18	0.38
0.00	0.00	0.00	0.19	0.45	1.59	1.03	1.26	2.93	3.42	7.20	6.53	0.54	0.34	0.02	0.04
0.00	0.00	0.00	0.19	0.22	0.26	0.34	0.42	0.59	0.85	1.20	6.53	0.20	0.14	0.01	0.01
0.00	0.00	0.00	0.00	0.00	0.26	0.34	0.42	0.00	0.00	0.00	0.00	0.05	0.04	0.00	0.01
0.00	0.00	0.00	0.39	0.22	0.53	0.34	0.84	1.17	1.71	1.20	2.18	0.24	0.17	0.01	0.02
0.21	0.88	0.83	1.55	2.89	4.24	5.17	10.91	13.48	12.82	23.98	15.23	2.49	1.67	0.08	0.20
0.00	0.00	0.00	0.00	0.00	0.00	0.00	0.00	0.00	0.00	0.00	0.00	0.00	0.00	0.00	0.00
0.21	0.00	0.00	0.58	0.67	2.12	2.07	6.29	6.45	6.84	6.00	13.06	1.08	0.73	0.03	0.09
0.21	0.44	0.42	0.39	0.45	0.79	0.34	0.84	2.35	2.56	1.20	10.88	0.54	0.43	0.02	0.04
0.21	0.22	0.42	0.97	1.11	1.32	3.10	5.87	11.14	8.55	13.19	10.88	1.48	1.04	0.04	0.13
0.85	0.66	1.25	1.55	0.89	1.85	4.48	4.20	5.86	6.84	16.79	23.93	1.76	1.31	0.07	0.12
0.85	1.54	1.67	1.55	4.45	8.74	13.43	20.56	29.32	38.46	44.37	56.57	5.46	3.75	0.17	0.42
0.00	0.00	0.00	0.00	0.45	0.26	0.00	0.00	0.59	0.85	3.60	0.00	0.13	0.07	0.00	0.01
0.21	0.00	0.00	0.00	0.00	1.06	1.38	2.10	2.93	5.13	4.80	10.88	0.55	0.36	0.01	0.04
11.46	18.21	33.14	70.42	144.67	284.59	439.04	785.82	1 132.74	1 358.03	1 929.49	2 939.58	197.10	130.05	5.10	14.69
11.46	18.21	33.14	70.04	144.67	284.06	437.32	783.72	1 129.22	1 352.90	1 922.29	2 913.47	196.38	129.59	5.09	14.65

表 6–15 河南省城市肿瘤登记地区

部位	ICD–10	病例数	构成(%)	年龄组						
				0~	1~	5~	10~	15~	20~	25~
唇	C00	2	0.03	0.00	0.00	0.00	0.00	0.00	0.00	0.00
舌	C01–C02	22	0.29	0.00	0.00	0.00	0.00	0.00	0.00	0.00
口	C03–C06	34	0.45	0.00	0.00	0.00	0.00	0.00	0.00	0.00
唾液腺	C07–C08	7	0.09	0.00	0.00	0.00	0.00	0.00	0.00	0.00
扁桃体	C09	3	0.04	0.00	0.00	0.00	0.00	0.00	0.00	0.00
其他的口咽	C10	4	0.05	0.00	0.00	0.27	0.00	0.00	0.00	0.00
鼻咽	C11	18	0.24	0.00	0.00	0.00	0.00	0.00	0.00	0.00
喉咽	C12–C13	0	0.00	0.00	0.00	0.00	0.00	0.00	0.00	0.00
咽，部位不明	C14	7	0.09	0.00	0.00	0.00	0.27	0.00	0.00	0.00
食管	C15	637	8.37	0.00	0.00	0.00	0.00	0.00	0.00	0.00
胃	C16	710	9.33	0.00	0.00	0.00	0.00	0.00	0.00	0.00
小肠	C17	41	0.54	0.00	0.00	0.00	0.00	0.00	0.00	0.00
结肠	C18	332	4.36	0.00	0.00	0.00	0.00	0.00	0.25	0.21
直肠	C19–C20	274	3.60	0.00	0.00	0.00	0.00	0.00	0.00	0.21
肛门	C21	10	0.13	0.00	0.00	0.00	0.00	0.00	0.00	0.00
肝脏	C22	756	9.94	0.00	0.35	0.00	0.00	0.28	0.25	0.00
胆囊及其他	C23–C24	271	3.56	0.00	0.00	0.00	0.00	0.00	0.00	0.21
胰腺	C25	321	4.22	0.00	0.00	0.27	0.00	0.00	0.00	0.00
鼻、鼻窦及其他	C30–C31	7	0.09	0.00	0.00	0.00	0.00	0.00	0.00	0.00
喉	C32	9	0.12	0.00	0.00	0.00	0.00	0.00	0.00	0.00
气管、支气管、肺	C33–C34	1 452	19.08	0.00	0.00	0.00	0.00	0.28	0.00	0.00
其他的胸腔器官	C37–C38	19	0.25	0.00	0.00	0.00	0.00	0.00	0.00	0.00
骨	C40–C41	51	0.67	0.00	0.00	0.27	0.27	0.00	0.00	0.00
皮肤的黑色素瘤	C43	8	0.11	0.00	0.00	0.00	0.00	0.00	0.00	0.00
其他的皮肤	C44	48	0.63	0.00	0.00	0.00	0.00	0.00	0.25	0.00
间皮瘤	C45	6	0.08	0.00	0.00	0.00	0.00	0.00	0.00	0.00
卡波西肉瘤	C46	0	0.00	0.00	0.00	0.00	0.00	0.00	0.00	0.00
周围神经、其他结缔组织、软组织	C47;C49	18	0.24	1.64	0.00	0.00	0.27	0.00	0.00	0.00
乳房	C50	709	9.32	0.00	0.00	0.00	0.00	0.00	0.00	0.63
外阴	C51	17	0.22	0.00	0.00	0.00	0.00	0.00	0.00	0.00
阴道	C52	9	0.12	0.00	0.00	0.00	0.00	0.00	0.00	0.00
子宫颈	C53	351	4.61	0.00	0.00	0.00	0.00	0.00	0.00	0.00
子宫体	C54	125	1.64	0.00	0.00	0.00	0.00	0.00	0.00	0.00
子宫，部位不明	C55	28	0.37	0.00	0.00	0.00	0.00	0.00	0.00	0.00
卵巢	C56	254	3.34	0.00	0.00	0.00	0.00	0.00	0.00	0.00
女性其他的生殖器	C57	8	0.11	0.00	0.00	0.00	0.00	0.00	0.00	0.00
胎盘	C58	0	0.00	0.00	0.00	0.00	0.00	0.00	0.00	0.00
阴茎	C60	0	0.00	0.00	0.00	0.00	0.00	0.00	0.00	0.00
前列腺	C61	0	0.00	0.00	0.00	0.00	0.00	0.00	0.00	0.00
睾丸	C62	0	0.00	0.00	0.00	0.00	0.00	0.00	0.00	0.00
男性其他的生殖器	C63	0	0.00	0.00	0.00	0.00	0.00	0.00	0.00	0.00
肾	C64	65	0.85	0.00	0.00	0.00	0.00	0.00	0.00	0.21
肾盂	C65	9	0.12	0.00	0.00	0.00	0.00	0.00	0.00	0.00
输尿管	C66	22	0.29	0.00	0.00	0.00	0.00	0.00	0.00	0.00
膀胱	C67	49	0.64	0.00	0.00	0.00	0.00	0.00	0.00	0.00
其他的泌尿器官	C68	5	0.07	0.00	0.00	0.00	0.00	0.00	0.00	0.00
眼	C69	3	0.04	0.00	0.00	0.00	0.00	0.00	0.00	0.00
脑、神经系统	C70–C72	206	2.71	0.00	0.35	1.92	0.55	0.28	1.52	0.00
甲状腺	C73	63	0.83	0.00	0.00	0.00	0.00	0.00	0.00	0.00
肾上腺	C74	6	0.08	0.00	0.00	0.00	0.00	0.00	0.00	0.00
其他的内分泌腺	C75	6	0.08	0.00	0.00	0.00	0.00	0.00	0.00	0.00
霍奇金病	C81	9	0.12	0.00	0.00	0.00	0.00	0.00	0.00	0.00
非霍奇金淋巴瘤	C82–C85;C96	125	1.64	0.00	0.00	0.00	0.00	0.85	0.00	0.00
免疫增生性疾病	C88	0	0.00	0.00	0.00	0.00	0.00	0.00	0.00	0.00
多发性骨髓瘤	C90	47	0.62	0.00	0.00	0.00	0.00	0.00	0.00	0.00
淋巴样白血病	C91	27	0.35	0.00	1.04	0.00	0.55	0.00	0.00	0.21
髓样白血病	C92–C94	52	0.68	0.00	0.35	0.00	0.55	0.00	0.25	0.00
白血病，未特指	C95	71	0.93	0.00	0.35	0.27	0.82	0.00	0.00	0.00
其他的或未指明部位	O&U	247	3.25	1.64	0.35	0.27	0.55	0.28	0.00	0.63
骨髓增殖性疾病	MPD	5	0.07	0.00	0.00	0.00	0.00	0.00	0.00	0.00
骨髓增生异常综合征	MDS	24	0.32	0.00	0.00	0.00	0.00	0.00	0.00	0.00
合计	ALL	7 609	100.00	3.27	2.76	3.30	3.84	1.98	2.53	2.30
C44 以外的部位	ALL but C44	7 561	99.37	3.27	2.76	3.30	3.84	1.98	2.28	2.30

2020 年女性死亡主要指标

30~	35~	40~	45~	50~	55~	60~	65~	70~	75~	80~	85+	粗率 (1/10^5)	世标率 (1/10^5)	累积率 (%) 0~64	0~74
0.00	0.21	0.00	0.00	0.00	0.00	0.34	0.00	0.00	0.00	0.00	0.00	0.03	0.03	0.00	0.00
0.20	0.00	0.00	0.19	0.68	0.26	0.34	0.79	1.04	1.42	4.43	7.85	0.36	0.20	0.01	0.02
0.00	0.00	0.20	0.19	0.23	0.00	0.68	1.97	2.59	2.13	11.08	9.42	0.55	0.30	0.01	0.03
0.00	0.00	0.00	0.00	0.00	0.26	0.68	0.00	0.52	0.00	3.32	0.00	0.11	0.06	0.00	0.01
0.00	0.00	0.00	0.38	0.00	0.00	0.34	0.00	0.00	0.00	0.00	0.00	0.05	0.04	0.00	0.00
0.00	0.00	0.00	0.00	0.00	0.26	0.00	0.00	0.00	1.42	0.00	0.00	0.06	0.05	0.00	0.00
0.20	0.21	0.00	0.38	0.23	0.00	0.68	1.58	1.04	1.42	2.22	1.57	0.29	0.19	0.01	0.02
0.00	0.00	0.00	0.00	0.00	0.00	0.00	0.00	0.00	0.00	0.00	0.00	0.00	0.00	0.00	0.00
0.00	0.00	0.00	0.00	0.00	0.00	0.34	0.00	0.00	1.42	2.22	1.57	0.11	0.07	0.00	0.00
0.00	0.00	0.61	0.38	0.90	4.72	16.21	29.97	57.60	93.17	144.08	179.03	10.34	5.54	0.11	0.55
1.00	1.25	2.25	4.62	6.31	8.91	14.52	35.89	49.30	85.35	139.65	199.45	11.53	6.41	0.19	0.62
0.00	0.00	0.00	0.19	0.68	1.05	0.34	1.18	1.56	4.98	11.08	14.13	0.67	0.34	0.01	0.02
0.40	0.00	1.02	2.12	2.93	4.72	10.13	15.77	17.64	39.12	76.47	83.24	5.39	3.01	0.11	0.28
0.40	0.00	0.82	1.73	3.83	5.24	6.08	13.80	15.05	27.03	50.98	86.38	4.45	2.51	0.09	0.24
0.00	0.00	0.00	0.19	0.23	0.26	0.00	0.00	0.52	0.71	0.00	7.85	0.16	0.09	0.00	0.01
0.60	1.46	2.25	5.00	9.02	15.46	26.68	48.11	63.83	70.41	93.10	157.05	12.27	7.45	0.31	0.87
0.20	0.21	0.20	0.19	2.93	3.93	6.08	13.01	21.28	27.03	58.74	86.38	4.40	2.42	0.07	0.24
0.00	0.21	0.00	1.92	3.16	6.29	10.47	13.41	26.99	36.27	59.85	76.95	5.21	2.97	0.11	0.31
0.00	0.00	0.20	0.00	0.00	0.26	0.00	0.00	0.52	1.42	2.22	0.00	0.11	0.06	0.00	0.00
0.00	0.00	0.20	0.00	0.23	0.00	0.34	0.00	0.52	0.00	1.11	6.28	0.15	0.08	0.00	0.01
0.80	0.63	4.08	10.01	17.58	24.63	41.87	79.26	110.02	140.11	272.64	345.50	23.58	13.57	0.50	1.45
0.00	0.00	0.00	0.00	0.23	0.26	1.35	0.00	1.56	1.42	2.22	9.42	0.31	0.18	0.01	0.02
0.20	0.42	0.20	0.19	0.23	0.52	1.35	3.15	2.08	3.56	8.87	18.85	0.83	0.51	0.02	0.04
0.00	0.00	0.20	0.00	0.23	0.26	0.00	0.00	1.04	0.00	2.22	1.57	0.13	0.07	0.00	0.01
0.00	0.00	0.41	0.58	0.45	0.52	1.01	0.39	4.15	3.56	5.54	25.13	0.78	0.45	0.02	0.04
0.00	0.00	0.00	0.00	0.23	0.00	0.00	0.39	1.56	0.00	1.11	0.00	0.10	0.06	0.00	0.01
0.00	0.00	0.00	0.00	0.00	0.00	0.00	0.00	0.00	0.00	0.00	0.00	0.00	0.00	0.00	0.00
0.20	0.21	0.00	0.19	0.45	0.52	0.34	0.39	1.04	1.42	2.22	1.57	0.29	0.22	0.01	0.02
1.79	2.92	6.54	12.31	20.06	23.32	24.65	32.73	35.29	42.67	70.93	95.80	11.51	7.33	0.46	0.80
0.00	0.21	0.20	0.00	0.00	0.79	1.01	0.79	0.00	1.42	2.22	4.71	0.28	0.17	0.01	0.02
0.00	0.00	0.20	0.00	0.00	0.26	0.00	0.79	0.52	0.71	1.11	3.14	0.15	0.09	0.00	0.01
1.59	1.46	2.86	5.39	10.59	11.53	12.16	18.14	24.91	18.49	31.03	29.84	5.70	3.69	0.23	0.44
0.20	0.42	0.82	0.58	1.35	3.93	5.74	7.10	10.38	12.09	13.30	15.70	2.03	1.26	0.07	0.15
0.00	0.00	0.20	0.19	0.45	1.83	2.03	0.79	0.52	0.71	2.22	7.85	0.45	0.29	0.02	0.03
0.60	0.21	1.63	2.89	6.76	9.43	11.48	11.44	15.57	12.80	32.14	32.98	4.12	2.60	0.17	0.30
0.00	0.00	0.20	0.00	0.23	0.26	0.00	0.79	0.00	0.00	2.22	1.57	0.13	0.08	0.00	0.01
0.00	0.00	0.00	0.00	0.00	0.00	0.00	0.00	0.00	0.00	0.00	0.00	0.00	0.00	0.00	0.00
0.00	0.00	0.00	0.00	0.00	0.00	0.00	0.00	0.00	0.00	0.00	0.00	0.00	0.00	0.00	0.00
0.00	0.00	0.00	0.00	0.00	0.00	0.00	0.00	0.00	0.00	0.00	0.00	0.00	0.00	0.00	0.00
0.00	0.00	0.00	0.00	0.00	0.00	0.00	0.00	0.00	0.00	0.00	0.00	0.00	0.00	0.00	0.00
0.00	0.00	0.00	0.00	0.00	0.00	0.00	0.00	0.00	0.00	0.00	0.00	0.00	0.00	0.00	0.00
0.00	0.21	0.41	0.19	0.45	1.05	2.36	2.76	4.15	6.40	15.52	14.13	1.06	0.60	0.02	0.06
0.00	0.00	0.00	0.00	0.00	0.00	0.34	0.00	1.04	1.42	2.22	3.14	0.15	0.08	0.00	0.01
0.00	0.00	0.00	0.19	0.00	0.00	0.34	0.79	1.04	2.13	9.97	6.28	0.36	0.17	0.00	0.01
0.00	0.00	0.00	0.19	0.45	0.79	1.01	1.97	1.56	2.13	14.41	25.13	0.80	0.42	0.01	0.03
0.00	0.00	0.00	0.00	0.00	0.00	0.34	0.79	0.00	0.00	1.11	1.57	0.08	0.05	0.00	0.01
0.00	0.00	0.00	0.19	0.00	0.00	0.00	0.00	0.52	0.71	0.00	0.00	0.05	0.03	0.00	0.00
0.20	0.42	1.23	2.12	3.83	5.76	5.07	9.86	19.20	15.65	19.95	20.42	3.34	2.32	0.12	0.26
0.20	0.00	0.41	0.96	0.90	1.83	1.35	3.15	3.11	4.98	11.08	14.13	1.02	0.60	0.03	0.06
0.00	0.00	0.00	0.19	0.00	0.00	0.00	0.00	0.00	0.00	4.43	1.57	0.10	0.04	0.00	0.00
0.40	0.00	0.00	0.00	0.00	0.00	0.00	0.00	1.04	0.00	2.22	0.00	0.10	0.06	0.00	0.01
0.00	0.21	0.00	0.00	0.00	0.00	0.00	0.39	2.08	0.00	1.11	3.14	0.15	0.09	0.00	0.01
0.00	0.00	0.61	1.35	1.80	1.83	2.03	8.28	11.42	17.07	9.97	23.56	2.03	1.25	0.04	0.14
0.00	0.00	0.00	0.00	0.00	0.00	0.00	0.00	0.00	0.00	0.00	0.00	0.00	0.00	0.00	0.00
0.00	0.00	0.20	0.38	0.68	1.05	1.35	2.76	3.11	3.56	7.76	12.56	0.76	0.45	0.02	0.05
0.00	0.00	0.00	0.58	0.23	0.00	0.68	1.18	1.56	2.13	2.22	6.28	0.44	0.37	0.02	0.03
0.20	0.21	0.41	0.58	0.90	1.05	2.70	3.94	2.59	3.56	2.22	4.71	0.84	0.62	0.04	0.07
0.20	0.00	1.02	0.77	1.13	1.57	1.69	4.34	3.63	6.40	5.54	12.56	1.15	0.80	0.04	0.08
0.20	0.21	1.84	1.35	2.48	4.45	8.44	11.83	15.05	33.43	38.79	40.83	4.01	2.46	0.11	0.24
0.00	0.00	0.00	0.00	0.00	0.00	0.00	0.79	0.00	0.00	1.11	3.14	0.08	0.04	0.00	0.00
0.20	0.00	0.00	0.00	0.68	0.26	1.01	1.58	2.59	2.13	1.11	4.71	0.39	0.25	0.01	0.03
9.96	11.25	31.45	58.88	103.68	149.34	225.91	386.07	542.31	734.00	1 261.25	1 708.68	123.54	73.09	3.04	7.68
9.96	11.25	31.04	58.30	103.23	148.81	224.90	385.68	538.16	730.44	1 255.71	1 683.55	122.77	72.64	3.02	7.64

表 6-16 河南省农村肿瘤登记地区

部位	ICD-10	病例数	构成(%)	年龄组						
				0~	1~	5~	10~	15~	20~	25~
唇	C00	34	0.07	0.00	0.00	0.00	0.00	0.00	0.00	0.04
舌	C01–C02	69	0.14	0.00	0.00	0.00	0.00	0.00	0.00	0.00
口	C03–C06	101	0.20	0.00	0.00	0.00	0.00	0.00	0.00	0.00
唾液腺	C07–C08	58	0.11	0.00	0.00	0.00	0.00	0.00	0.00	0.00
扁桃体	C09	14	0.03	0.00	0.00	0.00	0.00	0.00	0.00	0.00
其他的口咽	C10	36	0.07	0.00	0.00	0.00	0.00	0.00	0.00	0.00
鼻咽	C11	158	0.31	0.00	0.00	0.00	0.00	0.00	0.00	0.00
喉咽	C12–C13	47	0.09	0.00	0.00	0.00	0.00	0.00	0.00	0.00
咽，部位不明	C14	62	0.12	0.00	0.00	0.00	0.00	0.00	0.00	0.00
食管	C15	7 268	14.35	0.00	0.00	0.00	0.00	0.00	0.05	0.17
胃	C16	7 867	15.53	0.00	0.06	0.05	0.09	0.05	0.23	0.26
小肠	C17	208	0.41	0.00	0.00	0.00	0.00	0.00	0.00	0.00
结肠	C18	1 220	2.41	0.00	0.00	0.00	0.00	0.05	0.05	0.30
直肠	C19–C20	1 502	2.97	0.00	0.00	0.05	0.00	0.00	0.00	0.09
肛门	C21	154	0.30	0.00	0.00	0.00	0.00	0.00	0.00	0.00
肝脏	C22	6 769	13.37	0.00	0.13	0.14	0.13	0.10	0.09	0.26
胆囊及其他	C23–C24	1 020	2.01	0.00	0.00	0.00	0.00	0.00	0.00	0.04
胰腺	C25	1 107	2.19	0.00	0.00	0.00	0.00	0.00	0.05	0.00
鼻、鼻窦及其他	C30–C31	84	0.17	0.00	0.00	0.00	0.00	0.00	0.05	0.04
喉	C32	203	0.40	0.00	0.00	0.00	0.00	0.00	0.00	0.00
气管、支气管、肺	C33–C34	12 567	24.82	0.00	0.00	0.00	0.09	0.00	0.28	0.60
其他的胸腔器官	C37–C38	156	0.31	0.00	0.06	0.00	0.04	0.10	0.14	0.00
骨	C40–C41	421	0.83	0.00	0.06	0.24	0.36	0.44	0.60	0.34
皮肤的黑色素瘤	C43	45	0.09	0.00	0.00	0.00	0.00	0.00	0.00	0.00
其他的皮肤	C44	257	0.51	0.00	0.00	0.00	0.00	0.00	0.00	0.00
间皮瘤	C45	19	0.04	0.00	0.00	0.00	0.00	0.00	0.00	0.00
卡波西肉瘤	C46	1	0.00	0.00	0.00	0.00	0.00	0.00	0.00	0.00
周围神经、其他结缔组织、软组织	C47;C49	75	0.15	0.00	0.06	0.05	0.18	0.05	0.00	0.04
乳房	C50	1 414	2.79	0.00	0.00	0.00	0.00	0.00	0.19	0.18
外阴	C51	16	0.03	0.00	0.00	0.00	0.00	0.00	0.00	0.00
阴道	C52	22	0.04	0.00	0.00	0.00	0.00	0.00	0.00	0.00
子宫颈	C53	914	1.80	0.00	0.00	0.00	0.00	0.00	0.00	0.27
子宫体	C54	299	0.59	0.00	0.00	0.00	0.00	0.00	0.00	0.00
子宫，部位不明	C55	100	0.20	0.00	0.00	0.00	0.00	0.00	0.00	0.00
卵巢	C56	444	0.88	0.00	0.00	0.00	0.00	0.00	0.10	0.36
女性其他的生殖器	C57	19	0.04	0.00	0.00	0.10	0.00	0.00	0.00	0.00
胎盘	C58	0	0.00	0.00	0.00	0.00	0.00	0.00	0.00	0.00
阴茎	C60	31	0.06	0.00	0.00	0.00	0.00	0.00	0.00	0.00
前列腺	C61	450	0.89	0.00	0.00	0.00	0.00	0.00	0.09	0.00
睾丸	C62	18	0.04	0.00	0.00	0.00	0.00	0.00	0.00	0.00
男性其他的生殖器	C63	5	0.01	0.00	0.00	0.00	0.00	0.00	0.00	0.00
肾	C64	413	0.82	0.00	0.00	0.00	0.00	0.05	0.05	0.04
肾盂	C65	49	0.10	0.00	0.00	0.00	0.00	0.00	0.00	0.00
输尿管	C66	58	0.11	0.00	0.00	0.00	0.00	0.00	0.00	0.00
膀胱	C67	504	1.00	0.00	0.00	0.00	0.00	0.00	0.05	0.09
其他的泌尿器官	C68	10	0.02	0.00	0.00	0.00	0.00	0.00	0.00	0.00
眼	C69	22	0.04	0.00	0.06	0.00	0.00	0.00	0.00	0.04
脑、神经系统	C70–C72	1 359	2.68	0.31	0.32	1.55	0.89	0.39	0.96	0.65
甲状腺	C73	245	0.48	0.00	0.00	0.00	0.00	0.00	0.00	0.13
肾上腺	C74	56	0.11	0.00	0.00	0.09	0.00	0.00	0.00	0.04
其他的内分泌腺	C75	21	0.04	0.00	0.00	0.00	0.00	0.00	0.05	0.00
霍奇金病	C81	48	0.09	0.00	0.00	0.00	0.00	0.00	0.00	0.09
非霍奇金淋巴瘤	C82–C85;C96	507	1.00	0.00	0.00	0.09	0.40	0.19	0.41	0.22
免疫增生性疾病	C88	2	0.00	0.00	0.00	0.00	0.00	0.00	0.00	0.00
多发性骨髓瘤	C90	226	0.45	0.00	0.06	0.00	0.00	0.00	0.05	0.00
淋巴样白血病	C91	102	0.20	0.00	0.13	0.28	0.04	0.24	0.14	0.00
髓样白血病	C92–C94	250	0.49	0.00	0.51	0.14	0.18	0.29	0.23	0.30
白血病，未特指	C95	393	0.78	0.00	0.64	0.42	0.53	0.68	0.18	0.56
其他的或未指明部位	O&U	990	1.95	0.00	0.45	0.56	0.27	0.68	0.37	0.30
骨髓增殖性疾病	MPD	19	0.04	0.00	0.00	0.00	0.00	0.00	0.09	0.00
骨髓增生异常综合征	MDS	71	0.14	0.00	0.13	0.05	0.00	0.00	0.05	0.04
合计	ALL	50 641	100.00	0.31	2.68	3.76	3.20	3.29	4.31	5.08
C44 以外的部位	ALL but C44	50 384	99.49	0.31	2.68	3.76	3.20	3.29	4.31	5.08

2020 年合计死亡主要指标

30~	35~	40~	45~	50~	55~	60~	65~	70~	75~	80~	85+	粗率 ($1/10^5$)	世标率 ($1/10^5$)	累积率 (%) 0~64	累积率 (%) 0~74
0.00	0.00	0.05	0.09	0.00	0.16	0.27	0.31	0.68	0.35	1.70	1.87	0.11	0.07	0.00	0.01
0.12	0.05	0.18	0.13	0.09	0.27	0.54	1.02	0.91	1.57	2.54	1.50	0.22	0.15	0.01	0.02
0.04	0.00	0.05	0.04	0.32	0.60	0.40	1.65	2.16	3.48	3.11	1.12	0.33	0.21	0.01	0.03
0.04	0.05	0.09	0.13	0.41	0.22	0.27	0.71	1.14	0.52	1.13	2.99	0.19	0.13	0.01	0.02
0.00	0.00	0.00	0.04	0.05	0.11	0.00	0.39	0.11	0.35	0.57	0.00	0.05	0.03	0.00	0.00
0.00	0.00	0.05	0.04	0.14	0.22	0.20	0.24	1.14	0.35	1.41	1.50	0.12	0.08	0.00	0.01
0.20	0.23	0.09	0.48	0.78	0.88	1.41	1.73	2.04	2.79	3.96	4.12	0.51	0.35	0.02	0.04
0.00	0.05	0.05	0.00	0.14	0.05	0.07	0.39	1.25	1.57	2.54	2.25	0.15	0.09	0.00	0.01
0.12	0.00	0.09	0.04	0.09	0.22	0.47	0.86	0.91	2.09	1.41	2.62	0.20	0.13	0.01	0.01
0.28	0.64	0.96	3.15	8.03	19.65	42.68	95.81	167.58	235.22	289.39	339.77	23.56	14.94	0.38	1.69
1.16	1.50	2.71	6.43	14.96	30.00	50.14	112.36	166.21	220.60	266.78	319.94	25.50	16.56	0.54	1.93
0.08	0.05	0.05	0.53	0.59	1.04	1.68	3.61	3.29	5.05	3.96	6.36	0.67	0.46	0.02	0.05
0.12	0.77	0.64	1.88	3.19	5.64	7.19	14.75	20.90	34.13	42.39	50.89	3.95	2.58	0.10	0.28
0.40	0.36	0.96	2.23	3.56	5.86	9.81	19.07	26.02	38.83	56.80	68.10	4.87	3.16	0.12	0.34
0.00	0.14	0.18	0.39	0.41	0.99	0.67	1.26	3.07	3.48	5.65	6.74	0.50	0.33	0.01	0.04
2.48	4.04	7.61	16.67	27.41	41.61	51.42	90.86	109.98	124.31	145.54	214.04	21.94	14.98	0.76	1.76
0.04	0.09	0.46	0.66	1.87	3.56	6.65	16.40	20.56	26.29	35.04	45.28	3.31	2.15	0.07	0.25
0.32	0.32	0.92	1.01	3.51	5.31	8.00	15.69	22.15	26.29	30.52	37.79	3.59	2.38	0.10	0.29
0.12	0.09	0.00	0.18	0.55	0.33	0.74	0.63	0.57	2.26	2.26	3.74	0.27	0.18	0.01	0.02
0.04	0.05	0.09	0.04	0.32	0.77	1.34	3.69	3.18	6.79	5.09	9.35	0.66	0.43	0.01	0.05
1.12	2.09	4.81	13.57	31.97	57.86	83.14	178.04	261.08	334.46	371.35	471.12	40.73	26.73	0.98	3.17
0.20	0.14	0.09	0.26	0.73	0.82	0.94	1.41	2.50	3.48	4.80	4.12	0.51	0.35	0.02	0.04
0.32	0.27	0.23	0.66	1.37	2.08	2.08	4.79	6.59	8.18	11.02	14.59	1.36	0.99	0.05	0.10
0.04	0.09	0.00	0.00	0.32	0.27	0.27	0.39	1.02	1.04	1.13	0.75	0.15	0.10	0.00	0.01
0.08	0.18	0.05	0.13	0.73	0.82	0.87	2.28	3.29	5.92	11.87	25.82	0.83	0.51	0.01	0.04
0.04	0.05	0.00	0.04	0.09	0.16	0.20	0.31	0.34	0.00	0.28	0.00	0.06	0.04	0.00	0.01
0.00	0.05	0.00	0.00	0.00	0.00	0.00	0.00	0.00	0.00	0.00	0.00	0.00	0.00	0.00	0.00
0.16	0.18	0.18	0.18	0.14	0.33	0.47	0.47	0.91	1.39	1.41	2.99	0.24	0.18	0.01	0.02
1.16	3.04	4.34	10.72	17.05	23.41	24.76	36.16	33.23	36.93	28.93	41.50	9.46	6.44	0.42	0.77
0.00	0.00	0.00	0.09	0.09	0.11	0.41	0.16	0.66	0.33	0.00	3.01	0.11	0.07	0.00	0.01
0.08	0.00	0.00	0.09	0.19	0.33	0.54	0.00	0.44	0.66	2.49	1.20	0.15	0.09	0.01	0.01
1.74	1.71	3.59	6.25	9.97	11.82	14.01	22.70	25.09	26.70	24.94	34.28	6.11	4.10	0.25	0.49
0.25	0.28	0.57	1.16	4.47	4.53	4.08	6.42	6.60	11.21	9.98	18.04	2.00	1.28	0.08	0.14
0.17	0.00	0.00	0.54	0.93	1.33	0.95	2.82	2.20	5.28	6.48	3.61	0.67	0.41	0.02	0.04
0.58	1.04	1.51	2.59	4.19	7.07	5.58	11.11	14.53	12.20	15.46	12.63	2.97	1.98	0.12	0.24
0.00	0.00	0.00	0.09	0.19	0.22	0.27	0.63	0.44	0.66	0.50	1.20	0.13	0.09	0.00	0.01
0.00	0.00	0.00	0.00	0.00	0.00	0.00	0.00	0.00	0.00	0.00	0.00	0.00	0.00	0.00	0.00
0.00	0.00	0.00	0.09	0.18	0.22	0.13	0.63	1.64	2.58	1.96	3.96	0.19	0.14	0.00	0.01
0.08	0.09	0.00	0.60	0.18	1.09	2.66	7.87	20.67	31.73	63.25	86.17	2.83	1.93	0.02	0.17
0.15	0.00	0.00	0.09	0.09	0.22	0.40	0.31	0.70	0.74	0.65	0.99	0.11	0.08	0.00	0.01
0.00	0.00	0.00	0.00	0.09	0.00	0.13	0.00	0.47	0.00	0.00	0.99	0.03	0.02	0.00	0.00
0.16	0.23	0.55	0.74	1.64	1.86	3.09	5.41	7.61	9.40	9.89	11.60	1.34	0.91	0.04	0.11
0.00	0.05	0.05	0.09	0.05	0.16	0.67	0.31	1.02	1.39	1.13	2.25	0.16	0.11	0.01	0.01
0.04	0.05	0.00	0.00	0.00	0.33	0.34	0.78	1.02	1.92	2.83	1.87	0.19	0.12	0.00	0.01
0.00	0.14	0.32	0.35	0.73	1.42	2.49	5.49	6.82	17.41	20.35	38.17	1.63	1.02	0.03	0.09
0.04	0.00	0.00	0.00	0.00	0.05	0.00	0.16	0.23	0.00	0.28	1.12	0.03	0.02	0.00	0.00
0.00	0.00	0.00	0.04	0.14	0.05	0.20	0.08	0.11	0.87	0.00	1.87	0.07	0.05	0.00	0.00
1.72	1.32	1.88	3.28	4.88	6.19	8.47	14.67	24.20	26.81	23.46	31.81	4.40	3.23	0.16	0.36
0.48	0.18	0.23	0.44	0.91	1.15	1.48	3.69	3.98	4.70	7.07	5.24	0.79	0.54	0.02	0.06
0.04	0.05	0.09	0.31	0.05	0.33	0.34	0.39	1.36	1.04	0.85	1.50	0.18	0.13	0.01	0.02
0.00	0.00	0.00	0.04	0.09	0.16	0.13	0.08	0.34	0.52	0.85	0.75	0.07	0.05	0.00	0.00
0.00	0.09	0.09	0.09	0.18	0.27	0.27	0.47	0.80	1.92	0.28	0.75	0.16	0.11	0.01	0.01
0.24	0.41	0.78	0.92	1.55	2.79	2.55	6.43	10.57	10.97	10.17	10.48	1.64	1.16	0.05	0.14
0.00	0.00	0.00	0.00	0.00	0.00	0.00	0.16	0.00	0.00	0.00	0.00	0.01	0.00	0.00	0.00
0.04	0.05	0.09	0.22	0.59	1.70	1.08	4.63	6.36	4.70	2.26	1.87	0.73	0.51	0.02	0.07
0.04	0.18	0.14	0.22	0.46	0.66	1.01	0.63	1.14	1.74	1.13	1.12	0.33	0.27	0.02	0.03
0.24	0.45	0.50	0.61	0.87	1.31	1.55	2.67	3.07	4.00	4.80	3.37	0.81	0.64	0.04	0.06
0.64	0.36	0.46	0.92	0.91	1.92	2.15	5.26	4.66	6.44	8.20	5.61	1.27	1.01	0.05	0.10
0.64	1.00	1.38	1.40	3.51	4.32	5.04	12.40	17.16	19.33	28.26	31.81	3.21	2.26	0.10	0.25
0.00	0.00	0.00	0.00	0.00	0.05	0.20	0.39	0.00	0.35	0.85	1.12	0.06	0.04	0.00	0.00
0.04	0.05	0.14	0.13	0.09	0.27	0.40	0.47	1.82	1.92	1.70	2.25	0.23	0.17	0.01	0.02
13.90	18.99	32.23	69.81	137.05	230.04	330.20	678.88	976.60	1 273.44	1 508.56	1 901.68	164.13	109.03	4.27	12.55
13.82	18.81	32.19	69.68	136.32	229.21	329.33	676.60	973.30	1 267.52	1 496.69	1 875.86	163.30	108.52	4.26	12.51

表 6-17 河南省农村肿瘤登记地区

部位	ICD-10	病例数	构成 (%)	年龄组						
				0~	1~	5~	10~	15~	20~	25~
唇	C00	21	0.07	0	0.00	0.00	0.00	0.00	0.00	0.08
舌	C01–C02	37	0.12	0	0.00	0.00	0.00	0.00	0.00	0.00
口	C03–C06	54	0.17	0	0.00	0.00	0.00	0.00	0.00	0.00
唾液腺	C07–C08	40	0.13	0	0.00	0.00	0.00	0.00	0.00	0.00
扁桃体	C09	6	0.02	0	0.00	0.00	0.00	0.00	0.00	0.00
其他的口咽	C10	26	0.08	0	0.00	0.00	0.00	0.00	0.00	0.00
鼻咽	C11	104	0.33	0	0.00	0.00	0.00	0.00	0.00	0.00
喉咽	C12–C13	40	0.13	0	0.00	0.00	0.00	0.00	0.00	0.00
咽，部位不明	C14	42	0.13	0	0.00	0.00	0.00	0.00	0.00	0.00
食管	C15	4 552	14.60	0	0.00	0.00	0.00	0.00	0.00	0.00
胃	C16	5 531	17.73	0	0.12	0.09	0.00	0.00	0.18	0.08
小肠	C17	127	0.41	0	0.00	0.00	0.00	0.00	0.00	0.00
结肠	C18	638	2.05	0	0.00	0.00	0.00	0.09	0.09	0.33
直肠	C19–C20	833	2.67	0	0.00	0.09	0.00	0.00	0.00	0.16
肛门	C21	93	0.30	0	0.00	0.00	0.00	0.00	0.00	0.00
肝脏	C22	4 645	14.89	0	0.24	0.18	0.00	0.09	0.18	0.41
胆囊及其他	C23–C24	440	1.41	0	0.00	0.00	0.00	0.00	0.00	0.00
胰腺	C25	604	1.94	0	0.00	0.00	0.00	0.00	0.00	0.00
鼻、鼻窦及其他	C30–C31	46	0.15	0	0.00	0.00	0.00	0.00	0.00	0.00
喉	C32	172	0.55	0	0.00	0.00	0.00	0.00	0.00	0.00
气管、支气管、肺	C33–C34	8 918	28.59	0	0.00	0.00	0.08	0.00	0.44	0.91
其他的胸腔器官	C37–C38	80	0.26	0	0.00	0.00	0.00	0.18	0.26	0.00
骨	C40–C41	261	0.84	0	0.12	0.44	0.50	0.55	0.70	0.08
皮肤的黑色素瘤	C43	24	0.08	0	0.00	0.00	0.00	0.00	0.00	0.00
其他的皮肤	C44	142	0.46	0	0.00	0.00	0.00	0.00	0.00	0.00
间皮瘤	C45	11	0.04	0	0.00	0.00	0.00	0.00	0.00	0.00
卡波西肉瘤	C46	0	0.00	0	0.00	0.00	0.00	0.00	0.00	0.00
周围神经、其他结缔组织、软组织	C47;C49	40	0.13	0	0.12	0.00	0.17	0.00	0.00	0.00
乳房	C50	39	0.13	0	0.00	0.00	0.00	0.00	0.00	0.00
外阴	C51	0	0.00	0	0.00	0.00	0.00	0.00	0.00	0.00
阴道	C52	0	0.00	0	0.00	0.00	0.00	0.00	0.00	0.00
子宫颈	C53	1	0.00	0	0.00	0.00	0.00	0.00	0.00	0.00
子宫体	C54	0	0.00	0	0.00	0.00	0.00	0.00	0.00	0.00
子宫，部位不明	C55	1	0.00	0	0.00	0.00	0.00	0.00	0.00	0.00
卵巢	C56	0	0.00	0	0.00	0.00	0.00	0.00	0.00	0.00
女性其他的生殖器	C57	0	0.00	0	0.00	0.00	0.00	0.00	0.00	0.00
胎盘	C58	0	0.00	0	0.00	0.00	0.00	0.00	0.00	0.00
阴茎	C60	31	0.10	0	0.00	0.00	0.00	0.00	0.00	0.00
前列腺	C61	450	1.44	0	0.00	0.00	0.00	0.00	0.09	0.00
睾丸	C62	18	0.06	0	0.00	0.00	0.00	0.00	0.00	0.00
男性其他的生殖器	C63	5	0.02	0	0.00	0.00	0.00	0.00	0.00	0.00
肾	C64	263	0.84	0	0.00	0.00	0.00	0.09	0.09	0.08
肾盂	C65	31	0.10	0	0.00	0.00	0.00	0.00	0.00	0.00
输尿管	C66	41	0.13	0	0.00	0.00	0.00	0.00	0.00	0.00
膀胱	C67	386	1.24	0	0.00	0.00	0.00	0.00	0.00	0.16
其他的泌尿器官	C68	5	0.02	0	0.00	0.00	0.00	0.00	0.00	0.00
眼	C69	12	0.04	0	0.12	0.00	0.00	0.00	0.00	0.00
脑、神经系统	C70–C72	736	2.36	0	0.24	1.58	1.50	0.46	1.14	0.49
甲状腺	C73	79	0.25	0	0.00	0.00	0.00	0.00	0.00	0.00
肾上腺	C74	45	0.14	0	0.00	0.18	0.00	0.00	0.00	0.00
其他的内分泌腺	C75	13	0.04	0	0.00	0.00	0.00	0.00	0.09	0.00
霍奇金病	C81	24	0.08	0	0.00	0.00	0.00	0.00	0.00	0.08
非霍奇金淋巴瘤	C82–C85;C96	298	0.96	0	0.00	0.09	0.42	0.27	0.70	0.33
免疫增生性疾病	C88	2	0.01	0	0.00	0.00	0.00	0.00	0.00	0.00
多发性骨髓瘤	C90	137	0.44	0	0.12	0.00	0.00	0.00	0.09	0.00
淋巴样白血病	C91	62	0.20	0	0.12	0.26	0.08	0.37	0.18	0.00
髓样白血病	C92–C94	139	0.45	0	0.48	0.18	0.25	0.37	0.26	0.41
白血病，未特指	C95	210	0.67	0	0.48	0.18	0.33	0.55	0.26	0.82
其他的或未指明部位	O&U	581	1.86	0	0.48	0.44	0.42	0.73	0.53	0.49
骨髓增殖性疾病	MPD	8	0.03	0	0.00	0.00	0.00	0.00	0.09	0.00
骨髓增生异常综合征	MDS	44	0.14	0	0.12	0.09	0.00	0.00	0.00	0.00
合计	ALL	31 188	100.00	0	2.76	3.78	3.75	3.74	5.34	4.95
C44 以外的部位	ALL but C44	31 046	99.54	0	2.76	3.78	3.75	3.74	5.34	4.95

2020 年男性死亡主要指标

30~	35~	40~	45~	50~	55~	60~	65~	70~	75~	80~	85+	粗率 (1/10⁵)	世标率 (1/10⁵)	累积率 (%)	
														0~64	0~74
0.00	0.00	0.09	0.09	0.00	0.11	0.40	0.31	1.41	0.37	1.30	2.97	0.13	0.10	0.00	0.01
0.08	0.00	0.18	0.17	0.09	0.33	0.93	1.10	0.23	1.84	3.91	1.98	0.23	0.17	0.01	0.02
0.00	0.00	0.09	0.09	0.36	0.87	0.27	2.05	2.11	4.80	1.96	0.00	0.34	0.24	0.01	0.03
0.08	0.09	0.18	0.09	0.27	0.33	0.53	1.10	1.64	1.11	1.96	4.95	0.25	0.18	0.01	0.02
0.00	0.00	0.00	0.00	0.09	0.11	0.00	0.63	0.00	0.00	0.00	0.00	0.04	0.03	0.00	0.00
0.00	0.00	0.00	0.09	0.18	0.11	0.40	0.47	1.41	0.74	2.61	3.96	0.16	0.12	0.00	0.01
0.23	0.35	0.18	0.69	0.80	1.30	2.13	2.52	3.05	2.95	4.56	5.94	0.65	0.48	0.03	0.06
0.00	0.09	0.09	0.00	0.27	0.11	0.13	0.63	2.11	2.95	4.56	4.95	0.25	0.17	0.00	0.02
0.23	0.00	0.09	0.09	0.09	0.33	0.80	1.26	0.94	2.95	1.96	3.96	0.26	0.19	0.01	0.02
0.31	0.78	0.89	5.32	10.99	24.75	56.46	131.69	224.27	311.03	393.87	447.68	28.63	19.99	0.50	2.28
1.08	1.65	3.21	9.61	20.02	42.34	74.39	168.51	260.67	340.17	399.09	451.64	34.78	24.57	0.76	2.91
0.15	0.09	0.09	0.86	0.63	1.30	2.26	4.25	4.23	6.64	4.56	6.93	0.80	0.58	0.03	0.07
0.15	0.70	0.80	2.49	3.93	6.41	7.57	14.63	24.89	36.16	42.39	61.41	4.01	2.86	0.11	0.31
0.46	0.44	0.98	2.75	4.02	6.73	10.89	22.03	30.53	41.69	82.17	77.25	5.24	3.69	0.13	0.40
0.00	0.26	0.18	0.69	0.36	0.98	0.80	1.26	4.23	5.53	7.83	7.92	0.58	0.41	0.02	0.04
3.47	6.62	12.57	25.92	42.27	65.68	73.86	129.65	149.36	162.71	181.94	252.56	29.21	21.38	1.16	2.55
0.08	0.00	0.53	0.60	1.25	3.47	5.58	16.05	19.96	25.09	30.00	36.65	2.77	1.96	0.06	0.24
0.31	0.44	0.98	1.12	3.57	6.08	9.17	16.84	28.42	28.78	35.87	44.57	3.80	2.72	0.11	0.33
0.23	0.17	0.00	0.17	0.80	0.22	0.93	1.10	0.23	2.21	2.61	2.97	0.29	0.21	0.01	0.02
0.08	0.09	0.09	0.09	0.54	1.41	2.39	5.82	6.11	11.81	11.74	17.83	1.08	0.76	0.02	0.08
1.46	3.13	6.06	16.56	43.16	78.82	124.21	266.22	403.92	521.33	590.16	704.20	56.08	39.78	1.37	4.72
0.15	0.09	0.00	0.17	0.98	0.76	0.80	1.57	3.29	4.06	5.87	1.98	0.50	0.37	0.02	0.04
0.54	0.52	0.36	0.94	0.98	2.61	2.66	6.29	8.45	12.54	13.69	19.81	1.64	1.27	0.05	0.13
0.08	0.09	0.00	0.00	0.27	0.43	0.27	0.47	0.94	1.11	1.30	0.99	0.15	0.11	0.01	0.01
0.00	0.17	0.00	0.09	0.89	0.98	0.93	3.30	4.23	8.12	15.65	27.73	0.89	0.62	0.02	0.05
0.08	0.00	0.00	0.09	0.18	0.22	0.27	0.16	0.23	0.00	0.65	0.00	0.07	0.05	0.00	0.01
0.00	0.00	0.00	0.00	0.00	0.00	0.00	0.00	0.00	0.00	0.00	0.00	0.00	0.00	0.00	0.00
0.15	0.17	0.18	0.26	0.09	0.22	0.80	0.79	0.94	1.84	1.30	2.97	0.25	0.20	0.01	0.02
0.00	0.00	0.18	0.09	0.36	0.43	0.27	1.26	0.94	1.84	3.91	2.97	0.25	0.17	0.01	0.02
0.00	0.00	0.00	0.00	0.00	0.00	0.00	0.00	0.00	0.00	0.00	0.00	0.00	0.00	0.00	0.00
0.00	0.00	0.00	0.00	0.00	0.00	0.00	0.00	0.00	0.00	0.00	0.00	0.00	0.00	0.00	0.00
0.00	0.00	0.00	0.00	0.00	0.00	0.00	0.16	0.00	0.00	0.00	0.00	0.01	0.00	0.00	0.00
0.00	0.00	0.00	0.00	0.00	0.00	0.00	0.00	0.00	0.00	0.00	0.00	0.00	0.00	0.00	0.00
0.00	0.00	0.00	0.00	0.09	0.00	0.00	0.00	0.00	0.00	0.00	0.00	0.01	0.00	0.00	0.00
0.00	0.00	0.00	0.00	0.00	0.00	0.00	0.00	0.00	0.00	0.00	0.00	0.00	0.00	0.00	0.00
0.00	0.00	0.00	0.00	0.00	0.00	0.00	0.00	0.00	0.00	0.00	0.00	0.00	0.00	0.00	0.00
0.00	0.00	0.00	0.00	0.00	0.00	0.00	0.00	0.00	0.00	0.00	0.00	0.00	0.00	0.00	0.00
0.00	0.00	0.00	0.09	0.18	0.22	0.13	0.63	1.64	2.58	1.96	3.96	0.19	0.14	0.00	0.01
0.08	0.09	0.00	0.60	0.18	1.09	2.66	7.87	20.67	31.73	63.25	86.17	2.83	1.93	0.02	0.17
0.15	0.00	0.00	0.09	0.09	0.22	0.40	0.31	0.70	0.74	0.65	0.99	0.11	0.08	0.00	0.01
0.00	0.00	0.00	0.00	0.09	0.00	0.13	0.00	0.47	0.00	0.00	0.99	0.03	0.02	0.00	0.00
0.15	0.35	0.80	1.20	2.14	2.28	3.99	7.71	10.33	9.96	12.39	16.84	1.65	1.21	0.06	0.15
0.00	0.09	0.09	0.09	0.09	0.33	1.06	0.31	1.64	1.11	1.30	1.98	0.19	0.15	0.01	0.02
0.08	0.09	0.00	0.00	0.00	0.11	0.53	1.26	1.88	2.58	3.91	4.95	0.26	0.18	0.00	0.02
0.00	0.17	0.45	0.43	1.25	2.28	4.12	8.34	10.80	29.52	35.87	71.31	2.43	1.69	0.04	0.14
0.00	0.00	0.00	0.00	0.00	0.11	0.00	0.16	0.23	0.00	0.00	1.98	0.03	0.02	0.00	0.00
0.00	0.00	0.00	0.00	0.09	0.11	0.00	0.16	0.23	1.11	0.00	3.96	0.08	0.06	0.00	0.00
2.16	1.65	2.23	3.69	5.72	8.03	8.90	13.85	27.95	29.89	22.17	31.69	4.63	3.58	0.19	0.40
0.15	0.17	0.18	0.26	0.80	0.87	0.66	2.52	3.05	2.95	5.22	2.97	0.50	0.35	0.02	0.04
0.00	0.09	0.18	0.51	0.09	0.43	0.53	0.63	2.35	1.48	1.96	3.96	0.28	0.22	0.01	0.02
0.00	0.00	0.00	0.00	0.00	0.22	0.13	0.16	0.47	0.74	1.96	0.99	0.08	0.06	0.00	0.01
0.00	0.09	0.00	0.17	0.27	0.11	0.27	0.47	0.94	1.84	0.65	0.99	0.15	0.11	0.00	0.01
0.31	0.61	0.80	0.94	1.88	3.26	3.06	7.55	13.86	14.02	10.43	10.89	1.87	1.41	0.06	0.17
0.00	0.00	0.00	0.00	0.00	0.00	0.00	0.31	0.00	0.00	0.00	0.00	0.01	0.01	0.00	0.00
0.00	0.09	0.09	0.26	0.71	1.95	1.20	5.98	6.81	7.01	3.26	3.96	0.86	0.63	0.02	0.09
0.08	0.17	0.09	0.17	0.54	0.65	1.06	1.10	1.88	1.84	1.96	1.98	0.39	0.33	0.02	0.03
0.39	0.26	0.80	0.86	1.16	1.19	1.06	2.36	3.76	5.17	5.22	5.94	0.87	0.72	0.04	0.07
0.46	0.26	0.53	1.29	1.52	2.39	2.39	5.82	4.23	7.38	9.13	4.95	1.32	1.06	0.06	0.11
0.85	1.04	1.52	1.46	3.93	5.54	5.71	16.21	20.90	22.88	36.52	41.60	3.65	2.74	0.12	0.30
0.00	0.00	0.00	0.00	0.00	0.11	0.13	0.16	0.00	0.37	1.30	0.99	0.05	0.04	0.00	0.00
0.08	0.09	0.18	0.17	0.18	0.22	0.40	0.63	2.11	3.32	1.96	3.96	0.28	0.21	0.01	0.02
14.33	21.24	35.93	81.36	158.45	279.13	418.58	886.60	1 325.66	1 718.58	2 068.48	2 504.80	196.13	140.32	5.16	16.23
14.33	21.07	35.93	81.27	157.55	278.15	417.65	883.30	1 321.43	1 710.47	2 052.83	2 477.07	195.24	139.70	5.15	16.17

表 6-18 河南省农村肿瘤登记地区

部位	ICD-10	病例数	构成(%)	年龄组 0~	1~	5~	10~	15~	20~	25~
唇	C00	13	0.07	0.00	0.00	0.00	0.00	0.00	0.00	0.00
舌	C01–C02	32	0.16	0.00	0.00	0.00	0.00	0.00	0.00	0.00
口	C03–C06	47	0.24	0.00	0.00	0.00	0.00	0.00	0.00	0.00
唾液腺	C07–C08	18	0.09	0.00	0.00	0.00	0.00	0.00	0.00	0.00
扁桃体	C09	8	0.04	0.00	0.00	0.00	0.00	0.00	0.00	0.00
其他的口咽	C10	10	0.05	0.00	0.00	0.00	0.00	0.00	0.00	0.00
鼻咽	C11	54	0.28	0.00	0.00	0.00	0.00	0.00	0.00	0.00
喉咽	C12–C13	7	0.04	0.00	0.00	0.00	0.00	0.00	0.00	0.00
咽，部位不明	C14	20	0.10	0.00	0.00	0.00	0.00	0.00	0.00	0.00
食管	C15	2 716	13.96	0.00	0.00	0.00	0.00	0.00	0.10	0.36
胃	C16	2 336	12.01	0.00	0.00	0.00	0.19	0.10	0.29	0.45
小肠	C17	81	0.42	0.00	0.00	0.00	0.00	0.00	0.00	0.00
结肠	C18	582	2.99	0.00	0.00	0.00	0.00	0.00	0.00	0.27
直肠	C19–C20	669	3.44	0.00	0.00	0.00	0.00	0.00	0.00	0.00
肛门	C21	61	0.31	0.00	0.00	0.00	0.00	0.00	0.00	0.00
肝脏	C22	2 124	10.92	0.00	0.00	0.10	0.29	0.10	0.00	0.09
胆囊及其他	C23–C24	580	2.98	0.00	0.00	0.00	0.00	0.00	0.00	0.09
胰腺	C25	503	2.59	0.00	0.00	0.00	0.00	0.00	0.10	0.00
鼻、鼻窦及其他	C30–C31	38	0.20	0.00	0.00	0.00	0.00	0.00	0.10	0.09
喉	C32	31	0.16	0.00	0.00	0.00	0.00	0.00	0.00	0.00
气管、支气管、肺	C33–C34	3 649	18.76	0.00	0.00	0.00	0.10	0.00	0.10	0.27
其他的胸腔器官	C37–C38	76	0.39	0.00	0.14	0.00	0.10	0.00	0.00	0.00
骨	C40–C41	160	0.82	0.00	0.00	0.00	0.19	0.31	0.48	0.63
皮肤的黑色素瘤	C43	21	0.11	0.00	0.00	0.00	0.00	0.00	0.00	0.00
其他的皮肤	C44	115	0.59	0.00	0.00	0.00	0.00	0.00	0.00	0.00
间皮瘤	C45	8	0.04	0.00	0.00	0.00	0.00	0.00	0.00	0.00
卡波西肉瘤	C46	1	0.01	0.00	0.00	0.00	0.00	0.00	0.00	0.00
周围神经、其他结缔组织、软组织	C47;C49	35	0.18	0.00	0.00	0.10	0.19	0.10	0.00	0.09
乳房	C50	1 414	7.27	0.00	0.00	0.00	0.00	0.00	0.19	0.18
外阴	C51	16	0.08	0.00	0.00	0.00	0.00	0.00	0.00	0.00
阴道	C52	22	0.11	0.00	0.00	0.00	0.00	0.00	0.00	0.00
子宫颈	C53	914	4.70	0.00	0.00	0.00	0.00	0.00	0.00	0.27
子宫体	C54	299	1.54	0.00	0.00	0.00	0.00	0.00	0.00	0.00
子宫，部位不明	C55	100	0.51	0.00	0.00	0.00	0.00	0.00	0.00	0.00
卵巢	C56	444	2.28	0.00	0.00	0.00	0.00	0.00	0.10	0.36
女性其他的生殖器	C57	19	0.10	0.00	0.00	0.10	0.00	0.00	0.00	0.00
胎盘	C58	0	0.00	0.00	0.00	0.00	0.00	0.00	0.00	0.00
阴茎	C60	0	0.00	0.00	0.00	0.00	0.00	0.00	0.00	0.00
前列腺	C61	0	0.00	0.00	0.00	0.00	0.00	0.00	0.00	0.00
睾丸	C62	1	0.01	0.00	0.00	0.00	0.00	0.00	0.00	0.00
男性其他的生殖器	C63	0	0.00	0.00	0.00	0.00	0.00	0.00	0.00	0.00
肾	C64	150	0.77	0.00	0.00	0.00	0.00	0.00	0.00	0.00
肾盂	C65	18	0.09	0.00	0.00	0.00	0.00	0.00	0.00	0.00
输尿管	C66	17	0.09	0.00	0.00	0.00	0.00	0.00	0.00	0.00
膀胱	C67	118	0.61	0.00	0.00	0.00	0.00	0.00	0.10	0.00
其他的泌尿器官	C68	5	0.03	0.00	0.00	0.00	0.00	0.00	0.00	0.00
眼	C69	10	0.05	0.00	0.00	0.00	0.00	0.00	0.00	0.09
脑、神经系统	C70–C72	623	3.20	0.65	0.41	1.52	0.19	0.31	0.77	0.81
甲状腺	C73	166	0.85	0.00	0.00	0.00	0.00	0.00	0.00	0.27
肾上腺	C74	11	0.06	0.00	0.00	0.00	0.00	0.00	0.00	0.09
其他的内分泌腺	C75	8	0.04	0.00	0.00	0.00	0.00	0.00	0.00	0.00
霍奇金病	C81	24	0.12	0.00	0.00	0.00	0.00	0.00	0.00	0.09
非霍奇金淋巴瘤	C82–C85;C96	209	1.07	0.00	0.00	0.10	0.38	0.10	0.10	0.09
免疫增生性疾病	C88	0	0.00	0.00	0.00	0.00	0.00	0.00	0.00	0.00
多发性骨髓瘤	C90	89	0.46	0.00	0.00	0.00	0.00	0.00	0.00	0.00
淋巴样白血病	C91	40	0.21	0.00	0.14	0.30	0.00	0.10	0.10	0.00
髓样白血病	C92–C94	111	0.57	0.00	0.55	0.10	0.10	0.21	0.19	0.18
白血病，未特指	C95	183	0.94	0.00	0.82	0.71	0.76	0.83	0.10	0.27
其他的或未指明部位	O&U	409	2.10	0.00	0.41	0.71	0.10	0.62	0.19	0.09
骨髓增殖性疾病	MPD	11	0.06	0.00	0.00	0.00	0.00	0.00	0.10	0.00
骨髓增生异常综合征	MDS	27	0.14	0.00	0.14	0.00	0.00	0.00	0.10	0.09
合计	ALL	19 453	100.00	0.65	2.60	3.74	2.58	2.79	3.18	5.22
C44 以外的部位	ALL but C44	19 338	99.41	0.65	2.60	3.74	2.58	2.79	3.18	5.22

2020 年女性死亡主要指标

												粗率	世标率	累积率 (%)	
30~	35~	40~	45~	50~	55~	60~	65~	70~	75~	80~	85+	$(1/10^5)$	$(1/10^5)$	0~64	0~74
0.00	0.00	0.00	0.09	0.00	0.22	0.14	0.31	0.00	0.33	2.00	1.20	0.09	0.05	0.00	0.00
0.17	0.09	0.19	0.09	0.09	0.22	0.14	0.94	1.54	1.32	1.50	1.20	0.21	0.14	0.00	0.02
0.08	0.00	0.00	0.00	0.28	0.33	0.54	1.25	2.20	2.31	3.99	1.80	0.31	0.19	0.01	0.02
0.00	0.00	0.00	0.18	0.56	0.11	0.00	0.31	0.66	0.00	0.50	1.80	0.12	0.08	0.00	0.01
0.00	0.00	0.00	0.09	0.00	0.11	0.00	0.16	0.22	0.66	1.00	0.00	0.05	0.03	0.00	0.00
0.00	0.00	0.09	0.00	0.09	0.33	0.00	0.00	0.88	0.00	0.50	0.00	0.07	0.04	0.00	0.01
0.17	0.09	0.00	0.27	0.75	0.44	0.68	0.94	1.10	2.64	3.49	3.01	0.36	0.22	0.01	0.02
0.00	0.00	0.00	0.00	0.00	0.00	0.00	0.16	0.44	0.33	1.00	0.60	0.05	0.02	0.00	0.00
0.00	0.00	0.09	0.00	0.09	0.11	0.14	0.47	0.88	1.32	1.00	1.80	0.13	0.08	0.00	0.01
0.25	0.47	1.04	0.89	4.94	14.47	28.57	60.11	114.44	167.48	209.48	274.25	18.16	10.35	0.26	1.13
1.24	1.33	2.17	3.13	9.69	17.45	25.30	56.51	77.69	113.74	165.59	239.97	15.62	9.17	0.31	0.98
0.00	0.00	0.00	0.18	0.56	0.77	1.09	2.97	2.42	3.63	3.49	6.01	0.54	0.33	0.01	0.04
0.08	0.85	0.47	1.25	2.42	4.86	6.80	14.87	17.17	32.31	42.39	44.51	3.89	2.32	0.09	0.25
0.33	0.28	0.94	1.70	3.07	4.97	8.71	16.12	21.79	36.27	37.41	62.55	4.47	2.68	0.10	0.29
0.00	0.00	0.19	0.09	0.47	0.99	0.54	1.25	1.98	1.65	3.99	6.01	0.41	0.25	0.01	0.03
1.41	1.23	2.36	7.06	11.92	17.12	28.43	52.28	73.07	90.01	117.71	190.65	14.21	8.67	0.35	0.98
0.00	0.19	0.38	0.71	2.51	3.64	7.75	16.75	21.13	27.36	38.90	50.52	3.88	2.31	0.08	0.27
0.33	0.19	0.85	0.89	3.45	4.53	6.80	14.56	16.29	24.07	26.43	33.68	3.36	2.07	0.09	0.24
0.00	0.00	0.00	0.18	0.28	0.44	0.54	0.16	0.88	2.31	2.00	4.21	0.25	0.16	0.01	0.01
0.00	0.00	0.09	0.00	0.09	0.11	0.27	1.57	0.44	2.31	0.00	4.21	0.21	0.13	0.00	0.01
0.75	0.95	3.49	10.45	20.31	36.55	41.08	90.31	127.21	167.48	203.99	329.58	24.40	14.69	0.57	1.66
0.25	0.19	0.19	0.36	0.47	0.88	1.09	1.25	1.76	2.97	3.99	5.41	0.51	0.33	0.02	0.03
0.08	0.00	0.09	0.36	1.77	1.55	1.50	3.29	4.84	4.29	8.98	11.43	1.07	0.72	0.03	0.08
0.00	0.09	0.00	0.00	0.37	0.11	0.27	0.31	1.10	0.99	1.00	0.60	0.14	0.09	0.00	0.01
0.17	0.19	0.09	0.18	0.56	0.66	0.82	1.25	2.42	3.96	8.98	24.66	0.77	0.42	0.01	0.03
0.00	0.09	0.00	0.00	0.00	0.11	0.14	0.47	0.44	0.00	0.00	0.00	0.05	0.04	0.00	0.01
0.00	0.09	0.00	0.00	0.00	0.00	0.00	0.00	0.00	0.00	0.00	0.00	0.01	0.01	0.00	0.00
0.17	0.19	0.19	0.09	0.19	0.44	0.14	0.16	0.88	0.99	1.50	3.01	0.23	0.17	0.01	0.01
1.16	3.04	4.34	10.72	17.05	23.41	24.76	36.16	33.23	36.93	28.93	41.50	9.46	6.44	0.42	0.77
0.00	0.00	0.00	0.09	0.09	0.11	0.41	0.16	0.66	0.33	0.00	3.01	0.11	0.07	0.00	0.01
0.08	0.00	0.00	0.09	0.19	0.33	0.54	0.00	0.44	0.66	2.49	1.20	0.15	0.09	0.01	0.01
1.74	1.71	3.59	6.25	9.97	11.82	14.01	22.70	25.09	26.70	24.94	34.28	6.11	4.10	0.25	0.49
0.25	0.28	0.57	1.16	4.47	4.53	4.08	6.42	6.60	11.21	9.98	18.04	2.00	1.28	0.08	0.14
0.17	0.00	0.00	0.54	0.93	1.33	0.95	2.82	2.20	5.28	6.48	3.61	0.67	0.41	0.02	0.04
0.58	1.04	1.51	2.59	4.19	7.07	5.58	11.11	14.53	12.20	15.46	12.63	2.97	1.98	0.12	0.24
0.00	0.00	0.00	0.09	0.19	0.22	0.27	0.63	0.44	0.66	0.50	1.20	0.13	0.09	0.00	0.01
0.00	0.00	0.00	0.00	0.00	0.00	0.00	0.00	0.00	0.00	0.00	0.00	0.00	0.00	0.00	0.00
0.00	0.00	0.00	0.00	0.00	0.00	0.00	0.00	0.00	0.00	0.00	0.00	0.00	0.00	0.00	0.00
0.00	0.00	0.00	0.00	0.00	0.00	0.00	0.00	0.00	0.00	0.00	0.00	0.00	0.00	0.00	0.00
0.00	0.00	0.00	0.00	0.00	0.00	0.00	0.00	0.00	0.33	0.00	0.00	0.01	0.00	0.00	0.00
0.00	0.00	0.00	0.00	0.00	0.00	0.00	0.00	0.00	0.00	0.00	0.00	0.00	0.00	0.00	0.00
0.17	0.09	0.28	0.27	1.12	1.44	2.18	3.13	5.06	8.90	7.98	8.42	1.00	0.62	0.03	0.07
0.00	0.00	0.00	0.09	0.00	0.00	0.27	0.31	0.44	1.65	1.00	2.41	0.12	0.07	0.00	0.01
0.00	0.00	0.00	0.00	0.00	0.55	0.14	0.31	0.22	1.32	2.00	0.00	0.11	0.06	0.00	0.01
0.00	0.09	0.19	0.27	0.19	0.55	0.82	2.66	3.08	6.59	8.48	18.04	0.79	0.44	0.01	0.04
0.08	0.00	0.00	0.00	0.00	0.00	0.00	0.16	0.22	0.00	0.50	0.60	0.03	0.02	0.00	0.00
0.00	0.00	0.00	0.09	0.19	0.00	0.41	0.00	0.00	0.66	0.00	0.60	0.07	0.05	0.00	0.00
1.24	0.95	1.51	2.86	4.01	4.31	8.03	15.50	20.69	24.07	24.44	31.88	4.17	2.87	0.13	0.32
0.83	0.19	0.28	0.63	1.02	1.44	2.31	4.85	4.84	6.26	8.48	6.62	1.11	0.72	0.03	0.08
0.08	0.00	0.00	0.09	0.00	0.22	0.14	0.16	0.44	0.66	0.00	0.00	0.07	0.05	0.00	0.01
0.00	0.00	0.00	0.09	0.19	0.11	0.14	0.00	0.22	0.33	0.00	0.60	0.05	0.04	0.00	0.00
0.00	0.09	0.19	0.00	0.09	0.44	0.27	0.47	0.66	1.98	0.00	0.60	0.16	0.11	0.01	0.01
0.17	0.19	0.76	0.89	1.21	2.32	2.04	5.32	7.48	8.24	9.98	10.22	1.40	0.92	0.04	0.11
0.00	0.00	0.00	0.00	0.00	0.00	0.00	0.00	0.00	0.00	0.00	0.00	0.00	0.00	0.00	0.00
0.08	0.00	0.09	0.18	0.47	1.44	0.95	3.29	5.94	2.64	1.50	0.60	0.60	0.39	0.02	0.06
0.00	0.19	0.19	0.27	0.37	0.66	0.95	0.16	0.44	1.65	0.50	0.60	0.27	0.22	0.02	0.02
0.08	0.66	0.19	0.36	0.56	1.44	2.04	2.97	2.42	2.97	4.49	1.80	0.74	0.56	0.03	0.06
0.83	0.47	0.38	0.54	0.28	1.44	1.90	4.70	5.06	5.60	7.48	6.01	1.22	0.97	0.05	0.09
0.41	0.95	1.23	1.34	3.07	3.09	4.35	8.61	13.65	16.15	21.95	25.86	2.74	1.82	0.08	0.19
0.00	0.00	0.00	0.00	0.00	0.00	0.27	0.63	0.00	0.33	0.50	1.20	0.07	0.05	0.00	0.00
0.00	0.00	0.09	0.09	0.00	0.33	0.41	0.31	1.54	0.66	1.50	1.20	0.18	0.13	0.01	0.02
13.44	16.53	28.32	57.79	114.75	180.11	239.69	472.23	649.47	875.66	1 080.30	1 535.44	130.10	80.29	3.35	8.96
13.27	16.34	28.23	57.61	114.20	179.44	238.88	470.98	647.05	871.70	1 071.33	1 510.78	129.33	79.87	3.34	8.93

二、河南省肿瘤登记地区发病和死亡主要结果

2. Cancer incidence and mortality in each cancer registry in Henan province

表 6-19　2020 年河南省郑州市城区恶性肿瘤发病主要指标

部位	ICD-10	男性						女性					
		病例数	构成 (%)	粗率 (1/10^5)	世标率 (1/10^5)	累积率 (%) 0~64	累积率 (%) 0~74	病例数	构成 (%)	粗率 (1/10^5)	世标率 (1/10^5)	累积率 (%) 0~64	累积率 (%) 0~74
唇	C00	2	0.06	0.19	0.19	0.01	0.01	1	0.03	0.09	0.05	0.00	0.00
舌	C01–C02	14	0.43	1.33	0.95	0.05	0.10	5	0.13	0.44	0.41	0.01	0.04
口	C03–C06	15	0.46	1.43	1.09	0.06	0.10	9	0.23	0.80	0.52	0.02	0.04
唾液腺	C07–C08	6	0.18	0.57	0.39	0.02	0.02	8	0.21	0.71	0.50	0.03	0.06
扁桃体	C09	3	0.09	0.29	0.23	0.03	0.03	2	0.05	0.18	0.12	0.01	0.01
其他的口咽	C10	4	0.12	0.38	0.26	0.02	0.02	0	0.00	0.00	0.00	0.00	0.00
鼻咽	C11	6	0.18	0.57	0.44	0.04	0.06	5	0.13	0.44	0.30	0.01	0.03
喉咽	C12–C13	7	0.22	0.67	0.52	0.03	0.06	0	0.00	0.00	0.00	0.00	0.00
咽，部位不明	C14	0	0.00	0.00	0.00	0.00	0.00	0	0.00	0.00	0.00	0.00	0.00
食管	C15	133	4.09	12.65	9.82	0.43	1.14	66	1.70	5.84	3.81	0.11	0.39
胃	C16	254	7.82	24.16	18.44	0.83	2.33	111	2.86	9.83	6.95	0.37	0.75
小肠	C17	17	0.52	1.62	1.23	0.07	0.14	9	0.23	0.80	0.49	0.01	0.05
结肠	C18	192	5.91	18.26	13.63	0.70	1.42	139	3.58	12.30	8.50	0.41	0.89
直肠	C19–C20	158	4.86	15.03	11.49	0.72	1.43	99	2.55	8.76	6.23	0.39	0.68
肛门	C21	2	0.06	0.19	0.11	0.01	0.01	2	0.05	0.18	0.10	0.01	0.01
肝脏	C22	319	9.82	30.34	23.39	1.43	2.78	127	3.27	11.24	7.54	0.29	0.82
胆囊及其他	C23–C24	57	1.75	5.42	4.28	0.22	0.48	55	1.42	4.87	2.98	0.10	0.28
胰腺	C25	102	3.14	9.70	7.22	0.33	0.85	88	2.27	7.79	5.21	0.20	0.57
鼻、鼻窦及其他	C30–C31	4	0.12	0.38	0.30	0.02	0.04	4	0.10	0.35	0.37	0.01	0.04
喉	C32	44	1.35	4.19	3.17	0.28	0.34	2	0.05	0.18	0.14	0.01	0.02
气管、支气管、肺	C33–C34	755	23.24	71.82	55.64	2.46	6.86	533	13.73	47.18	34.11	2.18	3.83
其他的胸腔器官	C37–C38	14	0.43	1.33	1.05	0.05	0.10	8	0.21	0.71	0.52	0.03	0.06
骨	C40–C41	21	0.65	2.00	1.77	0.09	0.17	25	0.64	2.21	2.11	0.10	0.16
皮肤的黑色素瘤	C43	5	0.15	0.48	0.39	0.01	0.06	4	0.10	0.35	0.24	0.00	0.03
其他的皮肤	C44	33	1.02	3.14	2.41	0.06	0.23	31	0.80	2.74	1.89	0.06	0.25
间皮瘤	C45	0	0.00	0.00	0.00	0.00	0.00	1	0.03	0.09	0.07	0.01	0.01
卡波西肉瘤	C46	0	0.00	0.00	0.00	0.00	0.00	0	0.00	0.00	0.00	0.00	0.00
周围神经、其他结缔组织、软组织	C47;C49	12	0.37	1.14	0.83	0.06	0.08	19	0.49	1.68	1.46	0.10	0.13
乳房	C50	11	0.34	1.05	0.79	0.05	0.10	742	19.11	65.68	48.45	4.00	5.19
外阴	C51	0	0.00	0.00	0.00	0.00	0.00	5	0.13	0.44	0.33	0.03	0.04
阴道	C52	0	0.00	0.00	0.00	0.00	0.00	10	0.26	0.89	0.77	0.06	0.09
子宫颈	C53	0	0.00	0.00	0.00	0.00	0.00	207	5.33	18.32	13.58	1.11	1.48
子宫体	C54	0	0.00	0.00	0.00	0.00	0.00	151	3.89	13.37	10.19	0.87	1.20
子宫，部位不明	C55	0	0.00	0.00	0.00	0.00	0.00	14	0.36	1.24	0.94	0.08	0.10
卵巢	C56	0	0.00	0.00	0.00	0.00	0.00	87	2.24	7.70	5.85	0.45	0.64
女性其他的生殖器	C57	0	0.00	0.00	0.00	0.00	0.00	6	0.15	0.53	0.40	0.02	0.06
胎盘	C58	0	0.00	0.00	0.00	0.00	0.00	0	0.00	0.00	0.00	0.00	0.00
阴茎	C60	5	0.15	0.48	0.38	0.02	0.03	0	0.00	0.00	0.00	0.00	0.00
前列腺	C61	162	4.99	15.41	11.11	0.19	1.11	0	0.00	0.00	0.00	0.00	0.00
睾丸	C62	5	0.15	0.48	0.37	0.03	0.03	0	0.00	0.00	0.00	0.00	0.00
男性其他的生殖器	C63	3	0.09	0.29	0.18	0.02	0.02	0	0.00	0.00	0.00	0.00	0.00
肾	C64	95	2.92	9.04	7.16	0.48	0.93	46	1.18	4.07	3.03	0.18	0.33
肾盂	C65	6	0.18	0.57	0.40	0.01	0.03	3	0.08	0.27	0.18	0.02	0.02
输尿管	C66	11	0.34	1.05	0.85	0.02	0.12	11	0.28	0.97	0.62	0.02	0.06
膀胱	C67	111	3.42	10.56	8.16	0.35	0.88	31	0.80	2.74	1.82	0.10	0.18
其他的泌尿器官	C68	0	0.00	0.00	0.00	0.00	0.00	0	0.00	0.00	0.00	0.00	0.00
眼	C69	3	0.09	0.29	0.37	0.02	0.02	1	0.03	0.09	0.04	0.00	0.00
脑、神经系统	C70–C72	55	1.69	5.23	4.62	0.24	0.40	45	1.16	3.98	3.02	0.16	0.27
甲状腺	C73	367	11.30	34.91	26.97	2.29	2.61	947	24.39	83.82	61.80	5.27	5.99
肾上腺	C74	6	0.18	0.57	0.65	0.03	0.03	1	0.03	0.09	0.07	0.01	0.01
其他的内分泌腺	C75	0	0.00	0.00	0.00	0.00	0.00	1	0.03	0.09	0.07	0.01	0.01
霍奇金病	C81	4	0.12	0.38	0.27	0.03	0.03	1	0.03	0.09	0.06	0.00	0.00
非霍奇金淋巴瘤	C82–C85;C96	71	2.19	6.75	5.67	0.35	0.60	76	1.96	6.73	4.60	0.23	0.50
免疫增生性疾病	C88	0	0.00	0.00	0.00	0.00	0.00	0	0.00	0.00	0.00	0.00	0.00
多发性骨髓瘤	C90	23	0.71	2.19	1.71	0.09	0.23	26	0.67	2.30	1.60	0.09	0.16
淋巴样白血病	C91	11	0.34	1.05	1.26	0.05	0.06	2	0.05	0.18	0.23	0.01	0.02
髓样白血病	C92–C94	23	0.71	2.19	1.54	0.07	0.17	23	0.59	2.04	1.78	0.12	0.20
白血病，未特指	C95	30	0.92	2.85	2.84	0.16	0.23	26	0.67	2.30	1.93	0.10	0.16
其他的或未指明部位	O&U	65	2.00	6.18	4.86	0.29	0.43	67	1.73	5.93	4.26	0.23	0.37
骨髓增殖性疾病	MPD	3	0.09	0.29	0.19	0.01	0.03	1	0.03	0.09	0.06	0.00	0.02
骨髓增生异常综合征	MDS	0	0.00	0.00	0.00	0.00	0.00	0	0.00	0.00	0.00	0.00	0.00
合计	ALL	3 249	100.00	309.05	239.61	12.85	26.95	3 883	100.00	343.71	250.31	17.63	26.26
C44 以外的部位	ALL but C44	3 216	98.98	305.91	237.20	12.79	26.72	3 852	99.20	340.96	248.42	17.57	26.01

表 6-20 2020 年河南省郑州市城区恶性肿瘤死亡主要指标

部位	ICD-10	男性						女性					
		病例数	构成 (%)	粗率 ($1/10^5$)	世标率 ($1/10^5$)	累积率 (%)		病例数	构成 (%)	粗率 ($1/10^5$)	世标率 ($1/10^5$)	累积率 (%)	
						0～64	0～74					0～64	0～74
唇	C00	1	0.05	0.10	0.08	0.00	0.00	0	0.00	0.00	0.00	0.00	0.00
舌	C01–C02	5	0.27	0.48	0.42	0.01	0.04	1	0.09	0.09	0.06	0.00	0.02
口	C03–C06	6	0.32	0.57	0.46	0.02	0.05	5	0.43	0.44	0.31	0.00	0.04
唾液腺	C07–C08	2	0.11	0.19	0.12	0.01	0.01	1	0.09	0.09	0.04	0.00	0.00
扁桃体	C09	1	0.05	0.10	0.09	0.00	0.02	1	0.09	0.09	0.07	0.01	0.01
其他的口咽	C10	4	0.21	0.38	0.30	0.02	0.05	0	0.00	0.00	0.00	0.00	0.00
鼻咽	C11	9	0.48	0.86	0.67	0.03	0.08	6	0.51	0.53	0.37	0.03	0.03
喉咽	C12–C13	4	0.21	0.38	0.27	0.01	0.03	0	0.00	0.00	0.00	0.00	0.00
咽，部位不明	C14	1	0.05	0.10	0.07	0.01	0.01	1	0.09	0.09	0.04	0.00	0.00
食管	C15	120	6.43	11.41	8.50	0.31	0.95	45	3.84	3.98	2.42	0.05	0.21
胃	C16	173	9.27	16.46	12.01	0.38	1.19	80	6.83	7.08	4.14	0.13	0.34
小肠	C17	11	0.59	1.05	0.87	0.03	0.14	6	0.51	0.53	0.25	0.00	0.00
结肠	C18	92	4.93	8.75	6.39	0.14	0.50	51	4.35	4.51	2.85	0.09	0.24
直肠	C19–C20	70	3.75	6.66	5.18	0.22	0.54	49	4.18	4.34	2.69	0.06	0.20
肛门	C21	3	0.16	0.29	0.19	0.01	0.03	1	0.09	0.09	0.05	0.00	0.00
肝脏	C22	278	14.89	26.44	20.09	1.15	2.30	120	10.24	10.62	7.08	0.22	0.75
胆囊及其他	C23–C24	46	2.46	4.38	3.47	0.10	0.36	61	5.20	5.40	3.47	0.10	0.35
胰腺	C25	67	3.59	6.37	4.79	0.24	0.57	66	5.63	5.84	3.87	0.16	0.41
鼻、鼻窦及其他	C30–C31	1	0.05	0.10	0.09	0.01	0.01	2	0.17	0.18	0.10	0.01	0.01
喉	C32	27	1.45	2.57	1.97	0.13	0.24	0	0.00	0.00	0.00	0.00	0.00
气管、支气管、肺	C33–C34	562	30.10	53.46	39.87	1.31	4.13	222	18.94	19.65	12.42	0.39	1.22
其他的胸腔器官	C37–C38	7	0.37	0.67	0.44	0.01	0.04	5	0.43	0.44	0.32	0.02	0.03
骨	C40–C41	16	0.86	1.52	1.29	0.04	0.14	8	0.68	0.71	0.50	0.01	0.05
皮肤的黑色素瘤	C43	4	0.21	0.38	0.29	0.03	0.03	1	0.09	0.09	0.04	0.00	0.00
其他的皮肤	C44	8	0.43	0.76	0.62	0.02	0.03	12	1.02	1.06	0.62	0.02	0.03
间皮瘤	C45	3	0.16	0.29	0.21	0.01	0.03	1	0.09	0.09	0.07	0.01	0.01
卡波西肉瘤	C46	0	0.00	0.00	0.00	0.00	0.00	0	0.00	0.00	0.00	0.00	0.00
周围神经、其他结缔组织、软组织	C47;C49	6	0.32	0.57	0.53	0.03	0.05	6	0.51	0.53	0.46	0.03	0.03
乳房	C50	3	0.16	0.29	0.18	0.00	0.02	103	8.79	9.12	6.14	0.30	0.63
外阴	C51	0	0.00	0.00	0.00	0.00	0.00	3	0.26	0.27	0.21	0.02	0.02
阴道	C52	0	0.00	0.00	0.00	0.00	0.00	1	0.09	0.09	0.08	0.00	0.01
子宫颈	C53	0	0.00	0.00	0.00	0.00	0.00	46	3.92	4.07	2.93	0.19	0.31
子宫体	C54	0	0.00	0.00	0.00	0.00	0.00	24	2.05	2.12	1.42	0.06	0.19
子宫，部位不明	C55	0	0.00	0.00	0.00	0.00	0.00	2	0.17	0.18	0.13	0.01	0.01
卵巢	C56	0	0.00	0.00	0.00	0.00	0.00	39	3.33	3.45	2.49	0.20	0.25
女性其他的生殖器	C57	0	0.00	0.00	0.00	0.00	0.00	3	0.26	0.27	0.15	0.00	0.01
胎盘	C58	0	0.00	0.00	0.00	0.00	0.00	0	0.00	0.00	0.00	0.00	0.00
阴茎	C60	1	0.05	0.10	0.09	0.00	0.02	0	0.00	0.00	0.00	0.00	0.00
前列腺	C61	70	3.75	6.66	4.50	0.03	0.19	0	0.00	0.00	0.00	0.00	0.00
睾丸	C62	0	0.00	0.00	0.00	0.00	0.00	0	0.00	0.00	0.00	0.00	0.00
男性其他的生殖器	C63	2	0.11	0.19	0.09	0.00	0.00	0	0.00	0.00	0.00	0.00	0.00
肾	C64	23	1.23	2.19	1.69	0.06	0.21	13	1.11	1.15	0.69	0.01	0.06
肾盂	C65	3	0.16	0.29	0.18	0.00	0.02	4	0.34	0.35	0.20	0.00	0.02
输尿管	C66	8	0.43	0.76	0.55	0.02	0.06	7	0.60	0.62	0.34	0.01	0.01
膀胱	C67	38	2.04	3.61	2.59	0.04	0.09	11	0.94	0.97	0.59	0.01	0.04
其他的泌尿器官	C68	0	0.00	0.00	0.00	0.00	0.00	0	0.00	0.00	0.00	0.00	0.00
眼	C69	3	0.16	0.29	0.19	0.01	0.02	1	0.09	0.09	0.07	0.01	0.01
脑、神经系统	C70–C72	42	2.25	4.00	3.29	0.16	0.25	35	2.99	3.10	2.39	0.12	0.23
甲状腺	C73	6	0.32	0.57	0.43	0.03	0.04	11	0.94	0.97	0.61	0.04	0.05
肾上腺	C74	3	0.16	0.29	0.21	0.00	0.02	0	0.00	0.00	0.00	0.00	0.00
其他的内分泌腺	C75	0	0.00	0.00	0.00	0.00	0.00	1	0.09	0.09	0.04	0.00	0.00
霍奇金病	C81	3	0.16	0.29	0.16	0.01	0.01	2	0.17	0.18	0.10	0.00	0.02
非霍奇金淋巴瘤	C82–C85;C96	39	2.09	3.71	2.74	0.10	0.29	33	2.82	2.92	1.84	0.06	0.16
免疫增生性疾病	C88	0	0.00	0.00	0.00	0.00	0.00	0	0.00	0.00	0.00	0.00	0.00
多发性骨髓瘤	C90	9	0.48	0.86	0.65	0.01	0.07	10	0.85	0.89	0.57	0.02	0.07
淋巴样白血病	C91	3	0.16	0.29	0.28	0.01	0.01	4	0.34	0.35	0.37	0.01	0.04
髓样白血病	C92–C94	18	0.96	1.71	1.39	0.04	0.18	11	0.94	0.97	0.75	0.04	0.10
白血病，未特指	C95	28	1.50	2.66	2.25	0.11	0.21	14	1.19	1.24	0.90	0.02	0.07
其他的或未指明部位	O&U	28	1.50	2.66	1.99	0.11	0.22	35	2.99	3.10	2.02	0.05	0.14
骨髓增殖性疾病	MPD	2	0.11	0.19	0.14	0.02	0.02	0	0.00	0.00	0.00	0.00	0.00
骨髓增生异常综合征	MDS	8	0.43	0.76	0.52	0.00	0.03	8	0.68	0.71	0.50	0.03	0.05
合计	ALL	1 867	100.00	177.59	133.38	5.06	13.55	1 172	100.00	103.74	67.72	2.53	6.47
C44 以外的部位	ALL but C44	1 859	99.57	176.83	132.76	5.04	13.52	1 160	98.98	102.68	67.10	2.51	6.43

表 6-21 2020 年河南省中牟县恶性肿瘤发病主要指标

部位	ICD-10	男性						女性					
		病例数	构成(%)	粗率($1/10^5$)	世标率($1/10^5$)	累积率(%)		病例数	构成(%)	粗率($1/10^5$)	世标率($1/10^5$)	累积率(%)	
						0~64	0~74					0~64	0~74
唇	C00	1	0.15	0.37	0.34	0.00	0.08	1	0.13	0.41	0.31	0.00	0.08
舌	C01–C02	0	0.00	0.00	0.00	0.00	0.00	0	0.00	0.00	0.00	0.00	0.00
口	C03–C06	2	0.29	0.75	0.47	0.03	0.03	2	0.26	0.83	0.56	0.04	0.04
唾液腺	C07–C08	0	0.00	0.00	0.00	0.00	0.00	2	0.26	0.83	0.61	0.05	0.05
扁桃体	C09	0	0.00	0.00	0.00	0.00	0.00	1	0.13	0.41	0.27	0.00	0.05
其他的口咽	C10	0	0.00	0.00	0.00	0.00	0.00	1	0.13	0.41	0.28	0.02	0.02
鼻咽	C11	4	0.58	1.49	1.11	0.11	0.11	1	0.13	0.41	0.66	0.04	0.04
喉咽	C12–C13	0	0.00	0.00	0.00	0.00	0.00	0	0.00	0.00	0.00	0.00	0.00
咽，部位不明	C14	0	0.00	0.00	0.00	0.00	0.00	0	0.00	0.00	0.00	0.00	0.00
食管	C15	27	3.92	10.07	7.54	0.12	0.91	8	1.03	3.30	2.22	0.08	0.25
胃	C16	36	5.22	13.43	10.99	0.26	1.01	17	2.18	7.02	4.82	0.37	0.57
小肠	C17	9	1.31	3.36	2.73	0.13	0.46	4	0.51	1.65	1.10	0.06	0.14
结肠	C18	23	3.34	8.58	6.86	0.31	0.74	12	1.54	4.95	3.17	0.25	0.38
直肠	C19–C20	33	4.79	12.31	9.58	0.35	1.30	30	3.85	12.38	7.40	0.28	0.74
肛门	C21	0	0.00	0.00	0.00	0.00	0.00	1	0.13	0.41	0.28	0.02	0.02
肝脏	C22	132	19.16	49.25	38.07	2.58	4.44	45	5.77	18.57	12.70	0.70	1.31
胆囊及其他	C23–C24	9	1.31	3.36	2.63	0.08	0.27	11	1.41	4.54	3.12	0.09	0.26
胰腺	C25	13	1.89	4.85	4.17	0.13	0.52	19	2.44	7.84	5.00	0.26	0.63
鼻、鼻窦及其他	C30–C31	1	0.15	0.37	0.29	0.04	0.04	0	0.00	0.00	0.00	0.00	0.00
喉	C32	4	0.58	1.49	1.15	0.03	0.16	0	0.00	0.00	0.00	0.00	0.00
气管、支气管、肺	C33–C34	194	28.16	72.38	55.88	2.36	6.79	126	16.15	52.00	33.50	1.60	3.82
其他的胸腔器官	C37–C38	6	0.87	2.24	1.74	0.10	0.24	4	0.51	1.65	1.73	0.11	0.11
骨	C40–C41	3	0.44	1.12	1.24	0.08	0.08	5	0.64	2.06	1.59	0.11	0.16
皮肤的黑色素瘤	C43	2	0.29	0.75	0.60	0.03	0.07	1	0.13	0.41	0.37	0.02	0.02
其他的皮肤	C44	9	1.31	3.36	2.50	0.15	0.24	13	1.67	5.36	3.75	0.15	0.60
间皮瘤	C45	0	0.00	0.00	0.00	0.00	0.00	1	0.13	0.41	0.27	0.00	0.05
卡波西肉瘤	C46	0	0.00	0.00	0.00	0.00	0.00	0	0.00	0.00	0.00	0.00	0.00
周围神经、其他结缔组织、软组织	C47;C49	2	0.29	0.75	0.94	0.07	0.07	2	0.26	0.83	0.59	0.06	0.06
乳房	C50	1	0.15	0.37	0.34	0.00	0.08	145	18.59	59.84	43.83	3.69	4.73
外阴	C51	0	0.00	0.00	0.00	0.00	0.00	1	0.13	0.41	0.25	0.00	0.00
阴道	C52	0	0.00	0.00	0.00	0.00	0.00	0	0.00	0.00	0.00	0.00	0.00
子宫颈	C53	0	0.00	0.00	0.00	0.00	0.00	29	3.72	11.97	9.42	0.69	1.09
子宫体	C54	0	0.00	0.00	0.00	0.00	0.00	32	4.10	13.21	9.21	0.79	1.11
子宫，部位不明	C55	0	0.00	0.00	0.00	0.00	0.00	4	0.51	1.65	0.95	0.08	0.08
卵巢	C56	0	0.00	0.00	0.00	0.00	0.00	55	7.05	22.70	20.72	1.63	1.75
女性其他的生殖器	C57	0	0.00	0.00	0.00	0.00	0.00	1	0.13	0.41	0.31	0.04	0.04
胎盘	C58	0	0.00	0.00	0.00	0.00	0.00	1	0.13	0.41	0.50	0.03	0.03
阴茎	C60	0	0.00	0.00	0.00	0.00	0.00	0	0.00	0.00	0.00	0.00	0.00
前列腺	C61	21	3.05	7.83	6.20	0.14	1.05	0	0.00	0.00	0.00	0.00	0.00
睾丸	C62	0	0.00	0.00	0.00	0.00	0.00	0	0.00	0.00	0.00	0.00	0.00
男性其他的生殖器	C63	0	0.00	0.00	0.00	0.00	0.00	0	0.00	0.00	0.00	0.00	0.00
肾	C64	27	3.92	10.07	7.75	0.34	0.79	9	1.15	3.71	2.30	0.12	0.20
肾盂	C65	1	0.15	0.37	0.29	0.04	0.04	0	0.00	0.00	0.00	0.00	0.00
输尿管	C66	1	0.15	0.37	0.27	0.02	0.02	2	0.26	0.83	0.41	0.03	0.03
膀胱	C67	22	3.19	8.21	6.72	0.28	0.55	6	0.77	2.48	1.71	0.02	0.18
其他的泌尿器官	C68	0	0.00	0.00	0.00	0.00	0.00	0	0.00	0.00	0.00	0.00	0.00
眼	C69	0	0.00	0.00	0.00	0.00	0.00	0	0.00	0.00	0.00	0.00	0.00
脑、神经系统	C70–C72	15	2.18	5.60	4.90	0.32	0.41	12	1.54	4.95	4.75	0.31	0.31
甲状腺	C73	47	6.82	17.53	16.75	1.36	1.54	132	16.92	54.47	43.14	3.65	3.78
肾上腺	C74	1	0.15	0.37	0.28	0.00	0.05	0	0.00	0.00	0.00	0.00	0.00
其他的内分泌腺	C75	0	0.00	0.00	0.00	0.00	0.00	0	0.00	0.00	0.00	0.00	0.00
霍奇金病	C81	1	0.15	0.37	0.25	0.03	0.03	1	0.13	0.41	0.31	0.04	0.04
非霍奇金淋巴瘤	C82–C85;C96	17	2.47	6.34	5.49	0.21	0.60	14	1.79	5.78	3.83	0.23	0.35
免疫增生性疾病	C88	0	0.00	0.00	0.00	0.00	0.00	0	0.00	0.00	0.00	0.00	0.00
多发性骨髓瘤	C90	3	0.44	1.12	0.86	0.05	0.13	7	0.90	2.89	1.99	0.04	0.34
淋巴样白血病	C91	1	0.15	0.37	0.34	0.00	0.08	0	0.00	0.00	0.00	0.00	0.00
髓样白血病	C92–C94	4	0.58	1.49	1.44	0.08	0.12	4	0.51	1.65	1.36	0.14	0.14
白血病，未特指	C95	6	0.87	2.24	1.67	0.10	0.10	12	1.54	4.95	4.28	0.18	0.39
其他的或未指明部位	O&U	10	1.45	3.73	3.10	0.13	0.43	5	0.64	2.06	1.27	0.02	0.18
骨髓增殖性疾病	MPD	1	0.15	0.37	0.32	0.02	0.02	1	0.13	0.41	0.28	0.02	0.02
骨髓增生异常综合征	MDS	0	0.00	0.00	0.00	0.00	0.00	0	0.00	0.00	0.00	0.00	0.00
合计	ALL	689	100.00	257.05	205.79	10.07	23.60	780	100.00	321.89	235.10	16.07	24.16
C44 以外的部位	ALL but C44	680	98.69	253.69	203.29	9.92	23.36	767	98.33	316.53	231.35	15.92	23.56

表 6-22　2020 年河南省中牟县恶性肿瘤死亡主要指标

部位	ICD-10	男性						女性					
		病例数	构成(%)	粗率(1/10^5)	世标率(1/10^5)	累积率(%)		病例数	构成(%)	粗率(1/10^5)	世标率(1/10^5)	累积率(%)	
						0~64	0~74					0~64	0~74
唇	C00	1	0.24	0.37	0.27	0.03	0.03	0	0.00	0.00	0.00	0.00	0.00
舌	C01-C02	0	0.00	0.00	0.00	0.00	0.00	0	0.00	0.00	0.00	0.00	0.00
口	C03-C06	0	0.00	0.00	0.00	0.00	0.00	1	0.41	0.41	0.25	0.00	0.00
唾液腺	C07-C08	0	0.00	0.00	0.00	0.00	0.00	0	0.00	0.00	0.00	0.00	0.00
扁桃体	C09	0	0.00	0.00	0.00	0.00	0.00	0	0.00	0.00	0.00	0.00	0.00
其他的口咽	C10	0	0.00	0.00	0.00	0.00	0.00	0	0.00	0.00	0.00	0.00	0.00
鼻咽	C11	1	0.24	0.37	0.28	0.00	0.05	0	0.00	0.00	0.00	0.00	0.00
喉咽	C12-C13	0	0.00	0.00	0.00	0.00	0.00	0	0.00	0.00	0.00	0.00	0.00
咽，部位不明	C14	0	0.00	0.00	0.00	0.00	0.00	0	0.00	0.00	0.00	0.00	0.00
食管	C15	12	2.84	4.48	3.32	0.03	0.37	7	2.87	2.89	1.63	0.00	0.08
胃	C16	27	6.38	10.07	7.47	0.30	0.76	6	2.46	2.48	1.56	0.05	0.13
小肠	C17	5	1.18	1.87	1.39	0.08	0.08	5	2.05	2.06	1.03	0.03	0.03
结肠	C18	9	2.13	3.36	2.86	0.11	0.24	14	5.74	5.78	3.24	0.13	0.25
直肠	C19-C20	16	3.78	5.97	4.58	0.18	0.32	17	6.97	7.02	4.36	0.19	0.32
肛门	C21	0	0.00	0.00	0.00	0.00	0.00	0	0.00	0.00	0.00	0.00	0.00
肝脏	C22	113	26.71	42.16	32.37	2.10	3.99	31	12.70	12.79	7.97	0.30	0.74
胆囊及其他	C23-C24	4	0.95	1.49	1.12	0.07	0.12	6	2.46	2.48	1.44	0.00	0.12
胰腺	C25	7	1.65	2.61	2.27	0.06	0.31	10	4.10	4.13	2.33	0.10	0.18
鼻、鼻窦及其他	C30-C31	0	0.00	0.00	0.00	0.00	0.00	0	0.00	0.00	0.00	0.00	0.00
喉	C32	2	0.47	0.75	0.55	0.03	0.03	0	0.00	0.00	0.00	0.00	0.00
气管、支气管、肺	C33-C34	150	35.46	55.96	43.88	1.16	4.88	61	25.00	25.17	15.81	0.62	1.80
其他的胸腔器官	C37-C38	3	0.71	1.12	0.96	0.00	0.17	0	0.00	0.00	0.00	0.00	0.00
骨	C40-C41	3	0.71	1.12	0.88	0.06	0.15	1	0.41	0.41	0.25	0.00	0.00
皮肤的黑色素瘤	C43	0	0.00	0.00	0.00	0.00	0.00	0	0.00	0.00	0.00	0.00	0.00
其他的皮肤	C44	1	0.24	0.37	0.29	0.04	0.04	2	0.82	0.83	0.52	0.00	0.05
间皮瘤	C45	0	0.00	0.00	0.00	0.00	0.00	0	0.00	0.00	0.00	0.00	0.00
卡波西肉瘤	C46	0	0.00	0.00	0.00	0.00	0.00	0	0.00	0.00	0.00	0.00	0.00
周围神经、其他结缔组织、软组织	C47;C49	1	0.24	0.37	0.28	0.00	0.00	0	0.00	0.00	0.00	0.00	0.00
乳房	C50	0	0.00	0.00	0.00	0.00	0.00	20	8.20	8.25	5.84	0.43	0.71
外阴	C51	0	0.00	0.00	0.00	0.00	0.00	0	0.00	0.00	0.00	0.00	0.00
阴道	C52	0	0.00	0.00	0.00	0.00	0.00	0	0.00	0.00	0.00	0.00	0.00
子宫颈	C53	0	0.00	0.00	0.00	0.00	0.00	16	6.56	6.60	4.72	0.33	0.61
子宫体	C54	0	0.00	0.00	0.00	0.00	0.00	4	1.64	1.65	1.12	0.13	0.13
子宫，部位不明	C55	0	0.00	0.00	0.00	0.00	0.00	1	0.41	0.41	0.27	0.00	0.05
卵巢	C56	0	0.00	0.00	0.00	0.00	0.00	4	1.64	1.65	1.12	0.03	0.19
女性其他的生殖器	C57	0	0.00	0.00	0.00	0.00	0.00	0	0.00	0.00	0.00	0.00	0.00
胎盘	C58	0	0.00	0.00	0.00	0.00	0.00	0	0.00	0.00	0.00	0.00	0.00
阴茎	C60	2	0.47	0.75	0.48	0.00	0.00	0	0.00	0.00	0.00	0.00	0.00
前列腺	C61	13	3.07	4.85	3.74	0.07	0.37	0	0.00	0.00	0.00	0.00	0.00
睾丸	C62	0	0.00	0.00	0.00	0.00	0.00	0	0.00	0.00	0.00	0.00	0.00
男性其他的生殖器	C63	0	0.00	0.00	0.00	0.00	0.00	0	0.00	0.00	0.00	0.00	0.00
肾	C64	6	1.42	2.24	1.65	0.06	0.20	8	3.28	3.30	1.95	0.03	0.28
肾盂	C65	2	0.47	0.75	0.77	0.00	0.08	0	0.00	0.00	0.00	0.00	0.00
输尿管	C66	0	0.00	0.00	0.00	0.00	0.00	0	0.00	0.00	0.00	0.00	0.00
膀胱	C67	9	2.13	3.36	2.90	0.03	0.17	1	0.41	0.41	0.27	0.00	0.05
其他的泌尿器官	C68	0	0.00	0.00	0.00	0.00	0.00	0	0.00	0.00	0.00	0.00	0.00
眼	C69	0	0.00	0.00	0.00	0.00	0.00	0	0.00	0.00	0.00	0.00	0.00
脑、神经系统	C70-C72	9	2.13	3.36	3.07	0.15	0.19	5	2.05	2.06	1.29	0.09	0.09
甲状腺	C73	0	0.00	0.00	0.00	0.00	0.00	1	0.41	0.41	0.13	0.00	0.00
肾上腺	C74	1	0.24	0.37	0.29	0.04	0.04	0	0.00	0.00	0.00	0.00	0.00
其他的内分泌腺	C75	0	0.00	0.00	0.00	0.00	0.00	0	0.00	0.00	0.00	0.00	0.00
霍奇金病	C81	0	0.00	0.00	0.00	0.00	0.00	0	0.00	0.00	0.00	0.00	0.00
非霍奇金淋巴瘤	C82-C85;C96	5	1.18	1.87	1.52	0.09	0.17	8	3.28	3.30	2.01	0.02	0.22
免疫增生性疾病	C88	0	0.00	0.00	0.00	0.00	0.00	0	0.00	0.00	0.00	0.00	0.00
多发性骨髓瘤	C90	2	0.47	0.75	0.56	0.00	0.09	2	0.82	0.83	0.58	0.03	0.11
淋巴样白血病	C91	1	0.24	0.37	0.20	0.00	0.00	0	0.00	0.00	0.00	0.00	0.00
髓样白血病	C92-C94	1	0.24	0.37	0.35	0.02	0.02	1	0.41	0.41	0.50	0.03	0.03
白血病，未特指	C95	10	2.36	3.73	3.46	0.14	0.23	8	3.28	3.30	3.14	0.12	0.28
其他的或未指明部位	O&U	6	1.42	2.24	2.00	0.06	0.23	3	1.23	1.24	0.84	0.03	0.15
骨髓增殖性疾病	MPD	0	0.00	0.00	0.00	0.00	0.00	0	0.00	0.00	0.00	0.00	0.00
骨髓增生异常综合征	MDS	1	0.24	0.37	0.34	0.00	0.08	1	0.41	0.41	0.27	0.03	0.03
合计	ALL	423	100.00	157.81	124.08	4.90	13.41	244	100.00	100.69	64.45	2.73	6.62
C44 以外的部位	ALL but C44	422	99.76	157.44	123.79	4.87	13.38	242	99.18	99.87	63.93	2.73	6.58

表 6-23 2020 年河南省巩义市恶性肿瘤发病主要指标

部位	ICD-10	男性						女性					
		病例数	构成 (%)	粗率 (1/10^5)	世标率 (1/10^5)	累积率 (%) 0~64	累积率 (%) 0~74	病例数	构成 (%)	粗率 (1/10^5)	世标率 (1/10^5)	累积率 (%) 0~64	累积率 (%) 0~74
唇	C00	0	0.00	0.00	0.00	0.00	0.00	0	0.00	0.00	0.00	0.00	0.00
舌	C01–C02	1	0.10	0.23	0.18	0.02	0.02	3	0.32	0.72	0.49	0.04	0.04
口	C03–C06	5	0.51	1.16	0.85	0.02	0.11	1	0.11	0.24	0.24	0.00	0.04
唾液腺	C07–C08	1	0.10	0.23	0.20	0.03	0.03	0	0.00	0.00	0.00	0.00	0.00
扁桃体	C09	1	0.10	0.23	0.15	0.00	0.00	2	0.22	0.48	0.39	0.00	0.10
其他的口咽	C10	0	0.00	0.00	0.00	0.00	0.00	0	0.00	0.00	0.00	0.00	0.00
鼻咽	C11	4	0.41	0.92	0.72	0.08	0.08	4	0.43	0.96	0.71	0.04	0.09
喉咽	C12–C13	1	0.10	0.23	0.23	0.00	0.04	0	0.00	0.00	0.00	0.00	0.00
咽，部位不明	C14	2	0.20	0.46	0.39	0.04	0.04	0	0.00	0.00	0.00	0.00	0.00
食管	C15	93	9.44	21.48	17.82	0.44	2.25	58	6.28	13.90	9.28	0.30	1.06
胃	C16	152	15.43	35.12	28.40	0.91	3.89	52	5.63	12.46	9.56	0.22	1.42
小肠	C17	5	0.51	1.16	0.89	0.07	0.12	1	0.11	0.24	0.24	0.00	0.04
结肠	C18	35	3.55	8.09	6.37	0.24	0.60	23	2.49	5.51	4.34	0.33	0.49
直肠	C19–C20	33	3.35	7.62	6.30	0.32	0.77	36	3.90	8.63	6.61	0.30	0.87
肛门	C21	0	0.00	0.00	0.00	0.00	0.00	0	0.00	0.00	0.00	0.00	0.00
肝脏	C22	122	12.39	28.18	23.32	1.37	2.87	55	5.95	13.18	9.81	0.51	1.21
胆囊及其他	C23–C24	12	1.22	2.77	2.30	0.06	0.34	20	2.16	4.79	3.64	0.10	0.54
胰腺	C25	17	1.73	3.93	3.25	0.18	0.44	13	1.41	3.12	2.17	0.08	0.24
鼻、鼻窦及其他	C30–C31	2	0.20	0.46	0.38	0.02	0.06	2	0.22	0.48	0.45	0.03	0.07
喉	C32	7	0.71	1.62	1.34	0.04	0.12	3	0.32	0.72	0.52	0.02	0.06
气管、支气管、肺	C33–C34	252	25.58	58.22	47.63	1.92	5.93	159	17.21	38.10	27.77	1.32	3.32
其他的胸腔器官	C37–C38	5	0.51	1.16	0.92	0.07	0.07	1	0.11	0.24	0.13	0.00	0.00
骨	C40–C41	9	0.91	2.08	1.91	0.05	0.28	9	0.97	2.16	1.74	0.04	0.28
皮肤的黑色素瘤	C43	1	0.10	0.23	0.15	0.02	0.02	1	0.11	0.24	0.21	0.03	0.03
其他的皮肤	C44	9	0.91	2.08	1.86	0.03	0.13	11	1.19	2.64	1.79	0.04	0.21
间皮瘤	C45	0	0.00	0.00	0.00	0.00	0.00	0	0.00	0.00	0.00	0.00	0.00
卡波西肉瘤	C46	0	0.00	0.00	0.00	0.00	0.00	0	0.00	0.00	0.00	0.00	0.00
周围神经、其他结缔组织、软组织	C47;C49	3	0.30	0.69	0.52	0.03	0.07	4	0.43	0.96	1.10	0.09	0.09
乳房	C50	3	0.30	0.69	0.61	0.02	0.10	132	14.29	31.63	24.80	1.96	2.81
外阴	C51	0	0.00	0.00	0.00	0.00	0.00	1	0.11	0.24	0.19	0.02	0.02
阴道	C52	0	0.00	0.00	0.00	0.00	0.00	3	0.32	0.72	0.49	0.05	0.05
子宫颈	C53	0	0.00	0.00	0.00	0.00	0.00	93	10.06	22.29	17.42	1.38	2.04
子宫体	C54	0	0.00	0.00	0.00	0.00	0.00	42	4.55	10.07	8.03	0.61	0.95
子宫，部位不明	C55	0	0.00	0.00	0.00	0.00	0.00	5	0.54	1.20	0.95	0.03	0.11
卵巢	C56	0	0.00	0.00	0.00	0.00	0.00	23	2.49	5.51	4.58	0.36	0.52
女性其他的生殖器	C57	0	0.00	0.00	0.00	0.00	0.00	1	0.11	0.24	0.24	0.00	0.04
胎盘	C58	0	0.00	0.00	0.00	0.00	0.00	0	0.00	0.00	0.00	0.00	0.00
阴茎	C60	1	0.10	0.23	0.20	0.00	0.05	0	0.00	0.00	0.00	0.00	0.00
前列腺	C61	43	4.37	9.93	8.04	0.14	0.98	1	0.11	0.24	0.18	0.02	0.02
睾丸	C62	1	0.10	0.23	0.23	0.02	0.02	0	0.00	0.00	0.00	0.00	0.00
男性其他的生殖器	C63	0	0.00	0.00	0.00	0.00	0.00	0	0.00	0.00	0.00	0.00	0.00
肾	C64	21	2.13	4.85	3.80	0.22	0.44	9	0.97	2.16	1.84	0.09	0.25
肾盂	C65	2	0.20	0.46	0.28	0.01	0.01	2	0.22	0.48	0.45	0.03	0.07
输尿管	C66	1	0.10	0.23	0.20	0.03	0.03	0	0.00	0.00	0.00	0.00	0.00
膀胱	C67	24	2.44	5.54	4.37	0.10	0.50	5	0.54	1.20	0.84	0.02	0.11
其他的泌尿器官	C68	0	0.00	0.00	0.00	0.00	0.00	0	0.00	0.00	0.00	0.00	0.00
眼	C69	0	0.00	0.00	0.00	0.00	0.00	2	0.22	0.48	0.37	0.03	0.03
脑、神经系统	C70–C72	23	2.34	5.31	5.19	0.26	0.52	29	3.14	6.95	5.14	0.26	0.48
甲状腺	C73	17	1.73	3.93	3.34	0.24	0.40	64	6.93	15.34	13.17	1.05	1.17
肾上腺	C74	1	0.10	0.23	0.15	0.00	0.00	0	0.00	0.00	0.00	0.00	0.00
其他的内分泌腺	C75	0	0.00	0.00	0.00	0.00	0.00	0	0.00	0.00	0.00	0.00	0.00
霍奇金病	C81	0	0.00	0.00	0.00	0.00	0.00	0	0.00	0.00	0.00	0.00	0.00
非霍奇金淋巴瘤	C82–C85;C96	16	1.62	3.70	3.18	0.16	0.29	7	0.76	1.68	1.30	0.08	0.12
免疫增生性疾病	C88	0	0.00	0.00	0.00	0.00	0.00	0	0.00	0.00	0.00	0.00	0.00
多发性骨髓瘤	C90	4	0.41	0.92	0.84	0.04	0.12	2	0.22	0.48	0.39	0.02	0.06
淋巴样白血病	C91	0	0.00	0.00	0.00	0.00	0.00	0	0.00	0.00	0.00	0.00	0.00
髓样白血病	C92–C94	6	0.61	1.39	1.43	0.10	0.10	5	0.54	1.20	1.15	0.08	0.08
白血病，未特指	C95	5	0.51	1.16	1.13	0.04	0.15	3	0.32	0.72	0.59	0.02	0.11
其他的或未指明部位	O&U	45	4.57	10.40	8.63	0.49	0.80	36	3.90	8.63	7.84	0.38	1.03
骨髓增殖性疾病	MPD	0	0.00	0.00	0.00	0.00	0.00	1	0.11	0.24	0.24	0.00	0.04
骨髓增生异常综合征	MDS	0	0.00	0.00	0.00	0.00	0.00	0	0.00	0.00	0.00	0.00	0.00
合计	ALL	985	100.00	227.56	187.68	7.82	22.76	924	100.00	221.44	171.41	9.96	20.32
C44 以外的部位	ALL but C44	976	99.09	225.48	185.82	7.79	22.63	913	98.81	218.80	169.62	9.92	20.11

表 6-24 2020 年河南省巩义市恶性肿瘤死亡主要指标

部位	ICD-10	男性						女性					
		病例数	构成 (%)	粗率 ($1/10^5$)	世标率 ($1/10^5$)	累积率 (%) 0～64	累积率 (%) 0～74	病例数	构成 (%)	粗率 ($1/10^5$)	世标率 ($1/10^5$)	累积率 (%) 0～64	累积率 (%) 0～74
唇	C00	1	0.14	0.23	0.25	0.00	0.00	0	0.0	0.00	0.00	0.00	0.00
舌	C01–C02	0	0.00	0.00	0.00	0.00	0.00	0	0.0	0.00	0.00	0.00	0.00
口	C03–C06	1	0.14	0.23	0.23	0.00	0.04	1	0.2	0.24	0.13	0.00	0.00
唾液腺	C07–C08	0	0.00	0.00	0.00	0.00	0.00	0	0.0	0.00	0.00	0.00	0.00
扁桃体	C09	0	0.00	0.00	0.00	0.00	0.00	0	0.0	0.00	0.00	0.00	0.00
其他的口咽	C10	2	0.29	0.46	0.34	0.03	0.03	0	0.0	0.00	0.00	0.00	0.00
鼻咽	C11	2	0.29	0.46	0.33	0.03	0.03	2	0.4	0.48	0.26	0.00	0.00
喉咽	C12–C13	0	0.00	0.00	0.00	0.00	0.00	0	0.0	0.00	0.00	0.00	0.00
咽，部位不明	C14	1	0.14	0.23	0.15	0.02	0.02	1	0.2	0.24	0.13	0.00	0.00
食管	C15	61	8.83	14.09	11.61	0.16	1.13	57	11.4	13.66	8.75	0.19	0.92
胃	C16	118	17.08	27.26	22.29	0.45	3.03	49	9.8	11.74	8.56	0.17	1.22
小肠	C17	3	0.43	0.69	0.42	0.00	0.00	1	0.2	0.24	0.24	0.00	0.04
结肠	C18	16	2.32	3.70	3.02	0.09	0.32	15	3.0	3.59	2.89	0.10	0.45
直肠	C19–C20	29	4.20	6.70	5.36	0.13	0.46	19	3.8	4.55	3.26	0.05	0.46
肛门	C21	0	0.00	0.00	0.00	0.00	0.00	0	0.0	0.00	0.00	0.00	0.00
肝脏	C22	116	16.79	26.80	21.75	1.19	2.39	54	10.8	12.94	9.33	0.38	1.09
胆囊及其他	C23–C24	13	1.88	3.00	2.29	0.03	0.31	21	4.2	5.03	3.50	0.19	0.44
胰腺	C25	17	2.46	3.93	3.11	0.13	0.34	18	3.6	4.31	2.99	0.10	0.32
鼻、鼻窦及其他	C30–C31	0	0.00	0.00	0.00	0.00	0.00	0	0.0	0.00	0.00	0.00	0.00
喉	C32	6	0.87	1.39	1.17	0.02	0.14	1	0.2	0.24	0.13	0.00	0.00
气管、支气管、肺	C33–C34	198	28.65	45.74	38.05	1.12	4.39	87	17.4	20.85	14.59	0.53	1.66
其他的胸腔器官	C37–C38	0	0.00	0.00	0.00	0.00	0.00	3	0.6	0.72	0.48	0.04	0.04
骨	C40–C41	6	0.87	1.39	1.12	0.06	0.15	5	1.0	1.20	0.86	0.03	0.11
皮肤的黑色素瘤	C43	0	0.00	0.00	0.00	0.00	0.00	2	0.4	0.48	0.32	0.02	0.02
其他的皮肤	C44	4	0.58	0.92	0.74	0.02	0.10	9	1.8	2.16	1.27	0.02	0.12
间皮瘤	C45	1	0.14	0.23	0.23	0.02	0.02	1	0.2	0.24	0.21	0.03	0.03
卡波西肉瘤	C46	0	0.00	0.00	0.00	0.00	0.00	0	0.0	0.00	0.00	0.00	0.00
周围神经、其他结缔组织、软组织	C47;C49	0	0.00	0.00	0.00	0.00	0.00	0	0.0	0.00	0.00	0.00	0.00
乳房	C50	2	0.29	0.46	0.45	0.00	0.08	27	5.4	6.47	4.89	0.36	0.58
外阴	C51	0	0.00	0.00	0.00	0.00	0.00	2	0.4	0.48	0.38	0.02	0.07
阴道	C52	0	0.00	0.00	0.00	0.00	0.00	1	0.2	0.24	0.25	0.02	0.02
子宫颈	C53	0	0.00	0.00	0.00	0.00	0.00	37	7.4	8.87	6.82	0.32	0.99
子宫体	C54	0	0.00	0.00	0.00	0.00	0.00	10	2.0	2.40	1.75	0.08	0.16
子宫，部位不明	C55	0	0.00	0.00	0.00	0.00	0.00	2	0.4	0.48	0.29	0.00	0.05
卵巢	C56	0	0.00	0.00	0.00	0.00	0.00	6	1.2	1.44	1.06	0.06	0.15
女性其他的生殖器	C57	0	0.00	0.00	0.00	0.00	0.00	0	0.0	0.00	0.00	0.00	0.00
胎盘	C58	0	0.00	0.00	0.00	0.00	0.00	0	0.0	0.00	0.00	0.00	0.00
阴茎	C60	0	0.00	0.00	0.00	0.00	0.00	0	0.0	0.00	0.00	0.00	0.00
前列腺	C61	13	1.88	3.00	2.43	0.02	0.14	0	0.0	0.00	0.00	0.00	0.00
睾丸	C62	1	0.14	0.23	0.15	0.02	0.02	0	0.0	0.00	0.00	0.00	0.00
男性其他的生殖器	C63	0	0.00	0.00	0.00	0.00	0.00	0	0.0	0.00	0.00	0.00	0.00
肾	C64	5	0.72	1.16	1.01	0.04	0.13	4	0.8	0.96	0.77	0.07	0.07
肾盂	C65	0	0.00	0.00	0.00	0.00	0.00	0	0.0	0.00	0.00	0.00	0.00
输尿管	C66	0	0.00	0.00	0.00	0.00	0.00	0	0.0	0.00	0.00	0.00	0.00
膀胱	C67	14	2.03	3.23	2.49	0.03	0.07	4	0.8	0.96	0.71	0.00	0.15
其他的泌尿器官	C68	0	0.00	0.00	0.00	0.00	0.00	0	0.0	0.00	0.00	0.00	0.00
眼	C69	0	0.00	0.00	0.00	0.00	0.00	0	0.0	0.00	0.00	0.00	0.00
脑、神经系统	C70–C72	19	2.75	4.39	3.55	0.15	0.48	22	4.4	5.27	3.57	0.11	0.43
甲状腺	C73	1	0.14	0.23	0.18	0.02	0.02	5	1.0	1.20	1.01	0.05	0.14
肾上腺	C74	1	0.14	0.23	0.15	0.00	0.00	0	0.0	0.00	0.00	0.00	0.00
其他的内分泌腺	C75	0	0.00	0.00	0.00	0.00	0.00	0	0.0	0.00	0.00	0.00	0.00
霍奇金病	C81	0	0.00	0.00	0.00	0.00	0.00	0	0.0	0.00	0.00	0.00	0.00
非霍奇金淋巴瘤	C82–C85;C96	9	1.30	2.08	1.74	0.06	0.25	3	0.6	0.72	0.57	0.03	0.07
免疫增生性疾病	C88	0	0.00	0.00	0.00	0.00	0.00	0	0.0	0.00	0.00	0.00	0.00
多发性骨髓瘤	C90	1	0.14	0.23	0.23	0.00	0.04	3	0.6	0.72	0.63	0.00	0.14
淋巴样白血病	C91	1	0.14	0.23	0.20	0.00	0.05	0	0.0	0.00	0.00	0.00	0.00
髓样白血病	C92–C94	2	0.29	0.46	0.39	0.00	0.00	2	0.4	0.48	0.36	0.05	0.05
白血病，未特指	C95	5	0.72	1.16	1.11	0.03	0.15	3	0.6	0.72	0.64	0.04	0.08
其他的或未指明部位	O&U	21	3.04	4.85	4.27	0.26	0.39	23	4.6	5.51	4.06	0.29	0.44
骨髓增殖性疾病	MPD	0	0.00	0.00	0.00	0.00	0.00	0	0.0	0.00	0.00	0.00	0.00
骨髓增生异常综合征	MDS	1	0.14	0.23	0.18	0.02	0.02	0	0.0	0.00	0.00	0.00	0.00
合计	ALL	691	100.00	159.64	131.00	4.11	14.74	500	100.0	119.83	85.66	3.33	10.47
C44 以外的部位	ALL but C44	687	99.42	158.71	130.26	4.09	14.63	491	98.2	117.67	84.39	3.31	10.36

表 6-25　2020 年河南省荥阳市恶性肿瘤发病主要指标

部位	ICD-10	男性						女性					
		病例数	构成 (%)	粗率 (1/10^5)	世标率 (1/10^5)	累积率 (%)		病例数	构成 (%)	粗率 (1/10^5)	世标率 (1/10^5)	累积率 (%)	
						0~64	0~74					0~64	0~74
唇	C00	0	0.00	0.00	0.00	0.00	0.00	0	0.00	0.00	0.00	0.00	0.00
舌	C01-C02	1	0.11	0.28	0.17	0.00	0.03	0	0.00	0.00	0.00	0.00	0.00
口	C03-C06	4	0.45	1.12	0.71	0.05	0.13	4	0.45	1.13	0.61	0.02	0.05
唾液腺	C07-C08	1	0.11	0.28	0.17	0.00	0.03	1	0.11	0.28	0.16	0.00	0.03
扁桃体	C09	1	0.11	0.28	0.15	0.00	0.00	0	0.00	0.00	0.00	0.00	0.00
其他的口咽	C10	0	0.00	0.00	0.00	0.00	0.00	0	0.00	0.00	0.00	0.00	0.00
鼻咽	C11	4	0.45	1.12	0.87	0.08	0.08	0	0.00	0.00	0.00	0.00	0.00
喉咽	C12-C13	1	0.11	0.28	0.15	0.00	0.00	0	0.00	0.00	0.00	0.00	0.00
咽，部位不明	C14	2	0.22	0.56	0.33	0.02	0.06	1	0.11	0.28	0.19	0.02	0.02
食管	C15	91	10.19	25.51	15.35	0.49	1.78	68	7.64	19.27	10.62	0.33	1.15
胃	C16	143	16.01	40.08	24.49	0.78	2.89	40	4.49	11.33	6.55	0.18	0.71
小肠	C17	5	0.56	1.40	0.81	0.02	0.09	3	0.34	0.85	0.47	0.02	0.02
结肠	C18	33	3.70	9.25	6.12	0.43	0.72	38	4.27	10.77	6.40	0.30	0.72
直肠	C19-C20	38	4.26	10.65	6.51	0.22	0.60	26	2.92	7.37	4.52	0.26	0.61
肛门	C21	1	0.11	0.28	0.17	0.02	0.02	1	0.11	0.28	0.19	0.02	0.02
肝脏	C22	99	11.09	27.75	18.67	1.24	2.12	34	3.82	9.63	5.81	0.31	0.53
胆囊及其他	C23-C24	16	1.79	4.48	2.65	0.07	0.42	25	2.81	7.08	3.98	0.18	0.51
胰腺	C25	15	1.68	4.20	2.88	0.22	0.32	11	1.24	3.12	1.69	0.10	0.16
鼻、鼻窦及其他	C30-C31	1	0.11	0.28	0.17	0.00	0.04	2	0.22	0.57	0.26	0.00	0.00
喉	C32	7	0.78	1.96	1.30	0.08	0.21	0	0.00	0.00	0.00	0.00	0.00
气管、支气管、肺	C33-C34	200	22.40	56.06	34.92	1.63	4.39	96	10.79	27.20	16.14	0.93	1.80
其他的胸腔器官	C37-C38	2	0.22	0.56	0.30	0.00	0.03	6	0.67	1.70	1.14	0.08	0.11
骨	C40-C41	2	0.22	0.56	0.49	0.05	0.05	8	0.90	2.27	1.33	0.08	0.17
皮肤的黑色素瘤	C43	4	0.45	1.12	0.74	0.04	0.07	1	0.11	0.28	0.19	0.02	0.02
其他的皮肤	C44	5	0.56	1.40	0.84	0.00	0.04	14	1.57	3.97	2.10	0.06	0.21
间皮瘤	C45	0	0.00	0.00	0.00	0.00	0.00	1	0.11	0.28	0.16	0.00	0.03
卡波西肉瘤	C46	0	0.00	0.00	0.00	0.00	0.00	0	0.00	0.00	0.00	0.00	0.00
周围神经、其他结缔组织、软组织	C47;C49	1	0.11	0.28	0.17	0.00	0.03	1	0.11	0.28	0.14	0.00	0.00
乳房	C50	4	0.45	1.12	0.75	0.04	0.12	163	18.31	46.19	31.88	2.49	3.43
外阴	C51	0	0.00	0.00	0.00	0.00	0.00	3	0.34	0.85	0.49	0.02	0.05
阴道	C52	0	0.00	0.00	0.00	0.00	0.00	3	0.34	0.85	0.56	0.04	0.08
子宫颈	C53	0	0.00	0.00	0.00	0.00	0.00	60	6.74	17.00	11.41	0.94	1.20
子宫体	C54	0	0.00	0.00	0.00	0.00	0.00	49	5.51	13.89	8.53	0.61	1.01
子宫，部位不明	C55	0	0.00	0.00	0.00	0.00	0.00	4	0.45	1.13	0.76	0.07	0.09
卵巢	C56	0	0.00	0.00	0.00	0.00	0.00	25	2.81	7.08	5.04	0.34	0.53
女性其他的生殖器	C57	0	0.00	0.00	0.00	0.00	0.00	2	0.22	0.57	0.33	0.02	0.02
胎盘	C58	0	0.00	0.00	0.00	0.00	0.00	0	0.00	0.00	0.00	0.00	0.00
阴茎	C60	4	0.45	1.12	0.85	0.04	0.07	0	0.00	0.00	0.00	0.00	0.00
前列腺	C61	42	4.70	11.77	6.91	0.07	0.80	0	0.00	0.00	0.00	0.00	0.00
睾丸	C62	1	0.11	0.28	0.21	0.02	0.02	0	0.00	0.00	0.00	0.00	0.00
男性其他的生殖器	C63	0	0.00	0.00	0.00	0.00	0.00	0	0.00	0.00	0.00	0.00	0.00
肾	C64	23	2.58	6.45	3.93	0.22	0.47	9	1.01	2.55	2.16	0.12	0.21
肾盂	C65	1	0.11	0.28	0.17	0.02	0.02	1	0.11	0.28	0.16	0.00	0.03
输尿管	C66	2	0.22	0.56	0.32	0.02	0.02	3	0.34	0.85	0.47	0.00	0.05
膀胱	C67	24	2.69	6.73	4.19	0.19	0.57	10	1.12	2.83	1.75	0.14	0.27
其他的泌尿器官	C68	0	0.00	0.00	0.00	0.00	0.00	0	0.00	0.00	0.00	0.00	0.00
眼	C69	1	0.11	0.28	0.43	0.02	0.02	0	0.00	0.00	0.00	0.00	0.00
脑、神经系统	C70-C72	11	1.23	3.08	2.17	0.14	0.25	19	2.13	5.38	3.86	0.26	0.38
甲状腺	C73	45	5.04	12.61	9.18	0.76	0.86	109	12.25	30.89	22.96	1.97	2.17
肾上腺	C74	2	0.22	0.56	0.36	0.02	0.02	0	0.00	0.00	0.00	0.00	0.00
其他的内分泌腺	C75	1	0.11	0.28	0.43	0.02	0.02	0	0.00	0.00	0.00	0.00	0.00
霍奇金病	C81	1	0.11	0.28	0.17	0.00	0.04	0	0.00	0.00	0.00	0.00	0.00
非霍奇金淋巴瘤	C82-C85;C96	20	2.24	5.61	4.57	0.32	0.43	15	1.69	4.25	2.70	0.22	0.32
免疫增生性疾病	C88	0	0.00	0.00	0.00	0.00	0.00	0	0.00	0.00	0.00	0.00	0.00
多发性骨髓瘤	C90	7	0.78	1.96	1.25	0.09	0.17	6	0.67	1.70	1.10	0.05	0.14
淋巴样白血病	C91	4	0.45	1.12	0.94	0.04	0.13	0	0.00	0.00	0.00	0.00	0.00
髓样白血病	C92-C94	6	0.67	1.68	1.07	0.06	0.18	6	0.67	1.70	0.94	0.05	0.11
白血病，未特指	C95	6	0.67	1.68	1.55	0.05	0.14	5	0.56	1.42	1.14	0.04	0.14
其他的或未指明部位	O&U	10	1.12	2.80	1.86	0.06	0.13	17	1.91	4.82	2.97	0.12	0.30
骨髓增殖性疾病	MPD	1	0.11	0.28	0.15	0.00	0.00	0	0.00	0.00	0.00	0.00	0.00
骨髓增生异常综合征	MDS	0	0.00	0.00	0.00	0.00	0.00	0	0.00	0.00	0.00	0.00	0.00
合计	ALL	893	100.00	250.30	160.58	7.64	18.63	890	100.00	252.20	161.85	10.41	17.38
C44 以外的部位	ALL but C44	888	99.44	248.89	159.74	7.64	18.58	876	98.43	248.23	159.76	10.34	17.18

表 6-26　2020 年河南省荥阳市恶性肿瘤死亡主要指标

部位	ICD-10	男性						女性					
		病例数	构成 (%)	粗率 ($1/10^5$)	世标率 ($1/10^5$)	累积率 (%)		病例数	构成 (%)	粗率 ($1/10^5$)	世标率 ($1/10^5$)	累积率 (%)	
						0～64	0～74					0～64	0～74
唇	C00	0	0.00	0.00	0.00	0.00	0.00	0	0.00	0.00	0.00	0.00	0.00
舌	C01–C02	0	0.00	0.00	0.00	0.00	0.00	1	0.30	0.28	0.11	0.00	0.00
口	C03–C06	0	0.00	0.00	0.00	0.00	0.00	1	0.30	0.28	0.14	0.00	0.00
唾液腺	C07–C08	0	0.00	0.00	0.00	0.00	0.00	0	0.00	0.00	0.00	0.00	0.00
扁桃体	C09	0	0.00	0.00	0.00	0.00	0.00	0	0.00	0.00	0.00	0.00	0.00
其他的口咽	C10	0	0.00	0.00	0.00	0.00	0.00	0	0.00	0.00	0.00	0.00	0.00
鼻咽	C11	1	0.19	0.28	0.21	0.02	0.02	0	0.00	0.00	0.00	0.00	0.00
喉咽	C12–C13	1	0.19	0.28	0.13	0.00	0.00	0	0.00	0.00	0.00	0.00	0.00
咽，部位不明	C14	3	0.56	0.84	0.49	0.00	0.07	0	0.00	0.00	0.00	0.00	0.00
食管	C15	78	14.47	21.86	13.18	0.35	1.26	45	13.39	12.75	6.81	0.09	0.66
胃	C16	98	18.18	27.47	16.64	0.47	1.70	22	6.55	6.23	3.31	0.06	0.33
小肠	C17	3	0.56	0.84	0.51	0.00	0.10	0	0.00	0.00	0.00	0.00	0.00
结肠	C18	9	1.67	2.52	1.43	0.04	0.12	17	5.06	4.82	2.58	0.02	0.23
直肠	C19–C20	9	1.67	2.52	1.48	0.08	0.21	14	4.17	3.97	2.22	0.06	0.31
肛门	C21	0	0.00	0.00	0.00	0.00	0.00	0	0.00	0.00	0.00	0.00	0.00
肝脏	C22	88	16.33	24.67	15.94	1.01	1.89	37	11.01	10.48	5.75	0.29	0.56
胆囊及其他	C23–C24	12	2.23	3.36	1.93	0.02	0.16	10	2.98	2.83	1.54	0.07	0.15
胰腺	C25	11	2.04	3.08	2.00	0.10	0.24	9	2.68	2.55	1.39	0.06	0.12
鼻、鼻窦及其他	C30–C31	0	0.00	0.00	0.00	0.00	0.00	3	0.89	0.85	0.53	0.05	0.05
喉	C32	3	0.56	0.84	0.43	0.00	0.03	0	0.00	0.00	0.00	0.00	0.00
气管、支气管、肺	C33–C34	144	26.72	40.36	24.86	0.81	2.93	75	22.32	21.25	11.99	0.44	1.52
其他的胸腔器官	C37–C38	0	0.00	0.00	0.00	0.00	0.00	2	0.60	0.57	0.36	0.02	0.02
骨	C40–C41	3	0.56	0.84	0.82	0.05	0.05	6	1.79	1.70	0.98	0.06	0.13
皮肤的黑色素瘤	C43	1	0.19	0.28	0.17	0.02	0.02	0	0.00	0.00	0.00	0.00	0.00
其他的皮肤	C44	3	0.56	0.84	0.48	0.00	0.00	2	0.60	0.57	0.34	0.02	0.02
间皮瘤	C45	0	0.00	0.00	0.00	0.00	0.00	1	0.30	0.28	0.16	0.00	0.03
卡波西肉瘤	C46	0	0.00	0.00	0.00	0.00	0.00	0	0.00	0.00	0.00	0.00	0.00
周围神经、其他结缔组织、软组织	C47;C49	3	0.56	0.84	0.50	0.00	0.00	1	0.30	0.28	0.11	0.00	0.00
乳房	C50	0	0.00	0.00	0.00	0.00	0.00	23	6.85	6.52	4.10	0.33	0.50
外阴	C51	0	0.00	0.00	0.00	0.00	0.00	0	0.00	0.00	0.00	0.00	0.00
阴道	C52	0	0.00	0.00	0.00	0.00	0.00	0	0.00	0.00	0.00	0.00	0.00
子宫颈	C53	0	0.00	0.00	0.00	0.00	0.00	17	5.06	4.82	3.24	0.26	0.33
子宫体	C54	0	0.00	0.00	0.00	0.00	0.00	1	0.30	0.28	0.15	0.00	0.04
子宫，部位不明	C55	0	0.00	0.00	0.00	0.00	0.00	1	0.30	0.28	0.16	0.00	0.03
卵巢	C56	0	0.00	0.00	0.00	0.00	0.00	12	3.57	3.40	1.97	0.10	0.30
女性其他的生殖器	C57	0	0.00	0.00	0.00	0.00	0.00	2	0.60	0.57	0.36	0.04	0.04
胎盘	C58	0	0.00	0.00	0.00	0.00	0.00	0	0.00	0.00	0.00	0.00	0.00
阴茎	C60	0	0.00	0.00	0.00	0.00	0.00	0	0.00	0.00	0.00	0.00	0.00
前列腺	C61	20	3.71	5.61	3.38	0.05	0.31	0	0.00	0.00	0.00	0.00	0.00
睾丸	C62	0	0.00	0.00	0.00	0.00	0.00	0	0.00	0.00	0.00	0.00	0.00
男性其他的生殖器	C63	0	0.00	0.00	0.00	0.00	0.00	0	0.00	0.00	0.00	0.00	0.00
肾	C64	5	0.93	1.40	1.14	0.05	0.14	1	0.30	0.28	0.14	0.00	0.00
肾盂	C65	0	0.00	0.00	0.00	0.00	0.00	0	0.00	0.00	0.00	0.00	0.00
输尿管	C66	1	0.19	0.28	0.15	0.00	0.00	0	0.00	0.00	0.00	0.00	0.00
膀胱	C67	6	1.11	1.68	1.09	0.00	0.00	2	0.60	0.57	0.31	0.00	0.03
其他的泌尿器官	C68	0	0.00	0.00	0.00	0.00	0.00	0	0.00	0.00	0.00	0.00	0.00
眼	C69	1	0.19	0.28	0.21	0.00	0.00	0	0.00	0.00	0.00	0.00	0.00
脑、神经系统	C70–C72	2	0.37	0.56	0.60	0.04	0.04	11	3.27	3.12	1.95	0.14	0.24
甲状腺	C73	2	0.37	0.56	0.34	0.00	0.07	0	0.00	0.00	0.00	0.00	0.00
肾上腺	C74	1	0.19	0.28	0.21	0.02	0.02	0	0.00	0.00	0.00	0.00	0.00
其他的内分泌腺	C75	0	0.00	0.00	0.00	0.00	0.00	0	0.00	0.00	0.00	0.00	0.00
霍奇金病	C81	0	0.00	0.00	0.00	0.00	0.00	0	0.00	0.00	0.00	0.00	0.00
非霍奇金淋巴瘤	C82–C85;C96	9	1.67	2.52	2.31	0.13	0.24	8	2.38	2.27	1.22	0.00	0.12
免疫增生性疾病	C88	0	0.00	0.00	0.00	0.00	0.00	0	0.00	0.00	0.00	0.00	0.00
多发性骨髓瘤	C90	3	0.56	0.84	0.53	0.02	0.09	2	0.60	0.57	0.32	0.02	0.06
淋巴样白血病	C91	1	0.19	0.28	0.19	0.02	0.02	1	0.30	0.28	0.31	0.03	0.03
髓样白血病	C92–C94	4	0.74	1.12	0.94	0.04	0.08	2	0.60	0.57	0.43	0.03	0.03
白血病，未特指	C95	6	1.11	1.68	1.03	0.02	0.07	4	1.19	1.13	0.66	0.02	0.08
其他的或未指明部位	O&U	8	1.48	2.24	1.73	0.12	0.19	3	0.89	0.85	0.48	0.00	0.09
骨髓增殖性疾病	MPD	0	0.00	0.00	0.00	0.00	0.00	0	0.00	0.00	0.00	0.00	0.00
骨髓增生异常综合征	MDS	0	0.00	0.00	0.00	0.00	0.00	0	0.00	0.00	0.00	0.00	0.00
合计	ALL	539	100.00	151.07	95.05	3.48	10.06	336	100.00	95.21	54.13	2.21	6.05
C44 以外的部位	ALL but C44	536	99.44	150.23	94.57	3.48	10.06	334	99.40	94.65	53.80	2.18	6.02

表 6-27　2020 年河南省登封市恶性肿瘤发病主要指标

部位	ICD-10	男性						女性					
		病例数	构成 (%)	粗率 (1/10^5)	世标率 (1/10^5)	累积率 (%) 0~64	累积率 (%) 0~74	病例数	构成 (%)	粗率 (1/10^5)	世标率 (1/10^5)	累积率 (%) 0~64	累积率 (%) 0~74
唇	C00	4	0.48	1.03	0.91	0.03	0.18	1	0.12	0.28	0.28	0.00	0.00
舌	C01–C02	3	0.36	0.77	0.69	0.06	0.06	0	0.00	0.00	0.00	0.00	0.00
口	C03–C06	1	0.12	0.26	0.25	0.00	0.06	2	0.23	0.57	0.51	0.05	0.05
唾液腺	C07–C08	2	0.24	0.51	0.40	0.03	0.03	0	0.00	0.00	0.00	0.00	0.00
扁桃体	C09	0	0.00	0.00	0.00	0.00	0.00	0	0.00	0.00	0.00	0.00	0.00
其他的口咽	C10	0	0.00	0.00	0.00	0.00	0.00	0	0.00	0.00	0.00	0.00	0.00
鼻咽	C11	3	0.36	0.77	0.58	0.05	0.05	2	0.23	0.57	0.50	0.06	0.06
喉咽	C12–C13	1	0.12	0.26	0.20	0.02	0.02	0	0.00	0.00	0.00	0.00	0.00
咽，部位不明	C14	0	0.00	0.00	0.00	0.00	0.00	0	0.00	0.00	0.00	0.00	0.00
食管	C15	76	9.11	19.48	15.03	0.48	2.30	39	4.56	11.07	7.52	0.18	0.81
胃	C16	91	10.91	23.33	17.92	0.58	2.41	35	4.09	9.94	7.53	0.35	0.69
小肠	C17	3	0.36	0.77	0.61	0.05	0.08	7	0.82	1.99	1.47	0.10	0.18
结肠	C18	27	3.24	6.92	5.43	0.26	0.56	23	2.69	6.53	4.27	0.19	0.40
直肠	C19–C20	37	4.44	9.48	7.31	0.23	0.99	23	2.69	6.53	4.84	0.34	0.59
肛门	C21	0	0.00	0.00	0.00	0.00	0.00	2	0.23	0.57	0.36	0.02	0.02
肝脏	C22	86	10.31	22.04	17.09	1.23	1.92	36	4.21	10.22	7.27	0.35	0.79
胆囊及其他	C23–C24	22	2.64	5.64	3.92	0.16	0.48	24	2.81	6.81	4.94	0.27	0.55
胰腺	C25	17	2.04	4.36	2.97	0.11	0.38	14	1.64	3.97	2.63	0.10	0.22
鼻、鼻窦及其他	C30–C31	3	0.36	0.77	0.64	0.03	0.09	2	0.23	0.57	0.44	0.05	0.05
喉	C32	2	0.24	0.51	0.49	0.03	0.03	0	0.00	0.00	0.00	0.00	0.00
气管、支气管、肺	C33–C34	198	23.74	50.75	40.12	1.80	5.65	85	9.94	24.13	17.22	0.86	2.20
其他的胸腔器官	C37–C38	4	0.48	1.03	0.91	0.07	0.13	3	0.35	0.85	0.57	0.05	0.05
骨	C40–C41	5	0.60	1.28	1.06	0.07	0.10	2	0.23	0.57	0.42	0.02	0.07
皮肤的黑色素瘤	C43	2	0.24	0.51	0.36	0.04	0.04	1	0.12	0.28	0.22	0.03	0.03
其他的皮肤	C44	8	0.96	2.05	1.57	0.08	0.08	4	0.47	1.14	0.90	0.04	0.07
间皮瘤	C45	0	0.00	0.00	0.00	0.00	0.00	0	0.00	0.00	0.00	0.00	0.00
卡波西肉瘤	C46	0	0.00	0.00	0.00	0.00	0.00	0	0.00	0.00	0.00	0.00	0.00
周围神经、其他结缔组织、软组织	C47;C49	5	0.60	1.28	1.02	0.06	0.06	5	0.58	1.42	1.23	0.07	0.11
乳房	C50	0	0.00	0.00	0.00	0.00	0.00	137	16.02	38.89	31.09	2.63	3.47
外阴	C51	0	0.00	0.00	0.00	0.00	0.00	1	0.12	0.28	0.19	0.00	0.03
阴道	C52	0	0.00	0.00	0.00	0.00	0.00	0	0.00	0.00	0.00	0.00	0.00
子宫颈	C53	0	0.00	0.00	0.00	0.00	0.00	94	10.99	26.69	21.30	1.83	2.23
子宫体	C54	0	0.00	0.00	0.00	0.00	0.00	36	4.21	10.22	8.19	0.62	0.90
子宫，部位不明	C55	0	0.00	0.00	0.00	0.00	0.00	3	0.35	0.85	0.58	0.05	0.05
卵巢	C56	0	0.00	0.00	0.00	0.00	0.00	40	4.68	11.36	9.29	0.64	0.95
女性其他的生殖器	C57	0	0.00	0.00	0.00	0.00	0.00	1	0.12	0.28	0.29	0.04	0.04
胎盘	C58	0	0.00	0.00	0.00	0.00	0.00	0	0.00	0.00	0.00	0.00	0.00
阴茎	C60	4	0.48	1.03	0.82	0.06	0.09	0	0.00	0.00	0.00	0.00	0.00
前列腺	C61	41	4.92	10.51	7.88	0.17	0.75	0	0.00	0.00	0.00	0.00	0.00
睾丸	C62	1	0.12	0.26	0.21	0.02	0.02	0	0.00	0.00	0.00	0.00	0.00
男性其他的生殖器	C63	0	0.00	0.00	0.00	0.00	0.00	0	0.00	0.00	0.00	0.00	0.00
肾	C64	17	2.04	4.36	3.62	0.24	0.36	7	0.82	1.99	1.57	0.12	0.20
肾盂	C65	2	0.24	0.51	0.37	0.03	0.03	1	0.12	0.28	0.14	0.00	0.00
输尿管	C66	5	0.60	1.28	0.90	0.08	0.08	2	0.23	0.57	0.48	0.00	0.03
膀胱	C67	34	4.08	8.72	6.36	0.28	0.67	10	1.17	2.84	2.23	0.14	0.25
其他的泌尿器官	C68	0	0.00	0.00	0.00	0.00	0.00	0	0.00	0.00	0.00	0.00	0.00
眼	C69	0	0.00	0.00	0.00	0.00	0.00	0	0.00	0.00	0.00	0.00	0.00
脑、神经系统	C70–C72	26	3.12	6.66	5.94	0.32	0.71	15	1.75	4.26	3.51	0.24	0.38
甲状腺	C73	38	4.56	9.74	8.16	0.76	0.83	147	17.19	41.73	34.86	3.23	3.51
肾上腺	C74	0	0.00	0.00	0.00	0.00	0.00	0	0.00	0.00	0.00	0.00	0.00
其他的内分泌腺	C75	0	0.00	0.00	0.00	0.00	0.00	1	0.12	0.28	0.21	0.02	0.02
霍奇金病	C81	2	0.24	0.51	0.52	0.02	0.05	2	0.23	0.57	0.42	0.02	0.05
非霍奇金淋巴瘤	C82–C85;C96	17	2.04	4.36	3.63	0.31	0.31	15	1.75	4.26	3.34	0.26	0.37
免疫增生性疾病	C88	0	0.00	0.00	0.00	0.00	0.00	0	0.00	0.00	0.00	0.00	0.00
多发性骨髓瘤	C90	7	0.84	1.79	1.42	0.07	0.22	3	0.35	0.85	0.78	0.09	0.09
淋巴样白血病	C91	2	0.24	0.51	0.52	0.02	0.05	1	0.12	0.28	0.19	0.00	0.03
髓样白血病	C92–C94	9	1.08	2.31	1.99	0.14	0.23	6	0.70	1.70	2.12	0.14	0.14
白血病，未特指	C95	7	0.84	1.79	1.33	0.07	0.10	8	0.94	2.27	2.15	0.08	0.19
其他的或未指明部位	O&U	14	1.68	3.59	2.64	0.16	0.25	11	1.29	3.12	2.13	0.12	0.20
骨髓增殖性疾病	MPD	8	0.96	2.05	1.64	0.12	0.15	4	0.47	1.14	1.00	0.13	0.13
骨髓增生异常综合征	MDS	0	0.00	0.00	0.00	0.00	0.00	0	0.00	0.00	0.00	0.00	0.00
合计	ALL	834	100.00	213.78	167.45	8.34	20.60	855	100.00	242.74	189.19	13.50	20.18
C44 以外的部位	ALL but C44	826	99.04	211.73	165.88	8.26	20.51	851	99.53	241.60	188.29	13.46	20.11

表 6-28　2020 年河南省登封市恶性肿瘤死亡主要指标

部位	ICD-10	男性						女性					
		病例数	构成(%)	粗率(1/10^5)	世标率(1/10^5)	累积率(%)		病例数	构成(%)	粗率(1/10^5)	世标率(1/10^5)	累积率(%)	
						0~64	0~74					0~64	0~74
唇	C00	1	0.17	0.26	0.25	0.00	0.06	0	0.00	0.00	0.00	0.00	0.00
舌	C01-C02	1	0.17	0.26	0.17	0.00	0.03	0	0.00	0.00	0.00	0.00	0.00
口	C03-C06	0	0.00	0.00	0.00	0.00	0.00	0	0.00	0.00	0.00	0.00	0.00
唾液腺	C07-C08	2	0.33	0.51	0.35	0.02	0.05	0	0.00	0.00	0.00	0.00	0.00
扁桃体	C09	0	0.00	0.00	0.00	0.00	0.00	0	0.00	0.00	0.00	0.00	0.00
其他的口咽	C10	0	0.00	0.00	0.00	0.00	0.00	0	0.00	0.00	0.00	0.00	0.00
鼻咽	C11	2	0.33	0.51	0.34	0.04	0.04	1	0.28	0.28	0.19	0.00	0.03
喉咽	C12-C13	0	0.00	0.00	0.00	0.00	0.00	0	0.00	0.00	0.00	0.00	0.00
咽，部位不明	C14	2	0.33	0.51	0.37	0.00	0.06	2	0.56	0.57	0.28	0.00	0.00
食管	C15	68	11.37	17.43	13.47	0.47	1.77	33	9.17	9.37	6.26	0.15	0.63
胃	C16	87	14.55	22.30	16.80	0.44	1.74	32	8.89	9.08	6.99	0.15	0.43
小肠	C17	2	0.33	0.51	0.29	0.00	0.03	2	0.56	0.57	0.36	0.03	0.03
结肠	C18	16	2.68	4.10	2.99	0.11	0.20	11	3.06	3.12	2.41	0.08	0.14
直肠	C19-C20	13	2.17	3.33	2.36	0.15	0.18	16	4.44	4.54	3.84	0.15	0.21
肛门	C21	0	0.00	0.00	0.00	0.00	0.00	0	0.00	0.00	0.00	0.00	0.00
肝脏	C22	84	14.05	21.53	16.60	1.10	1.91	29	8.06	8.23	5.88	0.21	0.63
胆囊及其他	C23-C24	20	3.34	5.13	3.84	0.09	0.48	20	5.56	5.68	4.20	0.16	0.33
胰腺	C25	14	2.34	3.59	2.73	0.19	0.37	13	3.61	3.69	2.69	0.10	0.19
鼻、鼻窦及其他	C30-C31	0	0.00	0.00	0.00	0.00	0.00	1	0.28	0.28	0.40	0.03	0.03
喉	C32	2	0.33	0.51	0.36	0.00	0.00	1	0.28	0.28	0.18	0.00	0.04
气管、支气管、肺	C33-C34	175	29.26	44.86	34.08	1.24	4.34	69	19.17	19.59	14.02	0.53	1.51
其他的胸腔器官	C37-C38	0	0.00	0.00	0.00	0.00	0.00	1	0.28	0.28	0.22	0.03	0.03
骨	C40-C41	4	0.67	1.03	0.61	0.02	0.04	0	0.00	0.00	0.00	0.00	0.00
皮肤的黑色素瘤	C43	0	0.00	0.00	0.00	0.00	0.00	1	0.28	0.28	0.22	0.03	0.03
其他的皮肤	C44	6	1.00	1.54	1.22	0.06	0.06	5	1.39	1.42	1.18	0.00	0.03
间皮瘤	C45	0	0.00	0.00	0.00	0.00	0.00	0	0.00	0.00	0.00	0.00	0.00
卡波西肉瘤	C46	0	0.00	0.00	0.00	0.00	0.00	0	0.00	0.00	0.00	0.00	0.00
周围神经、其他结缔组织、软组织	C47;C49	2	0.33	0.51	0.37	0.03	0.03	1	0.28	0.28	0.28	0.00	0.00
乳房	C50	1	0.17	0.26	0.24	0.00	0.00	19	5.28	5.39	4.07	0.32	0.54
外阴	C51	0	0.00	0.00	0.00	0.00	0.00	0	0.00	0.00	0.00	0.00	0.00
阴道	C52	0	0.00	0.00	0.00	0.00	0.00	0	0.00	0.00	0.00	0.00	0.00
子宫颈	C53	0	0.00	0.00	0.00	0.00	0.00	26	7.22	7.38	5.79	0.47	0.66
子宫体	C54	0	0.00	0.00	0.00	0.00	0.00	6	1.67	1.70	1.32	0.10	0.15
子宫，部位不明	C55	0	0.00	0.00	0.00	0.00	0.00	1	0.28	0.28	0.19	0.00	0.03
卵巢	C56	0	0.00	0.00	0.00	0.00	0.00	17	4.72	4.83	4.08	0.23	0.42
女性其他的生殖器	C57	0	0.00	0.00	0.00	0.00	0.00	1	0.28	0.28	0.22	0.03	0.03
胎盘	C58	0	0.00	0.00	0.00	0.00	0.00	0	0.00	0.00	0.00	0.00	0.00
阴茎	C60	0	0.00	0.00	0.00	0.00	0.00	0	0.00	0.00	0.00	0.00	0.00
前列腺	C61	13	2.17	3.33	2.57	0.02	0.17	0	0.00	0.00	0.00	0.00	0.00
睾丸	C62	0	0.00	0.00	0.00	0.00	0.00	0	0.00	0.00	0.00	0.00	0.00
男性其他的生殖器	C63	0	0.00	0.00	0.00	0.00	0.00	0	0.00	0.00	0.00	0.00	0.00
肾	C64	5	0.84	1.28	0.97	0.04	0.13	1	0.28	0.28	0.19	0.00	0.03
肾盂	C65	0	0.00	0.00	0.00	0.00	0.00	1	0.28	0.28	0.14	0.00	0.00
输尿管	C66	2	0.33	0.51	0.35	0.02	0.05	1	0.28	0.28	0.14	0.00	0.00
膀胱	C67	13	2.17	3.33	2.70	0.02	0.32	7	1.94	1.99	1.36	0.00	0.08
其他的泌尿器官	C68	0	0.00	0.00	0.00	0.00	0.00	0	0.00	0.00	0.00	0.00	0.00
眼	C69	0	0.00	0.00	0.00	0.00	0.00	0	0.00	0.00	0.00	0.00	0.00
脑、神经系统	C70-C72	20	3.34	5.13	4.26	0.29	0.53	12	3.33	3.41	2.66	0.15	0.32
甲状腺	C73	2	0.33	0.51	0.50	0.03	0.09	3	0.83	0.85	0.51	0.00	0.08
肾上腺	C74	0	0.00	0.00	0.00	0.00	0.00	1	0.28	0.28	0.29	0.04	0.04
其他的内分泌腺	C75	0	0.00	0.00	0.00	0.00	0.00	0	0.00	0.00	0.00	0.00	0.00
霍奇金病	C81	1	0.17	0.26	0.12	0.00	0.00	0	0.00	0.00	0.00	0.00	0.00
非霍奇金淋巴瘤	C82-C85;C96	12	2.01	3.08	2.39	0.16	0.19	6	1.67	1.70	1.36	0.07	0.14
免疫增生性疾病	C88	0	0.00	0.00	0.00	0.00	0.00	0	0.00	0.00	0.00	0.00	0.00
多发性骨髓瘤	C90	3	0.50	0.77	0.62	0.03	0.09	1	0.28	0.28	0.18	0.00	0.04
淋巴样白血病	C91	1	0.17	0.26	0.25	0.00	0.06	1	0.28	0.28	0.22	0.03	0.03
髓样白血病	C92-C94	1	0.17	0.26	0.21	0.02	0.02	0	0.00	0.00	0.00	0.00	0.00
白血病，未特指	C95	4	0.67	1.03	0.76	0.06	0.06	6	1.67	1.70	1.52	0.06	0.13
其他的或未指明部位	O&U	12	2.01	3.08	2.42	0.12	0.27	11	3.06	3.12	2.03	0.05	0.09
骨髓增殖性疾病	MPD	2	0.33	0.51	0.37	0.03	0.03	0	0.00	0.00	0.00	0.00	0.00
骨髓增生异常综合征	MDS	5	0.84	1.28	0.84	0.07	0.07	1	0.28	0.28	0.18	0.00	0.04
合计	ALL	598	100.00	153.28	116.77	4.88	13.48	360	100.00	102.21	76.04	3.17	7.14
C44 以外的部位	ALL but C44	592	99.00	151.75	115.55	4.81	13.42	355	98.61	100.79	74.86	3.17	7.11

表 6-29　2020 年河南省开封市祥符区恶性肿瘤发病主要指标

部位	ICD-10	男性						女性					
		病例数	构成 (%)	粗率 ($1/10^5$)	世标率 ($1/10^5$)	累积率 (%) 0~64	累积率 (%) 0~74	病例数	构成 (%)	粗率 ($1/10^5$)	世标率 ($1/10^5$)	累积率 (%) 0~64	累积率 (%) 0~74
唇	C00	3	0.36	0.88	0.75	0.02	0.08	2	0.22	0.61	0.50	0.03	0.03
舌	C01–C02	3	0.36	0.88	1.02	0.05	0.13	0	0.00	0.00	0.00	0.00	0.00
口	C03–C06	3	0.36	0.88	0.76	0.06	0.11	2	0.22	0.61	0.54	0.06	0.06
唾液腺	C07–C08	1	0.12	0.29	0.18	0.02	0.02	1	0.11	0.30	0.26	0.02	0.02
扁桃体	C09	0	0.00	0.00	0.00	0.00	0.00	0	0.00	0.00	0.00	0.00	0.00
其他的口咽	C10	0	0.00	0.00	0.00	0.00	0.00	0	0.00	0.00	0.00	0.00	0.00
鼻咽	C11	6	0.73	1.76	1.76	0.10	0.15	1	0.11	0.30	0.32	0.00	0.05
喉咽	C12–C13	2	0.24	0.59	0.54	0.06	0.06	0	0.00	0.00	0.00	0.00	0.00
咽，部位不明	C14	2	0.24	0.59	0.45	0.05	0.05	0	0.00	0.00	0.00	0.00	0.00
食管	C15	31	3.76	9.11	8.43	0.18	1.20	21	2.34	6.36	4.71	0.12	0.58
胃	C16	53	6.43	15.58	14.03	0.47	1.81	25	2.78	7.57	6.53	0.41	0.84
小肠	C17	5	0.61	1.47	1.22	0.08	0.08	7	0.78	2.12	1.44	0.08	0.16
结肠	C18	28	3.40	8.23	7.23	0.38	0.65	32	3.56	9.70	7.97	0.47	1.05
直肠	C19–C20	42	5.10	12.34	10.98	0.60	1.43	30	3.34	9.09	7.31	0.46	0.80
肛门	C21	1	0.12	0.29	0.32	0.00	0.08	0	0.00	0.00	0.00	0.00	0.00
肝脏	C22	142	17.23	41.73	37.13	2.26	4.55	49	5.45	14.85	11.55	0.54	1.49
胆囊及其他	C23–C24	18	2.18	5.29	4.92	0.07	0.71	22	2.45	6.67	5.18	0.13	0.70
胰腺	C25	24	2.91	7.05	6.48	0.22	0.97	15	1.67	4.54	3.34	0.18	0.36
鼻、鼻窦及其他	C30–C31	0	0.00	0.00	0.00	0.00	0.00	2	0.22	0.61	0.47	0.00	0.05
喉	C32	11	1.33	3.23	3.10	0.07	0.47	2	0.22	0.61	0.53	0.05	0.05
气管、支气管、肺	C33–C34	231	28.03	67.89	61.59	2.12	8.26	132	14.68	39.99	28.94	1.37	3.59
其他的胸腔器官	C37–C38	4	0.49	1.18	1.08	0.07	0.15	1	0.11	0.30	0.26	0.03	0.03
骨	C40–C41	5	0.61	1.47	1.42	0.10	0.15	2	0.22	0.61	0.49	0.02	0.07
皮肤的黑色素瘤	C43	4	0.49	1.18	1.14	0.02	0.21	3	0.33	0.91	0.90	0.00	0.20
其他的皮肤	C44	12	1.46	3.53	3.17	0.05	0.29	16	1.78	4.85	3.58	0.12	0.46
间皮瘤	C45	0	0.00	0.00	0.00	0.00	0.00	1	0.11	0.30	0.16	0.00	0.00
卡波西肉瘤	C46	1	0.12	0.29	0.35	0.02	0.02	0	0.00	0.00	0.00	0.00	0.00
周围神经、其他结缔组织、软组织	C47;C49	5	0.61	1.47	1.39	0.11	0.17	4	0.44	1.21	1.04	0.04	0.19
乳房	C50	0	0.00	0.00	0.00	0.00	0.00	125	13.90	37.87	31.73	2.53	3.50
外阴	C51	0	0.00	0.00	0.00	0.00	0.00	1	0.11	0.30	0.26	0.03	0.03
阴道	C52	0	0.00	0.00	0.00	0.00	0.00	4	0.44	1.21	0.87	0.04	0.11
子宫颈	C53	0	0.00	0.00	0.00	0.00	0.00	77	8.57	23.33	20.21	1.65	2.10
子宫体	C54	0	0.00	0.00	0.00	0.00	0.00	32	3.56	9.70	7.36	0.54	0.96
子宫，部位不明	C55	0	0.00	0.00	0.00	0.00	0.00	6	0.67	1.82	1.55	0.04	0.22
卵巢	C56	0	0.00	0.00	0.00	0.00	0.00	35	3.89	10.60	8.52	0.64	0.97
女性其他的生殖器	C57	0	0.00	0.00	0.00	0.00	0.00	2	0.22	0.61	0.57	0.02	0.10
胎盘	C58	0	0.00	0.00	0.00	0.00	0.00	1	0.11	0.30	0.22	0.01	0.01
阴茎	C60	3	0.36	0.88	0.79	0.03	0.08	0	0.00	0.00	0.00	0.00	0.00
前列腺	C61	23	2.79	6.76	5.94	0.00	0.67	0	0.00	0.00	0.00	0.00	0.00
睾丸	C62	1	0.12	0.29	0.35	0.03	0.03	0	0.00	0.00	0.00	0.00	0.00
男性其他的生殖器	C63	1	0.12	0.29	0.26	0.03	0.03	0	0.00	0.00	0.00	0.00	0.00
肾	C64	16	1.94	4.70	4.40	0.33	0.55	10	1.11	3.03	3.21	0.07	0.48
肾盂	C65	1	0.12	0.29	0.32	0.00	0.05	2	0.22	0.61	0.47	0.02	0.10
输尿管	C66	0	0.00	0.00	0.00	0.00	0.00	1	0.11	0.30	0.32	0.00	0.05
膀胱	C67	23	2.79	6.76	6.36	0.17	0.83	8	0.89	2.42	2.07	0.15	0.28
其他的泌尿器官	C68	0	0.00	0.00	0.00	0.00	0.00	0	0.00	0.00	0.00	0.00	0.00
眼	C69	2	0.24	0.59	0.67	0.03	0.03	4	0.44	1.21	1.05	0.08	0.13
脑、神经系统	C70–C72	19	2.31	5.58	5.65	0.33	0.71	12	1.33	3.64	3.28	0.20	0.38
甲状腺	C73	33	4.00	9.70	9.23	0.72	0.96	137	15.24	41.51	36.87	2.86	3.82
肾上腺	C74	0	0.00	0.00	0.00	0.00	0.00	0	0.00	0.00	0.00	0.00	0.00
其他的内分泌腺	C75	0	0.00	0.00	0.00	0.00	0.00	0	0.00	0.00	0.00	0.00	0.00
霍奇金病	C81	0	0.00	0.00	0.00	0.00	0.00	1	0.11	0.30	0.26	0.03	0.03
非霍奇金淋巴瘤	C82–C85;C96	18	2.18	5.29	4.30	0.27	0.48	20	2.22	6.06	4.92	0.32	0.52
免疫增生性疾病	C88	0	0.00	0.00	0.00	0.00	0.00	1	0.11	0.30	0.18	0.02	0.02
多发性骨髓瘤	C90	10	1.21	2.94	2.73	0.11	0.29	8	0.89	2.42	2.04	0.14	0.34
淋巴样白血病	C91	3	0.36	0.88	0.99	0.03	0.11	5	0.56	1.51	1.96	0.07	0.19
髓样白血病	C92–C94	14	1.70	4.11	4.00	0.22	0.46	15	1.67	4.54	4.41	0.27	0.39
白血病，未特指	C95	4	0.49	1.18	1.15	0.05	0.13	2	0.22	0.61	0.27	0.00	0.00
其他的或未指明部位	O&U	15	1.82	4.41	3.60	0.13	0.48	14	1.56	4.24	3.11	0.26	0.26
骨髓增殖性疾病	MPD	1	0.12	0.29	0.32	0.00	0.05	3	0.33	0.91	0.53	0.03	0.03
骨髓增生异常综合征	MDS	0	0.00	0.00	0.00	0.00	0.00	3	0.33	0.91	0.64	0.03	0.03
合计	ALL	824	100.00	242.18	220.49	9.67	27.74	899	100.00	272.38	222.87	14.19	25.84
C44 以外的部位	ALL but C44	812	98.54	238.65	217.32	9.61	27.44	883	98.22	267.53	219.29	14.07	25.38

表 6-30 2020 年河南省开封市祥符区恶性肿瘤死亡主要指标

部位	ICD-10	男性						女性					
		病例数	构成 (%)	粗率 (1/10^5)	世标率 (1/10^5)	累积率 (%)		病例数	构成 (%)	粗率 (1/10^5)	世标率 (1/10^5)	累积率 (%)	
						0~64	0~74					0~64	0~74
唇	C00	0	0.00	0.00	0.00	0.00	0.00	0	0.00	0.00	0.00	0.00	0.00
舌	C01-C02	0	0.00	0.00	0.00	0.00	0.00	0	0.00	0.00	0.00	0.00	0.00
口	C03-C06	3	0.51	0.88	0.76	0.06	0.11	1	0.25	0.30	0.11	0.00	0.00
唾液腺	C07-C08	0	0.00	0.00	0.00	0.00	0.00	0	0.00	0.00	0.00	0.00	0.00
扁桃体	C09	0	0.00	0.00	0.00	0.00	0.00	0	0.00	0.00	0.00	0.00	0.00
其他的口咽	C10	1	0.17	0.29	0.16	0.00	0.00	0	0.00	0.00	0.00	0.00	0.00
鼻咽	C11	1	0.17	0.29	0.26	0.03	0.03	1	0.25	0.30	0.26	0.03	0.03
喉咽	C12-C13	0	0.00	0.00	0.00	0.00	0.00	1	0.25	0.30	0.29	0.00	0.07
咽，部位不明	C14	1	0.17	0.29	0.18	0.02	0.02	0	0.00	0.00	0.00	0.00	0.00
食管	C15	39	6.61	11.46	9.78	0.08	1.18	28	7.02	8.48	5.81	0.02	0.80
胃	C16	45	7.63	13.23	11.90	0.30	1.45	25	6.27	7.57	5.23	0.23	0.53
小肠	C17	13	2.20	3.82	3.48	0.12	0.25	6	1.50	1.82	1.39	0.11	0.16
结肠	C18	8	1.36	2.35	2.27	0.12	0.20	11	2.76	3.33	2.51	0.08	0.31
直肠	C19-C20	15	2.54	4.41	3.85	0.11	0.59	19	4.76	5.76	4.33	0.19	0.42
肛门	C21	1	0.17	0.29	0.32	0.00	0.05	1	0.25	0.30	0.15	0.00	0.00
肝脏	C22	103	17.46	30.27	28.19	1.42	3.99	44	11.03	13.33	10.58	0.37	1.47
胆囊及其他	C23-C24	28	4.75	8.23	7.44	0.20	0.97	21	5.26	6.36	5.20	0.08	0.78
胰腺	C25	17	2.88	5.00	4.82	0.09	0.84	14	3.51	4.24	3.11	0.06	0.39
鼻、鼻窦及其他	C30-C31	0	0.00	0.00	0.00	0.00	0.00	0	0.00	0.00	0.00	0.00	0.00
喉	C32	5	0.85	1.47	1.22	0.02	0.16	1	0.25	0.30	0.26	0.03	0.03
气管、支气管、肺	C33-C34	191	32.37	56.14	49.71	1.23	6.52	92	23.06	27.87	19.95	0.76	2.41
其他的胸腔器官	C37-C38	0	0.00	0.00	0.00	0.00	0.00	2	0.50	0.61	0.33	0.02	0.02
骨	C40-C41	1	0.17	0.29	0.23	0.01	0.01	2	0.50	0.61	0.44	0.05	0.05
皮肤的黑色素瘤	C43	2	0.34	0.59	0.34	0.02	0.02	2	0.50	0.61	0.59	0.00	0.15
其他的皮肤	C44	8	1.36	2.35	2.12	0.02	0.21	5	1.25	1.51	0.69	0.00	0.00
间皮瘤	C45	0	0.00	0.00	0.00	0.00	0.00	0	0.00	0.00	0.00	0.00	0.00
卡波西肉瘤	C46	0	0.00	0.00	0.00	0.00	0.00	0	0.00	0.00	0.00	0.00	0.00
周围神经、其他结缔组织、软组织	C47;C49	1	0.17	0.29	0.26	0.03	0.03	2	0.50	0.61	0.56	0.05	0.05
乳房	C50	1	0.17	0.29	0.31	0.00	0.00	26	6.52	7.88	6.05	0.37	0.78
外阴	C51	0	0.00	0.00	0.00	0.00	0.00	0	0.00	0.00	0.00	0.00	0.00
阴道	C52	0	0.00	0.00	0.00	0.00	0.00	0	0.00	0.00	0.00	0.00	0.00
子宫颈	C53	0	0.00	0.00	0.00	0.00	0.00	13	3.26	3.94	2.98	0.19	0.36
子宫体	C54	0	0.00	0.00	0.00	0.00	0.00	3	0.75	0.91	0.65	0.02	0.07
子宫，部位不明	C55	0	0.00	0.00	0.00	0.00	0.00	2	0.50	0.61	0.42	0.03	0.03
卵巢	C56	0	0.00	0.00	0.00	0.00	0.00	10	2.51	3.03	2.08	0.13	0.18
女性其他的生殖器	C57	0	0.00	0.00	0.00	0.00	0.00	0	0.00	0.00	0.00	0.00	0.00
胎盘	C58	0	0.00	0.00	0.00	0.00	0.00	0	0.00	0.00	0.00	0.00	0.00
阴茎	C60	2	0.34	0.59	0.64	0.00	0.16	0	0.00	0.00	0.00	0.00	0.00
前列腺	C61	13	2.20	3.82	3.04	0.03	0.14	0	0.00	0.00	0.00	0.00	0.00
睾丸	C62	0	0.00	0.00	0.00	0.00	0.00	0	0.00	0.00	0.00	0.00	0.00
男性其他的生殖器	C63	0	0.00	0.00	0.00	0.00	0.00	0	0.00	0.00	0.00	0.00	0.00
肾	C64	4	0.68	1.18	1.13	0.05	0.16	2	0.50	0.61	0.64	0.03	0.10
肾盂	C65	1	0.17	0.29	0.32	0.00	0.05	2	0.50	0.61	0.61	0.00	0.13
输尿管	C66	1	0.17	0.29	0.32	0.00	0.08	2	0.50	0.61	0.61	0.00	0.13
膀胱	C67	11	1.86	3.23	3.02	0.06	0.19	4	1.00	1.21	0.74	0.00	0.07
其他的泌尿器官	C68	0	0.00	0.00	0.00	0.00	0.00	0	0.00	0.00	0.00	0.00	0.00
眼	C69	0	0.00	0.00	0.00	0.00	0.00	0	0.00	0.00	0.00	0.00	0.00
脑、神经系统	C70-C72	11	1.86	3.23	2.79	0.15	0.37	5	1.25	1.51	1.41	0.08	0.23
甲状腺	C73	4	0.68	1.18	1.03	0.08	0.13	8	2.01	2.42	1.94	0.14	0.26
肾上腺	C74	1	0.17	0.29	0.32	0.02	0.02	0	0.00	0.00	0.00	0.00	0.00
其他的内分泌腺	C75	0	0.00	0.00	0.00	0.00	0.00	0	0.00	0.00	0.00	0.00	0.00
霍奇金病	C81	0	0.00	0.00	0.00	0.00	0.00	0	0.00	0.00	0.00	0.00	0.00
非霍奇金淋巴瘤	C82-C85;C96	16	2.71	4.70	4.07	0.21	0.50	14	3.51	4.24	3.18	0.12	0.47
免疫增生性疾病	C88	0	0.00	0.00	0.00	0.00	0.00	0	0.00	0.00	0.00	0.00	0.00
多发性骨髓瘤	C90	13	2.20	3.82	3.74	0.05	0.56	6	1.50	1.82	1.58	0.06	0.26
淋巴样白血病	C91	3	0.51	0.88	0.88	0.02	0.10	6	1.50	1.82	1.39	0.10	0.10
髓样白血病	C92-C94	10	1.69	2.94	2.60	0.09	0.27	8	2.01	2.42	2.01	0.02	0.27
白血病，未特指	C95	3	0.51	0.88	0.83	0.03	0.11	4	1.00	1.21	1.18	0.05	0.10
其他的或未指明部位	O&U	8	1.36	2.35	1.94	0.08	0.26	4	1.00	1.21	0.78	0.03	0.11
骨髓增殖性疾病	MPD	0	0.00	0.00	0.00	0.00	0.00	1	0.25	0.30	0.11	0.00	0.00
骨髓增生异常综合征	MDS	5	0.85	1.47	1.47	0.00	0.19	1	0.25	0.30	0.26	0.03	0.03
合计	ALL	590	100.00	173.40	155.73	4.76	19.93	399	100.00	120.89	90.40	3.50	11.36
C44 以外的部位	ALL but C44	582	98.64	171.05	153.61	4.74	19.72	394	98.75	119.37	89.70	3.50	11.36

表 6-31　2020 年河南省洛阳市城区恶性肿瘤发病主要指标

部位	ICD-10	男性						女性					
		病例数	构成 (%)	粗率 ($1/10^5$)	世标率 ($1/10^5$)	累积率 (%)		病例数	构成 (%)	粗率 ($1/10^5$)	世标率 ($1/10^5$)	累积率 (%)	
						0～64	0～74					0～64	0～74
唇	C00	0	0.00	0.00	0.00	0.00	0.00	0	0.00	0.00	0.00	0.00	0.00
舌	C01–C02	5	0.17	0.54	0.50	0.04	0.05	3	0.11	0.32	0.14	0.01	0.01
口	C03–C06	15	0.52	1.63	0.89	0.04	0.13	11	0.39	1.19	0.59	0.02	0.10
唾液腺	C07–C08	6	0.21	0.65	0.35	0.02	0.04	6	0.21	0.65	0.52	0.04	0.05
扁桃体	C09	3	0.10	0.33	0.18	0.02	0.03	0	0.00	0.00	0.00	0.00	0.00
其他的口咽	C10	3	0.10	0.33	0.20	0.01	0.03	0	0.00	0.00	0.00	0.00	0.00
鼻咽	C11	12	0.41	1.30	0.83	0.06	0.09	4	0.14	0.43	0.28	0.01	0.04
喉咽	C12–C13	18	0.62	1.96	1.24	0.08	0.14	5	0.18	0.54	0.37	0.04	0.04
咽，部位不明	C14	1	0.03	0.11	0.06	0.00	0.02	2	0.07	0.22	0.06	0.00	0.00
食管	C15	236	8.12	25.65	13.40	0.57	1.66	174	6.23	18.75	8.37	0.19	1.17
胃	C16	337	11.59	36.62	19.57	0.84	2.64	138	4.94	14.87	6.97	0.34	0.72
小肠	C17	17	0.58	1.85	1.05	0.08	0.12	12	0.43	1.29	0.66	0.05	0.06
结肠	C18	160	5.50	17.39	9.11	0.52	1.05	146	5.23	15.74	7.58	0.39	0.92
直肠	C19–C20	151	5.19	16.41	8.59	0.34	1.05	126	4.51	13.58	7.17	0.46	0.82
肛门	C21	4	0.14	0.43	0.28	0.03	0.03	3	0.11	0.32	0.18	0.01	0.01
肝脏	C22	259	8.91	28.14	16.56	1.07	2.00	110	3.94	11.86	5.57	0.31	0.60
胆囊及其他	C23–C24	59	2.03	6.41	3.07	0.07	0.31	71	2.54	7.65	3.48	0.14	0.43
胰腺	C25	63	2.17	6.85	3.93	0.23	0.46	61	2.19	6.57	2.84	0.09	0.32
鼻、鼻窦及其他	C30–C31	5	0.17	0.54	0.20	0.01	0.01	5	0.18	0.54	0.25	0.01	0.03
喉	C32	30	1.03	3.26	1.89	0.12	0.25	2	0.07	0.22	0.09	0.00	0.01
气管、支气管、肺	C33–C34	706	24.28	76.72	41.92	2.13	5.41	350	12.54	37.73	19.40	1.10	2.21
其他的胸腔器官	C37–C38	7	0.24	0.76	0.49	0.03	0.05	4	0.14	0.43	0.26	0.02	0.03
骨	C40–C41	10	0.34	1.09	0.80	0.05	0.09	7	0.25	0.75	0.65	0.04	0.04
皮肤的黑色素瘤	C43	2	0.07	0.22	0.10	0.01	0.01	4	0.14	0.43	0.21	0.01	0.01
其他的皮肤	C44	23	0.79	2.50	1.14	0.03	0.11	31	1.11	3.34	1.58	0.08	0.16
间皮瘤	C45	3	0.10	0.33	0.18	0.01	0.02	1	0.04	0.11	0.08	0.01	0.01
卡波西肉瘤	C46	0	0.00	0.00	0.00	0.00	0.00	0	0.00	0.00	0.00	0.00	0.00
周围神经、其他结缔组织、软组织	C47;C49	10	0.34	1.09	0.69	0.04	0.07	7	0.25	0.75	0.83	0.05	0.06
乳房	C50	6	0.21	0.65	0.38	0.02	0.04	525	18.81	56.59	35.59	2.97	3.86
外阴	C51	0	0.00	0.00	0.00	0.00	0.00	5	0.18	0.54	0.27	0.01	0.03
阴道	C52	0	0.00	0.00	0.00	0.00	0.00	2	0.07	0.22	0.10	0.01	0.01
子宫颈	C53	0	0.00	0.00	0.00	0.00	0.00	147	5.27	15.84	9.96	0.82	1.10
子宫体	C54	0	0.00	0.00	0.00	0.00	0.00	105	3.76	11.32	7.15	0.61	0.81
子宫，部位不明	C55	0	0.00	0.00	0.00	0.00	0.00	4	0.14	0.43	0.27	0.02	0.04
卵巢	C56	0	0.00	0.00	0.00	0.00	0.00	71	2.54	7.65	4.93	0.40	0.52
女性其他的生殖器	C57	0	0.00	0.00	0.00	0.00	0.00	5	0.18	0.54	0.36	0.03	0.04
胎盘	C58	0	0.00	0.00	0.00	0.00	0.00	2	0.07	0.22	0.22	0.02	0.02
阴茎	C60	3	0.10	0.33	0.17	0.01	0.03	0	0.00	0.00	0.00	0.00	0.00
前列腺	C61	179	6.16	19.45	9.24	0.22	1.11	0	0.00	0.00	0.00	0.00	0.00
睾丸	C62	1	0.03	0.11	0.09	0.01	0.01	0	0.00	0.00	0.00	0.00	0.00
男性其他的生殖器	C63	5	0.17	0.54	0.40	0.03	0.03	0	0.00	0.00	0.00	0.00	0.00
肾	C64	76	2.61	8.26	4.84	0.32	0.59	48	1.72	5.17	2.80	0.16	0.32
肾盂	C65	8	0.28	0.87	0.53	0.03	0.07	3	0.11	0.32	0.14	0.01	0.01
输尿管	C66	8	0.28	0.87	0.41	0.02	0.03	9	0.32	0.97	0.44	0.02	0.05
膀胱	C67	106	3.65	11.52	6.05	0.29	0.71	30	1.07	3.23	1.35	0.06	0.15
其他的泌尿器官	C68	2	0.07	0.22	0.11	0.01	0.01	1	0.04	0.11	0.03	0.00	0.00
眼	C69	3	0.10	0.33	0.22	0.01	0.03	2	0.07	0.22	0.12	0.01	0.02
脑、神经系统	C70–C72	51	1.75	5.54	3.57	0.20	0.40	68	2.44	7.33	4.54	0.23	0.47
甲状腺	C73	121	4.16	13.15	9.69	0.82	0.93	304	10.89	32.77	23.87	2.07	2.26
肾上腺	C74	3	0.10	0.33	0.18	0.01	0.03	0	0.00	0.00	0.00	0.00	0.00
其他的内分泌腺	C75	13	0.45	1.41	0.73	0.03	0.07	3	0.11	0.32	0.18	0.02	0.02
霍奇金病	C81	3	0.10	0.33	0.26	0.02	0.02	6	0.21	0.65	0.50	0.04	0.05
非霍奇金淋巴瘤	C82–C85;C96	44	1.51	4.78	2.72	0.22	0.32	39	1.40	4.20	2.96	0.16	0.35
免疫增生性疾病	C88	0	0.00	0.00	0.00	0.00	0.00	0	0.00	0.00	0.00	0.00	0.00
多发性骨髓瘤	C90	19	0.65	2.06	1.23	0.05	0.20	16	0.57	1.72	0.84	0.03	0.10
淋巴样白血病	C91	4	0.14	0.43	0.35	0.01	0.01	5	0.18	0.54	0.26	0.01	0.03
髓样白血病	C92–C94	25	0.86	2.72	1.82	0.10	0.21	13	0.47	1.40	1.18	0.07	0.12
白血病，未特指	C95	25	0.86	2.72	2.45	0.14	0.20	23	0.82	2.48	1.57	0.08	0.14
其他的或未指明部位	O&U	55	1.89	5.98	3.14	0.14	0.39	70	2.51	7.55	3.82	0.21	0.38
骨髓增殖性疾病	MPD	1	0.03	0.11	0.09	0.01	0.01	2	0.07	0.22	0.11	0.01	0.01
骨髓增生异常综合征	MDS	2	0.07	0.22	0.09	0.01	0.01	0	0.00	0.00	0.00	0.00	0.00
合计	ALL	2 908	100.00	316.00	176.01	9.17	21.34	2 791	100.00	300.83	171.67	11.47	18.77
C44 以外的部位	ALL but C44	2 885	99.21	313.50	174.87	9.13	21.23	2 760	98.89	297.49	170.09	11.39	18.61

表 6-32 2020 年河南省洛阳市城区恶性肿瘤死亡主要指标

部位	ICD-10	男性						女性					
		病例数	构成(%)	粗率(1/10⁵)	世标率(1/10⁵)	累积率(%) 0~64	累积率(%) 0~74	病例数	构成(%)	粗率(1/10⁵)	世标率(1/10⁵)	累积率(%) 0~64	累积率(%) 0~74
唇	C00	0	0.00	0.00	0.00	0.00	0.00	0	0.00	0.00	0.00	0.00	0.00
舌	C01–C02	2	0.10	0.22	0.29	0.01	0.02	3	0.23	0.32	0.16	0.01	0.02
口	C03–C06	6	0.30	0.65	0.30	0.00	0.05	8	0.61	0.86	0.31	0.01	0.02
唾液腺	C07–C08	4	0.20	0.43	0.28	0.03	0.04	0	0.00	0.00	0.00	0.00	0.00
扁桃体	C09	1	0.05	0.11	0.07	0.00	0.01	0	0.00	0.00	0.00	0.00	0.00
其他的口咽	C10	2	0.10	0.22	0.09	0.01	0.01	1	0.08	0.11	0.04	0.00	0.00
鼻咽	C11	10	0.49	1.09	0.65	0.05	0.06	1	0.08	0.11	0.03	0.00	0.00
喉咽	C12–C13	6	0.30	0.65	0.31	0.02	0.03	0	0.00	0.00	0.00	0.00	0.00
咽，部位不明	C14	1	0.05	0.11	0.03	0.00	0.00	2	0.15	0.22	0.06	0.00	0.00
食管	C15	221	10.88	24.02	11.46	0.36	1.24	145	11.02	15.63	6.32	0.10	0.66
胃	C16	260	12.80	28.25	13.66	0.43	1.62	107	8.13	11.53	4.67	0.14	0.35
小肠	C17	15	0.74	1.63	0.86	0.06	0.07	8	0.61	0.86	0.32	0.01	0.01
结肠	C18	87	4.28	9.45	4.21	0.09	0.37	63	4.79	6.79	3.14	0.15	0.33
直肠	C19–C20	81	3.99	8.80	4.40	0.21	0.48	57	4.33	6.14	2.72	0.10	0.30
肛门	C21	0	0.00	0.00	0.00	0.00	0.00	0	0.00	0.00	0.00	0.00	0.00
肝脏	C22	245	12.06	26.62	14.87	0.89	1.70	120	9.12	12.93	6.19	0.28	0.62
胆囊及其他	C23–C24	54	2.66	5.87	2.75	0.05	0.34	58	4.41	6.25	2.70	0.09	0.24
胰腺	C25	54	2.66	5.87	3.09	0.19	0.32	54	4.10	5.82	2.38	0.07	0.24
鼻、鼻窦及其他	C30–C31	1	0.05	0.11	0.04	0.00	0.00	0	0.00	0.00	0.00	0.00	0.00
喉	C32	22	1.08	2.39	1.26	0.07	0.13	2	0.15	0.22	0.07	0.00	0.00
气管、支气管、肺	C33–C34	592	29.13	64.33	32.42	1.23	3.92	239	18.16	25.76	11.06	0.40	1.14
其他的胸腔器官	C37–C38	10	0.49	1.09	0.66	0.03	0.07	3	0.23	0.32	0.12	0.01	0.01
骨	C40–C41	9	0.44	0.98	0.59	0.03	0.08	8	0.61	0.86	0.58	0.03	0.04
皮肤的黑色素瘤	C43	2	0.10	0.22	0.07	0.00	0.00	2	0.15	0.22	0.06	0.00	0.00
其他的皮肤	C44	8	0.39	0.87	0.41	0.02	0.04	7	0.53	0.75	0.25	0.00	0.01
间皮瘤	C45	4	0.20	0.43	0.26	0.03	0.03	2	0.15	0.22	0.11	0.00	0.03
卡波西肉瘤	C46	0	0.00	0.00	0.00	0.00	0.00	0	0.00	0.00	0.00	0.00	0.00
周围神经、其他结缔组织、软组织	C47;C49	8	0.39	0.87	0.40	0.03	0.03	2	0.15	0.22	0.07	0.00	0.00
乳房	C50	3	0.15	0.33	0.22	0.02	0.03	114	8.66	12.29	6.37	0.41	0.67
外阴	C51	0	0.00	0.00	0.00	0.00	0.00	3	0.23	0.32	0.13	0.00	0.01
阴道	C52	0	0.00	0.00	0.00	0.00	0.00	1	0.08	0.11	0.08	0.01	0.01
子宫颈	C53	0	0.00	0.00	0.00	0.00	0.00	53	4.03	5.71	3.17	0.21	0.36
子宫体	C54	0	0.00	0.00	0.00	0.00	0.00	16	1.22	1.72	0.97	0.06	0.12
子宫，部位不明	C55	0	0.00	0.00	0.00	0.00	0.00	4	0.30	0.43	0.22	0.02	0.02
卵巢	C56	0	0.00	0.00	0.00	0.00	0.00	47	3.57	5.07	2.59	0.16	0.30
女性其他的生殖器	C57	0	0.00	0.00	0.00	0.00	0.00	1	0.08	0.11	0.07	0.00	0.01
胎盘	C58	0	0.00	0.00	0.00	0.00	0.00	0	0.00	0.00	0.00	0.00	0.00
阴茎	C60	2	0.10	0.22	0.10	0.01	0.01	0	0.00	0.00	0.00	0.00	0.00
前列腺	C61	69	3.40	7.50	2.95	0.03	0.16	0	0.00	0.00	0.00	0.00	0.00
睾丸	C62	1	0.05	0.11	0.09	0.01	0.01	0	0.00	0.00	0.00	0.00	0.00
男性其他的生殖器	C63	2	0.10	0.22	0.06	0.00	0.00	0	0.00	0.00	0.00	0.00	0.00
肾	C64	36	1.77	3.91	1.96	0.09	0.21	13	0.99	1.40	0.60	0.03	0.07
肾盂	C65	2	0.10	0.22	0.10	0.01	0.01	3	0.23	0.32	0.14	0.01	0.01
输尿管	C66	4	0.20	0.43	0.22	0.01	0.03	8	0.61	0.86	0.29	0.00	0.02
膀胱	C67	44	2.17	4.78	1.90	0.04	0.10	11	0.84	1.19	0.49	0.01	0.05
其他的泌尿器官	C68	1	0.05	0.11	0.03	0.00	0.00	0	0.00	0.00	0.00	0.00	0.00
眼	C69	1	0.05	0.11	0.08	0.01	0.01	0	0.00	0.00	0.00	0.00	0.00
脑、神经系统	C70–C72	37	1.82	4.02	2.44	0.13	0.27	38	2.89	4.10	2.77	0.14	0.30
甲状腺	C73	3	0.15	0.33	0.16	0.02	0.02	5	0.38	0.54	0.30	0.02	0.04
肾上腺	C74	1	0.05	0.11	0.08	0.01	0.01	1	0.08	0.11	0.03	0.00	0.00
其他的内分泌腺	C75	1	0.05	0.11	0.08	0.01	0.01	1	0.08	0.11	0.08	0.01	0.01
霍奇金病	C81	2	0.10	0.22	0.11	0.00	0.01	0	0.00	0.00	0.00	0.00	0.00
非霍奇金淋巴瘤	C82–C85;C96	17	0.84	1.85	1.09	0.07	0.14	29	2.20	3.13	1.92	0.10	0.21
免疫增生性疾病	C88	0	0.00	0.00	0.00	0.00	0.00	0	0.00	0.00	0.00	0.00	0.00
多发性骨髓瘤	C90	18	0.89	1.96	0.99	0.04	0.12	12	0.91	1.29	0.68	0.02	0.09
淋巴样白血病	C91	0	0.00	0.00	0.00	0.00	0.00	4	0.30	0.43	0.43	0.03	0.03
髓样白血病	C92–C94	11	0.54	1.20	0.68	0.02	0.09	6	0.46	0.65	0.49	0.03	0.05
白血病，未特指	C95	27	1.33	2.93	1.66	0.10	0.16	15	1.14	1.62	1.15	0.06	0.10
其他的或未指明部位	O&U	38	1.87	4.13	1.98	0.05	0.19	36	2.74	3.88	1.74	0.07	0.19
骨髓增殖性疾病	MPD	0	0.00	0.00	0.00	0.00	0.00	2	0.15	0.22	0.09	0.00	0.01
骨髓增生异常综合征	MDS	7	0.34	0.76	0.42	0.02	0.06	1	0.08	0.11	0.05	0.00	0.01
合计	ALL	2 032	100.00	220.81	110.82	4.52	12.29	1 316	100.00	141.85	66.19	2.80	6.72
C44 以外的部位	ALL but C44	2 024	99.61	219.94	110.41	4.50	12.25	1 309	99.47	141.09	65.94	2.80	6.70

表 6-33　2020 年河南省洛阳市孟津区恶性肿瘤发病主要指标

部位	ICD-10	男性						女性					
		病例数	构成 (%)	粗率 ($1/10^5$)	世标率 ($1/10^5$)	累积率 (%)		病例数	构成 (%)	粗率 ($1/10^5$)	世标率 ($1/10^5$)	累积率 (%)	
						0~64	0~74					0~64	0~74
唇	C00	0	0.00	0.00	0.00	0.00	0.00	1	0.13	0.36	0.20	0.00	0.05
舌	C01–C02	1	0.12	0.36	0.25	0.03	0.03	2	0.26	0.73	0.65	0.06	0.06
口	C03–C06	6	0.70	2.16	1.36	0.08	0.21	3	0.38	1.09	0.48	0.00	0.04
唾液腺	C07–C08	8	0.94	2.88	1.96	0.13	0.21	1	0.13	0.36	0.41	0.03	0.03
扁桃体	C09	0	0.00	0.00	0.00	0.00	0.00	0	0.00	0.00	0.00	0.00	0.00
其他的口咽	C10	0	0.00	0.00	0.00	0.00	0.00	0	0.00	0.00	0.00	0.00	0.00
鼻咽	C11	2	0.23	0.72	0.56	0.06	0.06	0	0.00	0.00	0.00	0.00	0.00
喉咽	C12–C13	2	0.23	0.72	0.56	0.06	0.06	0	0.00	0.00	0.00	0.00	0.00
咽，部位不明	C14	1	0.12	0.36	0.18	0.00	0.00	1	0.13	0.36	0.41	0.03	0.03
食管	C15	102	11.97	36.69	21.89	0.63	2.83	84	10.74	30.49	15.43	0.28	2.20
胃	C16	121	14.20	43.53	25.98	0.80	3.46	52	6.65	18.88	10.24	0.30	1.31
小肠	C17	7	0.82	2.52	1.51	0.08	0.23	2	0.26	0.73	0.35	0.00	0.05
结肠	C18	28	3.29	10.07	6.33	0.24	0.88	28	3.58	10.16	5.80	0.29	0.70
直肠	C19–C20	38	4.46	13.67	8.37	0.47	0.91	28	3.58	10.16	5.73	0.35	0.75
肛门	C21	0	0.00	0.00	0.00	0.00	0.00	0	0.00	0.00	0.00	0.00	0.00
肝脏	C22	66	7.75	23.74	15.34	1.03	1.93	33	4.22	11.98	6.64	0.39	0.82
胆囊及其他	C23–C24	21	2.46	7.55	4.71	0.19	0.65	25	3.20	9.08	4.47	0.10	0.46
胰腺	C25	23	2.70	8.27	5.20	0.14	0.74	18	2.30	6.53	3.14	0.08	0.36
鼻、鼻窦及其他	C30–C31	3	0.35	1.08	0.68	0.06	0.11	0	0.00	0.00	0.00	0.00	0.00
喉	C32	4	0.47	1.44	0.87	0.06	0.10	0	0.00	0.00	0.00	0.00	0.00
气管、支气管、肺	C33–C34	194	22.77	69.79	43.19	1.85	5.75	83	10.61	30.13	16.51	0.84	2.12
其他的胸腔器官	C37–C38	6	0.70	2.16	1.43	0.11	0.15	3	0.38	1.09	0.74	0.05	0.05
骨	C40–C41	6	0.70	2.16	1.53	0.05	0.09	8	1.02	2.90	1.47	0.05	0.19
皮肤的黑色素瘤	C43	1	0.12	0.36	0.23	0.00	0.04	4	0.51	1.45	0.87	0.05	0.09
其他的皮肤	C44	13	1.53	4.68	2.80	0.15	0.19	7	0.90	2.54	1.29	0.06	0.19
间皮瘤	C45	1	0.12	0.36	0.22	0.03	0.03	0	0.00	0.00	0.00	0.00	0.00
卡波西肉瘤	C46	0	0.00	0.00	0.00	0.00	0.00	0	0.00	0.00	0.00	0.00	0.00
周围神经、其他结缔组织、软组织	C47;C49	1	0.12	0.36	0.31	0.03	0.03	2	0.26	0.73	1.05	0.06	0.06
乳房	C50	0	0.00	0.00	0.00	0.00	0.00	98	12.53	35.58	24.70	2.00	2.58
外阴	C51	0	0.00	0.00	0.00	0.00	0.00	2	0.26	0.73	0.52	0.05	0.05
阴道	C52	0	0.00	0.00	0.00	0.00	0.00	1	0.13	0.36	0.24	0.03	0.03
子宫颈	C53	0	0.00	0.00	0.00	0.00	0.00	54	6.91	19.60	13.03	0.94	1.55
子宫体	C54	0	0.00	0.00	0.00	0.00	0.00	49	6.27	17.79	11.48	0.90	1.34
子宫，部位不明	C55	0	0.00	0.00	0.00	0.00	0.00	2	0.26	0.73	0.42	0.05	0.05
卵巢	C56	0	0.00	0.00	0.00	0.00	0.00	19	2.43	6.90	4.89	0.28	0.51
女性其他的生殖器	C57	0	0.00	0.00	0.00	0.00	0.00	7	0.90	2.54	1.64	0.13	0.18
胎盘	C58	0	0.00	0.00	0.00	0.00	0.00	0	0.00	0.00	0.00	0.00	0.00
阴茎	C60	0	0.00	0.00	0.00	0.00	0.00	0	0.00	0.00	0.00	0.00	0.00
前列腺	C61	39	4.58	14.03	8.35	0.17	1.08	0	0.00	0.00	0.00	0.00	0.00
睾丸	C62	1	0.12	0.36	0.32	0.03	0.03	0	0.00	0.00	0.00	0.00	0.00
男性其他的生殖器	C63	0	0.00	0.00	0.00	0.00	0.00	0	0.00	0.00	0.00	0.00	0.00
肾	C64	19	2.23	6.83	4.14	0.18	0.52	11	1.41	3.99	2.38	0.19	0.24
肾盂	C65	0	0.00	0.00	0.00	0.00	0.00	0	0.00	0.00	0.00	0.00	0.00
输尿管	C66	0	0.00	0.00	0.00	0.00	0.00	0	0.00	0.00	0.00	0.00	0.00
膀胱	C67	22	2.58	7.91	4.80	0.20	0.69	6	0.77	2.18	1.37	0.08	0.22
其他的泌尿器官	C68	1	0.12	0.36	0.27	0.02	0.02	0	0.00	0.00	0.00	0.00	0.00
眼	C69	0	0.00	0.00	0.00	0.00	0.00	1	0.13	0.36	0.21	0.03	0.03
脑、神经系统	C70–C72	29	3.40	10.43	7.28	0.43	0.77	29	3.71	10.53	7.20	0.38	0.79
甲状腺	C73	21	2.46	7.55	6.07	0.46	0.57	64	8.18	23.23	17.63	1.47	1.60
肾上腺	C74	2	0.23	0.72	0.39	0.00	0.04	3	0.38	1.09	0.59	0.03	0.08
其他的内分泌腺	C75	2	0.23	0.72	0.49	0.06	0.06	1	0.13	0.36	0.33	0.03	0.03
霍奇金病	C81	0	0.00	0.00	0.00	0.00	0.00	0	0.00	0.00	0.00	0.00	0.00
非霍奇金淋巴瘤	C82–C85;C96	19	2.23	6.83	5.11	0.25	0.45	17	2.17	6.17	3.57	0.16	0.43
免疫增生性疾病	C88	1	0.12	0.36	0.18	0.00	0.00	0	0.00	0.00	0.00	0.00	0.00
多发性骨髓瘤	C90	8	0.94	2.88	1.86	0.13	0.22	3	0.38	1.09	0.64	0.05	0.09
淋巴样白血病	C91	3	0.35	1.08	1.47	0.06	0.06	2	0.26	0.73	1.26	0.07	0.07
髓样白血病	C92–C94	6	0.70	2.16	1.28	0.02	0.16	7	0.90	2.54	1.71	0.09	0.16
白血病，未特指	C95	6	0.70	2.16	2.53	0.11	0.21	6	0.77	2.18	1.26	0.03	0.15
其他的或未指明部位	O&U	9	1.06	3.24	2.78	0.14	0.26	12	1.53	4.36	3.39	0.22	0.22
骨髓增殖性疾病	MPD	1	0.12	0.36	0.25	0.03	0.03	0	0.00	0.00	0.00	0.00	0.00
骨髓增生异常综合征	MDS	8	0.94	2.88	2.66	0.11	0.19	3	0.38	1.09	1.26	0.08	0.08
合计	ALL	852	100.00	306.49	195.66	8.70	24.05	782	100.00	283.88	175.59	10.30	20.01
C44 以外的部位	ALL but C44	839	98.47	301.81	192.86	8.54	23.86	775	99.10	281.34	174.29	10.24	19.81

表 6-34 2020 年河南省洛阳市孟津区恶性肿瘤死亡主要指标

部位	ICD-10	男性						女性					
		病例数	构成 (%)	粗率 (1/10^5)	世标率 (1/10^5)	累积率 (%)		病例数	构成 (%)	粗率 (1/10^5)	世标率 (1/10^5)	累积率 (%)	
						0~64	0~74					0~64	0~74
唇	C00	2	0.35	0.72	0.38	0.00	0.06	0	0.00	0.00	0.00	0.00	0.00
舌	C01-C02	2	0.35	0.72	0.40	0.03	0.03	0	0.00	0.00	0.00	0.00	0.00
口	C03-C06	2	0.35	0.72	0.40	0.00	0.06	4	1.02	1.45	0.65	0.00	0.09
唾液腺	C07-C08	1	0.18	0.36	0.25	0.03	0.03	0	0.00	0.00	0.00	0.00	0.00
扁桃体	C09	0	0.00	0.00	0.00	0.00	0.00	2	0.51	0.73	0.49	0.02	0.06
其他的口咽	C10	0	0.00	0.00	0.00	0.00	0.00	0	0.00	0.00	0.00	0.00	0.00
鼻咽	C11	4	0.71	1.44	0.80	0.02	0.06	1	0.26	0.36	0.21	0.03	0.03
喉咽	C12-C13	1	0.18	0.36	0.18	0.00	0.00	0	0.00	0.00	0.00	0.00	0.00
咽，部位不明	C14	0	0.00	0.00	0.00	0.00	0.00	0	0.00	0.00	0.00	0.00	0.00
食管	C15	80	14.13	28.78	16.16	0.36	1.46	66	16.84	23.96	11.04	0.17	1.36
胃	C16	105	18.55	37.77	21.41	0.61	2.08	36	9.18	13.07	6.60	0.19	0.71
小肠	C17	2	0.35	0.72	0.56	0.06	0.06	3	0.77	1.09	0.71	0.05	0.10
结肠	C18	14	2.47	5.04	2.76	0.09	0.18	15	3.83	5.45	2.42	0.08	0.15
直肠	C19-C20	14	2.47	5.04	3.00	0.11	0.28	11	2.81	3.99	2.11	0.08	0.31
肛门	C21	0	0.00	0.00	0.00	0.00	0.00	0	0.00	0.00	0.00	0.00	0.00
肝脏	C22	60	10.60	21.58	13.49	0.75	1.67	28	7.14	10.16	5.11	0.19	0.54
胆囊及其他	C23-C24	17	3.00	6.12	3.66	0.11	0.46	23	5.87	8.35	3.98	0.13	0.44
胰腺	C25	16	2.83	5.76	3.41	0.08	0.34	15	3.83	5.45	3.06	0.16	0.39
鼻、鼻窦及其他	C30-C31	1	0.18	0.36	0.20	0.00	0.00	1	0.26	0.36	0.24	0.02	0.02
喉	C32	2	0.35	0.72	0.40	0.00	0.06	0	0.00	0.00	0.00	0.00	0.00
气管、支气管、肺	C33-C34	151	26.68	54.32	32.53	1.33	3.78	58	14.80	21.06	10.83	0.53	1.28
其他的胸腔器官	C37-C38	2	0.35	0.72	0.48	0.05	0.05	3	0.77	1.09	0.64	0.05	0.05
骨	C40-C41	4	0.71	1.44	0.78	0.02	0.02	7	1.79	2.54	1.23	0.03	0.06
皮肤的黑色素瘤	C43	1	0.18	0.36	0.25	0.03	0.03	1	0.26	0.36	0.24	0.02	0.02
其他的皮肤	C44	1	0.18	0.36	0.20	0.00	0.00	4	1.02	1.45	0.74	0.06	0.06
间皮瘤	C45	0	0.00	0.00	0.00	0.00	0.00	0	0.00	0.00	0.00	0.00	0.00
卡波西肉瘤	C46	0	0.00	0.00	0.00	0.00	0.00	0	0.00	0.00	0.00	0.00	0.00
周围神经、其他结缔组织、软组织	C47;C49	0	0.00	0.00	0.00	0.00	0.00	2	0.51	0.73	0.54	0.05	0.05
乳房	C50	0	0.00	0.00	0.00	0.00	0.00	20	5.10	7.26	4.67	0.34	0.47
外阴	C51	0	0.00	0.00	0.00	0.00	0.00	0	0.00	0.00	0.00	0.00	0.00
阴道	C52	0	0.00	0.00	0.00	0.00	0.00	1	0.26	0.36	0.24	0.03	0.03
子宫颈	C53	0	0.00	0.00	0.00	0.00	0.00	17	4.34	6.17	3.24	0.19	0.35
子宫体	C54	0	0.00	0.00	0.00	0.00	0.00	7	1.79	2.54	1.51	0.10	0.18
子宫，部位不明	C55	0	0.00	0.00	0.00	0.00	0.00	1	0.26	0.36	0.11	0.00	0.00
卵巢	C56	0	0.00	0.00	0.00	0.00	0.00	13	3.32	4.72	2.76	0.13	0.37
女性其他的生殖器	C57	0	0.00	0.00	0.00	0.00	0.00	1	0.26	0.36	0.22	0.00	0.04
胎盘	C58	0	0.00	0.00	0.00	0.00	0.00	0	0.00	0.00	0.00	0.00	0.00
阴茎	C60	1	0.18	0.36	0.20	0.00	0.00	0	0.00	0.00	0.00	0.00	0.00
前列腺	C61	11	1.94	3.96	1.95	0.00	0.04	0	0.00	0.00	0.00	0.00	0.00
睾丸	C62	0	0.00	0.00	0.00	0.00	0.00	0	0.00	0.00	0.00	0.00	0.00
男性其他的生殖器	C63	0	0.00	0.00	0.00	0.00	0.00	0	0.00	0.00	0.00	0.00	0.00
肾	C64	3	0.53	1.08	0.59	0.03	0.03	4	1.02	1.45	0.58	0.00	0.05
肾盂	C65	0	0.00	0.00	0.00	0.00	0.00	1	0.26	0.36	0.11	0.00	0.00
输尿管	C66	0	0.00	0.00	0.00	0.00	0.00	1	0.26	0.36	0.11	0.00	0.00
膀胱	C67	8	1.41	2.88	1.46	0.03	0.03	0	0.00	0.00	0.00	0.00	0.00
其他的泌尿器官	C68	0	0.00	0.00	0.00	0.00	0.00	0	0.00	0.00	0.00	0.00	0.00
眼	C69	1	0.18	0.36	0.18	0.00	0.00	1	0.26	0.36	0.24	0.02	0.02
脑、神经系统	C70-C72	17	3.00	6.12	3.87	0.21	0.38	17	4.34	6.17	3.71	0.15	0.47
甲状腺	C73	2	0.35	0.72	0.33	0.00	0.00	4	1.02	1.45	0.83	0.05	0.10
肾上腺	C74	1	0.18	0.36	0.22	0.03	0.03	0	0.00	0.00	0.00	0.00	0.00
其他的内分泌腺	C75	3	0.53	1.08	0.59	0.03	0.08	0	0.00	0.00	0.00	0.00	0.00
霍奇金病	C81	0	0.00	0.00	0.00	0.00	0.00	0	0.00	0.00	0.00	0.00	0.00
非霍奇金淋巴瘤	C82-C85;C96	7	1.24	2.52	1.67	0.07	0.13	5	1.28	1.82	0.97	0.05	0.09
免疫增生性疾病	C88	0	0.00	0.00	0.00	0.00	0.00	0	0.00	0.00	0.00	0.00	0.00
多发性骨髓瘤	C90	7	1.24	2.52	1.59	0.03	0.29	1	0.26	0.36	0.22	0.00	0.04
淋巴样白血病	C91	2	0.35	0.72	0.48	0.05	0.05	1	0.26	0.36	0.22	0.00	0.04
髓样白血病	C92-C94	4	0.71	1.44	0.91	0.03	0.08	6	1.53	2.18	1.58	0.11	0.20
白血病，未特指	C95	3	0.53	1.08	0.71	0.03	0.08	5	1.28	1.82	1.53	0.03	0.12
其他的或未指明部位	O&U	9	1.59	3.24	1.90	0.08	0.23	3	0.77	1.09	0.54	0.03	0.03
骨髓增殖性疾病	MPD	1	0.18	0.36	0.25	0.03	0.03	0	0.00	0.00	0.00	0.00	0.00
骨髓增生异常综合征	MDS	4	0.71	1.44	1.19	0.06	0.06	3	0.77	1.09	0.51	0.00	0.10
合计	ALL	566	100.00	203.61	119.73	4.36	12.24	392	100.00	142.30	74.74	3.11	8.40
C44 以外的部位	ALL but C44	565	99.82	203.25	119.53	4.36	12.24	388	98.98	140.85	74.01	3.05	8.35

表 6-35　2020 年河南省新安县恶性肿瘤发病主要指标

部位	ICD-10	男性						女性					
		病例数	构成(%)	粗率(1/10⁵)	世标率(1/10⁵)	累积率(%)		病例数	构成(%)	粗率(1/10⁵)	世标率(1/10⁵)	累积率(%)	
						0~64	0~74					0~64	0~74
唇	C00	0	0.00	0.00	0.00	0.00	0.00	0	0.00	0.00	0.00	0.00	0.00
舌	C01–C02	0	0.00	0.00	0.00	0.00	0.00	0	0.00	0.00	0.00	0.00	0.00
口	C03–C06	4	0.50	1.43	1.01	0.07	0.07	2	0.26	0.76	0.42	0.00	0.04
唾液腺	C07–C08	4	0.50	1.43	1.00	0.03	0.16	2	0.26	0.76	0.63	0.05	0.05
扁桃体	C09	0	0.00	0.00	0.00	0.00	0.00	1	0.13	0.38	0.52	0.03	0.03
其他的口咽	C10	0	0.00	0.00	0.00	0.00	0.00	0	0.00	0.00	0.00	0.00	0.00
鼻咽	C11	2	0.25	0.72	0.45	0.06	0.06	1	0.13	0.38	0.26	0.00	0.04
喉咽	C12–C13	0	0.00	0.00	0.00	0.00	0.00	0	0.00	0.00	0.00	0.00	0.00
咽，部位不明	C14	0	0.00	0.00	0.00	0.00	0.00	1	0.13	0.38	0.35	0.03	0.03
食管	C15	90	11.25	32.20	18.89	0.40	2.69	56	7.24	21.32	11.27	0.32	1.49
胃	C16	123	15.38	44.00	27.17	1.04	3.51	55	7.11	20.94	10.87	0.37	1.28
小肠	C17	7	0.88	2.50	1.76	0.12	0.26	1	0.13	0.38	0.30	0.03	0.03
结肠	C18	23	2.88	8.23	5.42	0.32	0.71	33	4.26	12.56	7.50	0.50	0.67
直肠	C19–C20	30	3.75	10.73	6.47	0.26	0.81	24	3.10	9.14	4.96	0.29	0.46
肛门	C21	0	0.00	0.00	0.00	0.00	0.00	0	0.00	0.00	0.00	0.00	0.00
肝脏	C22	83	10.38	29.69	19.73	1.03	2.48	44	5.68	16.75	8.90	0.39	1.03
胆囊及其他	C23–C24	15	1.88	5.37	2.94	0.09	0.33	18	2.33	6.85	4.26	0.25	0.56
胰腺	C25	12	1.50	4.29	2.89	0.13	0.25	11	1.42	4.19	2.30	0.06	0.33
鼻、鼻窦及其他	C30–C31	1	0.13	0.36	0.17	0.00	0.00	0	0.00	0.00	0.00	0.00	0.00
喉	C32	5	0.63	1.79	1.20	0.08	0.12	2	0.26	0.76	0.42	0.00	0.04
气管、支气管、肺	C33–C34	235	29.38	84.07	52.46	2.28	6.98	113	14.60	43.02	24.10	1.08	2.81
其他的胸腔器官	C37–C38	0	0.00	0.00	0.00	0.00	0.00	1	0.13	0.38	0.30	0.03	0.03
骨	C40–C41	11	1.38	3.94	2.80	0.14	0.32	7	0.90	2.67	2.36	0.16	0.20
皮肤的黑色素瘤	C43	1	0.13	0.36	0.28	0.02	0.02	1	0.13	0.38	0.26	0.00	0.04
其他的皮肤	C44	4	0.50	1.43	0.84	0.03	0.09	5	0.65	1.90	1.19	0.06	0.16
间皮瘤	C45	0	0.00	0.00	0.00	0.00	0.00	0	0.00	0.00	0.00	0.00	0.00
卡波西肉瘤	C46	0	0.00	0.00	0.00	0.00	0.00	0	0.00	0.00	0.00	0.00	0.00
周围神经、其他结缔组织、软组织	C47;C49	2	0.25	0.72	0.58	0.05	0.05	4	0.52	1.52	1.57	0.12	0.12
乳房	C50	2	0.25	0.72	0.53	0.05	0.05	114	14.73	43.40	32.11	2.56	3.35
外阴	C51	0	0.00	0.00	0.00	0.00	0.00	2	0.26	0.76	0.54	0.03	0.08
阴道	C52	0	0.00	0.00	0.00	0.00	0.00	2	0.26	0.76	0.47	0.03	0.09
子宫颈	C53	0	0.00	0.00	0.00	0.00	0.00	69	8.91	26.27	18.66	1.47	1.95
子宫体	C54	0	0.00	0.00	0.00	0.00	0.00	26	3.36	9.90	6.80	0.58	0.78
子宫，部位不明	C55	0	0.00	0.00	0.00	0.00	0.00	8	1.03	3.05	2.34	0.21	0.25
卵巢	C56	0	0.00	0.00	0.00	0.00	0.00	29	3.75	11.04	7.91	0.64	0.78
女性其他的生殖器	C57	0	0.00	0.00	0.00	0.00	0.00	3	0.39	1.14	0.84	0.09	0.09
胎盘	C58	0	0.00	0.00	0.00	0.00	0.00	0	0.00	0.00	0.00	0.00	0.00
阴茎	C60	0	0.00	0.00	0.00	0.00	0.00	0	0.00	0.00	0.00	0.00	0.00
前列腺	C61	30	3.75	10.73	5.75	0.18	0.51	0	0.00	0.00	0.00	0.00	0.00
睾丸	C62	1	0.13	0.36	0.14	0.00	0.00	0	0.00	0.00	0.00	0.00	0.00
男性其他的生殖器	C63	0	0.00	0.00	0.00	0.00	0.00	0	0.00	0.00	0.00	0.00	0.00
肾	C64	12	1.50	4.29	2.91	0.23	0.27	9	1.16	3.43	2.51	0.27	0.27
肾盂	C65	0	0.00	0.00	0.00	0.00	0.00	2	0.26	0.76	0.56	0.03	0.07
输尿管	C66	5	0.63	1.79	0.91	0.06	0.06	1	0.13	0.38	0.23	0.00	0.06
膀胱	C67	23	2.88	8.23	4.63	0.11	0.45	7	0.90	2.67	1.44	0.05	0.11
其他的泌尿器官	C68	0	0.00	0.00	0.00	0.00	0.00	0	0.00	0.00	0.00	0.00	0.00
眼	C69	1	0.13	0.36	0.27	0.03	0.03	1	0.13	0.38	0.94	0.04	0.04
脑、神经系统	C70–C72	18	2.25	6.44	4.00	0.22	0.40	22	2.84	8.38	5.68	0.39	0.57
甲状腺	C73	11	1.38	3.94	2.74	0.25	0.33	51	6.59	19.42	15.27	1.37	1.41
肾上腺	C74	1	0.13	0.36	0.27	0.03	0.03	2	0.26	0.76	0.52	0.06	0.06
其他的内分泌腺	C75	1	0.13	0.36	0.28	0.02	0.02	1	0.13	0.38	0.24	0.03	0.03
霍奇金病	C81	1	0.13	0.36	0.23	0.00	0.06	0	0.00	0.00	0.00	0.00	0.00
非霍奇金淋巴瘤	C82–C85;C96	13	1.63	4.65	3.67	0.22	0.38	8	1.03	3.05	1.57	0.03	0.19
免疫增生性疾病	C88	0	0.00	0.00	0.00	0.00	0.00	0	0.00	0.00	0.00	0.00	0.00
多发性骨髓瘤	C90	2	0.25	0.72	0.40	0.00	0.04	1	0.13	0.38	0.26	0.00	0.04
淋巴样白血病	C91	0	0.00	0.00	0.00	0.00	0.00	1	0.13	0.38	0.26	0.00	0.04
髓样白血病	C92–C94	3	0.38	1.07	1.10	0.03	0.13	4	0.52	1.52	1.53	0.07	0.07
白血病，未特指	C95	6	0.75	2.15	1.86	0.11	0.15	4	0.52	1.52	1.67	0.06	0.12
其他的或未指明部位	O&U	17	2.13	6.08	4.50	0.24	0.38	24	3.10	9.14	6.28	0.37	0.67
骨髓增殖性疾病	MPD	1	0.13	0.36	0.38	0.02	0.02	0	0.00	0.00	0.00	0.00	0.00
骨髓增生异常综合征	MDS	0	0.00	0.00	0.00	0.00	0.00	1	0.13	0.38	0.30	0.03	0.03
合计	ALL	800	100.00	286.21	180.61	7.98	22.22	774	100.00	294.70	191.67	12.13	20.58
C44 以外的部位	ALL but C44	796	99.50	284.78	179.77	7.94	22.13	769	99.35	292.79	190.48	12.07	20.42

表 6-36 2020 年河南省新安县恶性肿瘤死亡主要指标

部位	ICD-10	男性						女性					
		病例数	构成 (%)	粗率 $(1/10^5)$	世标率 $(1/10^5)$	累积率 (%)		病例数	构成 (%)	粗率 $(1/10^5)$	世标率 $(1/10^5)$	累积率 (%)	
						0~64	0~74					0~64	0~74
唇	C00	0	0.00	0.00	0.00	0.00	0.00	0	0.00	0.00	0.00	0.00	0.00
舌	C01-C02	1	0.15	0.36	0.25	0.00	0.04	0	0.00	0.00	0.00	0.00	0.00
口	C03-C06	2	0.30	0.72	0.40	0.03	0.03	0	0.00	0.00	0.00	0.00	0.00
唾液腺	C07-C08	0	0.00	0.00	0.00	0.00	0.00	0	0.00	0.00	0.00	0.00	0.00
扁桃体	C09	0	0.00	0.00	0.00	0.00	0.00	0	0.00	0.00	0.00	0.00	0.00
其他的口咽	C10	2	0.30	0.72	0.40	0.00	0.06	0	0.00	0.00	0.00	0.00	0.00
鼻咽	C11	1	0.15	0.36	0.15	0.00	0.00	1	0.25	0.38	0.26	0.00	0.04
喉咽	C12-C13	0	0.00	0.00	0.00	0.00	0.00	0	0.00	0.00	0.00	0.00	0.00
咽，部位不明	C14	0	0.00	0.00	0.00	0.00	0.00	0	0.00	0.00	0.00	0.00	0.00
食管	C15	79	12.04	28.26	16.02	0.26	2.06	49	12.22	18.66	9.33	0.10	1.15
胃	C16	134	20.43	47.94	27.42	0.75	2.61	46	11.47	17.51	7.97	0.16	0.89
小肠	C17	2	0.30	0.72	0.47	0.02	0.08	1	0.25	0.38	0.11	0.00	0.00
结肠	C18	10	1.52	3.58	2.18	0.05	0.29	17	4.24	6.47	3.03	0.12	0.24
直肠	C19-C20	18	2.74	6.44	3.52	0.06	0.34	11	2.74	4.19	2.07	0.06	0.20
肛门	C21	0	0.00	0.00	0.00	0.00	0.00	0	0.00	0.00	0.00	0.00	0.00
肝脏	C22	70	10.67	25.04	16.23	0.85	2.07	42	10.47	15.99	7.84	0.24	0.81
胆囊及其他	C23-C24	16	2.44	5.72	3.24	0.12	0.34	17	4.24	6.47	3.45	0.11	0.40
胰腺	C25	13	1.98	4.65	2.59	0.12	0.22	9	2.24	3.43	2.22	0.13	0.29
鼻、鼻窦及其他	C30-C31	0	0.00	0.00	0.00	0.00	0.00	0	0.00	0.00	0.00	0.00	0.00
喉	C32	4	0.61	1.43	1.01	0.07	0.16	0	0.00	0.00	0.00	0.00	0.00
气管、支气管、肺	C33-C34	226	34.45	80.85	47.74	1.28	5.91	91	22.69	34.65	16.69	0.63	1.80
其他的胸腔器官	C37-C38	0	0.00	0.00	0.00	0.00	0.00	0	0.00	0.00	0.00	0.00	0.00
骨	C40-C41	7	1.07	2.50	1.63	0.07	0.11	4	1.00	1.52	0.87	0.05	0.11
皮肤的黑色素瘤	C43	0	0.00	0.00	0.00	0.00	0.00	2	0.50	0.76	0.52	0.03	0.07
其他的皮肤	C44	1	0.15	0.36	0.17	0.00	0.00	3	0.75	1.14	0.47	0.03	0.03
间皮瘤	C45	0	0.00	0.00	0.00	0.00	0.00	0	0.00	0.00	0.00	0.00	0.00
卡波西肉瘤	C46	0	0.00	0.00	0.00	0.00	0.00	0	0.00	0.00	0.00	0.00	0.00
周围神经、其他结缔组织、软组织	C47;C49	0	0.00	0.00	0.00	0.00	0.00	0	0.00	0.00	0.00	0.00	0.00
乳房	C50	1	0.15	0.36	0.31	0.03	0.03	28	6.98	10.66	6.50	0.44	0.75
外阴	C51	0	0.00	0.00	0.00	0.00	0.00	1	0.25	0.38	0.24	0.03	0.03
阴道	C52	0	0.00	0.00	0.00	0.00	0.00	0	0.00	0.00	0.00	0.00	0.00
子宫颈	C53	0	0.00	0.00	0.00	0.00	0.00	23	5.74	8.76	5.39	0.27	0.58
子宫体	C54	0	0.00	0.00	0.00	0.00	0.00	2	0.50	0.76	0.52	0.06	0.06
子宫，部位不明	C55	0	0.00	0.00	0.00	0.00	0.00	3	0.75	1.14	0.47	0.00	0.06
卵巢	C56	0	0.00	0.00	0.00	0.00	0.00	5	1.25	1.90	1.38	0.11	0.16
女性其他的生殖器	C57	0	0.00	0.00	0.00	0.00	0.00	0	0.00	0.00	0.00	0.00	0.00
胎盘	C58	0	0.00	0.00	0.00	0.00	0.00	0	0.00	0.00	0.00	0.00	0.00
阴茎	C60	1	0.15	0.36	0.24	0.02	0.02	0	0.00	0.00	0.00	0.00	0.00
前列腺	C61	9	1.37	3.22	1.73	0.03	0.19	0	0.00	0.00	0.00	0.00	0.00
睾丸	C62	0	0.00	0.00	0.00	0.00	0.00	0	0.00	0.00	0.00	0.00	0.00
男性其他的生殖器	C63	0	0.00	0.00	0.00	0.00	0.00	0	0.00	0.00	0.00	0.00	0.00
肾	C64	4	0.61	1.43	0.93	0.05	0.10	6	1.50	2.28	1.20	0.06	0.12
肾盂	C65	1	0.15	0.36	0.23	0.03	0.03	0	0.00	0.00	0.00	0.00	0.00
输尿管	C66	1	0.15	0.36	0.14	0.00	0.00	1	0.25	0.38	0.26	0.00	0.04
膀胱	C67	10	1.52	3.58	2.10	0.09	0.22	3	0.75	1.14	0.73	0.03	0.07
其他的泌尿器官	C68	0	0.00	0.00	0.00	0.00	0.00	0	0.00	0.00	0.00	0.00	0.00
眼	C69	0	0.00	0.00	0.00	0.00	0.00	0	0.00	0.00	0.00	0.00	0.00
脑、神经系统	C70-C72	17	2.59	6.08	4.43	0.21	0.47	8	2.00	3.05	1.87	0.13	0.23
甲状腺	C73	0	0.00	0.00	0.00	0.00	0.00	2	0.50	0.76	0.39	0.00	0.06
肾上腺	C74	1	0.15	0.36	0.27	0.03	0.03	0	0.00	0.00	0.00	0.00	0.00
其他的内分泌腺	C75	0	0.00	0.00	0.00	0.00	0.00	1	0.25	0.38	0.23	0.00	0.06
霍奇金病	C81	0	0.00	0.00	0.00	0.00	0.00	0	0.00	0.00	0.00	0.00	0.00
非霍奇金淋巴瘤	C82-C85;C96	4	0.61	1.43	0.80	0.06	0.06	1	0.25	0.38	0.12	0.00	0.00
免疫增生性疾病	C88	0	0.00	0.00	0.00	0.00	0.00	0	0.00	0.00	0.00	0.00	0.00
多发性骨髓瘤	C90	2	0.30	0.72	0.38	0.03	0.03	0	0.00	0.00	0.00	0.00	0.00
淋巴样白血病	C91	0	0.00	0.00	0.00	0.00	0.00	0	0.00	0.00	0.00	0.00	0.00
髓样白血病	C92-C94	5	0.76	1.79	1.09	0.03	0.13	7	1.75	2.67	2.18	0.10	0.10
白血病，未特指	C95	4	0.61	1.43	0.87	0.09	0.09	4	1.00	1.52	1.11	0.06	0.17
其他的或未指明部位	O&U	7	1.07	2.50	1.63	0.06	0.10	11	2.74	4.19	2.79	0.10	0.26
骨髓增殖性疾病	MPD	0	0.00	0.00	0.00	0.00	0.00	0	0.00	0.00	0.00	0.00	0.00
骨髓增生异常综合征	MDS	3	0.46	1.07	0.81	0.05	0.11	2	0.50	0.76	0.54	0.03	0.08
合计	ALL	656	100.00	234.69	139.39	4.48	15.92	401	100.00	152.68	80.75	3.08	8.87
C44 以外的部位	ALL but C44	655	99.85	234.33	139.22	4.48	15.92	398	99.25	151.54	80.29	3.05	8.84

表 6-37 2020 年河南省栾川县恶性肿瘤发病主要指标

部位	ICD-10	男性						女性					
		病例数	构成 (%)	粗率 $(1/10^5)$	世标率 $(1/10^5)$	累积率 (%) 0~64	累积率 (%) 0~74	病例数	构成 (%)	粗率 $(1/10^5)$	世标率 $(1/10^5)$	累积率 (%) 0~64	累积率 (%) 0~74
唇	C00	0	0.00	0.00	0.00	0.00	0.00	0	0.00	0.00	0.00	0.00	0.00
舌	C01–C02	0	0.00	0.00	0.00	0.00	0.00	1	0.22	0.58	0.44	0.04	0.04
口	C03–C06	1	0.20	0.53	0.36	0.00	0.06	4	0.86	2.32	1.33	0.08	0.08
唾液腺	C07–C08	2	0.41	1.07	0.83	0.07	0.07	1	0.22	0.58	0.45	0.04	0.04
扁桃体	C09	0	0.00	0.00	0.00	0.00	0.00	1	0.22	0.58	0.52	0.04	0.04
其他的口咽	C10	0	0.00	0.00	0.00	0.00	0.00	0	0.00	0.00	0.00	0.00	0.00
鼻咽	C11	4	0.82	2.13	1.40	0.11	0.20	1	0.22	0.58	0.51	0.04	0.04
喉咽	C12–C13	1	0.20	0.53	0.23	0.00	0.00	0	0.00	0.00	0.00	0.00	0.00
咽，部位不明	C14	1	0.20	0.53	0.36	0.00	0.06	0	0.00	0.00	0.00	0.00	0.00
食管	C15	78	15.95	41.59	25.45	1.02	3.29	36	7.78	20.84	11.54	0.54	1.36
胃	C16	103	21.06	54.92	34.87	2.09	4.39	36	7.78	20.84	12.63	0.88	1.55
小肠	C17	3	0.61	1.60	1.01	0.07	0.13	0	0.00	0.00	0.00	0.00	0.00
结肠	C18	16	3.27	8.53	5.78	0.28	0.78	6	1.30	3.47	1.92	0.08	0.23
直肠	C19–C20	13	2.66	6.93	4.53	0.29	0.47	13	2.81	7.53	4.27	0.29	0.50
肛门	C21	0	0.00	0.00	0.00	0.00	0.00	0	0.00	0.00	0.00	0.00	0.00
肝脏	C22	59	12.07	31.46	21.08	1.34	2.67	18	3.89	10.42	6.17	0.35	0.69
胆囊及其他	C23–C24	8	1.64	4.27	2.65	0.11	0.26	12	2.59	6.95	4.24	0.25	0.49
胰腺	C25	13	2.66	6.93	5.21	0.25	0.70	12	2.59	6.95	3.85	0.13	0.47
鼻、鼻窦及其他	C30–C31	1	0.20	0.53	0.37	0.05	0.05	0	0.00	0.00	0.00	0.00	0.00
喉	C32	0	0.00	0.00	0.00	0.00	0.00	0	0.00	0.00	0.00	0.00	0.00
气管、支气管、肺	C33–C34	90	18.40	47.99	30.78	1.45	3.91	40	8.64	23.16	14.05	0.81	1.72
其他的胸腔器官	C37–C38	3	0.61	1.60	1.04	0.09	0.15	3	0.65	1.74	1.28	0.12	0.12
骨	C40–C41	8	1.64	4.27	3.64	0.24	0.36	7	1.51	4.05	4.38	0.19	0.31
皮肤的黑色素瘤	C43	0	0.00	0.00	0.00	0.00	0.00	1	0.22	0.58	0.39	0.05	0.05
其他的皮肤	C44	0	0.00	0.00	0.00	0.00	0.00	1	0.22	0.58	0.27	0.00	0.00
间皮瘤	C45	0	0.00	0.00	0.00	0.00	0.00	2	0.43	1.16	0.81	0.04	0.10
卡波西肉瘤	C46	0	0.00	0.00	0.00	0.00	0.00	0	0.00	0.00	0.00	0.00	0.00
周围神经、其他结缔组织、软组织	C47;C49	2	0.41	1.07	0.76	0.07	0.07	1	0.22	0.58	0.36	0.04	0.04
乳房	C50	3	0.61	1.60	1.01	0.03	0.09	72	15.55	41.69	29.06	2.48	3.01
外阴	C51	0	0.00	0.00	0.00	0.00	0.00	2	0.43	1.16	0.71	0.09	0.09
阴道	C52	0	0.00	0.00	0.00	0.00	0.00	1	0.22	0.58	0.76	0.05	0.05
子宫颈	C53	0	0.00	0.00	0.00	0.00	0.00	40	8.64	23.16	16.45	1.22	1.65
子宫体	C54	0	0.00	0.00	0.00	0.00	0.00	30	6.48	17.37	11.33	1.08	1.23
子宫，部位不明	C55	0	0.00	0.00	0.00	0.00	0.00	0	0.00	0.00	0.00	0.00	0.00
卵巢	C56	0	0.00	0.00	0.00	0.00	0.00	20	4.32	11.58	7.79	0.52	0.97
女性其他的生殖器	C57	0	0.00	0.00	0.00	0.00	0.00	2	0.43	1.16	1.32	0.10	0.10
胎盘	C58	0	0.00	0.00	0.00	0.00	0.00	0	0.00	0.00	0.00	0.00	0.00
阴茎	C60	4	0.82	2.13	1.42	0.08	0.23	0	0.00	0.00	0.00	0.00	0.00
前列腺	C61	6	1.23	3.20	2.08	0.14	0.31	0	0.00	0.00	0.00	0.00	0.00
睾丸	C62	1	0.20	0.53	0.47	0.04	0.04	0	0.00	0.00	0.00	0.00	0.00
男性其他的生殖器	C63	0	0.00	0.00	0.00	0.00	0.00	0	0.00	0.00	0.00	0.00	0.00
肾	C64	5	1.02	2.67	1.84	0.07	0.25	5	1.08	2.89	2.41	0.14	0.20
肾盂	C65	0	0.00	0.00	0.00	0.00	0.00	0	0.00	0.00	0.00	0.00	0.00
输尿管	C66	1	0.20	0.53	0.36	0.00	0.06	0	0.00	0.00	0.00	0.00	0.00
膀胱	C67	15	3.07	8.00	5.12	0.24	0.71	4	0.86	2.32	1.29	0.00	0.12
其他的泌尿器官	C68	0	0.00	0.00	0.00	0.00	0.00	0	0.00	0.00	0.00	0.00	0.00
眼	C69	0	0.00	0.00	0.00	0.00	0.00	0	0.00	0.00	0.00	0.00	0.00
脑、神经系统	C70–C72	7	1.43	3.73	3.06	0.23	0.23	18	3.89	10.42	7.56	0.57	0.78
甲状腺	C73	15	3.07	8.00	6.08	0.56	0.56	51	11.02	29.53	21.66	1.86	2.04
肾上腺	C74	1	0.20	0.53	0.35	0.00	0.09	0	0.00	0.00	0.00	0.00	0.00
其他的内分泌腺	C75	1	0.20	0.53	0.79	0.04	0.04	0	0.00	0.00	0.00	0.00	0.00
霍奇金病	C81	1	0.20	0.53	0.55	0.03	0.03	0	0.00	0.00	0.00	0.00	0.00
非霍奇金淋巴瘤	C82–C85;C96	5	1.02	2.67	1.57	0.08	0.08	6	1.30	3.47	2.22	0.11	0.35
免疫增生性疾病	C88	0	0.00	0.00	0.00	0.00	0.00	0	0.00	0.00	0.00	0.00	0.00
多发性骨髓瘤	C90	2	0.41	1.07	0.72	0.00	0.12	3	0.65	1.74	1.12	0.08	0.17
淋巴样白血病	C91	2	0.41	1.07	0.82	0.04	0.13	1	0.22	0.58	0.87	0.05	0.05
髓样白血病	C92–C94	3	0.61	1.60	1.10	0.09	0.15	3	0.65	1.74	1.57	0.08	0.15
白血病，未特指	C95	5	1.02	2.67	3.86	0.17	0.23	4	0.86	2.32	2.23	0.09	0.09
其他的或未指明部位	O&U	6	1.23	3.20	2.13	0.11	0.23	5	1.08	2.89	1.55	0.12	0.12
骨髓增殖性疾病	MPD	0	0.00	0.00	0.00	0.00	0.00	0	0.00	0.00	0.00	0.00	0.00
骨髓增生异常综合征	MDS	0	0.00	0.00	0.00	0.00	0.00	0	0.00	0.00	0.00	0.00	0.00
合计	ALL	489	100.00	260.74	173.69	9.48	21.19	463	100.00	268.07	179.34	12.64	19.05
C44 以外的部位	ALL but C44	489	100.00	260.74	173.69	9.48	21.19	462	99.78	267.49	179.07	12.64	19.05

表 6-38 2020 年河南省栾川县恶性肿瘤死亡主要指标

部位	ICD-10	男性						女性					
		病例数	构成(%)	粗率($1/10^5$)	世标率($1/10^5$)	累积率(%) 0~64	累积率(%) 0~74	病例数	构成(%)	粗率($1/10^5$)	世标率($1/10^5$)	累积率(%) 0~64	累积率(%) 0~74
唇	C00	0	0.00	0.00	0.00	0.00	0.00	2	0.88	1.16	0.44	0.00	0.00
舌	C01–C02	0	0.00	0.00	0.00	0.00	0.00	0	0.00	0.00	0.00	0.00	0.00
口	C03–C06	1	0.26	0.53	0.23	0.00	0.00	0	0.00	0.00	0.00	0.00	0.00
唾液腺	C07–C08	0	0.00	0.00	0.00	0.00	0.00	1	0.44	0.58	0.37	0.00	0.06
扁桃体	C09	0	0.00	0.00	0.00	0.00	0.00	0	0.00	0.00	0.00	0.00	0.00
其他的口咽	C10	0	0.00	0.00	0.00	0.00	0.00	0	0.00	0.00	0.00	0.00	0.00
鼻咽	C11	4	1.03	2.13	1.33	0.13	0.13	0	0.00	0.00	0.00	0.00	0.00
喉咽	C12–C13	0	0.00	0.00	0.00	0.00	0.00	0	0.00	0.00	0.00	0.00	0.00
咽，部位不明	C14	1	0.26	0.53	0.36	0.00	0.06	0	0.00	0.00	0.00	0.00	0.00
食管	C15	72	18.51	38.39	22.90	0.77	2.74	29	12.83	16.79	8.88	0.21	1.01
胃	C16	98	25.19	52.25	31.05	0.90	3.58	34	15.04	19.69	11.64	0.53	1.50
小肠	C17	3	0.77	1.60	1.12	0.07	0.13	0	0.00	0.00	0.00	0.00	0.00
结肠	C18	7	1.80	3.73	2.21	0.17	0.25	4	1.77	2.32	1.13	0.08	0.08
直肠	C19–C20	13	3.34	6.93	4.27	0.17	0.41	11	4.87	6.37	3.33	0.16	0.25
肛门	C21	0	0.00	0.00	0.00	0.00	0.00	1	0.44	0.58	0.37	0.00	0.06
肝脏	C22	48	12.34	25.59	16.80	0.84	1.93	11	4.87	6.37	3.53	0.17	0.32
胆囊及其他	C23–C24	5	1.29	2.67	1.57	0.03	0.18	5	2.21	2.89	1.51	0.05	0.14
胰腺	C25	9	2.31	4.80	3.08	0.11	0.44	10	4.42	5.79	3.29	0.13	0.34
鼻、鼻窦及其他	C30–C31	1	0.26	0.53	0.37	0.05	0.05	1	0.44	0.58	0.23	0.00	0.00
喉	C32	1	0.26	0.53	0.36	0.00	0.06	0	0.00	0.00	0.00	0.00	0.00
气管、支气管、肺	C33–C34	82	21.08	43.72	26.78	1.09	3.48	32	14.16	18.53	10.18	0.46	1.19
其他的胸腔器官	C37–C38	1	0.26	0.53	0.27	0.00	0.00	1	0.44	0.58	0.32	0.04	0.04
骨	C40–C41	3	0.77	1.60	1.12	0.04	0.10	1	0.44	0.58	0.27	0.00	0.00
皮肤的黑色素瘤	C43	0	0.00	0.00	0.00	0.00	0.00	0	0.00	0.00	0.00	0.00	0.00
其他的皮肤	C44	1	0.26	0.53	0.23	0.00	0.00	0	0.00	0.00	0.00	0.00	0.00
间皮瘤	C45	0	0.00	0.00	0.00	0.00	0.00	0	0.00	0.00	0.00	0.00	0.00
卡波西肉瘤	C46	0	0.00	0.00	0.00	0.00	0.00	0	0.00	0.00	0.00	0.00	0.00
周围神经、其他结缔组织、软组织	C47;C49	1	0.26	0.53	0.34	0.03	0.03	0	0.00	0.00	0.00	0.00	0.00
乳房	C50	2	0.51	1.07	0.78	0.03	0.09	10	4.42	5.79	3.57	0.31	0.40
外阴	C51	0	0.00	0.00	0.00	0.00	0.00	0	0.00	0.00	0.00	0.00	0.00
阴道	C52	0	0.00	0.00	0.00	0.00	0.00	0	0.00	0.00	0.00	0.00	0.00
子宫颈	C53	0	0.00	0.00	0.00	0.00	0.00	22	9.73	12.74	7.30	0.33	0.87
子宫体	C54	0	0.00	0.00	0.00	0.00	0.00	6	2.65	3.47	1.75	0.04	0.19
子宫，部位不明	C55	0	0.00	0.00	0.00	0.00	0.00	0	0.00	0.00	0.00	0.00	0.00
卵巢	C56	0	0.00	0.00	0.00	0.00	0.00	13	5.75	7.53	4.59	0.16	0.62
女性其他的生殖器	C57	0	0.00	0.00	0.00	0.00	0.00	0	0.00	0.00	0.00	0.00	0.00
胎盘	C58	0	0.00	0.00	0.00	0.00	0.00	0	0.00	0.00	0.00	0.00	0.00
阴茎	C60	0	0.00	0.00	0.00	0.00	0.00	0	0.00	0.00	0.00	0.00	0.00
前列腺	C61	5	1.29	2.67	1.65	0.09	0.15	0	0.00	0.00	0.00	0.00	0.00
睾丸	C62	1	0.26	0.53	0.28	0.00	0.00	0	0.00	0.00	0.00	0.00	0.00
男性其他的生殖器	C63	0	0.00	0.00	0.00	0.00	0.00	0	0.00	0.00	0.00	0.00	0.00
肾	C64	4	1.03	2.13	1.32	0.00	0.18	2	0.88	1.16	0.66	0.05	0.05
肾盂	C65	0	0.00	0.00	0.00	0.00	0.00	0	0.00	0.00	0.00	0.00	0.00
输尿管	C66	0	0.00	0.00	0.00	0.00	0.00	1	0.44	0.58	0.27	0.00	0.00
膀胱	C67	2	0.51	1.07	0.70	0.00	0.17	2	0.88	1.16	0.50	0.00	0.00
其他的泌尿器官	C68	1	0.26	0.53	0.31	0.04	0.04	0	0.00	0.00	0.00	0.00	0.00
眼	C69	0	0.00	0.00	0.00	0.00	0.00	0	0.00	0.00	0.00	0.00	0.00
脑、神经系统	C70–C72	7	1.80	3.73	2.96	0.19	0.28	13	5.75	7.53	4.79	0.28	0.49
甲状腺	C73	2	0.51	1.07	0.62	0.03	0.03	3	1.33	1.74	0.86	0.08	0.08
肾上腺	C74	1	0.26	0.53	0.35	0.00	0.09	0	0.00	0.00	0.00	0.00	0.00
其他的内分泌腺	C75	1	0.26	0.53	0.65	0.04	0.04	0	0.00	0.00	0.00	0.00	0.00
霍奇金病	C81	0	0.00	0.00	0.00	0.00	0.00	0	0.00	0.00	0.00	0.00	0.00
非霍奇金淋巴瘤	C82–C85;C96	2	0.51	1.07	0.58	0.04	0.04	2	0.88	1.16	0.57	0.00	0.09
免疫增生性疾病	C88	0	0.00	0.00	0.00	0.00	0.00	0	0.00	0.00	0.00	0.00	0.00
多发性骨髓瘤	C90	1	0.26	0.53	0.36	0.00	0.06	0	0.00	0.00	0.00	0.00	0.00
淋巴样白血病	C91	0	0.00	0.00	0.00	0.00	0.00	0	0.00	0.00	0.00	0.00	0.00
髓样白血病	C92–C94	2	0.51	1.07	0.70	0.03	0.09	1	0.44	0.58	0.37	0.00	0.06
白血病，未特指	C95	2	0.51	1.07	1.55	0.08	0.08	4	1.77	2.32	0.92	0.00	0.00
其他的或未指明部位	O&U	5	1.29	2.67	1.65	0.03	0.24	4	1.77	2.32	1.51	0.16	0.16
骨髓增殖性疾病	MPD	0	0.00	0.00	0.00	0.00	0.00	0	0.00	0.00	0.00	0.00	0.00
骨髓增生异常综合征	MDS	0	0.00	0.00	0.00	0.00	0.00	0	0.00	0.00	0.00	0.00	0.00
合计	ALL	389	100.00	207.42	128.84	5.03	15.17	226	100.00	130.85	73.17	3.25	8.02
C44 以外的部位	ALL but C44	388	99.74	206.88	128.61	5.03	15.17	226	100.00	130.85	73.17	3.25	8.02

表 6-39　2020 年河南省嵩县恶性肿瘤发病主要指标

部位	ICD-10	男性						女性					
		病例数	构成(%)	粗率($1/10^5$)	世标率($1/10^5$)	累积率(%)		病例数	构成(%)	粗率($1/10^5$)	世标率($1/10^5$)	累积率(%)	
						0～64	0～74					0～64	0～74
唇	C00	1	0.11	0.30	0.23	0.00	0.06	0	0.00	0.00	0.00	0.00	0.00
舌	C01–C02	4	0.43	1.18	0.77	0.06	0.06	1	0.13	0.33	0.25	0.00	0.06
口	C03–C06	2	0.21	0.59	0.44	0.03	0.03	1	0.13	0.33	0.25	0.00	0.06
唾液腺	C07–C08	1	0.11	0.30	0.38	0.02	0.02	1	0.13	0.33	0.20	0.00	0.03
扁桃体	C09	0	0.00	0.00	0.00	0.00	0.00	0	0.00	0.00	0.00	0.00	0.00
其他的口咽	C10	1	0.11	0.30	0.19	0.00	0.03	0	0.00	0.00	0.00	0.00	0.00
鼻咽	C11	5	0.53	1.48	0.98	0.07	0.13	0	0.00	0.00	0.00	0.00	0.00
喉咽	C12–C13	0	0.00	0.00	0.00	0.00	0.00	0	0.00	0.00	0.00	0.00	0.00
咽，部位不明	C14	0	0.00	0.00	0.00	0.00	0.00	0	0.00	0.00	0.00	0.00	0.00
食管	C15	228	24.23	67.49	46.29	2.30	5.45	149	19.05	48.47	28.44	0.92	3.03
胃	C16	227	24.12	67.20	46.70	2.12	5.84	93	11.89	30.26	18.51	0.67	1.91
小肠	C17	4	0.43	1.18	0.80	0.00	0.15	0	0.00	0.00	0.00	0.00	0.00
结肠	C18	34	3.61	10.06	7.02	0.53	0.69	32	4.09	10.41	7.32	0.40	1.01
直肠	C19–C20	40	4.25	11.84	7.95	0.58	0.89	26	3.32	8.46	5.26	0.17	0.65
肛门	C21	0	0.00	0.00	0.00	0.00	0.00	1	0.13	0.33	0.20	0.00	0.03
肝脏	C22	71	7.55	21.02	14.50	0.91	1.60	43	5.50	13.99	8.51	0.34	1.05
胆囊及其他	C23–C24	7	0.74	2.07	1.32	0.02	0.21	13	1.66	4.23	2.55	0.11	0.31
胰腺	C25	13	1.38	3.85	2.65	0.09	0.40	8	1.02	2.60	1.79	0.03	0.13
鼻、鼻窦及其他	C30–C31	5	0.53	1.48	1.34	0.06	0.09	4	0.51	1.30	0.65	0.04	0.04
喉	C32	7	0.74	2.07	1.43	0.16	0.16	2	0.26	0.65	0.46	0.03	0.07
气管、支气管、肺	C33–C34	153	16.26	45.29	31.28	1.55	4.00	78	9.97	25.38	16.19	0.86	1.87
其他的胸腔器官	C37–C38	4	0.43	1.18	0.79	0.02	0.14	3	0.38	0.98	0.60	0.02	0.06
骨	C40–C41	12	1.28	3.55	2.88	0.14	0.35	4	0.51	1.30	0.97	0.03	0.13
皮肤的黑色素瘤	C43	1	0.11	0.30	0.19	0.02	0.02	0	0.00	0.00	0.00	0.00	0.00
其他的皮肤	C44	6	0.64	1.78	1.30	0.05	0.14	5	0.64	1.63	0.90	0.00	0.10
间皮瘤	C45	0	0.00	0.00	0.00	0.00	0.00	0	0.00	0.00	0.00	0.00	0.00
卡波西肉瘤	C46	0	0.00	0.00	0.00	0.00	0.00	0	0.00	0.00	0.00	0.00	0.00
周围神经、其他结缔组织、软组织	C47;C49	2	0.21	0.59	0.33	0.02	0.02	1	0.13	0.33	0.26	0.03	0.03
乳房	C50	1	0.11	0.30	0.15	0.00	0.00	95	12.15	30.91	23.98	1.80	2.71
外阴	C51	0	0.00	0.00	0.00	0.00	0.00	1	0.13	0.33	0.20	0.00	0.03
阴道	C52	0	0.00	0.00	0.00	0.00	0.00	0	0.00	0.00	0.00	0.00	0.00
子宫颈	C53	0	0.00	0.00	0.00	0.00	0.00	86	11.00	27.98	20.27	1.48	2.19
子宫体	C54	0	0.00	0.00	0.00	0.00	0.00	23	2.94	7.48	5.76	0.53	0.66
子宫，部位不明	C55	0	0.00	0.00	0.00	0.00	0.00	1	0.13	0.33	0.43	0.03	0.03
卵巢	C56	0	0.00	0.00	0.00	0.00	0.00	19	2.43	6.18	4.33	0.32	0.58
女性其他的生殖器	C57	0	0.00	0.00	0.00	0.00	0.00	0	0.00	0.00	0.00	0.00	0.00
胎盘	C58	0	0.00	0.00	0.00	0.00	0.00	0	0.00	0.00	0.00	0.00	0.00
阴茎	C60	5	0.53	1.48	0.94	0.05	0.11	0	0.00	0.00	0.00	0.00	0.00
前列腺	C61	15	1.59	4.44	2.81	0.00	0.25	0	0.00	0.00	0.00	0.00	0.00
睾丸	C62	0	0.00	0.00	0.00	0.00	0.00	0	0.00	0.00	0.00	0.00	0.00
男性其他的生殖器	C63	0	0.00	0.00	0.00	0.00	0.00	0	0.00	0.00	0.00	0.00	0.00
肾	C64	9	0.96	2.66	2.16	0.13	0.25	8	1.02	2.60	1.88	0.16	0.22
肾盂	C65	0	0.00	0.00	0.00	0.00	0.00	1	0.13	0.33	0.25	0.00	0.06
输尿管	C66	5	0.53	1.48	1.09	0.08	0.11	0	0.00	0.00	0.00	0.00	0.00
膀胱	C67	12	1.28	3.55	2.71	0.11	0.38	4	0.51	1.30	0.72	0.02	0.06
其他的泌尿器官	C68	0	0.00	0.00	0.00	0.00	0.00	0	0.00	0.00	0.00	0.00	0.00
眼	C69	3	0.32	0.89	0.92	0.05	0.08	0	0.00	0.00	0.00	0.00	0.00
脑、神经系统	C70–C72	13	1.38	3.85	3.38	0.23	0.32	14	1.79	4.55	3.69	0.20	0.39
甲状腺	C73	17	1.81	5.03	3.92	0.30	0.36	43	5.50	13.99	10.19	0.97	1.04
肾上腺	C74	0	0.00	0.00	0.00	0.00	0.00	0	0.00	0.00	0.00	0.00	0.00
其他的内分泌腺	C75	1	0.11	0.30	0.34	0.03	0.03	0	0.00	0.00	0.00	0.00	0.00
霍奇金病	C81	0	0.00	0.00	0.00	0.00	0.00	0	0.00	0.00	0.00	0.00	0.00
非霍奇金淋巴瘤	C82–C85;C96	16	1.70	4.74	3.27	0.25	0.37	7	0.90	2.28	2.07	0.09	0.23
免疫增生性疾病	C88	1	0.11	0.30	0.57	0.02	0.02	0	0.00	0.00	0.00	0.00	0.00
多发性骨髓瘤	C90	2	0.21	0.59	0.38	0.02	0.05	3	0.38	0.98	0.60	0.05	0.08
淋巴样白血病	C91	0	0.00	0.00	0.00	0.00	0.00	0	0.00	0.00	0.00	0.00	0.00
髓样白血病	C92–C94	5	0.53	1.48	1.39	0.07	0.14	5	0.64	1.63	1.31	0.07	0.20
白血病，未特指	C95	4	0.43	1.18	1.33	0.06	0.09	3	0.38	0.98	0.93	0.05	0.05
其他的或未指明部位	O&U	4	0.43	1.18	0.89	0.03	0.06	4	0.51	1.30	0.98	0.08	0.14
骨髓增殖性疾病	MPD	0	0.00	0.00	0.00	0.00	0.00	0	0.00	0.00	0.00	0.00	0.00
骨髓增生异常综合征	MDS	0	0.00	0.00	0.00	0.00	0.00	0	0.00	0.00	0.00	0.00	0.00
合计	ALL	941	100.00	278.56	196.00	10.17	23.10	782	100.00	254.41	170.92	9.50	19.24
C44 以外的部位	ALL but C44	935	99.36	276.78	194.69	10.12	22.96	777	99.36	252.79	170.01	9.50	19.14

表 6-40 2020 年河南省嵩县恶性肿瘤死亡主要指标

部位	ICD-10	男性						女性					
		病例数	构成(%)	粗率(1/10^5)	世标率(1/10^5)	累积率(%) 0~64	累积率(%) 0~74	病例数	构成(%)	粗率(1/10^5)	世标率(1/10^5)	累积率(%) 0~64	累积率(%) 0~74
唇	C00	0	0.00	0.00	0.00	0.00	0.00	0	0.00	0.00	0.00	0.00	0.00
舌	C01-C02	0	0.00	0.00	0.00	0.00	0.00	0	0.00	0.00	0.00	0.00	0.00
口	C03-C06	2	0.27	0.59	0.40	0.02	0.02	1	0.23	0.33	0.11	0.00	0.00
唾液腺	C07-C08	1	0.13	0.30	0.19	0.00	0.00	0	0.00	0.00	0.00	0.00	0.00
扁桃体	C09	0	0.00	0.00	0.00	0.00	0.00	0	0.00	0.00	0.00	0.00	0.00
其他的口咽	C10	1	0.13	0.30	0.23	0.00	0.06	0	0.00	0.00	0.00	0.00	0.00
鼻咽	C11	1	0.13	0.30	0.18	0.02	0.02	0	0.00	0.00	0.00	0.00	0.00
喉咽	C12-C13	1	0.13	0.30	0.23	0.00	0.06	0	0.00	0.00	0.00	0.00	0.00
咽，部位不明	C14	0	0.00	0.00	0.00	0.00	0.00	0	0.00	0.00	0.00	0.00	0.00
食管	C15	207	27.53	61.28	41.74	1.53	4.78	119	26.86	38.71	23.45	0.90	2.87
胃	C16	199	26.46	58.91	40.12	1.43	4.67	72	16.25	23.42	13.79	0.37	1.72
小肠	C17	2	0.27	0.59	0.43	0.02	0.05	1	0.23	0.33	0.11	0.00	0.00
结肠	C18	13	1.73	3.85	2.72	0.18	0.21	15	3.39	4.88	3.34	0.15	0.47
直肠	C19-C20	16	2.13	4.74	3.37	0.20	0.20	17	3.84	5.53	3.43	0.19	0.42
肛门	C21	0	0.00	0.00	0.00	0.00	0.00	0	0.00	0.00	0.00	0.00	0.00
肝脏	C22	66	8.78	19.54	13.53	0.88	1.54	39	8.80	12.69	8.17	0.30	0.94
胆囊及其他	C23-C24	5	0.66	1.48	0.99	0.03	0.15	13	2.93	4.23	2.40	0.04	0.30
胰腺	C25	15	1.99	4.44	3.10	0.08	0.38	5	1.13	1.63	0.93	0.00	0.03
鼻、鼻窦及其他	C30-C31	0	0.00	0.00	0.00	0.00	0.00	1	0.23	0.33	0.26	0.03	0.03
喉	C32	5	0.66	1.48	0.92	0.07	0.11	0	0.00	0.00	0.00	0.00	0.00
气管、支气管、肺	C33-C34	142	18.88	42.04	28.99	1.18	3.52	61	13.77	19.85	12.44	0.67	1.60
其他的胸腔器官	C37-C38	0	0.00	0.00	0.00	0.00	0.00	1	0.23	0.33	0.12	0.00	0.00
骨	C40-C41	12	1.60	3.55	2.56	0.08	0.30	3	0.68	0.98	0.60	0.05	0.08
皮肤的黑色素瘤	C43	1	0.13	0.30	0.19	0.00	0.03	0	0.00	0.00	0.00	0.00	0.00
其他的皮肤	C44	2	0.27	0.59	0.43	0.00	0.06	3	0.68	0.98	0.43	0.00	0.00
间皮瘤	C45	0	0.00	0.00	0.00	0.00	0.00	0	0.00	0.00	0.00	0.00	0.00
卡波西肉瘤	C46	0	0.00	0.00	0.00	0.00	0.00	0	0.00	0.00	0.00	0.00	0.00
周围神经、其他结缔组织、软组织	C47;C49	0	0.00	0.00	0.00	0.00	0.00	1	0.23	0.33	0.36	0.02	0.02
乳房	C50	1	0.13	0.30	0.15	0.00	0.00	20	4.51	6.51	4.56	0.29	0.61
外阴	C51	0	0.00	0.00	0.00	0.00	0.00	0	0.00	0.00	0.00	0.00	0.00
阴道	C52	0	0.00	0.00	0.00	0.00	0.00	1	0.23	0.33	0.25	0.00	0.06
子宫颈	C53	0	0.00	0.00	0.00	0.00	0.00	21	4.74	6.83	4.76	0.19	0.55
子宫体	C54	0	0.00	0.00	0.00	0.00	0.00	9	2.03	2.93	1.72	0.11	0.15
子宫，部位不明	C55	0	0.00	0.00	0.00	0.00	0.00	1	0.23	0.33	0.12	0.00	0.00
卵巢	C56	0	0.00	0.00	0.00	0.00	0.00	13	2.93	4.23	2.74	0.16	0.44
女性其他的生殖器	C57	0	0.00	0.00	0.00	0.00	0.00	0	0.00	0.00	0.00	0.00	0.00
胎盘	C58	0	0.00	0.00	0.00	0.00	0.00	0	0.00	0.00	0.00	0.00	0.00
阴茎	C60	1	0.13	0.30	0.19	0.00	0.00	0	0.00	0.00	0.00	0.00	0.00
前列腺	C61	9	1.20	2.66	1.59	0.00	0.12	0	0.00	0.00	0.00	0.00	0.00
睾丸	C62	0	0.00	0.00	0.00	0.00	0.00	0	0.00	0.00	0.00	0.00	0.00
男性其他的生殖器	C63	0	0.00	0.00	0.00	0.00	0.00	0	0.00	0.00	0.00	0.00	0.00
肾	C64	7	0.93	2.07	1.35	0.04	0.10	3	0.68	0.98	0.51	0.02	0.02
肾盂	C65	0	0.00	0.00	0.00	0.00	0.00	0	0.00	0.00	0.00	0.00	0.00
输尿管	C66	1	0.13	0.30	0.21	0.00	0.00	0	0.00	0.00	0.00	0.00	0.00
膀胱	C67	8	1.06	2.37	1.83	0.06	0.17	1	0.23	0.33	0.11	0.00	0.00
其他的泌尿器官	C68	0	0.00	0.00	0.00	0.00	0.00	0	0.00	0.00	0.00	0.00	0.00
眼	C69	0	0.00	0.00	0.00	0.00	0.00	0	0.00	0.00	0.00	0.00	0.00
脑、神经系统	C70-C72	10	1.33	2.96	2.31	0.13	0.23	7	1.58	2.28	2.01	0.12	0.22
甲状腺	C73	3	0.40	0.89	0.56	0.02	0.09	0	0.00	0.00	0.00	0.00	0.00
肾上腺	C74	0	0.00	0.00	0.00	0.00	0.00	0	0.00	0.00	0.00	0.00	0.00
其他的内分泌腺	C75	0	0.00	0.00	0.00	0.00	0.00	0	0.00	0.00	0.00	0.00	0.00
霍奇金病	C81	0	0.00	0.00	0.00	0.00	0.00	0	0.00	0.00	0.00	0.00	0.00
非霍奇金淋巴瘤	C82-C85;C96	9	1.20	2.66	2.20	0.18	0.24	9	2.03	2.93	2.36	0.13	0.25
免疫增生性疾病	C88	0	0.00	0.00	0.00	0.00	0.00	0	0.00	0.00	0.00	0.00	0.00
多发性骨髓瘤	C90	2	0.27	0.59	0.40	0.00	0.03	0	0.00	0.00	0.00	0.00	0.00
淋巴样白血病	C91	0	0.00	0.00	0.00	0.00	0.00	1	0.23	0.33	0.40	0.03	0.03
髓样白血病	C92-C94	3	0.40	0.89	0.82	0.07	0.07	3	0.68	0.98	0.86	0.07	0.10
白血病，未特指	C95	4	0.53	1.18	1.17	0.07	0.10	1	0.23	0.33	0.20	0.02	0.02
其他的或未指明部位	O&U	3	0.40	0.89	0.75	0.03	0.06	1	0.23	0.33	0.21	0.00	0.00
骨髓增殖性疾病	MPD	0	0.00	0.00	0.00	0.00	0.00	0	0.00	0.00	0.00	0.00	0.00
骨髓增生异常综合征	MDS	0	0.00	0.00	0.00	0.00	0.00	0	0.00	0.00	0.00	0.00	0.00
合计	ALL	752	100.00	222.61	153.86	6.32	17.36	443	100.00	144.12	90.76	3.89	10.95
C44 以外的部位	ALL but C44	750	99.73	222.02	153.43	6.32	17.30	440	99.32	143.15	90.34	3.89	10.95

表 6-41 2020 年河南省汝阳县恶性肿瘤发病主要指标

部位	ICD-10	男性						女性					
		病例数	构成(%)	粗率(1/10^5)	世标率(1/10^5)	累积率(%) 0~64	累积率(%) 0~74	病例数	构成(%)	粗率(1/10^5)	世标率(1/10^5)	累积率(%) 0~64	累积率(%) 0~74
唇	C00	1	0.15	0.36	0.18	0.00	0.00	0	0.00	0.00	0.00	0.00	0.00
舌	C01–C02	0	0.00	0.00	0.00	0.00	0.00	1	0.15	0.39	0.29	0.00	0.07
口	C03–C06	2	0.29	0.73	0.56	0.00	0.14	0	0.00	0.00	0.00	0.00	0.00
唾液腺	C07–C08	10	1.46	3.63	3.09	0.21	0.39	1	0.15	0.39	0.14	0.00	0.00
扁桃体	C09	0	0.00	0.00	0.00	0.00	0.00	0	0.00	0.00	0.00	0.00	0.00
其他的口咽	C10	0	0.00	0.00	0.00	0.00	0.00	0	0.00	0.00	0.00	0.00	0.00
鼻咽	C11	4	0.58	1.45	0.95	0.00	0.11	1	0.15	0.39	0.34	0.03	0.03
喉咽	C12–C13	0	0.00	0.00	0.00	0.00	0.00	0	0.00	0.00	0.00	0.00	0.00
咽，部位不明	C14	2	0.29	0.73	0.72	0.06	0.06	0	0.00	0.00	0.00	0.00	0.00
食管	C15	109	15.94	39.62	28.09	1.01	3.88	73	10.81	28.41	16.61	0.66	1.74
胃	C16	141	20.61	51.25	35.71	1.41	4.24	44	6.52	17.12	11.05	0.46	1.32
小肠	C17	8	1.17	2.91	2.31	0.21	0.35	3	0.44	1.17	0.76	0.04	0.09
结肠	C18	13	1.90	4.73	3.81	0.20	0.43	22	3.26	8.56	6.20	0.37	0.73
直肠	C19–C20	34	4.97	12.36	9.55	0.53	1.05	24	3.56	9.34	5.92	0.28	0.70
肛门	C21	0	0.00	0.00	0.00	0.00	0.00	0	0.00	0.00	0.00	0.00	0.00
肝脏	C22	55	8.04	19.99	14.97	0.98	1.60	25	3.70	9.73	6.49	0.32	0.65
胆囊及其他	C23–C24	6	0.88	2.18	1.47	0.06	0.17	10	1.48	3.89	2.27	0.05	0.31
胰腺	C25	5	0.73	1.82	1.11	0.03	0.07	14	2.07	5.45	3.86	0.18	0.50
鼻、鼻窦及其他	C30–C31	3	0.44	1.09	1.16	0.08	0.08	1	0.15	0.39	0.49	0.03	0.03
喉	C32	2	0.29	0.73	0.51	0.06	0.06	0	0.00	0.00	0.00	0.00	0.00
气管、支气管、肺	C33–C34	169	24.71	61.43	44.29	2.15	5.44	77	11.41	29.96	19.88	1.06	2.32
其他的胸腔器官	C37–C38	1	0.15	0.36	0.25	0.00	0.04	2	0.30	0.78	0.54	0.06	0.06
骨	C40–C41	9	1.32	3.27	3.03	0.19	0.26	3	0.44	1.17	0.93	0.09	0.09
皮肤的黑色素瘤	C43	0	0.00	0.00	0.00	0.00	0.00	0	0.00	0.00	0.00	0.00	0.00
其他的皮肤	C44	6	0.88	2.18	1.55	0.05	0.12	5	0.74	1.95	1.07	0.03	0.07
间皮瘤	C45	1	0.15	0.36	0.38	0.02	0.02	0	0.00	0.00	0.00	0.00	0.00
卡波西肉瘤	C46	0	0.00	0.00	0.00	0.00	0.00	0	0.00	0.00	0.00	0.00	0.00
周围神经、其他结缔组织、软组织	C47;C49	0	0.00	0.00	0.00	0.00	0.00	5	0.74	1.95	1.60	0.06	0.25
乳房	C50	1	0.15	0.36	0.25	0.00	0.04	110	16.30	42.81	35.05	3.08	3.47
外阴	C51	0	0.00	0.00	0.00	0.00	0.00	1	0.15	0.39	0.16	0.00	0.00
阴道	C52	0	0.00	0.00	0.00	0.00	0.00	2	0.30	0.78	0.42	0.00	0.04
子宫颈	C53	0	0.00	0.00	0.00	0.00	0.00	59	8.74	22.96	19.65	1.60	1.80
子宫体	C54	0	0.00	0.00	0.00	0.00	0.00	25	3.70	9.73	7.69	0.69	0.90
子宫，部位不明	C55	0	0.00	0.00	0.00	0.00	0.00	1	0.15	0.39	0.28	0.03	0.03
卵巢	C56	0	0.00	0.00	0.00	0.00	0.00	15	2.22	5.84	4.94	0.31	0.47
女性其他的生殖器	C57	0	0.00	0.00	0.00	0.00	0.00	5	0.74	1.95	1.70	0.15	0.15
胎盘	C58	0	0.00	0.00	0.00	0.00	0.00	0	0.00	0.00	0.00	0.00	0.00
阴茎	C60	0	0.00	0.00	0.00	0.00	0.00	0	0.00	0.00	0.00	0.00	0.00
前列腺	C61	12	1.75	4.36	3.08	0.04	0.37	0	0.00	0.00	0.00	0.00	0.00
睾丸	C62	2	0.29	0.73	0.49	0.02	0.06	0	0.00	0.00	0.00	0.00	0.00
男性其他的生殖器	C63	1	0.15	0.36	0.25	0.00	0.04	0	0.00	0.00	0.00	0.00	0.00
肾	C64	7	1.02	2.54	1.77	0.11	0.15	7	1.04	2.72	1.75	0.10	0.15
肾盂	C65	0	0.00	0.00	0.00	0.00	0.00	0	0.00	0.00	0.00	0.00	0.00
输尿管	C66	1	0.15	0.36	0.25	0.00	0.04	0	0.00	0.00	0.00	0.00	0.00
膀胱	C67	9	1.32	3.27	2.39	0.13	0.30	3	0.44	1.17	1.02	0.08	0.08
其他的泌尿器官	C68	0	0.00	0.00	0.00	0.00	0.00	0	0.00	0.00	0.00	0.00	0.00
眼	C69	0	0.00	0.00	0.00	0.00	0.00	2	0.30	0.78	0.67	0.02	0.02
脑、神经系统	C70–C72	19	2.78	6.91	5.51	0.29	0.72	24	3.56	9.34	7.77	0.35	0.68
甲状腺	C73	14	2.05	5.09	4.14	0.34	0.34	70	10.37	27.24	22.65	2.06	2.19
肾上腺	C74	1	0.15	0.36	0.18	0.00	0.00	1	0.15	0.39	0.26	0.00	0.04
其他的内分泌腺	C75	1	0.15	0.36	0.40	0.03	0.03	0	0.00	0.00	0.00	0.00	0.00
霍奇金病	C81	1	0.15	0.36	0.26	0.03	0.03	0	0.00	0.00	0.00	0.00	0.00
非霍奇金淋巴瘤	C82–C85;C96	3	0.44	1.09	0.91	0.06	0.06	14	2.07	5.45	4.03	0.20	0.47
免疫增生性疾病	C88	0	0.00	0.00	0.00	0.00	0.00	0	0.00	0.00	0.00	0.00	0.00
多发性骨髓瘤	C90	6	0.88	2.18	1.62	0.05	0.19	3	0.44	1.17	0.88	0.10	0.10
淋巴样白血病	C91	0	0.00	0.00	0.00	0.00	0.00	1	0.15	0.39	0.14	0.00	0.00
髓样白血病	C92–C94	1	0.15	0.36	0.38	0.02	0.02	5	0.74	1.95	1.34	0.10	0.10
白血病，未特指	C95	11	1.61	4.00	3.33	0.25	0.33	7	1.04	2.72	3.33	0.14	0.18
其他的或未指明部位	O&U	13	1.90	4.73	4.98	0.29	0.40	8	1.19	3.11	2.88	0.24	0.24
骨髓增殖性疾病	MPD	0	0.00	0.00	0.00	0.00	0.00	0	0.00	0.00	0.00	0.00	0.00
骨髓增生异常综合征	MDS	0	0.00	0.00	0.00	0.00	0.00	1	0.15	0.39	0.26	0.00	0.04
合计	ALL	684	100.00	248.63	183.90	8.90	21.65	675	100.00	262.68	195.28	12.96	20.12
C44 以外的部位	ALL but C44	678	99.12	246.45	182.35	8.85	21.52	670	99.26	260.73	194.21	12.93	20.05

表 6-42 2020 年河南省汝阳县恶性肿瘤死亡主要指标

部位	ICD-10	男性						女性					
		病例数	构成 (%)	粗率 (1/10⁵)	世标率 (1/10⁵)	累积率 (%)		病例数	构成 (%)	粗率 (1/10⁵)	世标率 (1/10⁵)	累积率 (%)	
						0~64	0~74					0~64	0~74
唇	C00	0	0.00	0.00	0.00	0.00	0.00	0	0.00	0.00	0.00	0.00	0.00
舌	C01–C02	1	0.20	0.36	0.18	0.00	0.00	1	0.31	0.39	0.43	0.04	0.04
口	C03–C06	0	0.00	0.00	0.00	0.00	0.00	1	0.31	0.39	0.26	0.00	0.04
唾液腺	C07–C08	0	0.00	0.00	0.00	0.00	0.00	0	0.00	0.00	0.00	0.00	0.00
扁桃体	C09	0	0.00	0.00	0.00	0.00	0.00	0	0.00	0.00	0.00	0.00	0.00
其他的口咽	C10	1	0.20	0.36	0.28	0.00	0.07	0	0.00	0.00	0.00	0.00	0.00
鼻咽	C11	6	1.21	2.18	1.61	0.06	0.17	0	0.00	0.00	0.00	0.00	0.00
喉咽	C12–C13	2	0.40	0.73	0.45	0.00	0.00	0	0.00	0.00	0.00	0.00	0.00
咽，部位不明	C14	0	0.00	0.00	0.00	0.00	0.00	0	0.00	0.00	0.00	0.00	0.00
食管	C15	96	19.39	34.90	23.76	0.56	2.50	53	16.36	20.63	11.30	0.08	1.07
胃	C16	113	22.83	41.07	28.57	0.90	3.49	43	13.27	16.73	9.89	0.27	1.08
小肠	C17	0	0.00	0.00	0.00	0.00	0.00	1	0.31	0.39	0.26	0.00	0.04
结肠	C18	9	1.82	3.27	2.49	0.09	0.35	15	4.63	5.84	3.59	0.23	0.36
直肠	C19–C20	7	1.41	2.54	1.87	0.03	0.29	12	3.70	4.67	3.31	0.23	0.31
肛门	C21	0	0.00	0.00	0.00	0.00	0.00	0	0.00	0.00	0.00	0.00	0.00
肝脏	C22	55	11.11	19.99	14.75	0.78	1.60	23	7.10	8.95	5.46	0.25	0.54
胆囊及其他	C23–C24	5	1.01	1.82	1.23	0.06	0.17	9	2.78	3.50	2.32	0.03	0.42
胰腺	C25	6	1.21	2.18	1.56	0.09	0.16	12	3.70	4.67	3.11	0.07	0.43
鼻、鼻窦及其他	C30–C31	3	0.61	1.09	0.72	0.02	0.09	0	0.00	0.00	0.00	0.00	0.00
喉	C32	1	0.20	0.36	0.25	0.00	0.04	0	0.00	0.00	0.00	0.00	0.00
气管、支气管、肺	C33–C34	124	25.05	45.07	31.35	1.30	3.17	56	17.28	21.79	13.75	0.59	1.56
其他的胸腔器官	C37–C38	1	0.20	0.36	0.28	0.00	0.07	3	0.93	1.17	0.96	0.08	0.08
骨	C40–C41	2	0.40	0.73	0.45	0.00	0.00	0	0.00	0.00	0.00	0.00	0.00
皮肤的黑色素瘤	C43	0	0.00	0.00	0.00	0.00	0.00	1	0.31	0.39	0.28	0.03	0.03
其他的皮肤	C44	2	0.40	0.73	0.49	0.00	0.00	2	0.62	0.78	0.40	0.00	0.00
间皮瘤	C45	0	0.00	0.00	0.00	0.00	0.00	0	0.00	0.00	0.00	0.00	0.00
卡波西肉瘤	C46	0	0.00	0.00	0.00	0.00	0.00	0	0.00	0.00	0.00	0.00	0.00
周围神经、其他结缔组织、软组织	C47;C49	3	0.61	1.09	0.87	0.07	0.07	1	0.31	0.39	0.14	0.00	0.00
乳房	C50	0	0.00	0.00	0.00	0.00	0.00	24	7.41	9.34	6.85	0.43	0.79
外阴	C51	0	0.00	0.00	0.00	0.00	0.00	1	0.31	0.39	0.29	0.00	0.07
阴道	C52	0	0.00	0.00	0.00	0.00	0.00	0	0.00	0.00	0.00	0.00	0.00
子宫颈	C53	0	0.00	0.00	0.00	0.00	0.00	17	5.25	6.62	4.52	0.21	0.60
子宫体	C54	0	0.00	0.00	0.00	0.00	0.00	4	1.23	1.56	1.07	0.03	0.07
子宫，部位不明	C55	0	0.00	0.00	0.00	0.00	0.00	0	0.00	0.00	0.00	0.00	0.00
卵巢	C56	0	0.00	0.00	0.00	0.00	0.00	7	2.16	2.72	1.90	0.11	0.19
女性其他的生殖器	C57	0	0.00	0.00	0.00	0.00	0.00	0	0.00	0.00	0.00	0.00	0.00
胎盘	C58	0	0.00	0.00	0.00	0.00	0.00	0	0.00	0.00	0.00	0.00	0.00
阴茎	C60	2	0.40	0.73	0.50	0.00	0.08	0	0.00	0.00	0.00	0.00	0.00
前列腺	C61	6	1.21	2.18	1.38	0.00	0.07	0	0.00	0.00	0.00	0.00	0.00
睾丸	C62	0	0.00	0.00	0.00	0.00	0.00	0	0.00	0.00	0.00	0.00	0.00
男性其他的生殖器	C63	0	0.00	0.00	0.00	0.00	0.00	0	0.00	0.00	0.00	0.00	0.00
肾	C64	2	0.40	0.73	0.63	0.05	0.05	1	0.31	0.39	0.14	0.00	0.00
肾盂	C65	0	0.00	0.00	0.00	0.00	0.00	0	0.00	0.00	0.00	0.00	0.00
输尿管	C66	0	0.00	0.00	0.00	0.00	0.00	0	0.00	0.00	0.00	0.00	0.00
膀胱	C67	9	1.82	3.27	2.19	0.10	0.14	2	0.62	0.78	0.43	0.00	0.07
其他的泌尿器官	C68	0	0.00	0.00	0.00	0.00	0.00	0	0.00	0.00	0.00	0.00	0.00
眼	C69	0	0.00	0.00	0.00	0.00	0.00	0	0.00	0.00	0.00	0.00	0.00
脑、神经系统	C70–C72	13	2.63	4.73	3.75	0.14	0.57	12	3.70	4.67	3.19	0.19	0.28
甲状腺	C73	3	0.61	1.09	0.72	0.00	0.11	2	0.62	0.78	0.40	0.00	0.04
肾上腺	C74	1	0.20	0.36	0.18	0.00	0.00	0	0.00	0.00	0.00	0.00	0.00
其他的内分泌腺	C75	0	0.00	0.00	0.00	0.00	0.00	0	0.00	0.00	0.00	0.00	0.00
霍奇金病	C81	0	0.00	0.00	0.00	0.00	0.00	0	0.00	0.00	0.00	0.00	0.00
非霍奇金淋巴瘤	C82–C85;C96	5	1.01	1.82	1.52	0.07	0.19	4	1.23	1.56	1.05	0.04	0.16
免疫增生性疾病	C88	0	0.00	0.00	0.00	0.00	0.00	0	0.00	0.00	0.00	0.00	0.00
多发性骨髓瘤	C90	5	1.01	1.82	1.19	0.00	0.07	1	0.31	0.39	0.34	0.04	0.04
淋巴样白血病	C91	1	0.20	0.36	0.38	0.02	0.02	1	0.31	0.39	0.26	0.03	0.03
髓样白血病	C92–C94	0	0.00	0.00	0.00	0.00	0.00	5	1.54	1.95	1.20	0.06	0.15
白血病，未特指	C95	3	0.61	1.09	0.92	0.03	0.07	3	0.93	1.17	0.95	0.05	0.09
其他的或未指明部位	O&U	1	0.20	0.36	0.31	0.04	0.04	3	0.93	1.17	0.96	0.04	0.11
骨髓增殖性疾病	MPD	1	0.20	0.36	0.21	0.00	0.00	0	0.00	0.00	0.00	0.00	0.00
骨髓增生异常综合征	MDS	6	1.21	2.18	1.94	0.03	0.17	4	1.23	1.56	0.79	0.00	0.04
合计	ALL	495	100.00	179.93	126.99	4.44	13.83	324	100.00	126.09	79.78	3.12	8.76
C44 以外的部位	ALL but C44	493	99.60	179.20	126.50	4.44	13.83	322	99.38	125.31	79.39	3.12	8.76

表 6-43　2020 年河南省宜阳县恶性肿瘤发病主要指标

部位	ICD-10	男性						女性					
		病例数	构成 (%)	粗率 (1/10⁵)	世标率 (1/10⁵)	累积率 (%)		病例数	构成 (%)	粗率 (1/10⁵)	世标率 (1/10⁵)	累积率 (%)	
						0~64	0~74					0~64	0~74
唇	C00	1	0.09	0.27	0.12	0.00	0.00	1	0.10	0.29	0.09	0.00	0.00
舌	C01–C02	1	0.09	0.27	0.23	0.02	0.02	0	0.00	0.00	0.00	0.00	0.00
口	C03–C06	2	0.19	0.54	0.42	0.02	0.05	4	0.42	1.16	0.84	0.05	0.12
唾液腺	C07–C08	3	0.28	0.81	0.46	0.03	0.03	2	0.21	0.58	0.36	0.00	0.09
扁桃体	C09	1	0.09	0.27	0.19	0.00	0.05	0	0.00	0.00	0.00	0.00	0.00
其他的口咽	C10	0	0.00	0.00	0.00	0.00	0.00	0	0.00	0.00	0.00	0.00	0.00
鼻咽	C11	1	0.09	0.27	0.20	0.00	0.03	1	0.10	0.29	0.24	0.02	0.02
喉咽	C12–C13	0	0.00	0.00	0.00	0.00	0.00	0	0.00	0.00	0.00	0.00	0.00
咽，部位不明	C14	1	0.09	0.27	0.20	0.00	0.03	1	0.10	0.29	0.08	0.00	0.00
食管	C15	219	20.56	58.89	38.70	1.34	5.08	163	16.94	47.25	26.07	0.83	3.20
胃	C16	203	19.06	54.59	36.94	1.68	4.69	87	9.04	25.22	14.12	0.55	1.52
小肠	C17	1	0.09	0.27	0.24	0.02	0.02	2	0.21	0.58	0.25	0.00	0.00
结肠	C18	27	2.54	7.26	5.13	0.32	0.56	23	2.39	6.67	3.95	0.24	0.43
直肠	C19–C20	24	2.25	6.45	4.30	0.17	0.55	44	4.57	12.75	7.55	0.28	1.05
肛门	C21	0	0.00	0.00	0.00	0.00	0.00	2	0.21	0.58	0.37	0.02	0.02
肝脏	C22	94	8.83	25.28	18.09	0.95	2.29	50	5.20	14.49	8.71	0.37	1.17
胆囊及其他	C23–C24	8	0.75	2.15	1.35	0.07	0.12	32	3.33	9.28	5.33	0.25	0.60
胰腺	C25	18	1.69	4.84	3.27	0.23	0.31	10	1.04	2.90	1.79	0.12	0.24
鼻、鼻窦及其他	C30–C31	0	0.00	0.00	0.00	0.00	0.00	2	0.21	0.58	0.41	0.02	0.05
喉	C32	7	0.66	1.88	1.19	0.05	0.13	0	0.00	0.00	0.00	0.00	0.00
气管、支气管、肺	C33–C34	246	23.10	66.15	43.59	2.04	4.91	106	11.02	30.72	18.47	0.94	2.26
其他的胸腔器官	C37–C38	0	0.00	0.00	0.00	0.00	0.00	1	0.10	0.29	0.09	0.00	0.00
骨	C40–C41	6	0.56	1.61	1.49	0.11	0.14	6	0.62	1.74	1.10	0.09	0.09
皮肤的黑色素瘤	C43	0	0.00	0.00	0.00	0.00	0.00	2	0.21	0.58	0.39	0.02	0.07
其他的皮肤	C44	4	0.38	1.08	0.61	0.00	0.03	5	0.52	1.45	0.50	0.00	0.00
间皮瘤	C45	0	0.00	0.00	0.00	0.00	0.00	0	0.00	0.00	0.00	0.00	0.00
卡波西肉瘤	C46	0	0.00	0.00	0.00	0.00	0.00	0	0.00	0.00	0.00	0.00	0.00
周围神经、其他结缔组织、软组织	C47;C49	5	0.47	1.34	0.99	0.11	0.11	4	0.42	1.16	0.86	0.04	0.12
乳房	C50	0	0.00	0.00	0.00	0.00	0.00	116	12.06	33.62	25.44	2.14	2.67
外阴	C51	0	0.00	0.00	0.00	0.00	0.00	1	0.10	0.29	0.27	0.02	0.02
阴道	C52	0	0.00	0.00	0.00	0.00	0.00	0	0.00	0.00	0.00	0.00	0.00
子宫颈	C53	0	0.00	0.00	0.00	0.00	0.00	71	7.38	20.58	15.36	1.24	1.64
子宫体	C54	0	0.00	0.00	0.00	0.00	0.00	26	2.70	7.54	5.73	0.49	0.65
子宫，部位不明	C55	0	0.00	0.00	0.00	0.00	0.00	9	0.94	2.61	1.89	0.20	0.20
卵巢	C56	0	0.00	0.00	0.00	0.00	0.00	25	2.60	7.25	5.19	0.41	0.60
女性其他的生殖器	C57	0	0.00	0.00	0.00	0.00	0.00	0	0.00	0.00	0.00	0.00	0.00
胎盘	C58	0	0.00	0.00	0.00	0.00	0.00	2	0.21	0.58	0.54	0.04	0.04
阴茎	C60	1	0.09	0.27	0.12	0.00	0.00	0	0.00	0.00	0.00	0.00	0.00
前列腺	C61	17	1.60	4.57	2.95	0.07	0.33	0	0.00	0.00	0.00	0.00	0.00
睾丸	C62	0	0.00	0.00	0.00	0.00	0.00	0	0.00	0.00	0.00	0.00	0.00
男性其他的生殖器	C63	0	0.00	0.00	0.00	0.00	0.00	0	0.00	0.00	0.00	0.00	0.00
肾	C64	21	1.97	5.65	4.38	0.36	0.49	10	1.04	2.90	1.95	0.13	0.16
肾盂	C65	0	0.00	0.00	0.00	0.00	0.00	0	0.00	0.00	0.00	0.00	0.00
输尿管	C66	2	0.19	0.54	0.41	0.00	0.07	3	0.31	0.87	0.50	0.02	0.07
膀胱	C67	18	1.69	4.84	3.57	0.18	0.56	7	0.73	2.03	1.39	0.04	0.24
其他的泌尿器官	C68	0	0.00	0.00	0.00	0.00	0.00	0	0.00	0.00	0.00	0.00	0.00
眼	C69	1	0.09	0.27	0.19	0.00	0.05	2	0.21	0.58	0.78	0.03	0.07
脑、神经系统	C70–C72	27	2.54	7.26	6.04	0.34	0.73	32	3.33	9.28	6.71	0.31	0.72
甲状腺	C73	22	2.07	5.92	4.82	0.39	0.46	49	5.09	14.20	11.17	0.83	1.09
肾上腺	C74	2	0.19	0.54	0.40	0.02	0.05	2	0.21	0.58	0.52	0.05	0.05
其他的内分泌腺	C75	2	0.19	0.54	0.31	0.02	0.02	3	0.31	0.87	0.73	0.07	0.07
霍奇金病	C81	4	0.38	1.08	0.88	0.09	0.09	0	0.00	0.00	0.00	0.00	0.00
非霍奇金淋巴瘤	C82–C85;C96	21	1.97	5.65	3.93	0.18	0.54	5	0.52	1.45	0.97	0.05	0.12
免疫增生性疾病	C88	0	0.00	0.00	0.00	0.00	0.00	0	0.00	0.00	0.00	0.00	0.00
多发性骨髓瘤	C90	8	0.75	2.15	1.50	0.07	0.19	9	0.94	2.61	1.75	0.12	0.20
淋巴样白血病	C91	6	0.56	1.61	1.95	0.11	0.15	2	0.21	0.58	0.72	0.04	0.04
髓样白血病	C92–C94	14	1.31	3.76	2.93	0.23	0.32	10	1.04	2.90	2.26	0.13	0.25
白血病，未特指	C95	12	1.13	3.23	2.72	0.22	0.30	18	1.87	5.22	4.60	0.28	0.42
其他的或未指明部位	O&U	14	1.31	3.76	3.12	0.16	0.25	10	1.04	2.90	2.40	0.12	0.27
骨髓增殖性疾病	MPD	1	0.09	0.27	0.26	0.02	0.02	2	0.21	0.58	0.43	0.03	0.06
骨髓增生异常综合征	MDS	0	0.00	0.00	0.00	0.00	0.00	0	0.00	0.00	0.00	0.00	0.00
合计	ALL	1 065	100.00	286.40	198.23	9.59	23.77	962	100.00	278.83	182.86	10.61	20.69
C44 以外的部位	ALL but C44	1 061	99.62	285.32	197.62	9.59	23.74	957	99.48	277.38	182.35	10.61	20.69

表 6-44 2020 年河南省宜阳县恶性肿瘤死亡主要指标

部位	ICD-10	男性						女性					
		病例数	构成(%)	粗率($1/10^5$)	世标率($1/10^5$)	累积率(%)		病例数	构成(%)	粗率($1/10^5$)	世标率($1/10^5$)	累积率(%)	
						0~64	0~74					0~64	0~74
唇	C00	0	0.00	0.00	0.00	0.00	0.00	1	0.20	0.29	0.09	0.00	0.00
舌	C01-C02	0	0.00	0.00	0.00	0.00	0.00	0	0.00	0.00	0.00	0.00	0.00
口	C03-C06	1	0.13	0.27	0.22	0.03	0.03	3	0.59	0.87	0.51	0.00	0.08
唾液腺	C07-C08	1	0.13	0.27	0.12	0.00	0.00	1	0.20	0.29	0.21	0.02	0.02
扁桃体	C09	0	0.00	0.00	0.00	0.00	0.00	0	0.00	0.00	0.00	0.00	0.00
其他的口咽	C10	0	0.00	0.00	0.00	0.00	0.00	0	0.00	0.00	0.00	0.00	0.00
鼻咽	C11	1	0.13	0.27	0.22	0.03	0.03	0	0.00	0.00	0.00	0.00	0.00
喉咽	C12-C13	1	0.13	0.27	0.12	0.00	0.00	0	0.00	0.00	0.00	0.00	0.00
咽，部位不明	C14	1	0.13	0.27	0.20	0.00	0.03	0	0.00	0.00	0.00	0.00	0.00
食管	C15	174	21.83	46.79	28.63	0.64	3.27	116	22.92	33.62	16.84	0.25	2.04
胃	C16	154	19.32	41.41	26.34	0.61	3.31	59	11.66	17.10	8.35	0.14	0.83
小肠	C17	0	0.00	0.00	0.00	0.00	0.00	1	0.20	0.29	0.13	0.00	0.00
结肠	C18	13	1.63	3.50	1.97	0.03	0.11	12	2.37	3.48	1.80	0.07	0.14
直肠	C19-C20	13	1.63	3.50	2.35	0.16	0.24	17	3.36	4.93	2.94	0.17	0.36
肛门	C21	1	0.13	0.27	0.12	0.00	0.00	1	0.20	0.29	0.13	0.00	0.00
肝脏	C22	83	10.41	22.32	15.16	0.74	1.68	44	8.70	12.75	7.70	0.35	0.85
胆囊及其他	C23-C24	7	0.88	1.88	1.23	0.05	0.19	21	4.15	6.09	3.25	0.12	0.35
胰腺	C25	14	1.76	3.76	2.49	0.06	0.35	10	1.98	2.90	1.73	0.09	0.22
鼻、鼻窦及其他	C30-C31	0	0.00	0.00	0.00	0.00	0.00	1	0.20	0.29	0.18	0.00	0.04
喉	C32	3	0.38	0.81	0.47	0.00	0.03	0	0.00	0.00	0.00	0.00	0.00
气管、支气管、肺	C33-C34	199	24.97	53.51	35.08	1.34	4.31	89	17.59	25.80	14.45	0.69	1.80
其他的胸腔器官	C37-C38	0	0.00	0.00	0.00	0.00	0.00	1	0.20	0.29	0.18	0.00	0.04
骨	C40-C41	3	0.38	0.81	0.59	0.02	0.09	4	0.79	1.16	0.76	0.04	0.04
皮肤的黑色素瘤	C43	1	0.13	0.27	0.20	0.00	0.03	1	0.20	0.29	0.18	0.00	0.04
其他的皮肤	C44	2	0.25	0.54	0.41	0.00	0.07	3	0.59	0.87	0.45	0.00	0.09
间皮瘤	C45	0	0.00	0.00	0.00	0.00	0.00	0	0.00	0.00	0.00	0.00	0.00
卡波西肉瘤	C46	0	0.00	0.00	0.00	0.00	0.00	0	0.00	0.00	0.00	0.00	0.00
周围神经、其他结缔组织、软组织	C47;C49	2	0.25	0.54	0.77	0.05	0.05	1	0.20	0.29	0.13	0.00	0.00
乳房	C50	1	0.13	0.27	0.14	0.00	0.00	24	4.74	6.96	4.33	0.30	0.49
外阴	C51	0	0.00	0.00	0.00	0.00	0.00	0	0.00	0.00	0.00	0.00	0.00
阴道	C52	0	0.00	0.00	0.00	0.00	0.00	0	0.00	0.00	0.00	0.00	0.00
子宫颈	C53	0	0.00	0.00	0.00	0.00	0.00	23	4.55	6.67	3.95	0.17	0.47
子宫体	C54	0	0.00	0.00	0.00	0.00	0.00	7	1.38	2.03	1.32	0.09	0.17
子宫，部位不明	C55	0	0.00	0.00	0.00	0.00	0.00	2	0.40	0.58	0.45	0.04	0.04
卵巢	C56	0	0.00	0.00	0.00	0.00	0.00	9	1.78	2.61	1.84	0.18	0.18
女性其他的生殖器	C57	0	0.00	0.00	0.00	0.00	0.00	0	0.00	0.00	0.00	0.00	0.00
胎盘	C58	0	0.00	0.00	0.00	0.00	0.00	0	0.00	0.00	0.00	0.00	0.00
阴茎	C60	0	0.00	0.00	0.00	0.00	0.00	0	0.00	0.00	0.00	0.00	0.00
前列腺	C61	15	1.88	4.03	2.37	0.04	0.25	0	0.00	0.00	0.00	0.00	0.00
睾丸	C62	0	0.00	0.00	0.00	0.00	0.00	0	0.00	0.00	0.00	0.00	0.00
男性其他的生殖器	C63	0	0.00	0.00	0.00	0.00	0.00	0	0.00	0.00	0.00	0.00	0.00
肾	C64	8	1.00	2.15	1.53	0.09	0.19	2	0.40	0.58	0.39	0.02	0.02
肾盂	C65	0	0.00	0.00	0.00	0.00	0.00	0	0.00	0.00	0.00	0.00	0.00
输尿管	C66	2	0.25	0.54	0.39	0.00	0.08	0	0.00	0.00	0.00	0.00	0.00
膀胱	C67	10	1.25	2.69	1.59	0.05	0.16	1	0.20	0.29	0.08	0.00	0.00
其他的泌尿器官	C68	0	0.00	0.00	0.00	0.00	0.00	0	0.00	0.00	0.00	0.00	0.00
眼	C69	0	0.00	0.00	0.00	0.00	0.00	0	0.00	0.00	0.00	0.00	0.00
脑、神经系统	C70-C72	23	2.89	6.19	4.60	0.16	0.50	17	3.36	4.93	3.11	0.10	0.32
甲状腺	C73	5	0.63	1.34	0.92	0.07	0.10	2	0.40	0.58	0.42	0.02	0.07
肾上腺	C74	1	0.13	0.27	0.12	0.00	0.00	1	0.20	0.29	0.29	0.02	0.02
其他的内分泌腺	C75	1	0.13	0.27	0.12	0.00	0.00	0	0.00	0.00	0.00	0.00	0.00
霍奇金病	C81	2	0.25	0.54	0.40	0.04	0.04	0	0.00	0.00	0.00	0.00	0.00
非霍奇金淋巴瘤	C82-C85;C96	12	1.51	3.23	2.11	0.05	0.30	6	1.19	1.74	1.07	0.02	0.10
免疫增生性疾病	C88	0	0.00	0.00	0.00	0.00	0.00	0	0.00	0.00	0.00	0.00	0.00
多发性骨髓瘤	C90	6	0.75	1.61	1.12	0.07	0.15	7	1.38	2.03	1.27	0.05	0.21
淋巴样白血病	C91	4	0.50	1.08	0.76	0.05	0.13	1	0.20	0.29	0.24	0.02	0.02
髓样白血病	C92-C94	9	1.13	2.42	2.00	0.12	0.20	4	0.79	1.16	0.92	0.04	0.12
白血病，未特指	C95	8	1.00	2.15	1.28	0.07	0.12	8	1.58	2.32	1.91	0.11	0.15
其他的或未指明部位	O&U	15	1.88	4.03	2.86	0.11	0.34	3	0.59	0.87	0.35	0.00	0.04
骨髓增殖性疾病	MPD	0	0.00	0.00	0.00	0.00	0.00	1	0.20	0.29	0.22	0.03	0.03
骨髓增生异常综合征	MDS	1	0.13	0.27	0.14	0.00	0.00	2	0.40	0.58	0.78	0.03	0.07
合计	ALL	797	100.00	214.33	139.15	4.68	16.42	506	100.00	146.66	82.96	3.20	9.47
C44 以外的部位	ALL but C44	795	99.75	213.79	138.74	4.68	16.35	503	99.41	145.79	82.50	3.20	9.38

表 6-45　2020 年河南省洛宁县恶性肿瘤发病主要指标

部位	ICD-10	男性						女性					
		病例数	构成(%)	粗率($1/10^5$)	世标率($1/10^5$)	累积率(%)		病例数	构成(%)	粗率($1/10^5$)	世标率($1/10^5$)	累积率(%)	
						0~64	0~74					0~64	0~74
唇	C00	0	0.00	0.00	0.00	0.00	0.00	0	0.00	0.00	0.00	0.00	0.00
舌	C01–C02	3	0.39	1.13	0.79	0.05	0.13	0	0.00	0.00	0.00	0.00	0.00
口	C03–C06	7	0.90	2.63	1.90	0.02	0.30	4	0.64	1.63	1.18	0.09	0.09
唾液腺	C07–C08	1	0.13	0.38	0.25	0.00	0.04	0	0.00	0.00	0.00	0.00	0.00
扁桃体	C09	0	0.00	0.00	0.00	0.00	0.00	0	0.00	0.00	0.00	0.00	0.00
其他的口咽	C10	0	0.00	0.00	0.00	0.00	0.00	0	0.00	0.00	0.00	0.00	0.00
鼻咽	C11	2	0.26	0.75	0.61	0.06	0.06	0	0.00	0.00	0.00	0.00	0.00
喉咽	C12–C13	1	0.13	0.38	0.26	0.00	0.00	0	0.00	0.00	0.00	0.00	0.00
咽，部位不明	C14	1	0.13	0.38	0.25	0.00	0.04	0	0.00	0.00	0.00	0.00	0.00
食管	C15	174	22.37	65.41	49.11	2.52	6.75	116	18.50	47.18	30.47	1.25	3.87
胃	C16	163	20.95	61.28	45.58	2.23	5.76	61	9.73	24.81	15.89	0.75	1.93
小肠	C17	8	1.03	3.01	2.13	0.15	0.23	5	0.80	2.03	1.30	0.11	0.15
结肠	C18	28	3.60	10.53	7.51	0.43	0.91	13	2.07	5.29	3.46	0.26	0.38
直肠	C19–C20	23	2.96	8.65	6.48	0.30	1.08	17	2.71	6.91	4.62	0.32	0.51
肛门	C21	0	0.00	0.00	0.00	0.00	0.00	0	0.00	0.00	0.00	0.00	0.00
肝脏	C22	56	7.20	21.05	15.64	0.82	1.89	31	4.94	12.61	8.54	0.42	1.17
胆囊及其他	C23–C24	23	2.96	8.65	6.68	0.28	0.64	34	5.42	13.83	8.88	0.51	0.86
胰腺	C25	11	1.41	4.14	2.99	0.18	0.42	9	1.44	3.66	2.43	0.16	0.31
鼻、鼻窦及其他	C30–C31	0	0.00	0.00	0.00	0.00	0.00	1	0.16	0.41	0.24	0.00	0.04
喉	C32	6	0.77	2.26	1.59	0.10	0.22	0	0.00	0.00	0.00	0.00	0.00
气管、支气管、肺	C33–C34	138	17.74	51.88	38.45	2.15	5.12	58	9.25	23.59	15.68	0.83	1.98
其他的胸腔器官	C37–C38	0	0.00	0.00	0.00	0.00	0.00	1	0.16	0.41	0.40	0.03	0.03
骨	C40–C41	7	0.90	2.63	1.94	0.20	0.20	3	0.48	1.22	1.05	0.07	0.11
皮肤的黑色素瘤	C43	0	0.00	0.00	0.00	0.00	0.00	1	0.16	0.41	0.26	0.03	0.03
其他的皮肤	C44	7	0.90	2.63	1.85	0.10	0.26	5	0.80	2.03	1.22	0.03	0.18
间皮瘤	C45	0	0.00	0.00	0.00	0.00	0.00	0	0.00	0.00	0.00	0.00	0.00
卡波西肉瘤	C46	0	0.00	0.00	0.00	0.00	0.00	0	0.00	0.00	0.00	0.00	0.00
周围神经、其他结缔组织、软组织	C47;C49	2	0.26	0.75	0.75	0.06	0.06	0	0.00	0.00	0.00	0.00	0.00
乳房	C50	1	0.13	0.38	0.30	0.04	0.04	84	13.40	34.16	27.05	2.30	2.64
外阴	C51	0	0.00	0.00	0.00	0.00	0.00	1	0.16	0.41	0.26	0.03	0.03
阴道	C52	0	0.00	0.00	0.00	0.00	0.00	1	0.16	0.41	0.33	0.03	0.03
子宫颈	C53	0	0.00	0.00	0.00	0.00	0.00	53	8.45	21.56	15.86	1.19	1.87
子宫体	C54	0	0.00	0.00	0.00	0.00	0.00	12	1.91	4.88	3.73	0.28	0.40
子宫，部位不明	C55	0	0.00	0.00	0.00	0.00	0.00	2	0.32	0.81	0.50	0.03	0.07
卵巢	C56	0	0.00	0.00	0.00	0.00	0.00	17	2.71	6.91	5.93	0.50	0.61
女性其他的生殖器	C57	0	0.00	0.00	0.00	0.00	0.00	0	0.00	0.00	0.00	0.00	0.00
胎盘	C58	0	0.00	0.00	0.00	0.00	0.00	0	0.00	0.00	0.00	0.00	0.00
阴茎	C60	1	0.13	0.38	0.25	0.00	0.04	0	0.00	0.00	0.00	0.00	0.00
前列腺	C61	9	1.16	3.38	2.42	0.07	0.27	0	0.00	0.00	0.00	0.00	0.00
睾丸	C62	0	0.00	0.00	0.00	0.00	0.00	0	0.00	0.00	0.00	0.00	0.00
男性其他的生殖器	C63	2	0.26	0.75	0.54	0.04	0.08	0	0.00	0.00	0.00	0.00	0.00
肾	C64	18	2.31	6.77	4.74	0.22	0.71	10	1.59	4.07	2.59	0.08	0.31
肾盂	C65	2	0.26	0.75	0.50	0.02	0.02	1	0.16	0.41	0.24	0.00	0.04
输尿管	C66	1	0.13	0.38	0.24	0.02	0.02	0	0.00	0.00	0.00	0.00	0.00
膀胱	C67	16	2.06	6.01	4.44	0.21	0.64	4	0.64	1.63	1.15	0.11	0.11
其他的泌尿器官	C68	0	0.00	0.00	0.00	0.00	0.00	0	0.00	0.00	0.00	0.00	0.00
眼	C69	1	0.13	0.38	0.31	0.00	0.08	2	0.32	0.81	1.10	0.07	0.07
脑、神经系统	C70–C72	11	1.41	4.14	3.77	0.26	0.30	11	1.75	4.47	2.98	0.18	0.34
甲状腺	C73	9	1.16	3.38	2.53	0.19	0.27	26	4.15	10.57	8.43	0.72	0.80
肾上腺	C74	2	0.26	0.75	0.62	0.00	0.15	2	0.32	0.81	0.50	0.03	0.07
其他的内分泌腺	C75	5	0.64	1.88	1.74	0.11	0.16	5	0.80	2.03	1.59	0.15	0.15
霍奇金病	C81	1	0.13	0.38	0.39	0.02	0.02	1	0.16	0.41	0.42	0.03	0.03
非霍奇金淋巴瘤	C82–C85;C96	13	1.67	4.89	3.62	0.20	0.36	14	2.23	5.69	4.35	0.27	0.40
免疫增生性疾病	C88	0	0.00	0.00	0.00	0.00	0.00	0	0.00	0.00	0.00	0.00	0.00
多发性骨髓瘤	C90	3	0.39	1.13	0.84	0.07	0.12	0	0.00	0.00	0.00	0.00	0.00
淋巴样白血病	C91	2	0.26	0.75	0.59	0.06	0.06	3	0.48	1.22	0.88	0.06	0.13
髓样白血病	C92–C94	5	0.64	1.88	1.79	0.12	0.20	7	1.12	2.85	2.17	0.20	0.20
白血病，未特指	C95	3	0.39	1.13	0.98	0.02	0.10	5	0.80	2.03	1.34	0.03	0.18
其他的或未指明部位	O&U	11	1.41	4.14	3.12	0.19	0.31	7	1.12	2.85	2.42	0.21	0.21
骨髓增殖性疾病	MPD	1	0.13	0.38	0.25	0.00	0.04	0	0.00	0.00	0.00	0.00	0.00
骨髓增生异常综合征	MDS	0	0.00	0.00	0.00	0.00	0.00	0	0.00	0.00	0.00	0.00	0.00
合计	ALL	778	100.00	292.47	218.75	11.56	28.11	627	100.00	255.01	179.45	11.34	20.31
C44 以外的部位	ALL but C44	771	99.10	289.84	216.90	11.46	27.85	622	99.20	252.98	178.23	11.32	20.13

表 6-46 2020 年河南省洛宁县恶性肿瘤死亡主要指标

部位	ICD-10	男性						女性					
		病例数	构成 (%)	粗率 ($1/10^5$)	世标率 ($1/10^5$)	累积率 (%) 0~64	累积率 (%) 0~74	病例数	构成 (%)	粗率 ($1/10^5$)	世标率 ($1/10^5$)	累积率 (%) 0~64	累积率 (%) 0~74
唇	C00	0	0.00	0.00	0.00	0.00	0.00	0	0.00	0.00	0.00	0.00	0.00
舌	C01–C02	0	0.00	0.00	0.00	0.00	0.00	0	0.00	0.00	0.00	0.00	0.00
口	C03–C06	2	0.36	0.75	0.50	0.03	0.03	1	0.32	0.41	0.19	0.00	0.00
唾液腺	C07–C08	1	0.18	0.38	0.31	0.00	0.08	1	0.32	0.41	0.26	0.03	0.03
扁桃体	C09	0	0.00	0.00	0.00	0.00	0.00	0	0.00	0.00	0.00	0.00	0.00
其他的口咽	C10	0	0.00	0.00	0.00	0.00	0.00	0	0.00	0.00	0.00	0.00	0.00
鼻咽	C11	0	0.00	0.00	0.00	0.00	0.00	0	0.00	0.00	0.00	0.00	0.00
喉咽	C12–C13	0	0.00	0.00	0.00	0.00	0.00	0	0.00	0.00	0.00	0.00	0.00
咽，部位不明	C14	0	0.00	0.00	0.00	0.00	0.00	0	0.00	0.00	0.00	0.00	0.00
食管	C15	151	26.82	56.77	44.10	1.54	5.31	75	23.73	30.50	19.84	0.81	2.06
胃	C16	134	23.80	50.37	37.61	1.54	4.29	50	15.82	20.34	12.67	0.46	1.16
小肠	C17	3	0.53	1.13	0.85	0.07	0.14	5	1.58	2.03	1.38	0.08	0.16
结肠	C18	16	2.84	6.01	4.61	0.33	0.45	6	1.90	2.44	1.51	0.03	0.27
直肠	C19–C20	12	2.13	4.51	3.52	0.12	0.40	9	2.85	3.66	2.49	0.10	0.40
肛门	C21	0	0.00	0.00	0.00	0.00	0.00	0	0.00	0.00	0.00	0.00	0.00
肝脏	C22	58	10.30	21.80	16.39	0.77	2.00	22	6.96	8.95	6.13	0.31	0.88
胆囊及其他	C23–C24	19	3.37	7.14	5.75	0.14	0.41	25	7.91	10.17	6.51	0.25	0.79
胰腺	C25	7	1.24	2.63	1.84	0.06	0.26	7	2.22	2.85	1.87	0.02	0.32
鼻、鼻窦及其他	C30–C31	0	0.00	0.00	0.00	0.00	0.00	0	0.00	0.00	0.00	0.00	0.00
喉	C32	3	0.53	1.13	0.81	0.02	0.10	0	0.00	0.00	0.00	0.00	0.00
气管、支气管、肺	C33–C34	98	17.41	36.84	28.23	1.13	3.50	41	12.97	16.68	10.86	0.60	1.29
其他的胸腔器官	C37–C38	1	0.18	0.38	0.30	0.04	0.04	0	0.00	0.00	0.00	0.00	0.00
骨	C40–C41	6	1.07	2.26	2.04	0.12	0.19	2	0.63	0.81	0.49	0.03	0.03
皮肤的黑色素瘤	C43	1	0.18	0.38	0.33	0.00	0.00	0	0.00	0.00	0.00	0.00	0.00
其他的皮肤	C44	2	0.36	0.75	0.50	0.02	0.02	2	0.63	0.81	0.47	0.00	0.04
间皮瘤	C45	0	0.00	0.00	0.00	0.00	0.00	0	0.00	0.00	0.00	0.00	0.00
卡波西肉瘤	C46	0	0.00	0.00	0.00	0.00	0.00	0	0.00	0.00	0.00	0.00	0.00
周围神经、其他结缔组织、软组织	C47;C49	0	0.00	0.00	0.00	0.00	0.00	0	0.00	0.00	0.00	0.00	0.00
乳房	C50	1	0.18	0.38	0.25	0.00	0.04	13	4.11	5.29	3.53	0.27	0.46
外阴	C51	0	0.00	0.00	0.00	0.00	0.00	0	0.00	0.00	0.00	0.00	0.00
阴道	C52	0	0.00	0.00	0.00	0.00	0.00	1	0.32	0.41	0.31	0.04	0.04
子宫颈	C53	0	0.00	0.00	0.00	0.00	0.00	12	3.80	4.88	3.03	0.06	0.52
子宫体	C54	0	0.00	0.00	0.00	0.00	0.00	0	0.00	0.00	0.00	0.00	0.00
子宫，部位不明	C55	0	0.00	0.00	0.00	0.00	0.00	1	0.32	0.41	0.24	0.00	0.04
卵巢	C56	0	0.00	0.00	0.00	0.00	0.00	6	1.90	2.44	1.70	0.09	0.24
女性其他的生殖器	C57	0	0.00	0.00	0.00	0.00	0.00	0	0.00	0.00	0.00	0.00	0.00
胎盘	C58	0	0.00	0.00	0.00	0.00	0.00	0	0.00	0.00	0.00	0.00	0.00
阴茎	C60	0	0.00	0.00	0.00	0.00	0.00	0	0.00	0.00	0.00	0.00	0.00
前列腺	C61	4	0.71	1.50	1.07	0.00	0.12	0	0.00	0.00	0.00	0.00	0.00
睾丸	C62	0	0.00	0.00	0.00	0.00	0.00	0	0.00	0.00	0.00	0.00	0.00
男性其他的生殖器	C63	1	0.18	0.38	0.30	0.04	0.04	0	0.00	0.00	0.00	0.00	0.00
肾	C64	5	0.89	1.88	1.34	0.07	0.23	3	0.95	1.22	0.61	0.00	0.04
肾盂	C65	0	0.00	0.00	0.00	0.00	0.00	1	0.32	0.41	0.28	0.00	0.00
输尿管	C66	1	0.18	0.38	0.30	0.04	0.04	0	0.00	0.00	0.00	0.00	0.00
膀胱	C67	2	0.36	0.75	0.50	0.02	0.02	2	0.63	0.81	0.43	0.00	0.04
其他的泌尿器官	C68	0	0.00	0.00	0.00	0.00	0.00	0	0.00	0.00	0.00	0.00	0.00
眼	C69	0	0.00	0.00	0.00	0.00	0.00	1	0.32	0.41	0.26	0.03	0.03
脑、神经系统	C70–C72	5	0.89	1.88	1.51	0.09	0.09	5	1.58	2.03	1.47	0.06	0.17
甲状腺	C73	0	0.00	0.00	0.00	0.00	0.00	1	0.32	0.41	0.24	0.00	0.04
肾上腺	C74	1	0.18	0.38	0.29	0.02	0.02	2	0.63	0.81	0.60	0.04	0.11
其他的内分泌腺	C75	1	0.18	0.38	0.43	0.00	0.00	0	0.00	0.00	0.00	0.00	0.00
霍奇金病	C81	0	0.00	0.00	0.00	0.00	0.00	0	0.00	0.00	0.00	0.00	0.00
非霍奇金淋巴瘤	C82–C85;C96	11	1.95	4.14	3.39	0.19	0.46	10	3.16	4.07	2.65	0.14	0.30
免疫增生性疾病	C88	0	0.00	0.00	0.00	0.00	0.00	0	0.00	0.00	0.00	0.00	0.00
多发性骨髓瘤	C90	1	0.18	0.38	0.25	0.00	0.04	1	0.32	0.41	0.29	0.00	0.07
淋巴样白血病	C91	0	0.00	0.00	0.00	0.00	0.00	1	0.32	0.41	0.29	0.00	0.07
髓样白血病	C92–C94	2	0.36	0.75	0.79	0.03	0.11	2	0.63	0.81	0.47	0.00	0.00
白血病，未特指	C95	3	0.53	1.13	1.09	0.07	0.07	5	1.58	2.03	1.38	0.03	0.18
其他的或未指明部位	O&U	9	1.60	3.38	3.13	0.09	0.25	3	0.95	1.22	0.97	0.03	0.03
骨髓增殖性疾病	MPD	2	0.36	0.75	0.57	0.00	0.04	0	0.00	0.00	0.00	0.00	0.00
骨髓增生异常综合征	MDS	0	0.00	0.00	0.00	0.00	0.00	0	0.00	0.00	0.00	0.00	0.00
合计	ALL	563	100.00	211.65	162.89	6.59	18.80	316	100.00	128.52	83.43	3.51	9.81
C44 以外的部位	ALL but C44	561	99.64	210.90	162.39	6.57	18.78	314	99.37	127.71	82.96	3.51	9.77

表 6-47　2020 年河南省伊川县恶性肿瘤发病主要指标

部位	ICD-10	男性						女性					
		病例数	构成 (%)	粗率 ($1/10^5$)	世标率 ($1/10^5$)	累积率 (%) 0~64	累积率 (%) 0~74	病例数	构成 (%)	粗率 ($1/10^5$)	世标率 ($1/10^5$)	累积率 (%) 0~64	累积率 (%) 0~74
唇	C00	3	0.28	0.62	0.74	0.03	0.06	2	0.18	0.44	0.25	0.02	0.02
舌	C01–C02	1	0.09	0.21	0.19	0.02	0.02	1	0.09	0.22	0.16	0.00	0.04
口	C03–C06	4	0.38	0.83	0.68	0.03	0.10	5	0.44	1.10	0.81	0.02	0.05
唾液腺	C07–C08	8	0.75	1.66	1.34	0.10	0.14	4	0.35	0.88	0.73	0.07	0.07
扁桃体	C09	1	0.09	0.21	0.16	0.00	0.04	0	0.00	0.00	0.00	0.00	0.00
其他的口咽	C10	0	0.00	0.00	0.00	0.00	0.00	0	0.00	0.00	0.00	0.00	0.00
鼻咽	C11	5	0.47	1.04	0.80	0.09	0.09	2	0.18	0.44	0.33	0.00	0.07
喉咽	C12–C13	3	0.28	0.62	0.51	0.04	0.07	0	0.00	0.00	0.00	0.00	0.00
咽，部位不明	C14	0	0.00	0.00	0.00	0.00	0.00	3	0.27	0.66	0.36	0.02	0.02
食管	C15	224	21.07	46.57	34.45	1.20	4.59	170	15.06	37.41	24.47	0.57	3.38
胃	C16	167	15.71	34.72	25.88	1.00	3.30	81	7.17	17.82	11.94	0.49	1.56
小肠	C17	6	0.56	1.25	0.93	0.08	0.08	7	0.62	1.54	0.98	0.06	0.10
结肠	C18	31	2.92	6.44	5.09	0.30	0.68	26	2.30	5.72	4.06	0.19	0.46
直肠	C19–C20	45	4.23	9.36	7.21	0.46	0.81	29	2.57	6.38	4.33	0.26	0.46
肛门	C21	2	0.19	0.42	0.33	0.02	0.05	0	0.00	0.00	0.00	0.00	0.00
肝脏	C22	91	8.56	18.92	15.09	1.02	1.76	53	4.69	11.66	8.30	0.44	0.98
胆囊及其他	C23–C24	9	0.85	1.87	1.45	0.08	0.18	11	0.97	2.42	1.59	0.04	0.22
胰腺	C25	16	1.51	3.33	2.48	0.14	0.25	11	0.97	2.42	1.73	0.13	0.21
鼻、鼻窦及其他	C30–C31	4	0.38	0.83	0.75	0.05	0.05	3	0.27	0.66	0.39	0.02	0.02
喉	C32	5	0.47	1.04	0.95	0.01	0.14	2	0.18	0.44	0.23	0.00	0.04
气管、支气管、肺	C33–C34	214	20.13	44.49	33.07	1.15	4.43	111	9.83	24.43	16.87	0.86	2.06
其他的胸腔器官	C37–C38	9	0.85	1.87	1.69	0.11	0.18	2	0.18	0.44	0.26	0.00	0.03
骨	C40–C41	8	0.75	1.66	1.62	0.12	0.12	9	0.80	1.98	1.58	0.10	0.15
皮肤的黑色素瘤	C43	1	0.09	0.21	0.18	0.02	0.02	1	0.09	0.22	0.16	0.02	0.02
其他的皮肤	C44	3	0.28	0.62	0.42	0.02	0.02	5	0.44	1.10	0.52	0.00	0.03
间皮瘤	C45	0	0.00	0.00	0.00	0.00	0.00	0	0.00	0.00	0.00	0.00	0.00
卡波西肉瘤	C46	1	0.09	0.21	0.17	0.00	0.03	0	0.00	0.00	0.00	0.00	0.00
周围神经、其他结缔组织、软组织	C47;C49	2	0.19	0.42	0.42	0.03	0.03	4	0.35	0.88	1.08	0.07	0.07
乳房	C50	5	0.47	1.04	0.85	0.06	0.13	185	16.39	40.71	32.91	2.66	3.37
外阴	C51	0	0.00	0.00	0.00	0.00	0.00	1	0.09	0.22	0.09	0.00	0.00
阴道	C52	0	0.00	0.00	0.00	0.00	0.00	2	0.18	0.44	0.26	0.02	0.02
子宫颈	C53	0	0.00	0.00	0.00	0.00	0.00	84	7.44	18.48	14.76	1.20	1.57
子宫体	C54	0	0.00	0.00	0.00	0.00	0.00	37	3.28	8.14	6.50	0.56	0.78
子宫，部位不明	C55	0	0.00	0.00	0.00	0.00	0.00	14	1.24	3.08	2.43	0.20	0.23
卵巢	C56	0	0.00	0.00	0.00	0.00	0.00	49	4.34	10.78	9.46	0.63	1.02
女性其他的生殖器	C57	0	0.00	0.00	0.00	0.00	0.00	3	0.27	0.66	0.53	0.02	0.07
胎盘	C58	0	0.00	0.00	0.00	0.00	0.00	0	0.00	0.00	0.00	0.00	0.00
阴茎	C60	6	0.56	1.25	0.98	0.06	0.11	0	0.00	0.00	0.00	0.00	0.00
前列腺	C61	29	2.73	6.03	4.20	0.05	0.49	0	0.00	0.00	0.00	0.00	0.00
睾丸	C62	2	0.19	0.42	0.36	0.04	0.04	0	0.00	0.00	0.00	0.00	0.00
男性其他的生殖器	C63	0	0.00	0.00	0.00	0.00	0.00	0	0.00	0.00	0.00	0.00	0.00
肾	C64	13	1.22	2.70	2.25	0.10	0.33	11	0.97	2.42	1.78	0.09	0.22
肾盂	C65	1	0.09	0.21	0.16	0.02	0.02	0	0.00	0.00	0.00	0.00	0.00
输尿管	C66	1	0.09	0.21	0.17	0.00	0.03	1	0.09	0.22	0.16	0.00	0.04
膀胱	C67	18	1.69	3.74	3.01	0.16	0.25	6	0.53	1.32	0.84	0.06	0.09
其他的泌尿器官	C68	0	0.00	0.00	0.00	0.00	0.00	0	0.00	0.00	0.00	0.00	0.00
眼	C69	1	0.09	0.21	0.18	0.02	0.02	0	0.00	0.00	0.00	0.00	0.00
脑、神经系统	C70–C72	27	2.54	5.61	4.67	0.31	0.47	30	2.66	6.60	4.73	0.35	0.50
甲状腺	C73	21	1.98	4.37	3.72	0.34	0.38	61	5.40	13.42	10.98	0.90	1.20
肾上腺	C74	0	0.00	0.00	0.00	0.00	0.00	0	0.00	0.00	0.00	0.00	0.00
其他的内分泌腺	C75	2	0.19	0.42	0.28	0.02	0.02	0	0.00	0.00	0.00	0.00	0.00
霍奇金病	C81	1	0.09	0.21	0.13	0.00	0.00	3	0.27	0.66	0.52	0.05	0.05
非霍奇金淋巴瘤	C82–C85;C96	14	1.32	2.91	2.30	0.14	0.27	22	1.95	4.84	3.61	0.17	0.47
免疫增生性疾病	C88	0	0.00	0.00	0.00	0.00	0.00	1	0.09	0.22	0.45	0.02	0.02
多发性骨髓瘤	C90	2	0.19	0.42	0.33	0.02	0.04	3	0.27	0.66	0.58	0.06	0.06
淋巴样白血病	C91	1	0.09	0.21	0.16	0.00	0.04	0	0.00	0.00	0.00	0.00	0.00
髓样白血病	C92–C94	10	0.94	2.08	1.89	0.11	0.21	15	1.33	3.30	2.75	0.22	0.26
白血病，未特指	C95	12	1.13	2.49	2.74	0.17	0.21	10	0.89	2.20	1.94	0.05	0.26
其他的或未指明部位	O&U	33	3.10	6.86	5.34	0.25	0.60	48	4.25	10.56	8.12	0.47	0.75
骨髓增殖性疾病	MPD	1	0.09	0.21	0.15	0.02	0.02	1	0.09	0.22	0.12	0.00	0.00
骨髓增生异常综合征	MDS	0	0.00	0.00	0.00	0.00	0.00	0	0.00	0.00	0.00	0.00	0.00
合计	ALL	1 063	100.00	220.99	170.49	7.99	20.88	1 129	100.00	248.43	184.64	11.10	21.03
C44 以外的部位	ALL but C44	1 060	99.72	220.36	170.07	7.97	20.87	1 124	99.56	247.33	184.12	11.10	21.01

表 6-48 2020 年河南省伊川县恶性肿瘤死亡主要指标

部位	ICD-10	男性						女性					
		病例数	构成 (%)	粗率 ($1/10^5$)	世标率 ($1/10^5$)	累积率 (%)		病例数	构成 (%)	粗率 ($1/10^5$)	世标率 ($1/10^5$)	累积率 (%)	
						0~64	0~74					0~64	0~74
唇	C00	0	0.00	0.00	0.00	0.00	0.00	1	0.18	0.22	0.09	0.00	0.00
舌	C01–C02	1	0.12	0.21	0.13	0.00	0.00	1	0.18	0.22	0.17	0.01	0.01
口	C03–C06	3	0.37	0.62	0.47	0.00	0.06	1	0.18	0.22	0.16	0.00	0.04
唾液腺	C07–C08	1	0.12	0.21	0.16	0.00	0.04	1	0.18	0.22	0.20	0.02	0.02
扁桃体	C09	0	0.00	0.00	0.00	0.00	0.00	0	0.00	0.00	0.00	0.00	0.00
其他的口咽	C10	1	0.12	0.21	0.12	0.00	0.00	1	0.18	0.22	0.09	0.00	0.00
鼻咽	C11	1	0.12	0.21	0.16	0.00	0.04	2	0.37	0.44	0.20	0.00	0.00
喉咽	C12–C13	0	0.00	0.00	0.00	0.00	0.00	0	0.00	0.00	0.00	0.00	0.00
咽，部位不明	C14	1	0.12	0.21	0.13	0.00	0.00	0	0.00	0.00	0.00	0.00	0.00
食管	C15	149	18.17	30.98	21.57	0.38	2.56	126	23.03	27.73	15.43	0.39	1.78
胃	C16	143	17.44	29.73	20.74	0.62	2.15	58	10.60	12.76	7.30	0.16	0.74
小肠	C17	0	0.00	0.00	0.00	0.00	0.00	4	0.73	0.88	0.53	0.02	0.05
结肠	C18	18	2.20	3.74	2.84	0.16	0.33	17	3.11	3.74	2.41	0.12	0.25
直肠	C19–C20	32	3.90	6.65	4.84	0.23	0.41	14	2.56	3.08	1.59	0.04	0.12
肛门	C21	3	0.37	0.62	0.44	0.02	0.06	0	0.00	0.00	0.00	0.00	0.00
肝脏	C22	85	10.37	17.67	13.70	0.72	1.59	41	7.50	9.02	5.66	0.21	0.61
胆囊及其他	C23–C24	8	0.98	1.66	1.22	0.03	0.12	11	2.01	2.42	1.37	0.02	0.11
胰腺	C25	16	1.95	3.33	2.34	0.12	0.26	13	2.38	2.86	1.93	0.10	0.25
鼻、鼻窦及其他	C30–C31	1	0.12	0.21	0.13	0.00	0.00	3	0.55	0.66	0.30	0.00	0.00
喉	C32	5	0.61	1.04	0.75	0.00	0.09	2	0.37	0.44	0.26	0.02	0.02
气管、支气管、肺	C33–C34	230	28.05	47.81	34.48	0.86	4.43	88	16.09	19.36	12.04	0.41	1.48
其他的胸腔器官	C37–C38	1	0.12	0.21	0.24	0.01	0.01	0	0.00	0.00	0.00	0.00	0.00
骨	C40–C41	5	0.61	1.04	0.92	0.06	0.06	3	0.55	0.66	0.53	0.03	0.07
皮肤的黑色素瘤	C43	1	0.12	0.21	0.18	0.02	0.02	1	0.18	0.22	0.16	0.02	0.02
其他的皮肤	C44	2	0.24	0.42	0.24	0.00	0.00	5	0.91	1.10	0.49	0.00	0.04
间皮瘤	C45	0	0.00	0.00	0.00	0.00	0.00	0	0.00	0.00	0.00	0.00	0.00
卡波西肉瘤	C46	0	0.00	0.00	0.00	0.00	0.00	0	0.00	0.00	0.00	0.00	0.00
周围神经、其他结缔组织、软组织	C47;C49	0	0.00	0.00	0.00	0.00	0.00	1	0.18	0.22	0.16	0.02	0.02
乳房	C50	0	0.00	0.00	0.00	0.00	0.00	30	5.48	6.60	4.81	0.25	0.65
外阴	C51	0	0.00	0.00	0.00	0.00	0.00	1	0.18	0.22	0.07	0.00	0.00
阴道	C52	0	0.00	0.00	0.00	0.00	0.00	0	0.00	0.00	0.00	0.00	0.00
子宫颈	C53	0	0.00	0.00	0.00	0.00	0.00	40	7.31	8.80	6.67	0.48	0.83
子宫体	C54	0	0.00	0.00	0.00	0.00	0.00	6	1.10	1.32	0.71	0.04	0.08
子宫，部位不明	C55	0	0.00	0.00	0.00	0.00	0.00	2	0.37	0.44	0.34	0.02	0.05
卵巢	C56	0	0.00	0.00	0.00	0.00	0.00	9	1.65	1.98	1.57	0.10	0.25
女性其他的生殖器	C57	0	0.00	0.00	0.00	0.00	0.00	0	0.00	0.00	0.00	0.00	0.00
胎盘	C58	0	0.00	0.00	0.00	0.00	0.00	0	0.00	0.00	0.00	0.00	0.00
阴茎	C60	0	0.00	0.00	0.00	0.00	0.00	0	0.00	0.00	0.00	0.00	0.00
前列腺	C61	17	2.07	3.53	2.26	0.02	0.22	0	0.00	0.00	0.00	0.00	0.00
睾丸	C62	1	0.12	0.21	0.16	0.01	0.01	0	0.00	0.00	0.00	0.00	0.00
男性其他的生殖器	C63	0	0.00	0.00	0.00	0.00	0.00	0	0.00	0.00	0.00	0.00	0.00
肾	C64	6	0.73	1.25	0.91	0.02	0.11	4	0.73	0.88	0.58	0.04	0.07
肾盂	C65	1	0.12	0.21	0.11	0.00	0.00	0	0.00	0.00	0.00	0.00	0.00
输尿管	C66	1	0.12	0.21	0.17	0.00	0.03	1	0.18	0.22	0.09	0.00	0.00
膀胱	C67	14	1.71	2.91	2.03	0.11	0.14	3	0.55	0.66	0.42	0.00	0.06
其他的泌尿器官	C68	0	0.00	0.00	0.00	0.00	0.00	0	0.00	0.00	0.00	0.00	0.00
眼	C69	0	0.00	0.00	0.00	0.00	0.00	0	0.00	0.00	0.00	0.00	0.00
脑、神经系统	C70–C72	22	2.68	4.57	3.89	0.24	0.33	19	3.47	4.18	2.77	0.19	0.25
甲状腺	C73	4	0.49	0.83	0.62	0.02	0.08	6	1.10	1.32	0.96	0.06	0.09
肾上腺	C74	1	0.12	0.21	0.17	0.00	0.03	0	0.00	0.00	0.00	0.00	0.00
其他的内分泌腺	C75	0	0.00	0.00	0.00	0.00	0.00	1	0.18	0.22	0.12	0.00	0.00
霍奇金病	C81	1	0.12	0.21	0.16	0.02	0.02	1	0.18	0.22	0.19	0.02	0.02
非霍奇金淋巴瘤	C82–C85;C96	12	1.46	2.49	1.96	0.15	0.24	10	1.83	2.20	1.63	0.12	0.19
免疫增生性疾病	C88	0	0.00	0.00	0.00	0.00	0.00	0	0.00	0.00	0.00	0.00	0.00
多发性骨髓瘤	C90	3	0.37	0.62	0.48	0.03	0.03	2	0.37	0.44	0.34	0.00	0.06
淋巴样白血病	C91	2	0.24	0.42	0.34	0.01	0.05	0	0.00	0.00	0.00	0.00	0.00
髓样白血病	C92–C94	7	0.85	1.46	1.26	0.09	0.13	4	0.73	0.88	0.53	0.04	0.04
白血病，未特指	C95	4	0.49	0.83	0.71	0.07	0.07	4	0.73	0.88	0.69	0.03	0.07
其他的或未指明部位	O&U	17	2.07	3.53	2.46	0.07	0.18	9	1.65	1.98	1.42	0.07	0.18
骨髓增殖性疾病	MPD	0	0.00	0.00	0.00	0.00	0.00	0	0.00	0.00	0.00	0.00	0.00
骨髓增生异常综合征	MDS	0	0.00	0.00	0.00	0.00	0.00	1	0.18	0.22	0.23	0.01	0.01
合计	ALL	820	100.00	170.47	123.48	4.06	13.91	547	100.00	120.37	75.18	3.08	8.51
C44 以外的部位	ALL but C44	818	99.76	170.05	123.24	4.06	13.91	542	99.09	119.27	74.69	3.08	8.47

表 6-49　2020 年河南省洛阳市偃师区恶性肿瘤发病主要指标

部位	ICD-10	男性						女性					
		病例数	构成(%)	粗率(1/10^5)	世标率(1/10^5)	累积率(%)		病例数	构成(%)	粗率(1/10^5)	世标率(1/10^5)	累积率(%)	
						0~64	0~74					0~64	0~74
唇	C00	1	0.11	0.31	0.09	0.00	0.00	0	0.00	0.00	0.00	0.00	0.00
舌	C01–C02	1	0.11	0.31	0.20	0.03	0.03	1	0.11	0.32	0.19	0.02	0.02
口	C03–C06	8	0.91	2.45	1.43	0.11	0.18	3	0.34	0.97	0.47	0.02	0.02
唾液腺	C07–C08	5	0.57	1.53	1.07	0.09	0.13	3	0.34	0.97	0.46	0.00	0.09
扁桃体	C09	0	0.00	0.00	0.00	0.00	0.00	0	0.00	0.00	0.00	0.00	0.00
其他的口咽	C10	0	0.00	0.00	0.00	0.00	0.00	0	0.00	0.00	0.00	0.00	0.00
鼻咽	C11	1	0.11	0.31	0.18	0.00	0.03	2	0.23	0.64	0.24	0.00	0.03
喉咽	C12–C13	0	0.00	0.00	0.00	0.00	0.00	0	0.00	0.00	0.00	0.00	0.00
咽，部位不明	C14	0	0.00	0.00	0.00	0.00	0.00	1	0.11	0.32	0.08	0.00	0.00
食管	C15	109	12.34	33.40	16.49	0.48	2.25	66	7.54	21.28	9.53	0.44	1.14
胃	C16	136	15.40	41.67	20.62	0.76	2.60	56	6.40	18.05	8.22	0.32	0.94
小肠	C17	3	0.34	0.92	0.56	0.05	0.08	6	0.69	1.93	0.88	0.05	0.10
结肠	C18	36	4.08	11.03	6.32	0.35	0.75	32	3.66	10.32	5.31	0.32	0.74
直肠	C19–C20	36	4.08	11.03	6.25	0.41	0.68	31	3.54	9.99	5.08	0.30	0.72
肛门	C21	0	0.00	0.00	0.00	0.00	0.00	0	0.00	0.00	0.00	0.00	0.00
肝脏	C22	81	9.17	24.82	15.09	1.06	1.81	39	4.46	12.57	5.64	0.27	0.66
胆囊及其他	C23–C24	28	3.17	8.58	4.68	0.24	0.57	33	3.77	10.64	4.39	0.09	0.57
胰腺	C25	16	1.81	4.90	2.57	0.12	0.29	18	2.06	5.80	2.86	0.08	0.35
鼻、鼻窦及其他	C30–C31	4	0.45	1.23	0.72	0.04	0.07	0	0.00	0.00	0.00	0.00	0.00
喉	C32	12	1.36	3.68	2.18	0.11	0.27	1	0.11	0.32	0.18	0.02	0.02
气管、支气管、肺	C33–C34	162	18.35	49.64	26.40	1.48	3.33	118	13.49	38.04	18.43	1.03	2.39
其他的胸腔器官	C37–C38	5	0.57	1.53	1.03	0.04	0.13	6	0.69	1.93	0.92	0.04	0.10
骨	C40–C41	7	0.79	2.14	2.67	0.13	0.16	4	0.46	1.29	0.80	0.09	0.09
皮肤的黑色素瘤	C43	1	0.11	0.31	0.18	0.02	0.02	2	0.23	0.64	0.34	0.02	0.05
其他的皮肤	C44	9	1.02	2.76	1.66	0.09	0.18	8	0.91	2.58	1.46	0.10	0.13
间皮瘤	C45	0	0.00	0.00	0.00	0.00	0.00	1	0.11	0.32	0.10	0.00	0.00
卡波西肉瘤	C46	0	0.00	0.00	0.00	0.00	0.00	0	0.00	0.00	0.00	0.00	0.00
周围神经、其他结缔组织、软组织	C47;C49	5	0.57	1.53	0.85	0.02	0.08	4	0.46	1.29	0.85	0.09	0.09
乳房	C50	1	0.11	0.31	0.11	0.00	0.00	159	18.17	51.26	33.50	2.75	3.67
外阴	C51	0	0.00	0.00	0.00	0.00	0.00	0	0.00	0.00	0.00	0.00	0.00
阴道	C52	0	0.00	0.00	0.00	0.00	0.00	2	0.23	0.64	0.41	0.05	0.05
子宫颈	C53	0	0.00	0.00	0.00	0.00	0.00	41	4.69	13.22	7.95	0.66	0.87
子宫体	C54	0	0.00	0.00	0.00	0.00	0.00	36	4.11	11.61	7.07	0.66	0.81
子宫，部位不明	C55	0	0.00	0.00	0.00	0.00	0.00	3	0.34	0.97	0.67	0.04	0.07
卵巢	C56	0	0.00	0.00	0.00	0.00	0.00	29	3.31	9.35	6.17	0.42	0.69
女性其他的生殖器	C57	0	0.00	0.00	0.00	0.00	0.00	1	0.11	0.32	0.08	0.00	0.00
胎盘	C58	0	0.00	0.00	0.00	0.00	0.00	1	0.11	0.32	0.24	0.02	0.02
阴茎	C60	2	0.23	0.61	0.35	0.03	0.06	0	0.00	0.00	0.00	0.00	0.00
前列腺	C61	40	4.53	12.26	5.77	0.12	0.72	0	0.00	0.00	0.00	0.00	0.00
睾丸	C62	3	0.34	0.92	1.96	0.09	0.09	0	0.00	0.00	0.00	0.00	0.00
男性其他的生殖器	C63	2	0.23	0.61	0.33	0.00	0.07	0	0.00	0.00	0.00	0.00	0.00
肾	C64	12	1.36	3.68	2.32	0.13	0.30	6	0.69	1.93	1.06	0.07	0.16
肾盂	C65	1	0.11	0.31	0.18	0.00	0.03	0	0.00	0.00	0.00	0.00	0.00
输尿管	C66	2	0.23	0.61	0.22	0.00	0.00	2	0.23	0.64	0.21	0.00	0.03
膀胱	C67	31	3.51	9.50	5.08	0.26	0.62	6	0.69	1.93	0.67	0.02	0.06
其他的泌尿器官	C68	0	0.00	0.00	0.00	0.00	0.00	0	0.00	0.00	0.00	0.00	0.00
眼	C69	2	0.23	0.61	0.26	0.00	0.04	0	0.00	0.00	0.00	0.00	0.00
脑、神经系统	C70–C72	18	2.04	5.52	3.98	0.23	0.41	20	2.29	6.45	4.32	0.25	0.42
甲状腺	C73	20	2.27	6.13	4.28	0.39	0.42	75	8.57	24.18	18.86	1.59	1.69
肾上腺	C74	4	0.45	1.23	0.76	0.07	0.07	2	0.23	0.64	0.34	0.02	0.05
其他的内分泌腺	C75	0	0.00	0.00	0.00	0.00	0.00	2	0.23	0.64	0.34	0.02	0.05
霍奇金病	C81	1	0.11	0.31	0.18	0.00	0.03	0	0.00	0.00	0.00	0.00	0.00
非霍奇金淋巴瘤	C82–C85;C96	33	3.74	10.11	7.79	0.53	0.66	14	1.60	4.51	2.66	0.21	0.35
免疫增生性疾病	C88	0	0.00	0.00	0.00	0.00	0.00	0	0.00	0.00	0.00	0.00	0.00
多发性骨髓瘤	C90	5	0.57	1.53	0.71	0.05	0.05	8	0.91	2.58	1.28	0.07	0.19
淋巴样白血病	C91	2	0.23	0.61	0.51	0.02	0.06	2	0.23	0.64	0.70	0.05	0.05
髓样白血病	C92–C94	17	1.93	5.21	4.31	0.28	0.40	11	1.26	3.55	2.23	0.20	0.23
白血病，未特指	C95	11	1.25	3.37	2.26	0.12	0.24	11	1.26	3.55	2.02	0.16	0.22
其他的或未指明部位	O&U	10	1.13	3.06	1.65	0.09	0.12	9	1.03	2.90	1.58	0.05	0.16
骨髓增殖性疾病	MPD	0	0.00	0.00	0.00	0.00	0.00	0	0.00	0.00	0.00	0.00	0.00
骨髓增生异常综合征	MDS	0	0.00	0.00	0.00	0.00	0.00	0	0.00	0.00	0.00	0.00	0.00
合计	ALL	883	100.00	270.55	154.23	8.06	18.02	875	100.00	282.08	158.77	10.61	18.10
C44 以外的部位	ALL but C44	874	98.98	267.79	152.57	7.96	17.84	867	99.09	279.50	157.32	10.52	17.97

表 6-50 2020 年河南省洛阳市偃师区恶性肿瘤死亡主要指标

部位	ICD-10	男性						女性					
		病例数	构成 (%)	粗率 $(1/10^5)$	世标率 $(1/10^5)$	累积率 (%)		病例数	构成 (%)	粗率 $(1/10^5)$	世标率 $(1/10^5)$	累积率 (%)	
						0～64	0～74					0～64	0～74
唇	C00	0	0.00	0.00	0.00	0.00	0.00	0	0.00	0.00	0.00	0.00	0.00
舌	C01–C02	1	0.16	0.31	0.09	0.00	0.00	0	0.00	0.00	0.00	0.00	0.00
口	C03–C06	0	0.00	0.00	0.00	0.00	0.00	2	0.42	0.64	0.26	0.00	0.03
唾液腺	C07–C08	1	0.16	0.31	0.09	0.00	0.00	1	0.21	0.32	0.09	0.00	0.00
扁桃体	C09	0	0.00	0.00	0.00	0.00	0.00	0	0.00	0.00	0.00	0.00	0.00
其他的口咽	C10	0	0.00	0.00	0.00	0.00	0.00	0	0.00	0.00	0.00	0.00	0.00
鼻咽	C11	3	0.47	0.92	0.53	0.03	0.09	0	0.00	0.00	0.00	0.00	0.00
喉咽	C12–C13	1	0.16	0.31	0.09	0.00	0.00	0	0.00	0.00	0.00	0.00	0.00
咽，部位不明	C14	0	0.00	0.00	0.00	0.00	0.00	0	0.00	0.00	0.00	0.00	0.00
食管	C15	98	15.36	30.03	14.02	0.26	1.60	58	12.24	18.70	6.79	0.10	0.76
胃	C16	121	18.97	37.07	17.61	0.60	1.83	51	10.76	16.44	6.46	0.27	0.60
小肠	C17	3	0.47	0.92	0.51	0.05	0.05	2	0.42	0.64	0.15	0.00	0.00
结肠	C18	14	2.19	4.29	2.32	0.13	0.19	18	3.80	5.80	2.48	0.09	0.31
直肠	C19–C20	15	2.35	4.60	2.35	0.13	0.19	23	4.85	7.41	2.75	0.09	0.22
肛门	C21	0	0.00	0.00	0.00	0.00	0.00	0	0.00	0.00	0.00	0.00	0.00
肝脏	C22	71	11.13	21.75	12.32	0.93	1.36	34	7.17	10.96	5.46	0.32	0.71
胆囊及其他	C23–C24	22	3.45	6.74	3.38	0.10	0.47	32	6.75	10.32	4.12	0.11	0.51
胰腺	C25	20	3.13	6.13	3.21	0.16	0.26	19	4.01	6.13	2.66	0.09	0.37
鼻、鼻窦及其他	C30–C31	3	0.47	0.92	0.58	0.04	0.04	1	0.21	0.32	0.10	0.00	0.00
喉	C32	4	0.63	1.23	0.63	0.02	0.05	0	0.00	0.00	0.00	0.00	0.00
气管、支气管、肺	C33–C34	133	20.85	40.75	20.68	0.83	2.66	76	16.03	24.50	10.27	0.30	1.27
其他的胸腔器官	C37–C38	3	0.47	0.92	0.85	0.05	0.08	5	1.05	1.61	1.50	0.06	0.08
骨	C40–C41	6	0.94	1.84	1.85	0.06	0.09	1	0.21	0.32	0.09	0.00	0.00
皮肤的黑色素瘤	C43	1	0.16	0.31	0.15	0.00	0.04	3	0.63	0.97	0.40	0.00	0.06
其他的皮肤	C44	3	0.47	0.92	0.39	0.00	0.03	2	0.42	0.64	0.16	0.00	0.00
间皮瘤	C45	0	0.00	0.00	0.00	0.00	0.00	0	0.00	0.00	0.00	0.00	0.00
卡波西肉瘤	C46	0	0.00	0.00	0.00	0.00	0.00	0	0.00	0.00	0.00	0.00	0.00
周围神经、其他结缔组织、软组织	C47;C49	2	0.31	0.61	0.24	0.00	0.04	2	0.42	0.64	0.53	0.04	0.04
乳房	C50	0	0.00	0.00	0.00	0.00	0.00	42	8.86	13.54	6.94	0.43	0.85
外阴	C51	0	0.00	0.00	0.00	0.00	0.00	0	0.00	0.00	0.00	0.00	0.00
阴道	C52	0	0.00	0.00	0.00	0.00	0.00	1	0.21	0.32	0.14	0.00	0.03
子宫颈	C53	0	0.00	0.00	0.00	0.00	0.00	14	2.95	4.51	2.42	0.18	0.27
子宫体	C54	0	0.00	0.00	0.00	0.00	0.00	6	1.27	1.93	0.89	0.05	0.14
子宫，部位不明	C55	0	0.00	0.00	0.00	0.00	0.00	0	0.00	0.00	0.00	0.00	0.00
卵巢	C56	0	0.00	0.00	0.00	0.00	0.00	11	2.32	3.55	1.95	0.13	0.29
女性其他的生殖器	C57	0	0.00	0.00	0.00	0.00	0.00	0	0.00	0.00	0.00	0.00	0.00
胎盘	C58	0	0.00	0.00	0.00	0.00	0.00	0	0.00	0.00	0.00	0.00	0.00
阴茎	C60	0	0.00	0.00	0.00	0.00	0.00	0	0.00	0.00	0.00	0.00	0.00
前列腺	C61	16	2.51	4.90	2.11	0.03	0.17	0	0.00	0.00	0.00	0.00	0.00
睾丸	C62	0	0.00	0.00	0.00	0.00	0.00	0	0.00	0.00	0.00	0.00	0.00
男性其他的生殖器	C63	0	0.00	0.00	0.00	0.00	0.00	0	0.00	0.00	0.00	0.00	0.00
肾	C64	10	1.57	3.06	1.42	0.05	0.15	5	1.05	1.61	0.70	0.00	0.12
肾盂	C65	0	0.00	0.00	0.00	0.00	0.00	1	0.21	0.32	0.19	0.02	0.02
输尿管	C66	0	0.00	0.00	0.00	0.00	0.00	0	0.00	0.00	0.00	0.00	0.00
膀胱	C67	12	1.88	3.68	1.65	0.03	0.17	2	0.42	0.64	0.18	0.00	0.00
其他的泌尿器官	C68	0	0.00	0.00	0.00	0.00	0.00	0	0.00	0.00	0.00	0.00	0.00
眼	C69	2	0.31	0.61	0.96	0.04	0.04	0	0.00	0.00	0.00	0.00	0.00
脑、神经系统	C70–C72	20	3.13	6.13	3.49	0.23	0.50	18	3.80	5.80	2.42	0.09	0.32
甲状腺	C73	1	0.16	0.31	0.09	0.00	0.00	7	1.48	2.26	0.86	0.02	0.05
肾上腺	C74	1	0.16	0.31	0.20	0.03	0.03	2	0.42	0.64	0.40	0.02	0.05
其他的内分泌腺	C75	2	0.31	0.61	0.29	0.00	0.03	0	0.00	0.00	0.00	0.00	0.00
霍奇金病	C81	0	0.00	0.00	0.00	0.00	0.00	0	0.00	0.00	0.00	0.00	0.00
非霍奇金淋巴瘤	C82–C85;C96	11	1.72	3.37	1.74	0.11	0.14	9	1.90	2.90	1.48	0.09	0.21
免疫增生性疾病	C88	0	0.00	0.00	0.00	0.00	0.00	0	0.00	0.00	0.00	0.00	0.00
多发性骨髓瘤	C90	8	1.25	2.45	1.08	0.00	0.13	2	0.42	0.64	0.36	0.02	0.05
淋巴样白血病	C91	2	0.31	0.61	0.45	0.05	0.05	0	0.00	0.00	0.00	0.00	0.00
髓样白血病	C92–C94	8	1.25	2.45	1.55	0.08	0.18	7	1.48	2.26	1.45	0.14	0.17
白血病，未特指	C95	10	1.57	3.06	2.02	0.10	0.23	6	1.27	1.93	0.86	0.05	0.10
其他的或未指明部位	O&U	7	1.10	2.14	0.93	0.05	0.05	11	2.32	3.55	1.46	0.02	0.16
骨髓增殖性疾病	MPD	0	0.00	0.00	0.00	0.00	0.00	0	0.00	0.00	0.00	0.00	0.00
骨髓增生异常综合征	MDS	3	0.47	0.92	0.41	0.00	0.08	0	0.00	0.00	0.00	0.00	0.00
合计	ALL	638	100.00	195.48	100.30	4.17	11.00	474	100.00	152.81	66.94	2.73	7.82
C44 以外的部位	ALL but C44	635	99.53	194.56	99.90	4.17	10.97	472	99.58	152.16	66.78	2.73	7.82

表 6-51　2020 年河南省平顶山市城区恶性肿瘤发病主要指标

部位	ICD-10	男性						女性					
		病例数	构成 (%)	粗率 (1/10^5)	世标率 (1/10^5)	累积率 (%) 0~64	累积率 (%) 0~74	病例数	构成 (%)	粗率 (1/10^5)	世标率 (1/10^5)	累积率 (%) 0~64	累积率 (%) 0~74
唇	C00	1	0.07	0.22	0.09	0.00	0.00	2	0.13	0.43	0.20	0.00	0.03
舌	C01–C02	5	0.36	1.09	0.76	0.04	0.04	2	0.13	0.43	0.20	0.00	0.03
口	C03–C06	7	0.50	1.52	0.91	0.06	0.08	6	0.40	1.29	0.80	0.08	0.08
唾液腺	C07–C08	2	0.14	0.43	0.25	0.03	0.03	0	0.00	0.00	0.00	0.00	0.00
扁桃体	C09	0	0.00	0.00	0.00	0.00	0.00	0	0.00	0.00	0.00	0.00	0.00
其他的口咽	C10	4	0.29	0.87	0.56	0.05	0.05	0	0.00	0.00	0.00	0.00	0.00
鼻咽	C11	4	0.29	0.87	0.90	0.07	0.09	1	0.07	0.22	0.11	0.01	0.01
喉咽	C12–C13	4	0.29	0.87	0.51	0.05	0.05	0	0.00	0.00	0.00	0.00	0.00
咽，部位不明	C14	1	0.07	0.22	0.11	0.01	0.01	1	0.07	0.22	0.09	0.00	0.00
食管	C15	82	5.89	17.83	11.44	0.56	1.49	43	2.87	9.27	5.14	0.14	0.70
胃	C16	106	7.61	23.05	14.23	0.57	1.62	41	2.74	8.84	5.64	0.28	0.54
小肠	C17	7	0.50	1.52	1.01	0.06	0.11	8	0.53	1.73	0.96	0.05	0.15
结肠	C18	65	4.67	14.13	8.59	0.34	0.94	50	3.34	10.78	6.07	0.31	0.68
直肠	C19–C20	64	4.59	13.91	8.73	0.52	1.08	47	3.14	10.13	5.98	0.33	0.64
肛门	C21	1	0.07	0.22	0.13	0.00	0.03	3	0.20	0.65	0.27	0.00	0.03
肝脏	C22	134	9.62	29.13	18.41	1.23	2.09	49	3.27	10.57	5.89	0.18	0.69
胆囊及其他	C23–C24	22	1.58	4.78	3.19	0.12	0.30	26	1.74	5.61	2.81	0.07	0.24
胰腺	C25	33	2.37	7.17	4.47	0.12	0.62	38	2.54	8.19	4.45	0.14	0.49
鼻、鼻窦及其他	C30–C31	5	0.36	1.09	0.70	0.05	0.11	2	0.13	0.43	0.23	0.00	0.02
喉	C32	19	1.36	4.13	2.60	0.18	0.26	0	0.00	0.00	0.00	0.00	0.00
气管、支气管、肺	C33–C34	417	29.94	90.66	56.30	2.61	6.53	236	15.75	50.89	29.09	1.73	3.33
其他的胸腔器官	C37–C38	4	0.29	0.87	0.47	0.01	0.04	4	0.27	0.86	0.42	0.03	0.03
骨	C40–C41	8	0.57	1.74	1.16	0.05	0.09	6	0.40	1.29	0.81	0.05	0.07
皮肤的黑色素瘤	C43	2	0.14	0.43	0.46	0.03	0.03	3	0.20	0.65	0.45	0.04	0.04
其他的皮肤	C44	9	0.65	1.96	1.14	0.05	0.11	12	0.80	2.59	1.36	0.02	0.13
间皮瘤	C45	0	0.00	0.00	0.00	0.00	0.00	0	0.00	0.00	0.00	0.00	0.00
卡波西肉瘤	C46	0	0.00	0.00	0.00	0.00	0.00	0	0.00	0.00	0.00	0.00	0.00
周围神经、其他结缔组织、软组织	C47;C49	6	0.43	1.30	0.88	0.04	0.10	7	0.47	1.51	0.93	0.07	0.10
乳房	C50	3	0.22	0.65	0.45	0.02	0.05	276	18.42	59.51	36.33	2.94	3.93
外阴	C51	0	0.00	0.00	0.00	0.00	0.00	2	0.13	0.43	0.26	0.00	0.05
阴道	C52	0	0.00	0.00	0.00	0.00	0.00	1	0.07	0.22	0.13	0.02	0.02
子宫颈	C53	0	0.00	0.00	0.00	0.00	0.00	94	6.28	20.27	12.83	0.99	1.53
子宫体	C54	0	0.00	0.00	0.00	0.00	0.00	51	3.40	11.00	6.78	0.53	0.84
子宫，部位不明	C55	0	0.00	0.00	0.00	0.00	0.00	2	0.13	0.43	0.23	0.01	0.01
卵巢	C56	0	0.00	0.00	0.00	0.00	0.00	35	2.34	7.55	4.62	0.35	0.50
女性其他的生殖器	C57	0	0.00	0.00	0.00	0.00	0.00	4	0.27	0.86	0.77	0.07	0.07
胎盘	C58	0	0.00	0.00	0.00	0.00	0.00	0	0.00	0.00	0.00	0.00	0.00
阴茎	C60	2	0.14	0.43	0.27	0.00	0.00	0	0.00	0.00	0.00	0.00	0.00
前列腺	C61	66	4.74	14.35	8.31	0.15	0.87	0	0.00	0.00	0.00	0.00	0.00
睾丸	C62	2	0.14	0.43	0.66	0.04	0.04	0	0.00	0.00	0.00	0.00	0.00
男性其他的生殖器	C63	1	0.07	0.22	0.11	0.00	0.00	0	0.00	0.00	0.00	0.00	0.00
肾	C64	33	2.37	7.17	4.36	0.26	0.49	10	0.67	2.16	1.15	0.06	0.12
肾盂	C65	2	0.14	0.43	0.22	0.01	0.01	3	0.20	0.65	0.43	0.04	0.04
输尿管	C66	1	0.07	0.22	0.16	0.00	0.03	3	0.20	0.65	0.27	0.00	0.03
膀胱	C67	51	3.66	11.09	7.12	0.42	0.75	12	0.80	2.59	1.46	0.11	0.14
其他的泌尿器官	C68	1	0.07	0.22	0.11	0.01	0.01	0	0.00	0.00	0.00	0.00	0.00
眼	C69	1	0.07	0.22	0.11	0.01	0.01	2	0.13	0.43	0.52	0.02	0.02
脑、神经系统	C70–C72	17	1.22	3.70	3.17	0.19	0.25	36	2.40	7.76	4.87	0.35	0.48
甲状腺	C73	81	5.81	17.61	13.60	1.11	1.20	276	18.42	59.51	40.37	3.60	3.88
肾上腺	C74	1	0.07	0.22	0.11	0.01	0.01	0	0.00	0.00	0.00	0.00	0.00
其他的内分泌腺	C75	1	0.07	0.22	0.30	0.02	0.02	0	0.00	0.00	0.00	0.00	0.00
霍奇金病	C81	3	0.22	0.65	0.61	0.03	0.06	1	0.07	0.22	0.45	0.03	0.03
非霍奇金淋巴瘤	C82–C85;C96	30	2.15	6.52	4.51	0.26	0.58	25	1.67	5.39	3.19	0.13	0.35
免疫增生性疾病	C88	0	0.00	0.00	0.00	0.00	0.00	0	0.00	0.00	0.00	0.00	0.00
多发性骨髓瘤	C90	10	0.72	2.17	1.36	0.02	0.19	11	0.73	2.37	1.42	0.08	0.20
淋巴样白血病	C91	6	0.43	1.30	1.02	0.09	0.09	5	0.33	1.08	1.77	0.09	0.09
髓样白血病	C92–C94	17	1.22	3.70	2.44	0.15	0.27	13	0.87	2.80	1.84	0.15	0.21
白血病，未特指	C95	5	0.36	1.09	0.57	0.03	0.06	2	0.13	0.43	0.52	0.03	0.03
其他的或未指明部位	O&U	43	3.09	9.35	6.71	0.39	0.59	46	3.07	9.92	6.23	0.40	0.57
骨髓增殖性疾病	MPD	3	0.22	0.65	0.36	0.01	0.01	1	0.07	0.22	0.45	0.03	0.03
骨髓增生异常综合征	MDS	1	0.07	0.22	0.19	0.02	0.02	0	0.00	0.00	0.00	0.00	0.00
合计	ALL	1 393	100.00	302.85	194.82	10.12	21.53	1 498	100.00	323.01	198.79	13.54	21.21
C44 以外的部位	ALL but C44	1 384	99.35	300.89	193.68	10.08	21.42	1 486	99.20	320.43	197.43	13.52	21.08

表 6-52 2020 年河南省平顶山市城区恶性肿瘤死亡主要指标

部位	ICD-10	男性						女性					
		病例数	构成 (%)	粗率 $(1/10^5)$	世标率 $(1/10^5)$	累积率 (%)		病例数	构成 (%)	粗率 $(1/10^5)$	世标率 $(1/10^5)$	累积率 (%)	
						0~64	0~74					0~64	0~74
唇	C00	0	0.00	0.00	0.00	0.00	0.00	0	0.00	0.00	0.00	0.00	0.00
舌	C01–C02	1	0.12	0.22	0.16	0.00	0.00	2	0.36	0.43	0.26	0.00	0.02
口	C03–C06	0	0.00	0.00	0.00	0.00	0.00	2	0.36	0.43	0.24	0.01	0.04
唾液腺	C07–C08	2	0.24	0.43	0.27	0.01	0.04	1	0.18	0.22	0.07	0.00	0.00
扁桃体	C09	0	0.00	0.00	0.00	0.00	0.00	1	0.18	0.22	0.12	0.01	0.01
其他的口咽	C10	0	0.00	0.00	0.00	0.00	0.00	1	0.18	0.22	0.13	0.02	0.02
鼻咽	C11	0	0.00	0.00	0.00	0.00	0.00	0	0.00	0.00	0.00	0.00	0.00
喉咽	C12–C13	1	0.12	0.22	0.13	0.02	0.02	0	0.00	0.00	0.00	0.00	0.00
咽，部位不明	C14	2	0.24	0.43	0.32	0.00	0.03	0	0.00	0.00	0.00	0.00	0.00
食管	C15	60	7.06	13.04	8.00	0.25	0.74	31	5.57	6.68	3.12	0.00	0.23
胃	C16	81	9.53	17.61	10.48	0.23	1.26	32	5.75	6.90	3.85	0.13	0.35
小肠	C17	3	0.35	0.65	0.45	0.02	0.05	4	0.72	0.86	0.37	0.00	0.03
结肠	C18	30	3.53	6.52	3.67	0.09	0.24	19	3.41	4.10	1.93	0.06	0.14
直肠	C19–C20	30	3.53	6.52	4.01	0.12	0.44	18	3.23	3.88	2.22	0.10	0.22
肛门	C21	0	0.00	0.00	0.00	0.00	0.00	1	0.18	0.22	0.12	0.00	0.03
肝脏	C22	112	13.18	24.35	15.14	0.91	1.67	52	9.34	11.21	6.16	0.21	0.58
胆囊及其他	C23–C24	15	1.76	3.26	1.96	0.05	0.13	16	2.87	3.45	1.70	0.02	0.16
胰腺	C25	32	3.76	6.96	4.34	0.13	0.48	31	5.57	6.68	3.53	0.16	0.35
鼻、鼻窦及其他	C30–C31	7	0.82	1.52	0.91	0.05	0.12	0	0.00	0.00	0.00	0.00	0.00
喉	C32	6	0.71	1.30	0.88	0.02	0.11	0	0.00	0.00	0.00	0.00	0.00
气管、支气管、肺	C33–C34	320	37.65	69.57	41.44	1.33	4.02	130	23.34	28.03	15.24	0.66	1.47
其他的胸腔器官	C37–C38	1	0.12	0.22	0.13	0.00	0.03	2	0.36	0.43	0.25	0.02	0.02
骨	C40–C41	6	0.71	1.30	1.16	0.06	0.10	6	1.08	1.29	0.64	0.02	0.05
皮肤的黑色素瘤	C43	2	0.24	0.43	0.30	0.00	0.03	0	0.00	0.00	0.00	0.00	0.00
其他的皮肤	C44	2	0.24	0.43	0.24	0.00	0.03	2	0.36	0.43	0.24	0.00	0.03
间皮瘤	C45	0	0.00	0.00	0.00	0.00	0.00	0	0.00	0.00	0.00	0.00	0.00
卡波西肉瘤	C46	0	0.00	0.00	0.00	0.00	0.00	0	0.00	0.00	0.00	0.00	0.00
周围神经、其他结缔组织、软组织	C47;C49	3	0.35	0.65	0.44	0.02	0.02	1	0.18	0.22	0.09	0.00	0.00
乳房	C50	0	0.00	0.00	0.00	0.00	0.00	58	10.41	12.51	7.17	0.49	0.71
外阴	C51	0	0.00	0.00	0.00	0.00	0.00	1	0.18	0.22	0.18	0.02	0.02
阴道	C52	0	0.00	0.00	0.00	0.00	0.00	0	0.00	0.00	0.00	0.00	0.00
子宫颈	C53	0	0.00	0.00	0.00	0.00	0.00	25	4.49	5.39	2.99	0.16	0.38
子宫体	C54	0	0.00	0.00	0.00	0.00	0.00	6	1.08	1.29	0.67	0.01	0.07
子宫，部位不明	C55	0	0.00	0.00	0.00	0.00	0.00	4	0.72	0.86	0.54	0.04	0.06
卵巢	C56	0	0.00	0.00	0.00	0.00	0.00	15	2.69	3.23	1.82	0.11	0.19
女性其他的生殖器	C57	0	0.00	0.00	0.00	0.00	0.00	0	0.00	0.00	0.00	0.00	0.00
胎盘	C58	0	0.00	0.00	0.00	0.00	0.00	0	0.00	0.00	0.00	0.00	0.00
阴茎	C60	1	0.12	0.22	0.16	0.00	0.00	0	0.00	0.00	0.00	0.00	0.00
前列腺	C61	24	2.82	5.22	3.09	0.00	0.03	0	0.00	0.00	0.00	0.00	0.00
睾丸	C62	0	0.00	0.00	0.00	0.00	0.00	0	0.00	0.00	0.00	0.00	0.00
男性其他的生殖器	C63	0	0.00	0.00	0.00	0.00	0.00	0	0.00	0.00	0.00	0.00	0.00
肾	C64	14	1.65	3.04	1.88	0.04	0.19	7	1.26	1.51	0.75	0.03	0.03
肾盂	C65	1	0.12	0.22	0.11	0.00	0.00	1	0.18	0.22	0.09	0.00	0.00
输尿管	C66	3	0.35	0.65	0.41	0.01	0.01	1	0.18	0.22	0.07	0.00	0.00
膀胱	C67	11	1.29	2.39	1.25	0.00	0.03	2	0.36	0.43	0.25	0.02	0.02
其他的泌尿器官	C68	0	0.00	0.00	0.00	0.00	0.00	1	0.18	0.22	0.12	0.00	0.00
眼	C69	0	0.00	0.00	0.00	0.00	0.00	1	0.18	0.22	0.09	0.00	0.00
脑、神经系统	C70–C72	20	2.35	4.35	3.14	0.13	0.29	21	3.77	4.53	2.59	0.16	0.33
甲状腺	C73	1	0.12	0.22	0.09	0.00	0.00	4	0.72	0.86	0.47	0.01	0.03
肾上腺	C74	0	0.00	0.00	0.00	0.00	0.00	0	0.00	0.00	0.00	0.00	0.00
其他的内分泌腺	C75	0	0.00	0.00	0.00	0.00	0.00	2	0.36	0.43	0.20	0.00	0.03
霍奇金病	C81	1	0.12	0.22	0.30	0.02	0.02	0	0.00	0.00	0.00	0.00	0.00
非霍奇金淋巴瘤	C82–C85;C96	16	1.88	3.48	2.07	0.11	0.30	13	2.33	2.80	1.42	0.03	0.13
免疫增生性疾病	C88	0	0.00	0.00	0.00	0.00	0.00	0	0.00	0.00	0.00	0.00	0.00
多发性骨髓瘤	C90	4	0.47	0.87	0.64	0.05	0.05	2	0.36	0.43	0.17	0.00	0.00
淋巴样白血病	C91	1	0.12	0.22	0.16	0.01	0.01	4	0.72	0.86	0.48	0.02	0.05
髓样白血病	C92–C94	9	1.06	1.96	1.11	0.05	0.11	4	0.72	0.86	0.67	0.07	0.07
白血病，未特指	C95	4	0.47	0.87	0.45	0.02	0.05	0	0.00	0.00	0.00	0.00	0.00
其他的或未指明部位	O&U	22	2.59	4.78	2.80	0.11	0.27	33	5.92	7.12	4.03	0.20	0.43
骨髓增殖性疾病	MPD	0	0.00	0.00	0.00	0.00	0.00	0	0.00	0.00	0.00	0.00	0.00
骨髓增生异常综合征	MDS	2	0.24	0.43	0.34	0.02	0.05	0	0.00	0.00	0.00	0.00	0.00
合计	ALL	850	100.00	184.80	112.45	3.89	10.97	557	100.00	120.11	65.07	2.80	6.33
C44 以外的部位	ALL but C44	848	99.76	184.36	112.21	3.89	10.93	555	99.64	119.68	64.83	2.80	6.30

表 6-53　2020 年河南省鲁山县恶性肿瘤发病主要指标

部位	ICD-10	男性						女性					
		病例数	构成(%)	粗率($1/10^5$)	世标率($1/10^5$)	累积率(%)		病例数	构成(%)	粗率($1/10^5$)	世标率($1/10^5$)	累积率(%)	
						0~64	0~74					0~64	0~74
唇	C00	0	0.00	0.00	0.00	0.00	0.00	1	0.10	0.22	0.20	0.02	0.02
舌	C01–C02	2	0.17	0.40	0.34	0.03	0.03	2	0.19	0.43	0.44	0.05	0.05
口	C03–C06	3	0.25	0.60	0.54	0.02	0.06	2	0.19	0.43	0.48	0.03	0.07
唾液腺	C07–C08	2	0.17	0.40	0.33	0.01	0.05	1	0.10	0.22	0.26	0.03	0.03
扁桃体	C09	0	0.00	0.00	0.00	0.00	0.00	0	0.00	0.00	0.00	0.00	0.00
其他的口咽	C10	0	0.00	0.00	0.00	0.00	0.00	0	0.00	0.00	0.00	0.00	0.00
鼻咽	C11	4	0.34	0.80	0.71	0.08	0.08	3	0.29	0.65	0.47	0.02	0.06
喉咽	C12–C13	0	0.00	0.00	0.00	0.00	0.00	0	0.00	0.00	0.00	0.00	0.00
咽，部位不明	C14	0	0.00	0.00	0.00	0.00	0.00	2	0.19	0.43	0.64	0.01	0.01
食管	C15	130	10.89	25.92	27.68	0.64	2.72	66	6.27	14.35	13.43	0.30	1.39
胃	C16	221	18.51	44.07	43.29	1.86	5.26	75	7.13	16.31	15.57	0.51	1.06
小肠	C17	1	0.08	0.20	0.22	0.03	0.03	4	0.38	0.87	0.70	0.03	0.07
结肠	C18	45	3.77	8.97	8.46	0.44	0.88	32	3.04	6.96	6.26	0.36	0.72
直肠	C19–C20	41	3.43	8.18	7.97	0.41	0.89	29	2.76	6.31	6.06	0.19	0.74
肛门	C21	0	0.00	0.00	0.00	0.00	0.00	0	0.00	0.00	0.00	0.00	0.00
肝脏	C22	114	9.55	22.73	22.65	1.25	2.29	77	7.32	16.75	15.59	0.83	1.67
胆囊及其他	C23–C24	19	1.59	3.79	3.77	0.11	0.48	13	1.24	2.83	2.54	0.12	0.36
胰腺	C25	20	1.68	3.99	4.06	0.10	0.42	17	1.62	3.70	3.49	0.19	0.43
鼻、鼻窦及其他	C30–C31	0	0.00	0.00	0.00	0.00	0.00	0	0.00	0.00	0.00	0.00	0.00
喉	C32	6	0.50	1.20	1.53	0.06	0.14	2	0.19	0.43	0.38	0.03	0.03
气管、支气管、肺	C33–C34	316	26.47	63.01	68.76	2.44	6.87	142	13.50	30.88	28.61	1.15	2.54
其他的胸腔器官	C37–C38	3	0.25	0.60	0.59	0.03	0.07	5	0.48	1.09	0.85	0.04	0.12
骨	C40–C41	11	0.92	2.19	2.40	0.03	0.23	14	1.33	3.04	2.70	0.13	0.26
皮肤的黑色素瘤	C43	0	0.00	0.00	0.00	0.00	0.00	1	0.10	0.22	0.20	0.02	0.02
其他的皮肤	C44	14	1.17	2.79	3.38	0.12	0.20	6	0.57	1.30	1.28	0.01	0.12
间皮瘤	C45	0	0.00	0.00	0.00	0.00	0.00	0	0.00	0.00	0.00	0.00	0.00
卡波西肉瘤	C46	0	0.00	0.00	0.00	0.00	0.00	0	0.00	0.00	0.00	0.00	0.00
周围神经、其他结缔组织、软组织	C47;C49	1	0.08	0.20	0.16	0.00	0.04	2	0.19	0.43	0.53	0.02	0.02
乳房	C50	1	0.08	0.20	0.19	0.02	0.02	121	11.50	26.32	23.18	1.93	2.59
外阴	C51	0	0.00	0.00	0.00	0.00	0.00	3	0.29	0.65	0.53	0.05	0.05
阴道	C52	0	0.00	0.00	0.00	0.00	0.00	0	0.00	0.00	0.00	0.00	0.00
子宫颈	C53	0	0.00	0.00	0.00	0.00	0.00	120	11.41	26.10	23.15	1.78	2.61
子宫体	C54	0	0.00	0.00	0.00	0.00	0.00	44	4.18	9.57	8.85	0.84	0.99
子宫，部位不明	C55	0	0.00	0.00	0.00	0.00	0.00	7	0.67	1.52	1.28	0.05	0.17
卵巢	C56	0	0.00	0.00	0.00	0.00	0.00	20	1.90	4.35	3.74	0.31	0.43
女性其他的生殖器	C57	0	0.00	0.00	0.00	0.00	0.00	1	0.10	0.22	0.18	0.02	0.02
胎盘	C58	0	0.00	0.00	0.00	0.00	0.00	0	0.00	0.00	0.00	0.00	0.00
阴茎	C60	3	0.25	0.60	0.61	0.04	0.08	0	0.00	0.00	0.00	0.00	0.00
前列腺	C61	29	2.43	5.78	6.84	0.00	0.48	0	0.00	0.00	0.00	0.00	0.00
睾丸	C62	4	0.34	0.80	0.62	0.04	0.04	0	0.00	0.00	0.00	0.00	0.00
男性其他的生殖器	C63	0	0.00	0.00	0.00	0.00	0.00	0	0.00	0.00	0.00	0.00	0.00
肾	C64	19	1.59	3.79	3.45	0.20	0.40	12	1.14	2.61	2.11	0.11	0.19
肾盂	C65	1	0.08	0.20	0.16	0.00	0.04	4	0.38	0.87	0.88	0.03	0.08
输尿管	C66	2	0.17	0.40	0.38	0.05	0.05	0	0.00	0.00	0.00	0.00	0.00
膀胱	C67	25	2.09	4.99	6.70	0.23	0.51	8	0.76	1.74	1.51	0.09	0.16
其他的泌尿器官	C68	0	0.00	0.00	0.00	0.00	0.00	0	0.00	0.00	0.00	0.00	0.00
眼	C69	0	0.00	0.00	0.00	0.00	0.00	0	0.00	0.00	0.00	0.00	0.00
脑、神经系统	C70–C72	33	2.76	6.58	6.80	0.28	0.59	33	3.14	7.18	6.23	0.44	0.67
甲状腺	C73	30	2.51	5.98	5.51	0.44	0.60	112	10.65	24.36	21.21	1.92	2.08
肾上腺	C74	2	0.17	0.40	0.38	0.03	0.07	0	0.00	0.00	0.00	0.00	0.00
其他的内分泌腺	C75	0	0.00	0.00	0.00	0.00	0.00	1	0.10	0.22	0.22	0.00	0.04
霍奇金病	C81	2	0.17	0.40	0.36	0.01	0.01	0	0.00	0.00	0.00	0.00	0.00
非霍奇金淋巴瘤	C82–C85;C96	20	1.68	3.99	3.60	0.22	0.47	7	0.67	1.52	1.45	0.06	0.15
免疫增生性疾病	C88	0	0.00	0.00	0.00	0.00	0.00	1	0.10	0.22	0.26	0.03	0.03
多发性骨髓瘤	C90	11	0.92	2.19	2.09	0.07	0.35	6	0.57	1.30	1.19	0.02	0.22
淋巴样白血病	C91	5	0.42	1.00	1.14	0.04	0.12	1	0.10	0.22	0.16	0.01	0.01
髓样白血病	C92–C94	11	0.92	2.19	2.01	0.11	0.31	10	0.95	2.17	1.92	0.14	0.22
白血病，未特指	C95	3	0.25	0.60	0.63	0.07	0.07	1	0.10	0.22	0.18	0.02	0.02
其他的或未指明部位	O&U	39	3.27	7.78	8.00	0.44	0.80	44	4.18	9.57	8.79	0.46	0.88
骨髓增殖性疾病	MPD	1	0.08	0.20	0.22	0.03	0.03	0	0.00	0.00	0.00	0.00	0.00
骨髓增生异常综合征	MDS	0	0.00	0.00	0.00	0.00	0.00	0	0.00	0.00	0.00	0.00	0.00
合计	ALL	1 194	100.00	238.10	246.51	9.98	25.76	1 052	100.00	228.79	207.70	12.42	21.39
C44 以外的部位	ALL but C44	1 180	98.83	235.31	243.13	9.86	25.56	1 046	99.43	227.49	206.42	12.41	21.27

表 6-54 2020 年河南省鲁山县恶性肿瘤死亡主要指标

部位	ICD-10	男性						女性					
		病例数	构成(%)	粗率(1/10^5)	世标率(1/10^5)	累积率(%)		病例数	构成(%)	粗率(1/10^5)	世标率(1/10^5)	累积率(%)	
						0~64	0~74					0~64	0~74
唇	C00	0	0.00	0.00	0.00	0.00	0.00	0	0.00	0.00	0.00	0.00	0.00
舌	C01-C02	0	0.00	0.00	0.00	0.00	0.00	0	0.00	0.00	0.00	0.00	0.00
口	C03-C06	0	0.00	0.00	0.00	0.00	0.00	1	0.21	0.22	0.22	0.00	0.04
唾液腺	C07-C08	0	0.00	0.00	0.00	0.00	0.00	0	0.00	0.00	0.00	0.00	0.00
扁桃体	C09	0	0.00	0.00	0.00	0.00	0.00	0	0.00	0.00	0.00	0.00	0.00
其他的口咽	C10	1	0.11	0.20	0.16	0.00	0.04	0	0.00	0.00	0.00	0.00	0.00
鼻咽	C11	2	0.23	0.40	0.33	0.03	0.03	2	0.41	0.43	0.24	0.00	0.00
喉咽	C12-C13	3	0.34	0.60	0.54	0.00	0.08	1	0.21	0.22	0.11	0.00	0.00
咽，部位不明	C14	1	0.11	0.20	0.63	0.00	0.00	1	0.21	0.22	0.18	0.02	0.02
食管	C15	139	15.72	27.72	31.78	0.50	2.57	54	11.09	11.74	11.55	0.22	0.70
胃	C16	184	20.81	36.69	43.28	0.78	3.82	62	12.73	13.48	13.94	0.36	0.75
小肠	C17	1	0.11	0.20	0.16	0.00	0.04	1	0.21	0.22	0.22	0.00	0.04
结肠	C18	15	1.70	2.99	3.20	0.15	0.27	15	3.08	3.26	2.73	0.11	0.24
直肠	C19-C20	19	2.15	3.79	4.69	0.08	0.27	14	2.87	3.04	2.68	0.03	0.16
肛门	C21	2	0.23	0.40	0.33	0.00	0.08	0	0.00	0.00	0.00	0.00	0.00
肝脏	C22	106	11.99	21.14	22.58	0.94	2.13	67	13.76	14.57	13.89	0.50	1.20
胆囊及其他	C23-C24	16	1.81	3.19	3.75	0.11	0.35	8	1.64	1.74	1.41	0.03	0.19
胰腺	C25	13	1.47	2.59	2.29	0.05	0.25	11	2.26	2.39	1.89	0.10	0.18
鼻、鼻窦及其他	C30-C31	0	0.00	0.00	0.00	0.00	0.00	1	0.21	0.22	0.17	0.00	0.04
喉	C32	3	0.34	0.60	1.42	0.00	0.04	0	0.00	0.00	0.00	0.00	0.00
气管、支气管、肺	C33-C34	247	27.94	49.25	58.52	1.55	4.22	108	22.18	23.49	22.40	0.70	1.78
其他的胸腔器官	C37-C38	4	0.45	0.80	1.19	0.02	0.10	1	0.21	0.22	0.16	0.01	0.01
骨	C40-C41	6	0.68	1.20	1.52	0.03	0.11	8	1.64	1.74	1.44	0.06	0.10
皮肤的黑色素瘤	C43	0	0.00	0.00	0.00	0.00	0.00	0	0.00	0.00	0.00	0.00	0.00
其他的皮肤	C44	7	0.79	1.40	2.12	0.00	0.08	4	0.82	0.87	1.26	0.00	0.04
间皮瘤	C45	0	0.00	0.00	0.00	0.00	0.00	0	0.00	0.00	0.00	0.00	0.00
卡波西肉瘤	C46	0	0.00	0.00	0.00	0.00	0.00	0	0.00	0.00	0.00	0.00	0.00
周围神经、其他结缔组织、软组织	C47;C49	0	0.00	0.00	0.00	0.00	0.00	1	0.21	0.22	0.18	0.02	0.02
乳房	C50	2	0.23	0.40	0.33	0.02	0.06	26	5.34	5.65	4.92	0.43	0.47
外阴	C51	0	0.00	0.00	0.00	0.00	0.00	0	0.00	0.00	0.00	0.00	0.00
阴道	C52	0	0.00	0.00	0.00	0.00	0.00	0	0.00	0.00	0.00	0.00	0.00
子宫颈	C53	0	0.00	0.00	0.00	0.00	0.00	30	6.16	6.52	6.42	0.39	0.74
子宫体	C54	0	0.00	0.00	0.00	0.00	0.00	8	1.64	1.74	1.96	0.11	0.19
子宫，部位不明	C55	0	0.00	0.00	0.00	0.00	0.00	3	0.62	0.65	0.38	0.00	0.04
卵巢	C56	0	0.00	0.00	0.00	0.00	0.00	11	2.26	2.39	1.91	0.11	0.22
女性其他的生殖器	C57	0	0.00	0.00	0.00	0.00	0.00	0	0.00	0.00	0.00	0.00	0.00
胎盘	C58	0	0.00	0.00	0.00	0.00	0.00	0	0.00	0.00	0.00	0.00	0.00
阴茎	C60	0	0.00	0.00	0.00	0.00	0.00	0	0.00	0.00	0.00	0.00	0.00
前列腺	C61	9	1.02	1.79	2.36	0.00	0.08	0	0.00	0.00	0.00	0.00	0.00
睾丸	C62	0	0.00	0.00	0.00	0.00	0.00	0	0.00	0.00	0.00	0.00	0.00
男性其他的生殖器	C63	0	0.00	0.00	0.00	0.00	0.00	0	0.00	0.00	0.00	0.00	0.00
肾	C64	4	0.45	0.80	0.68	0.00	0.04	4	0.82	0.87	0.78	0.00	0.04
肾盂	C65	1	0.11	0.20	0.16	0.00	0.04	2	0.41	0.43	0.37	0.03	0.03
输尿管	C66	0	0.00	0.00	0.00	0.00	0.00	0	0.00	0.00	0.00	0.00	0.00
膀胱	C67	19	2.15	3.79	4.75	0.11	0.35	0	0.00	0.00	0.00	0.00	0.00
其他的泌尿器官	C68	0	0.00	0.00	0.00	0.00	0.00	0	0.00	0.00	0.00	0.00	0.00
眼	C69	0	0.00	0.00	0.00	0.00	0.00	0	0.00	0.00	0.00	0.00	0.00
脑、神经系统	C70-C72	27	3.05	5.38	4.73	0.29	0.61	23	4.72	5.00	4.36	0.21	0.41
甲状腺	C73	2	0.23	0.40	0.37	0.00	0.04	3	0.62	0.65	0.53	0.04	0.08
肾上腺	C74	2	0.23	0.40	0.40	0.00	0.08	0	0.00	0.00	0.00	0.00	0.00
其他的内分泌腺	C75	0	0.00	0.00	0.00	0.00	0.00	0	0.00	0.00	0.00	0.00	0.00
霍奇金病	C81	0	0.00	0.00	0.00	0.00	0.00	0	0.00	0.00	0.00	0.00	0.00
非霍奇金淋巴瘤	C82-C85;C96	7	0.79	1.40	1.20	0.08	0.20	0	0.00	0.00	0.00	0.00	0.00
免疫增生性疾病	C88	1	0.11	0.20	0.23	0.00	0.04	0	0.00	0.00	0.00	0.00	0.00
多发性骨髓瘤	C90	7	0.79	1.40	1.28	0.03	0.24	3	0.62	0.65	0.47	0.02	0.06
淋巴样白血病	C91	5	0.57	1.00	0.95	0.05	0.10	1	0.21	0.22	0.17	0.01	0.01
髓样白血病	C92-C94	7	0.79	1.40	1.79	0.07	0.11	1	0.21	0.22	0.11	0.00	0.00
白血病，未特指	C95	2	0.23	0.40	0.40	0.00	0.04	0	0.00	0.00	0.00	0.00	0.00
其他的或未指明部位	O&U	19	2.15	3.79	3.73	0.06	0.34	11	2.26	2.39	1.87	0.12	0.21
骨髓增殖性疾病	MPD	1	0.11	0.20	0.16	0.00	0.00	1	0.21	0.22	0.22	0.00	0.04
骨髓增生异常综合征	MDS	0	0.00	0.00	0.00	0.00	0.00	0	0.00	0.00	0.00	0.00	0.00
合计	ALL	884	100.00	176.28	202.01	4.94	16.84	487	100.00	105.91	99.14	3.63	8.04
C44 以外的部位	ALL but C44	877	99.21	174.88	199.89	4.94	16.76	483	99.18	105.04	97.89	3.63	8.00

表 6-55 2020 年河南省郏县恶性肿瘤发病主要指标

部位	ICD-10	男性						女性					
		病例数	构成 (%)	粗率 (1/10^5)	世标率 (1/10^5)	累积率 (%) 0~64	累积率 (%) 0~74	病例数	构成 (%)	粗率 (1/10^5)	世标率 (1/10^5)	累积率 (%) 0~64	累积率 (%) 0~74
唇	C00	0	0.00	0.00	0.00	0.00	0.00	0	0.00	0.00	0.00	0.00	0.00
舌	C01–C02	1	0.13	0.29	0.43	0.03	0.03	1	0.14	0.33	0.15	0.00	0.00
口	C03–C06	3	0.40	0.88	0.93	0.03	0.15	3	0.41	0.98	0.74	0.06	0.06
唾液腺	C07–C08	1	0.13	0.29	0.21	0.03	0.03	1	0.14	0.33	0.24	0.03	0.03
扁桃体	C09	0	0.00	0.00	0.00	0.00	0.00	0	0.00	0.00	0.00	0.00	0.00
其他的口咽	C10	1	0.13	0.29	0.25	0.00	0.06	0	0.00	0.00	0.00	0.00	0.00
鼻咽	C11	5	0.67	1.47	1.21	0.06	0.06	4	0.55	1.31	0.99	0.10	0.10
喉咽	C12–C13	2	0.27	0.59	0.56	0.00	0.11	0	0.00	0.00	0.00	0.00	0.00
咽，部位不明	C14	0	0.00	0.00	0.00	0.00	0.00	1	0.14	0.33	0.30	0.03	0.03
食管	C15	50	6.73	14.72	13.05	0.44	1.66	38	5.25	12.48	8.90	0.33	1.05
胃	C16	76	10.23	22.37	18.54	0.67	2.20	28	3.87	9.19	6.12	0.20	0.43
小肠	C17	2	0.27	0.59	0.56	0.02	0.07	2	0.28	0.66	0.63	0.04	0.09
结肠	C18	22	2.96	6.48	5.45	0.22	0.67	11	1.52	3.61	2.87	0.22	0.36
直肠	C19–C20	40	5.38	11.78	9.28	0.37	1.12	21	2.90	6.89	5.35	0.18	0.72
肛门	C21	0	0.00	0.00	0.00	0.00	0.00	1	0.14	0.33	0.18	0.00	0.00
肝脏	C22	73	9.83	21.49	18.26	0.85	1.98	43	5.94	14.12	9.94	0.15	1.28
胆囊及其他	C23–C24	9	1.21	2.65	2.35	0.07	0.29	12	1.66	3.94	2.95	0.06	0.42
胰腺	C25	23	3.10	6.77	5.16	0.38	0.56	11	1.52	3.61	2.90	0.09	0.38
鼻、鼻窦及其他	C30–C31	1	0.13	0.29	0.27	0.03	0.03	0	0.00	0.00	0.00	0.00	0.00
喉	C32	5	0.67	1.47	1.14	0.07	0.12	0	0.00	0.00	0.00	0.00	0.00
气管、支气管、肺	C33–C34	274	36.88	80.67	65.77	2.59	8.45	112	15.47	36.77	27.42	1.12	3.50
其他的胸腔器官	C37–C38	0	0.00	0.00	0.00	0.00	0.00	4	0.55	1.31	1.20	0.06	0.17
骨	C40–C41	5	0.67	1.47	1.32	0.05	0.18	6	0.83	1.97	2.06	0.17	0.17
皮肤的黑色素瘤	C43	1	0.13	0.29	0.21	0.03	0.03	0	0.00	0.00	0.00	0.00	0.00
其他的皮肤	C44	4	0.54	1.18	1.10	0.00	0.11	2	0.28	0.66	0.48	0.00	0.06
间皮瘤	C45	0	0.00	0.00	0.00	0.00	0.00	0	0.00	0.00	0.00	0.00	0.00
卡波西肉瘤	C46	0	0.00	0.00	0.00	0.00	0.00	0	0.00	0.00	0.00	0.00	0.00
周围神经、其他结缔组织、软组织	C47;C49	2	0.27	0.59	0.52	0.05	0.05	2	0.28	0.66	0.51	0.04	0.04
乳房	C50	1	0.13	0.29	0.31	0.00	0.05	157	21.69	51.54	42.31	3.55	4.92
外阴	C51	0	0.00	0.00	0.00	0.00	0.00	0	0.00	0.00	0.00	0.00	0.00
阴道	C52	0	0.00	0.00	0.00	0.00	0.00	0	0.00	0.00	0.00	0.00	0.00
子宫颈	C53	0	0.00	0.00	0.00	0.00	0.00	54	7.46	17.73	14.21	1.19	1.61
子宫体	C54	0	0.00	0.00	0.00	0.00	0.00	41	5.66	13.46	11.57	1.01	1.42
子宫，部位不明	C55	0	0.00	0.00	0.00	0.00	0.00	1	0.14	0.33	0.30	0.03	0.03
卵巢	C56	0	0.00	0.00	0.00	0.00	0.00	17	2.35	5.58	5.05	0.29	0.47
女性其他的生殖器	C57	0	0.00	0.00	0.00	0.00	0.00	3	0.41	0.98	0.86	0.06	0.13
胎盘	C58	0	0.00	0.00	0.00	0.00	0.00	0	0.00	0.00	0.00	0.00	0.00
阴茎	C60	2	0.27	0.59	0.62	0.00	0.06	0	0.00	0.00	0.00	0.00	0.00
前列腺	C61	19	2.56	5.59	4.61	0.03	0.58	0	0.00	0.00	0.00	0.00	0.00
睾丸	C62	3	0.40	0.88	0.79	0.02	0.08	0	0.00	0.00	0.00	0.00	0.00
男性其他的生殖器	C63	0	0.00	0.00	0.00	0.00	0.00	0	0.00	0.00	0.00	0.00	0.00
肾	C64	5	0.67	1.47	1.25	0.07	0.18	4	0.55	1.31	1.08	0.04	0.11
肾盂	C65	1	0.13	0.29	0.37	0.00	0.00	0	0.00	0.00	0.00	0.00	0.00
输尿管	C66	2	0.27	0.59	0.37	0.02	0.02	0	0.00	0.00	0.00	0.00	0.00
膀胱	C67	12	1.62	3.53	3.05	0.11	0.36	4	0.55	1.31	0.92	0.04	0.09
其他的泌尿器官	C68	0	0.00	0.00	0.00	0.00	0.00	0	0.00	0.00	0.00	0.00	0.00
眼	C69	1	0.13	0.29	0.37	0.00	0.00	0	0.00	0.00	0.00	0.00	0.00
脑、神经系统	C70–C72	23	3.10	6.77	5.36	0.33	0.61	18	2.49	5.91	4.78	0.35	0.52
甲状腺	C73	13	1.75	3.83	3.04	0.27	0.40	51	7.04	16.74	13.89	1.18	1.35
肾上腺	C74	2	0.27	0.59	0.41	0.04	0.04	0	0.00	0.00	0.00	0.00	0.00
其他的内分泌腺	C75	0	0.00	0.00	0.00	0.00	0.00	0	0.00	0.00	0.00	0.00	0.00
霍奇金病	C81	0	0.00	0.00	0.00	0.00	0.00	0	0.00	0.00	0.00	0.00	0.00
非霍奇金淋巴瘤	C82–C85;C96	5	0.67	1.47	1.24	0.08	0.08	14	1.93	4.60	3.88	0.27	0.45
免疫增生性疾病	C88	0	0.00	0.00	0.00	0.00	0.00	0	0.00	0.00	0.00	0.00	0.00
多发性骨髓瘤	C90	4	0.54	1.18	0.87	0.08	0.14	3	0.41	0.98	0.89	0.10	0.10
淋巴样白血病	C91	1	0.13	0.29	0.27	0.03	0.03	1	0.14	0.33	0.30	0.04	0.04
髓样白血病	C92–C94	10	1.35	2.94	2.42	0.13	0.25	7	0.97	2.30	1.82	0.12	0.18
白血病，未特指	C95	0	0.00	0.00	0.00	0.00	0.00	1	0.14	0.33	0.58	0.03	0.03
其他的或未指明部位	O&U	39	5.25	11.48	10.17	0.44	1.01	45	6.22	14.77	12.37	0.77	1.27
骨髓增殖性疾病	MPD	0	0.00	0.00	0.00	0.00	0.00	0	0.00	0.00	0.00	0.00	0.00
骨髓增生异常综合征	MDS	0	0.00	0.00	0.00	0.00	0.00	0	0.00	0.00	0.00	0.00	0.00
合计	ALL	743	100.00	218.74	182.07	7.62	21.85	724	100.00	237.70	188.72	11.96	21.59
C44 以外的部位	ALL but C44	739	99.46	217.57	180.97	7.62	21.73	722	99.72	237.04	188.24	11.96	21.53

表 6-56　2020 年河南省郏县恶性肿瘤死亡主要指标

部位	ICD-10	男性						女性					
		病例数	构成 (%)	粗率 (1/10⁵)	世标率 (1/10⁵)	累积率 (%) 0~64	累积率 (%) 0~74	病例数	构成 (%)	粗率 (1/10⁵)	世标率 (1/10⁵)	累积率 (%) 0~64	累积率 (%) 0~74
唇	C00	1	0.15	0.29	0.25	0.00	0.06	0	0.00	0.00	0.00	0.00	0.00
舌	C01–C02	3	0.46	0.88	0.70	0.07	0.07	2	0.52	0.66	0.44	0.00	0.07
口	C03–C06	0	0.00	0.00	0.00	0.00	0.00	2	0.52	0.66	0.33	0.00	0.00
唾液腺	C07–C08	1	0.15	0.29	0.31	0.00	0.05	0	0.00	0.00	0.00	0.00	0.00
扁桃体	C09	0	0.00	0.00	0.00	0.00	0.00	0	0.00	0.00	0.00	0.00	0.00
其他的口咽	C10	0	0.00	0.00	0.00	0.00	0.00	0	0.00	0.00	0.00	0.00	0.00
鼻咽	C11	2	0.31	0.59	0.63	0.02	0.02	1	0.26	0.33	0.18	0.00	0.00
喉咽	C12–C13	0	0.00	0.00	0.00	0.00	0.00	0	0.00	0.00	0.00	0.00	0.00
咽，部位不明	C14	0	0.00	0.00	0.00	0.00	0.00	0	0.00	0.00	0.00	0.00	0.00
食管	C15	58	8.94	17.08	15.31	0.20	1.70	31	8.03	10.18	6.43	0.08	0.71
胃	C16	78	12.02	22.96	19.67	0.43	2.40	30	7.77	9.85	6.62	0.12	0.65
小肠	C17	0	0.00	0.00	0.00	0.00	0.00	1	0.26	0.33	0.33	0.00	0.06
结肠	C18	12	1.85	3.53	3.07	0.02	0.37	7	1.81	2.30	1.50	0.06	0.13
直肠	C19–C20	21	3.24	6.18	4.17	0.14	0.20	18	4.66	5.91	4.20	0.15	0.45
肛门	C21	1	0.15	0.29	0.25	0.00	0.06	2	0.52	0.66	0.33	0.00	0.00
肝脏	C22	81	12.48	23.85	19.78	0.84	2.49	52	13.47	17.07	12.31	0.44	1.47
胆囊及其他	C23–C24	6	0.92	1.77	1.60	0.03	0.14	15	3.89	4.92	3.77	0.13	0.49
胰腺	C25	20	3.08	5.89	4.31	0.28	0.41	8	2.07	2.63	2.00	0.08	0.19
鼻、鼻窦及其他	C30–C31	1	0.15	0.29	0.17	0.00	0.00	0	0.00	0.00	0.00	0.00	0.00
喉	C32	9	1.39	2.65	2.22	0.07	0.29	0	0.00	0.00	0.00	0.00	0.00
气管、支气管、肺	C33–C34	245	37.75	72.13	59.40	1.57	6.68	102	26.42	33.49	24.08	0.84	2.85
其他的胸腔器官	C37–C38	1	0.15	0.29	0.19	0.00	0.00	1	0.26	0.33	0.24	0.03	0.03
骨	C40–C41	5	0.77	1.47	1.22	0.07	0.12	1	0.26	0.33	0.58	0.03	0.03
皮肤的黑色素瘤	C43	0	0.00	0.00	0.00	0.00	0.00	0	0.00	0.00	0.00	0.00	0.00
其他的皮肤	C44	1	0.15	0.29	0.37	0.00	0.00	2	0.52	0.66	0.36	0.00	0.00
间皮瘤	C45	0	0.00	0.00	0.00	0.00	0.00	0	0.00	0.00	0.00	0.00	0.00
卡波西肉瘤	C46	0	0.00	0.00	0.00	0.00	0.00	0	0.00	0.00	0.00	0.00	0.00
周围神经、其他结缔组织、软组织	C47;C49	0	0.00	0.00	0.00	0.00	0.00	0	0.00	0.00	0.00	0.00	0.00
乳房	C50	2	0.31	0.59	0.37	0.02	0.02	26	6.74	8.54	6.47	0.45	0.68
外阴	C51	0	0.00	0.00	0.00	0.00	0.00	2	0.52	0.66	0.63	0.04	0.09
阴道	C52	0	0.00	0.00	0.00	0.00	0.00	2	0.52	0.66	0.33	0.00	0.00
子宫颈	C53	0	0.00	0.00	0.00	0.00	0.00	17	4.40	5.58	4.12	0.21	0.52
子宫体	C54	0	0.00	0.00	0.00	0.00	0.00	3	0.78	0.98	0.82	0.06	0.12
子宫，部位不明	C55	0	0.00	0.00	0.00	0.00	0.00	1	0.26	0.33	0.24	0.03	0.03
卵巢	C56	0	0.00	0.00	0.00	0.00	0.00	10	2.59	3.28	2.56	0.10	0.27
女性其他的生殖器	C57	0	0.00	0.00	0.00	0.00	0.00	1	0.26	0.33	0.26	0.00	0.07
胎盘	C58	0	0.00	0.00	0.00	0.00	0.00	0	0.00	0.00	0.00	0.00	0.00
阴茎	C60	1	0.15	0.29	0.17	0.00	0.00	0	0.00	0.00	0.00	0.00	0.00
前列腺	C61	6	0.92	1.77	1.91	0.03	0.03	0	0.00	0.00	0.00	0.00	0.00
睾丸	C62	3	0.46	0.88	0.83	0.03	0.15	0	0.00	0.00	0.00	0.00	0.00
男性其他的生殖器	C63	0	0.00	0.00	0.00	0.00	0.00	0	0.00	0.00	0.00	0.00	0.00
肾	C64	4	0.62	1.18	0.90	0.07	0.12	3	0.78	0.98	0.72	0.03	0.09
肾盂	C65	2	0.31	0.59	0.44	0.03	0.03	1	0.26	0.33	0.18	0.00	0.00
输尿管	C66	4	0.62	1.18	0.81	0.03	0.09	0	0.00	0.00	0.00	0.00	0.00
膀胱	C67	7	1.08	2.06	1.71	0.05	0.17	6	1.55	1.97	1.43	0.00	0.18
其他的泌尿器官	C68	2	0.31	0.59	0.62	0.00	0.06	0	0.00	0.00	0.00	0.00	0.00
眼	C69	1	0.15	0.29	0.37	0.00	0.00	0	0.00	0.00	0.00	0.00	0.00
脑、神经系统	C70–C72	22	3.39	6.48	5.23	0.22	0.53	12	3.11	3.94	2.72	0.14	0.26
甲状腺	C73	0	0.00	0.00	0.00	0.00	0.00	2	0.52	0.66	0.41	0.00	0.07
肾上腺	C74	3	0.46	0.88	0.74	0.04	0.04	0	0.00	0.00	0.00	0.00	0.00
其他的内分泌腺	C75	1	0.15	0.29	0.27	0.03	0.03	0	0.00	0.00	0.00	0.00	0.00
霍奇金病	C81	1	0.15	0.29	0.17	0.00	0.00	0	0.00	0.00	0.00	0.00	0.00
非霍奇金淋巴瘤	C82–C85;C96	1	0.15	0.29	0.31	0.00	0.05	1	0.26	0.33	0.15	0.00	0.00
免疫增生性疾病	C88	0	0.00	0.00	0.00	0.00	0.00	0	0.00	0.00	0.00	0.00	0.00
多发性骨髓瘤	C90	3	0.46	0.88	0.78	0.05	0.11	1	0.26	0.33	0.30	0.04	0.04
淋巴样白血病	C91	1	0.15	0.29	0.19	0.02	0.02	0	0.00	0.00	0.00	0.00	0.00
髓样白血病	C92–C94	4	0.62	1.18	0.90	0.02	0.02	2	0.52	0.66	0.41	0.00	0.07
白血病，未特指	C95	0	0.00	0.00	0.00	0.00	0.00	1	0.26	0.33	0.15	0.00	0.00
其他的或未指明部位	O&U	35	5.39	10.30	9.44	0.39	0.80	20	5.18	6.57	5.31	0.16	0.71
骨髓增殖性疾病	MPD	0	0.00	0.00	0.00	0.00	0.00	0	0.00	0.00	0.00	0.00	0.00
骨髓增生异常综合征	MDS	0	0.00	0.00	0.00	0.00	0.00	0	0.00	0.00	0.00	0.00	0.00
合计	ALL	649	100.00	191.07	159.78	4.77	17.32	386	100.00	126.73	90.91	3.23	10.29
C44 以外的部位	ALL but C44	648	99.85	190.77	159.41	4.77	17.32	384	99.48	126.07	90.55	3.23	10.29

表 6-57　2020 年河南省舞钢市恶性肿瘤发病主要指标

部位	ICD-10	男性						女性					
		病例数	构成 (%)	粗率 (1/10^5)	世标率 (1/10^5)	累积率 (%) 0~64	累积率 (%) 0~74	病例数	构成 (%)	粗率 (1/10^5)	世标率 (1/10^5)	累积率 (%) 0~64	累积率 (%) 0~74
唇	C00	0	0.00	0.00	0.00	0.00	0.00	0	0.00	0.00	0.00	0.00	0.00
舌	C01–C02	0	0.00	0.00	0.00	0.00	0.00	3	0.70	1.85	1.29	0.09	0.16
口	C03–C06	4	0.71	2.37	1.43	0.09	0.09	0	0.00	0.00	0.00	0.00	0.00
唾液腺	C07–C08	2	0.35	1.19	0.84	0.08	0.08	1	0.23	0.62	0.40	0.00	0.07
扁桃体	C09	0	0.00	0.00	0.00	0.00	0.00	0	0.00	0.00	0.00	0.00	0.00
其他的口咽	C10	0	0.00	0.00	0.00	0.00	0.00	0	0.00	0.00	0.00	0.00	0.00
鼻咽	C11	2	0.35	1.19	0.70	0.05	0.10	1	0.23	0.62	0.35	0.03	0.03
喉咽	C12–C13	0	0.00	0.00	0.00	0.00	0.00	1	0.23	0.62	0.35	0.00	0.09
咽，部位不明	C14	0	0.00	0.00	0.00	0.00	0.00	0	0.00	0.00	0.00	0.00	0.00
食管	C15	76	13.43	45.10	24.80	0.87	3.27	40	9.37	24.71	11.78	0.32	1.61
胃	C16	78	13.78	46.28	26.08	1.02	3.53	18	4.22	11.12	5.39	0.25	0.49
小肠	C17	3	0.53	1.78	1.06	0.09	0.18	0	0.00	0.00	0.00	0.00	0.00
结肠	C18	14	2.47	8.31	4.72	0.16	0.81	9	2.11	5.56	3.68	0.30	0.45
直肠	C19–C20	28	4.95	16.61	9.14	0.36	1.29	19	4.45	11.74	6.37	0.36	0.73
肛门	C21	2	0.35	1.19	0.74	0.03	0.09	0	0.00	0.00	0.00	0.00	0.00
肝脏	C22	74	13.07	43.91	26.06	1.47	3.05	31	7.26	19.15	11.05	0.37	1.73
胆囊及其他	C23–C24	3	0.53	1.78	0.97	0.03	0.09	2	0.47	1.24	0.51	0.00	0.00
胰腺	C25	8	1.41	4.75	2.87	0.22	0.31	8	1.87	4.94	2.68	0.12	0.28
鼻、鼻窦及其他	C30–C31	0	0.00	0.00	0.00	0.00	0.00	2	0.47	1.24	0.75	0.00	0.15
喉	C32	8	1.41	4.75	2.74	0.18	0.38	0	0.00	0.00	0.00	0.00	0.00
气管、支气管、肺	C33–C34	147	25.97	87.23	48.00	1.77	5.99	46	10.77	28.41	15.54	0.56	2.10
其他的胸腔器官	C37–C38	2	0.35	1.19	0.53	0.00	0.06	1	0.23	0.62	0.37	0.05	0.05
骨	C40–C41	2	0.35	1.19	1.09	0.07	0.07	1	0.23	0.62	0.16	0.00	0.00
皮肤的黑色素瘤	C43	1	0.18	0.59	0.34	0.00	0.06	0	0.00	0.00	0.00	0.00	0.00
其他的皮肤	C44	13	2.30	7.71	4.18	0.16	0.41	14	3.28	8.65	4.31	0.12	0.42
间皮瘤	C45	0	0.00	0.00	0.00	0.00	0.00	0	0.00	0.00	0.00	0.00	0.00
卡波西肉瘤	C46	0	0.00	0.00	0.00	0.00	0.00	0	0.00	0.00	0.00	0.00	0.00
周围神经、其他结缔组织、软组织	C47;C49	1	0.18	0.59	0.35	0.03	0.03	2	0.47	1.24	1.05	0.09	0.09
乳房	C50	1	0.18	0.59	0.51	0.04	0.04	61	14.29	37.68	23.86	1.93	2.50
外阴	C51	0	0.00	0.00	0.00	0.00	0.00	1	0.23	0.62	0.29	0.00	0.00
阴道	C52	0	0.00	0.00	0.00	0.00	0.00	0	0.00	0.00	0.00	0.00	0.00
子宫颈	C53	0	0.00	0.00	0.00	0.00	0.00	43	10.07	26.56	16.56	1.21	1.94
子宫体	C54	0	0.00	0.00	0.00	0.00	0.00	9	2.11	5.56	3.69	0.32	0.41
子宫，部位不明	C55	0	0.00	0.00	0.00	0.00	0.00	0	0.00	0.00	0.00	0.00	0.00
卵巢	C56	0	0.00	0.00	0.00	0.00	0.00	10	2.34	6.18	3.73	0.24	0.46
女性其他的生殖器	C57	0	0.00	0.00	0.00	0.00	0.00	2	0.47	1.24	0.76	0.05	0.11
胎盘	C58	0	0.00	0.00	0.00	0.00	0.00	0	0.00	0.00	0.00	0.00	0.00
阴茎	C60	2	0.35	1.19	0.69	0.03	0.09	0	0.00	0.00	0.00	0.00	0.00
前列腺	C61	16	2.83	9.49	4.83	0.09	0.40	0	0.00	0.00	0.00	0.00	0.00
睾丸	C62	0	0.00	0.00	0.00	0.00	0.00	0	0.00	0.00	0.00	0.00	0.00
男性其他的生殖器	C63	0	0.00	0.00	0.00	0.00	0.00	0	0.00	0.00	0.00	0.00	0.00
肾	C64	9	1.59	5.34	3.74	0.30	0.41	4	0.94	2.47	1.48	0.16	0.16
肾盂	C65	1	0.18	0.59	0.36	0.05	0.05	1	0.23	0.62	0.29	0.00	0.00
输尿管	C66	1	0.18	0.59	0.34	0.00	0.06	0	0.00	0.00	0.00	0.00	0.00
膀胱	C67	14	2.47	8.31	4.27	0.17	0.40	3	0.70	1.85	1.09	0.03	0.19
其他的泌尿器官	C68	0	0.00	0.00	0.00	0.00	0.00	0	0.00	0.00	0.00	0.00	0.00
眼	C69	0	0.00	0.00	0.00	0.00	0.00	1	0.23	0.62	0.35	0.00	0.09
脑、神经系统	C70–C72	19	3.36	11.27	8.15	0.44	0.75	4	0.94	2.47	1.46	0.08	0.23
甲状腺	C73	18	3.18	10.68	7.86	0.64	0.78	61	14.29	37.68	29.12	2.41	2.63
肾上腺	C74	1	0.18	0.59	1.07	0.04	0.04	0	0.00	0.00	0.00	0.00	0.00
其他的内分泌腺	C75	0	0.00	0.00	0.00	0.00	0.00	0	0.00	0.00	0.00	0.00	0.00
霍奇金病	C81	0	0.00	0.00	0.00	0.00	0.00	0	0.00	0.00	0.00	0.00	0.00
非霍奇金淋巴瘤	C82–C85;C96	4	0.71	2.37	1.53	0.13	0.19	7	1.64	4.32	3.37	0.22	0.35
免疫增生性疾病	C88	0	0.00	0.00	0.00	0.00	0.00	0	0.00	0.00	0.00	0.00	0.00
多发性骨髓瘤	C90	2	0.35	1.19	0.67	0.00	0.11	3	0.70	1.85	1.12	0.12	0.12
淋巴样白血病	C91	0	0.00	0.00	0.00	0.00	0.00	0	0.00	0.00	0.00	0.00	0.00
髓样白血病	C92–C94	1	0.18	0.59	0.28	0.00	0.00	1	0.23	0.62	0.37	0.05	0.05
白血病，未特指	C95	0	0.00	0.00	0.00	0.00	0.00	2	0.47	1.24	0.66	0.05	0.05
其他的或未指明部位	O&U	9	1.59	5.34	2.93	0.08	0.23	15	3.51	9.27	4.88	0.21	0.60
骨髓增殖性疾病	MPD	0	0.00	0.00	0.00	0.00	0.00	0	0.00	0.00	0.00	0.00	0.00
骨髓增生异常综合征	MDS	0	0.00	0.00	0.00	0.00	0.00	0	0.00	0.00	0.00	0.00	0.00
合计	ALL	566	100.00	335.85	193.86	8.72	23.43	427	100.00	263.76	159.11	9.73	18.34
C44 以外的部位	ALL but C44	553	97.70	328.14	189.68	8.56	23.02	413	96.72	255.11	154.80	9.61	17.92

表 6-58 2020 年河南省舞钢市恶性肿瘤死亡主要指标

部位	ICD-10	男性						女性					
		病例数	构成(%)	粗率(1/10^5)	世标率(1/10^5)	累积率(%)		病例数	构成(%)	粗率(1/10^5)	世标率(1/10^5)	累积率(%)	
						0~64	0~74					0~64	0~74
唇	C00	0	0.00	0.00	0.00	0.00	0.00	0	0.00	0.00	0.00	0.00	0.00
舌	C01–C02	0	0.00	0.00	0.00	0.00	0.00	2	1.38	1.24	0.74	0.09	0.09
口	C03–C06	0	0.00	0.00	0.00	0.00	0.00	1	0.69	0.62	0.35	0.00	0.09
唾液腺	C07–C08	0	0.00	0.00	0.00	0.00	0.00	0	0.00	0.00	0.00	0.00	0.00
扁桃体	C09	0	0.00	0.00	0.00	0.00	0.00	0	0.00	0.00	0.00	0.00	0.00
其他的口咽	C10	0	0.00	0.00	0.00	0.00	0.00	0	0.00	0.00	0.00	0.00	0.00
鼻咽	C11	1	0.34	0.59	0.34	0.00	0.06	3	2.07	1.85	0.96	0.03	0.10
喉咽	C12–C13	0	0.00	0.00	0.00	0.00	0.00	0	0.00	0.00	0.00	0.00	0.00
咽、部位不明	C14	0	0.00	0.00	0.00	0.00	0.00	0	0.00	0.00	0.00	0.00	0.00
食管	C15	45	15.10	26.70	13.25	0.08	1.04	13	8.97	8.03	3.47	0.05	0.29
胃	C16	42	14.09	24.92	13.13	0.28	1.52	14	9.66	8.65	3.91	0.13	0.28
小肠	C17	0	0.00	0.00	0.00	0.00	0.00	1	0.69	0.62	0.29	0.00	0.00
结肠	C18	4	1.34	2.37	1.44	0.08	0.25	4	2.76	2.47	1.34	0.00	0.20
直肠	C19–C20	12	4.03	7.12	3.66	0.05	0.33	5	3.45	3.09	1.22	0.00	0.07
肛门	C21	1	0.34	0.59	0.40	0.03	0.03	0	0.00	0.00	0.00	0.00	0.00
肝脏	C22	45	15.10	26.70	15.40	0.77	1.81	15	10.34	9.27	5.26	0.28	0.70
胆囊及其他	C23–C24	1	0.34	0.59	0.34	0.00	0.08	4	2.76	2.47	1.02	0.00	0.09
胰腺	C25	4	1.34	2.37	1.45	0.12	0.12	6	4.14	3.71	2.04	0.05	0.18
鼻、鼻窦及其他	C30–C31	0	0.00	0.00	0.00	0.00	0.00	0	0.00	0.00	0.00	0.00	0.00
喉	C32	4	1.34	2.37	1.29	0.00	0.20	0	0.00	0.00	0.00	0.00	0.00
气管、支气管、肺	C33–C34	87	29.19	51.62	27.26	0.68	2.68	34	23.45	21.00	10.23	0.30	1.11
其他的胸腔器官	C37–C38	1	0.34	0.59	0.36	0.05	0.05	0	0.00	0.00	0.00	0.00	0.00
骨	C40–C41	7	2.35	4.15	2.67	0.12	0.34	2	1.38	1.24	0.75	0.00	0.15
皮肤的黑色素瘤	C43	1	0.34	0.59	0.34	0.00	0.06	0	0.00	0.00	0.00	0.00	0.00
其他的皮肤	C44	3	1.01	1.78	0.96	0.00	0.17	1	0.69	0.62	0.16	0.00	0.00
间皮瘤	C45	0	0.00	0.00	0.00	0.00	0.00	0	0.00	0.00	0.00	0.00	0.00
卡波西肉瘤	C46	0	0.00	0.00	0.00	0.00	0.00	0	0.00	0.00	0.00	0.00	0.00
周围神经、其他结缔组织、软组织	C47;C49	0	0.00	0.00	0.00	0.00	0.00	0	0.00	0.00	0.00	0.00	0.00
乳房	C50	0	0.00	0.00	0.00	0.00	0.00	12	8.28	7.41	4.31	0.30	0.44
外阴	C51	0	0.00	0.00	0.00	0.00	0.00	0	0.00	0.00	0.00	0.00	0.00
阴道	C52	0	0.00	0.00	0.00	0.00	0.00	0	0.00	0.00	0.00	0.00	0.00
子宫颈	C53	0	0.00	0.00	0.00	0.00	0.00	4	2.76	2.47	1.51	0.08	0.23
子宫体	C54	0	0.00	0.00	0.00	0.00	0.00	1	0.69	0.62	0.40	0.00	0.07
子宫，部位不明	C55	0	0.00	0.00	0.00	0.00	0.00	0	0.00	0.00	0.00	0.00	0.00
卵巢	C56	0	0.00	0.00	0.00	0.00	0.00	6	4.14	3.71	2.15	0.14	0.40
女性其他的生殖器	C57	0	0.00	0.00	0.00	0.00	0.00	0	0.00	0.00	0.00	0.00	0.00
胎盘	C58	0	0.00	0.00	0.00	0.00	0.00	0	0.00	0.00	0.00	0.00	0.00
阴茎	C60	1	0.34	0.59	0.28	0.00	0.00	0	0.00	0.00	0.00	0.00	0.00
前列腺	C61	6	2.01	3.56	2.01	0.00	0.28	0	0.00	0.00	0.00	0.00	0.00
睾丸	C62	0	0.00	0.00	0.00	0.00	0.00	0	0.00	0.00	0.00	0.00	0.00
男性其他的生殖器	C63	0	0.00	0.00	0.00	0.00	0.00	0	0.00	0.00	0.00	0.00	0.00
肾	C64	3	1.01	1.78	1.03	0.05	0.16	2	1.38	1.24	0.72	0.09	0.09
肾盂	C65	0	0.00	0.00	0.00	0.00	0.00	0	0.00	0.00	0.00	0.00	0.00
输尿管	C66	1	0.34	0.59	0.20	0.00	0.00	0	0.00	0.00	0.00	0.00	0.00
膀胱	C67	3	1.01	1.78	0.89	0.05	0.05	1	0.69	0.62	0.40	0.00	0.07
其他的泌尿器官	C68	0	0.00	0.00	0.00	0.00	0.00	0	0.00	0.00	0.00	0.00	0.00
眼	C69	0	0.00	0.00	0.00	0.00	0.00	0	0.00	0.00	0.00	0.00	0.00
脑、神经系统	C70–C72	9	3.02	5.34	2.67	0.10	0.19	7	4.83	4.32	2.67	0.18	0.33
甲状腺	C73	0	0.00	0.00	0.00	0.00	0.00	0	0.00	0.00	0.00	0.00	0.00
肾上腺	C74	0	0.00	0.00	0.00	0.00	0.00	0	0.00	0.00	0.00	0.00	0.00
其他的内分泌腺	C75	0	0.00	0.00	0.00	0.00	0.00	0	0.00	0.00	0.00	0.00	0.00
霍奇金病	C81	0	0.00	0.00	0.00	0.00	0.00	0	0.00	0.00	0.00	0.00	0.00
非霍奇金淋巴瘤	C82–C85;C96	5	1.68	2.97	1.71	0.05	0.30	1	0.69	0.62	0.37	0.05	0.05
免疫增生性疾病	C88	0	0.00	0.00	0.00	0.00	0.00	0	0.00	0.00	0.00	0.00	0.00
多发性骨髓瘤	C90	4	1.34	2.37	1.36	0.03	0.23	0	0.00	0.00	0.00	0.00	0.00
淋巴样白血病	C91	0	0.00	0.00	0.00	0.00	0.00	0	0.00	0.00	0.00	0.00	0.00
髓样白血病	C92–C94	1	0.34	0.59	0.36	0.05	0.05	0	0.00	0.00	0.00	0.00	0.00
白血病，未特指	C95	2	0.67	1.19	0.67	0.00	0.11	2	1.38	1.24	0.66	0.05	0.05
其他的或未指明部位	O&U	5	1.68	2.97	1.53	0.00	0.11	4	2.76	2.47	1.34	0.00	0.20
骨髓增殖性疾病	MPD	0	0.00	0.00	0.00	0.00	0.00	0	0.00	0.00	0.00	0.00	0.00
骨髓增生异常综合征	MDS	0	0.00	0.00	0.00	0.00	0.00	0	0.00	0.00	0.00	0.00	0.00
合计	ALL	298	100.00	176.83	95.00	2.58	10.21	145	100.00	89.57	46.28	1.81	5.26
C44 以外的部位	ALL but C44	295	98.99	175.05	94.04	2.58	10.04	144	99.31	88.95	46.12	1.81	5.26

表 6-59 2020 年河南省林州市恶性肿瘤发病主要指标

部位	ICD-10	男性						女性					
		病例数	构成 (%)	粗率 (1/10^5)	世标率 (1/10^5)	累积率 (%)		病例数	构成 (%)	粗率 (1/10^5)	世标率 (1/10^5)	累积率 (%)	
						0~64	0~74					0~64	0~74
唇	C00	0	0.00	0.00	0.00	0.00	0.00	3	0.16	0.54	0.35	0.03	0.03
舌	C01–C02	7	0.35	1.21	0.88	0.04	0.11	8	0.42	1.45	0.90	0.06	0.11
口	C03–C06	11	0.56	1.89	1.25	0.07	0.18	5	0.26	0.91	0.50	0.03	0.09
唾液腺	C07–C08	3	0.15	0.52	0.30	0.01	0.05	1	0.05	0.18	0.09	0.01	0.01
扁桃体	C09	0	0.00	0.00	0.00	0.00	0.00	0	0.00	0.00	0.00	0.00	0.00
其他的口咽	C10	2	0.10	0.34	0.22	0.01	0.01	0	0.00	0.00	0.00	0.00	0.00
鼻咽	C11	6	0.30	1.03	1.32	0.07	0.07	0	0.00	0.00	0.00	0.00	0.00
喉咽	C12–C13	6	0.30	1.03	0.72	0.06	0.09	2	0.10	0.36	0.30	0.02	0.03
咽，部位不明	C14	1	0.05	0.17	0.10	0.00	0.02	0	0.00	0.00	0.00	0.00	0.00
食管	C15	449	22.76	77.30	51.13	2.29	6.16	345	18.06	62.59	34.11	1.56	4.24
胃	C16	589	29.85	101.40	66.80	3.80	8.88	303	15.86	54.97	30.96	1.62	3.73
小肠	C17	8	0.41	1.38	0.98	0.06	0.09	3	0.16	0.54	0.30	0.02	0.04
结肠	C18	67	3.40	11.53	7.64	0.46	1.00	60	3.14	10.88	6.26	0.35	0.79
直肠	C19–C20	74	3.75	12.74	8.23	0.47	1.10	69	3.61	12.52	7.01	0.42	0.98
肛门	C21	0	0.00	0.00	0.00	0.00	0.00	0	0.00	0.00	0.00	0.00	0.00
肝脏	C22	137	6.94	23.59	16.24	0.90	1.85	65	3.40	11.79	6.46	0.30	0.74
胆囊及其他	C23–C24	23	1.17	3.96	2.69	0.10	0.32	32	1.68	5.81	3.05	0.11	0.36
胰腺	C25	18	0.91	3.10	2.43	0.13	0.21	23	1.20	4.17	2.37	0.14	0.30
鼻、鼻窦及其他	C30–C31	1	0.05	0.17	0.11	0.01	0.01	2	0.10	0.36	0.19	0.01	0.03
喉	C32	22	1.12	3.79	2.25	0.06	0.33	1	0.05	0.18	0.15	0.01	0.01
气管、支气管、肺	C33–C34	244	12.37	42.01	28.77	1.43	3.41	173	9.06	31.38	18.11	1.07	2.23
其他的胸腔器官	C37–C38	3	0.15	0.52	0.34	0.02	0.03	6	0.31	1.09	0.64	0.06	0.08
骨	C40–C41	14	0.71	2.41	2.08	0.12	0.20	12	0.63	2.18	1.28	0.04	0.14
皮肤的黑色素瘤	C43	1	0.05	0.17	0.13	0.00	0.00	5	0.26	0.91	0.72	0.03	0.07
其他的皮肤	C44	8	0.41	1.38	1.14	0.03	0.06	6	0.31	1.09	0.54	0.01	0.08
间皮瘤	C45	1	0.05	0.17	0.10	0.00	0.02	2	0.10	0.36	0.21	0.02	0.04
卡波西肉瘤	C46	0	0.00	0.00	0.00	0.00	0.00	0	0.00	0.00	0.00	0.00	0.00
周围神经、其他结缔组织、软组织	C47;C49	6	0.30	1.03	0.64	0.04	0.06	3	0.16	0.54	0.42	0.04	0.04
乳房	C50	1	0.05	0.17	0.10	0.00	0.02	225	11.78	40.82	29.65	2.49	2.96
外阴	C51	0	0.00	0.00	0.00	0.00	0.00	3	0.16	0.54	0.27	0.01	0.05
阴道	C52	0	0.00	0.00	0.00	0.00	0.00	2	0.10	0.36	0.18	0.00	0.01
子宫颈	C53	0	0.00	0.00	0.00	0.00	0.00	180	9.42	32.65	23.26	2.08	2.43
子宫体	C54	0	0.00	0.00	0.00	0.00	0.00	38	1.99	6.89	4.65	0.41	0.52
子宫，部位不明	C55	0	0.00	0.00	0.00	0.00	0.00	18	0.94	3.27	2.16	0.20	0.20
卵巢	C56	0	0.00	0.00	0.00	0.00	0.00	46	2.41	8.34	5.57	0.42	0.59
女性其他的生殖器	C57	0	0.00	0.00	0.00	0.00	0.00	6	0.31	1.09	0.64	0.03	0.06
胎盘	C58	0	0.00	0.00	0.00	0.00	0.00	0	0.00	0.00	0.00	0.00	0.00
阴茎	C60	5	0.25	0.86	0.58	0.05	0.08	0	0.00	0.00	0.00	0.00	0.00
前列腺	C61	29	1.47	4.99	3.17	0.08	0.43	0	0.00	0.00	0.00	0.00	0.00
睾丸	C62	1	0.05	0.17	0.42	0.02	0.02	0	0.00	0.00	0.00	0.00	0.00
男性其他的生殖器	C63	0	0.00	0.00	0.00	0.00	0.00	0	0.00	0.00	0.00	0.00	0.00
肾	C64	16	0.81	2.75	2.22	0.13	0.26	9	0.47	1.63	1.11	0.08	0.12
肾盂	C65	3	0.15	0.52	0.33	0.00	0.02	0	0.00	0.00	0.00	0.00	0.00
输尿管	C66	1	0.05	0.17	0.10	0.00	0.02	1	0.05	0.18	0.10	0.01	0.01
膀胱	C67	21	1.06	3.62	2.38	0.10	0.27	12	0.63	2.18	1.23	0.08	0.11
其他的泌尿器官	C68	0	0.00	0.00	0.00	0.00	0.00	0	0.00	0.00	0.00	0.00	0.00
眼	C69	2	0.10	0.34	0.32	0.01	0.03	0	0.00	0.00	0.00	0.00	0.00
脑、神经系统	C70–C72	52	2.64	8.95	6.94	0.43	0.74	67	3.51	12.15	8.64	0.61	0.94
甲状腺	C73	20	1.01	3.44	2.75	0.24	0.27	87	4.55	15.78	11.95	1.09	1.18
肾上腺	C74	0	0.00	0.00	0.00	0.00	0.00	0	0.00	0.00	0.00	0.00	0.00
其他的内分泌腺	C75	2	0.10	0.34	0.21	0.02	0.02	0	0.00	0.00	0.00	0.00	0.00
霍奇金病	C81	2	0.10	0.34	0.36	0.03	0.03	2	0.10	0.36	0.18	0.01	0.02
非霍奇金淋巴瘤	C82–C85;C96	38	1.93	6.54	4.87	0.23	0.50	21	1.10	3.81	2.73	0.16	0.30
免疫增生性疾病	C88	0	0.00	0.00	0.00	0.00	0.00	0	0.00	0.00	0.00	0.00	0.00
多发性骨髓瘤	C90	11	0.56	1.89	1.15	0.06	0.18	14	0.73	2.54	1.55	0.15	0.19
淋巴样白血病	C91	4	0.20	0.69	1.09	0.05	0.05	3	0.16	0.54	0.68	0.05	0.05
髓样白血病	C92–C94	9	0.46	1.55	1.09	0.06	0.09	8	0.42	1.45	1.05	0.06	0.10
白血病，未特指	C95	31	1.57	5.34	4.91	0.33	0.43	19	0.99	3.45	2.92	0.15	0.25
其他的或未指明部位	O&U	24	1.22	4.13	3.07	0.21	0.30	20	1.05	3.63	2.80	0.21	0.29
骨髓增殖性疾病	MPD	0	0.00	0.00	0.00	0.00	0.00	0	0.00	0.00	0.00	0.00	0.00
骨髓增生异常综合征	MDS	0	0.00	0.00	0.00	0.00	0.00	0	0.00	0.00	0.00	0.00	0.00
合计	ALL	1 973	100.00	339.66	232.56	12.22	28.03	1 910	100.00	346.49	216.24	14.25	24.55
C44 以外的部位	ALL but C44	1 965	99.59	338.28	231.42	12.19	27.97	1 904	99.69	345.40	215.71	14.24	24.46

表 6-60 2020 年河南省林州市恶性肿瘤死亡主要指标

部位	ICD-10	男性						女性					
		病例数	构成 (%)	粗率 (1/10^5)	世标率 (1/10^5)	累积率 (%)		病例数	构成 (%)	粗率 (1/10^5)	世标率 (1/10^5)	累积率 (%)	
						0~64	0~74					0~64	0~74
唇	C00	0	0.00	0.00	0.00	0.00	0.00	0	0.00	0.00	0.00	0.00	0.00
舌	C01–C02	0	0.00	0.00	0.00	0.00	0.00	3	0.29	0.54	0.26	0.00	0.05
口	C03–C06	4	0.28	0.69	0.39	0.00	0.09	4	0.39	0.73	0.45	0.04	0.06
唾液腺	C07–C08	4	0.28	0.69	0.40	0.01	0.07	1	0.10	0.18	0.11	0.01	0.01
扁桃体	C09	1	0.07	0.17	0.10	0.00	0.02	0	0.00	0.00	0.00	0.00	0.00
其他的口咽	C10	1	0.07	0.17	0.10	0.00	0.02	0	0.00	0.00	0.00	0.00	0.00
鼻咽	C11	3	0.21	0.52	0.35	0.01	0.01	1	0.10	0.18	0.10	0.01	0.01
喉咽	C12–C13	3	0.21	0.52	0.42	0.00	0.04	0	0.00	0.00	0.00	0.00	0.00
咽，部位不明	C14	1	0.07	0.17	0.10	0.00	0.02	0	0.00	0.00	0.00	0.00	0.00
食管	C15	349	24.49	60.08	41.77	1.16	4.12	296	28.74	53.70	27.17	0.45	2.67
胃	C16	474	33.26	81.60	52.84	1.60	6.65	207	20.10	37.55	19.54	0.51	2.11
小肠	C17	5	0.35	0.86	0.54	0.02	0.07	2	0.19	0.36	0.24	0.03	0.03
结肠	C18	37	2.60	6.37	4.34	0.12	0.46	43	4.17	7.80	4.26	0.15	0.42
直肠	C19–C20	45	3.16	7.75	5.50	0.14	0.54	31	3.01	5.62	2.79	0.03	0.37
肛门	C21	1	0.07	0.17	0.14	0.01	0.01	0	0.00	0.00	0.00	0.00	0.00
肝脏	C22	139	9.75	23.93	17.51	0.81	1.59	45	4.37	8.16	4.35	0.17	0.47
胆囊及其他	C23–C24	19	1.33	3.27	2.23	0.07	0.24	33	3.20	5.99	3.21	0.12	0.33
胰腺	C25	16	1.12	2.75	1.91	0.05	0.22	22	2.14	3.99	2.20	0.09	0.23
鼻、鼻窦及其他	C30–C31	2	0.14	0.34	0.24	0.01	0.03	2	0.19	0.36	0.21	0.03	0.03
喉	C32	8	0.56	1.38	0.85	0.01	0.09	2	0.19	0.36	0.17	0.00	0.04
气管、支气管、肺	C33–C34	162	11.37	27.89	19.11	0.74	2.14	119	11.55	21.59	11.92	0.55	1.36
其他的胸腔器官	C37–C38	5	0.35	0.86	0.53	0.03	0.06	3	0.29	0.54	0.30	0.02	0.02
骨	C40–C41	9	0.63	1.55	1.12	0.04	0.14	10	0.97	1.81	1.56	0.06	0.15
皮肤的黑色素瘤	C43	2	0.14	0.34	0.24	0.01	0.01	0	0.00	0.00	0.00	0.00	0.00
其他的皮肤	C44	6	0.42	1.03	0.64	0.01	0.07	5	0.49	0.91	0.47	0.00	0.04
间皮瘤	C45	0	0.00	0.00	0.00	0.00	0.00	2	0.19	0.36	0.17	0.00	0.04
卡波西肉瘤	C46	0	0.00	0.00	0.00	0.00	0.00	1	0.10	0.18	0.18	0.01	0.01
周围神经、其他结缔组织、软组织	C47;C49	3	0.21	0.52	0.53	0.02	0.02	2	0.19	0.36	0.30	0.02	0.02
乳房	C50	1	0.07	0.17	0.23	0.00	0.00	50	4.85	9.07	5.48	0.37	0.60
外阴	C51	0	0.00	0.00	0.00	0.00	0.00	0	0.00	0.00	0.00	0.00	0.00
阴道	C52	0	0.00	0.00	0.00	0.00	0.00	0	0.00	0.00	0.00	0.00	0.00
子宫颈	C53	0	0.00	0.00	0.00	0.00	0.00	21	2.04	3.81	2.21	0.13	0.25
子宫体	C54	0	0.00	0.00	0.00	0.00	0.00	4	0.39	0.73	0.41	0.04	0.05
子宫，部位不明	C55	0	0.00	0.00	0.00	0.00	0.00	5	0.49	0.91	0.50	0.01	0.03
卵巢	C56	0	0.00	0.00	0.00	0.00	0.00	25	2.43	4.54	2.65	0.14	0.30
女性其他的生殖器	C57	0	0.00	0.00	0.00	0.00	0.00	4	0.39	0.73	0.37	0.00	0.04
胎盘	C58	0	0.00	0.00	0.00	0.00	0.00	0	0.00	0.00	0.00	0.00	0.00
阴茎	C60	1	0.07	0.17	0.23	0.00	0.00	0	0.00	0.00	0.00	0.00	0.00
前列腺	C61	15	1.05	2.58	1.97	0.05	0.14	0	0.00	0.00	0.00	0.00	0.00
睾丸	C62	0	0.00	0.00	0.00	0.00	0.00	0	0.00	0.00	0.00	0.00	0.00
男性其他的生殖器	C63	0	0.00	0.00	0.00	0.00	0.00	0	0.00	0.00	0.00	0.00	0.00
肾	C64	12	0.84	2.07	1.40	0.09	0.17	5	0.49	0.91	0.48	0.04	0.08
肾盂	C65	2	0.14	0.34	0.24	0.01	0.01	0	0.00	0.00	0.00	0.00	0.00
输尿管	C66	4	0.28	0.69	0.48	0.01	0.04	2	0.19	0.36	0.24	0.03	0.03
膀胱	C67	7	0.49	1.21	1.00	0.01	0.05	8	0.78	1.45	0.82	0.03	0.05
其他的泌尿器官	C68	0	0.00	0.00	0.00	0.00	0.00	0	0.00	0.00	0.00	0.00	0.00
眼	C69	0	0.00	0.00	0.00	0.00	0.00	1	0.10	0.18	0.13	0.02	0.02
脑、神经系统	C70–C72	33	2.32	5.68	4.72	0.29	0.48	29	2.82	5.26	3.60	0.17	0.40
甲状腺	C73	2	0.14	0.34	0.24	0.01	0.03	4	0.39	0.73	0.42	0.03	0.06
肾上腺	C74	0	0.00	0.00	0.00	0.00	0.00	1	0.10	0.18	0.10	0.01	0.01
其他的内分泌腺	C75	0	0.00	0.00	0.00	0.00	0.00	2	0.19	0.36	0.26	0.02	0.02
霍奇金病	C81	0	0.00	0.00	0.00	0.00	0.00	0	0.00	0.00	0.00	0.00	0.00
非霍奇金淋巴瘤	C82–C85;C96	12	0.84	2.07	1.52	0.04	0.16	7	0.68	1.27	0.75	0.03	0.10
免疫增生性疾病	C88	0	0.00	0.00	0.00	0.00	0.00	0	0.00	0.00	0.00	0.00	0.00
多发性骨髓瘤	C90	6	0.42	1.03	0.61	0.03	0.10	8	0.78	1.45	0.70	0.01	0.12
淋巴样白血病	C91	5	0.35	0.86	0.87	0.06	0.06	1	0.10	0.18	0.10	0.01	0.01
髓样白血病	C92–C94	2	0.14	0.34	0.25	0.02	0.02	3	0.29	0.54	0.35	0.03	0.03
白血病，未特指	C95	14	0.98	2.41	1.84	0.12	0.18	9	0.87	1.63	1.05	0.07	0.11
其他的或未指明部位	O&U	8	0.56	1.38	1.03	0.06	0.08	5	0.49	0.91	0.58	0.03	0.05
骨髓增殖性疾病	MPD	0	0.00	0.00	0.00	0.00	0.00	1	0.10	0.18	0.09	0.00	0.01
骨髓增生异常综合征	MDS	2	0.14	0.34	0.22	0.00	0.00	1	0.10	0.18	0.21	0.02	0.02
合计	ALL	1 425	100.00	245.32	168.71	5.70	18.25	1 030	100.00	186.85	101.47	3.54	10.87
C44 以外的部位	ALL but C44	1 419	99.58	244.29	168.07	5.69	18.18	1 025	99.51	185.94	101.01	3.54	10.82

表 6-61　2020 年河南省鹤壁市城区恶性肿瘤发病主要指标

部位	ICD-10	男性						女性					
		病例数	构成(%)	粗率($1/10^5$)	世标率($1/10^5$)	累积率(%)		病例数	构成(%)	粗率($1/10^5$)	世标率($1/10^5$)	累积率(%)	
						0~64	0~74					0~64	0~74
唇	C00	4	0.41	1.19	0.86	0.03	0.07	3	0.34	0.92	0.61	0.03	0.08
舌	C01–C02	7	0.72	2.09	1.36	0.06	0.20	7	0.79	2.15	1.41	0.06	0.17
口	C03–C06	4	0.41	1.19	0.92	0.04	0.08	6	0.68	1.84	1.38	0.07	0.15
唾液腺	C07–C08	2	0.21	0.60	0.46	0.05	0.05	4	0.45	1.23	0.70	0.02	0.10
扁桃体	C09	2	0.21	0.60	0.47	0.05	0.05	0	0.00	0.00	0.00	0.00	0.00
其他的口咽	C10	2	0.21	0.60	0.38	0.00	0.03	2	0.23	0.61	0.37	0.02	0.07
鼻咽	C11	6	0.62	1.79	1.19	0.11	0.16	2	0.23	0.61	0.37	0.02	0.07
喉咽	C12–C13	4	0.41	1.19	0.78	0.04	0.15	2	0.23	0.61	0.29	0.00	0.05
咽，部位不明	C14	4	0.41	1.19	0.75	0.02	0.08	0	0.00	0.00	0.00	0.00	0.00
食管	C15	152	15.72	45.31	30.58	1.29	4.15	97	10.95	29.81	16.97	0.47	2.48
胃	C16	141	14.58	42.03	27.93	1.31	3.47	71	8.01	21.82	12.81	0.54	1.59
小肠	C17	15	1.55	4.47	2.86	0.18	0.22	9	1.02	2.77	1.57	0.05	0.25
结肠	C18	36	3.72	10.73	7.17	0.35	0.88	40	4.51	12.29	7.35	0.43	0.84
直肠	C19–C20	32	3.31	9.54	6.31	0.33	0.82	19	2.14	5.84	3.86	0.20	0.53
肛门	C21	0	0.00	0.00	0.00	0.00	0.00	1	0.11	0.31	0.18	0.02	0.02
肝脏	C22	105	10.86	31.30	21.23	1.51	2.21	42	4.74	12.91	7.30	0.36	0.71
胆囊及其他	C23–C24	24	2.48	7.15	4.69	0.16	0.70	11	1.24	3.38	2.18	0.10	0.34
胰腺	C25	14	1.45	4.17	2.83	0.20	0.27	19	2.14	5.84	2.91	0.16	0.23
鼻、鼻窦及其他	C30–C31	0	0.00	0.00	0.00	0.00	0.00	1	0.11	0.31	0.28	0.03	0.03
喉	C32	7	0.72	2.09	1.42	0.03	0.23	3	0.34	0.92	0.53	0.00	0.07
气管、支气管、肺	C33–C34	224	23.16	66.78	43.77	2.31	5.04	107	12.08	32.88	18.75	0.94	2.10
其他的胸腔器官	C37–C38	7	0.72	2.09	1.52	0.07	0.20	3	0.34	0.92	0.82	0.05	0.08
骨	C40–C41	8	0.83	2.38	2.12	0.09	0.12	9	1.02	2.77	2.20	0.13	0.18
皮肤的黑色素瘤	C43	0	0.00	0.00	0.00	0.00	0.00	4	0.45	1.23	0.86	0.04	0.12
其他的皮肤	C44	5	0.52	1.49	0.97	0.09	0.09	5	0.56	1.54	0.98	0.07	0.10
间皮瘤	C45	1	0.10	0.30	0.36	0.02	0.02	0	0.00	0.00	0.00	0.00	0.00
卡波西肉瘤	C46	0	0.00	0.00	0.00	0.00	0.00	0	0.00	0.00	0.00	0.00	0.00
周围神经、其他结缔组织、软组织	C47;C49	3	0.31	0.89	0.50	0.02	0.06	2	0.23	0.61	0.56	0.06	0.06
乳房	C50	0	0.00	0.00	0.00	0.00	0.00	135	15.24	41.49	29.76	2.14	3.10
外阴	C51	0	0.00	0.00	0.00	0.00	0.00	3	0.34	0.92	0.47	0.02	0.06
阴道	C52	0	0.00	0.00	0.00	0.00	0.00	2	0.23	0.61	0.40	0.00	0.08
子宫颈	C53	0	0.00	0.00	0.00	0.00	0.00	72	8.13	22.13	16.28	1.38	1.68
子宫体	C54	0	0.00	0.00	0.00	0.00	0.00	39	4.40	11.99	7.95	0.58	0.98
子宫，部位不明	C55	0	0.00	0.00	0.00	0.00	0.00	0	0.00	0.00	0.00	0.00	0.00
卵巢	C56	0	0.00	0.00	0.00	0.00	0.00	23	2.60	7.07	4.80	0.37	0.55
女性其他的生殖器	C57	0	0.00	0.00	0.00	0.00	0.00	2	0.23	0.61	0.41	0.02	0.07
胎盘	C58	0	0.00	0.00	0.00	0.00	0.00	0	0.00	0.00	0.00	0.00	0.00
阴茎	C60	2	0.21	0.60	0.38	0.00	0.03	0	0.00	0.00	0.00	0.00	0.00
前列腺	C61	21	2.17	6.26	3.77	0.00	0.40	0	0.00	0.00	0.00	0.00	0.00
睾丸	C62	2	0.21	0.60	0.41	0.00	0.07	0	0.00	0.00	0.00	0.00	0.00
男性其他的生殖器	C63	0	0.00	0.00	0.00	0.00	0.00	0	0.00	0.00	0.00	0.00	0.00
肾	C64	10	1.03	2.98	2.03	0.10	0.28	5	0.56	1.54	0.97	0.08	0.11
肾盂	C65	3	0.31	0.89	0.55	0.02	0.05	0	0.00	0.00	0.00	0.00	0.00
输尿管	C66	5	0.52	1.49	0.99	0.08	0.08	0	0.00	0.00	0.00	0.00	0.00
膀胱	C67	10	1.03	2.98	2.00	0.09	0.09	4	0.45	1.23	0.54	0.04	0.04
其他的泌尿器官	C68	0	0.00	0.00	0.00	0.00	0.00	0	0.00	0.00	0.00	0.00	0.00
眼	C69	0	0.00	0.00	0.00	0.00	0.00	0	0.00	0.00	0.00	0.00	0.00
脑、神经系统	C70–C72	22	2.28	6.56	4.90	0.27	0.58	18	2.03	5.53	3.67	0.20	0.48
甲状腺	C73	20	2.07	5.96	4.85	0.45	0.45	73	8.24	22.43	16.27	1.29	1.70
肾上腺	C74	4	0.41	1.19	0.68	0.06	0.06	0	0.00	0.00	0.00	0.00	0.00
其他的内分泌腺	C75	0	0.00	0.00	0.00	0.00	0.00	2	0.23	0.61	0.42	0.03	0.03
霍奇金病	C81	7	0.72	2.09	1.78	0.04	0.21	1	0.11	0.31	0.18	0.02	0.02
非霍奇金淋巴瘤	C82–C85;C96	8	0.83	2.38	1.90	0.12	0.18	4	0.45	1.23	0.85	0.05	0.12
免疫增生性疾病	C88	0	0.00	0.00	0.00	0.00	0.00	0	0.00	0.00	0.00	0.00	0.00
多发性骨髓瘤	C90	6	0.62	1.79	1.30	0.07	0.21	5	0.56	1.54	0.90	0.06	0.10
淋巴样白血病	C91	9	0.93	2.68	2.18	0.11	0.24	9	1.02	2.77	2.07	0.12	0.17
髓样白血病	C92–C94	13	1.34	3.88	3.14	0.16	0.32	6	0.68	1.84	1.33	0.10	0.15
白血病，未特指	C95	13	1.34	3.88	2.57	0.10	0.17	10	1.13	3.07	1.68	0.06	0.09
其他的或未指明部位	O&U	3	0.31	0.89	0.66	0.03	0.09	4	0.45	1.23	1.07	0.09	0.09
骨髓增殖性疾病	MPD	0	0.00	0.00	0.00	0.00	0.00	0	0.00	0.00	0.00	0.00	0.00
骨髓增生异常综合征	MDS	0	0.00	0.00	0.00	0.00	0.00	0	0.00	0.00	0.00	0.00	0.00
合计	ALL	967	100.00	288.28	195.47	10.07	22.85	886	100.00	272.28	175.25	10.53	20.04
C44 以外的部位	ALL but C44	962	99.48	286.79	194.50	9.98	22.77	881	99.44	270.74	174.27	10.46	19.94

表 6-62　2020 年河南省鹤壁市城区恶性肿瘤死亡主要指标

部位	ICD-10	男性						女性					
		病例数	构成 (%)	粗率 (1/10^5)	世标率 (1/10^5)	累积率 (%) 0~64	累积率 (%) 0~74	病例数	构成 (%)	粗率 (1/10^5)	世标率 (1/10^5)	累积率 (%) 0~64	累积率 (%) 0~74
唇	C00	1	0.14	0.30	0.20	0.00	0.00	1	0.24	0.31	0.32	0.03	0.03
舌	C01–C02	4	0.54	1.19	0.90	0.05	0.05	4	0.96	1.23	0.50	0.02	0.02
口	C03–C06	2	0.27	0.60	0.42	0.00	0.09	3	0.72	0.92	0.68	0.02	0.11
唾液腺	C07–C08	0	0.00	0.00	0.00	0.00	0.00	2	0.48	0.61	0.37	0.03	0.03
扁桃体	C09	1	0.14	0.30	0.18	0.00	0.00	0	0.00	0.00	0.00	0.00	0.00
其他的口咽	C10	0	0.00	0.00	0.00	0.00	0.00	1	0.24	0.31	0.13	0.00	0.00
鼻咽	C11	1	0.14	0.30	0.17	0.02	0.02	1	0.24	0.31	0.09	0.00	0.00
喉咽	C12–C13	1	0.14	0.30	0.21	0.02	0.02	0	0.00	0.00	0.00	0.00	0.00
咽，部位不明	C14	2	0.27	0.60	0.34	0.04	0.04	0	0.00	0.00	0.00	0.00	0.00
食管	C15	126	17.07	37.56	24.43	0.71	2.98	70	16.83	21.51	11.50	0.40	1.32
胃	C16	110	14.91	32.79	21.15	0.72	1.86	47	11.30	14.44	7.87	0.31	0.81
小肠	C17	5	0.68	1.49	1.02	0.04	0.04	1	0.24	0.31	0.18	0.02	0.02
结肠	C18	28	3.79	8.35	5.50	0.31	0.56	14	3.37	4.30	2.08	0.07	0.15
直肠	C19–C20	18	2.44	5.37	3.58	0.15	0.34	8	1.92	2.46	1.45	0.04	0.16
肛门	C21	0	0.00	0.00	0.00	0.00	0.00	0	0.00	0.00	0.00	0.00	0.00
肝脏	C22	97	13.14	28.92	19.72	1.22	2.18	32	7.69	9.83	5.22	0.23	0.52
胆囊及其他	C23–C24	12	1.63	3.58	2.56	0.16	0.27	9	2.16	2.77	1.30	0.04	0.09
胰腺	C25	11	1.49	3.28	2.04	0.09	0.18	16	3.85	4.92	2.28	0.11	0.16
鼻、鼻窦及其他	C30–C31	0	0.00	0.00	0.00	0.00	0.00	0	0.00	0.00	0.00	0.00	0.00
喉	C32	4	0.54	1.19	0.71	0.02	0.11	1	0.24	0.31	0.09	0.00	0.00
气管、支气管、肺	C33–C34	204	27.64	60.82	39.69	1.77	4.04	62	14.90	19.05	10.03	0.38	1.05
其他的胸腔器官	C37–C38	5	0.68	1.49	0.88	0.00	0.14	1	0.24	0.31	0.11	0.00	0.00
骨	C40–C41	5	0.68	1.49	0.97	0.05	0.05	3	0.72	0.92	0.67	0.03	0.13
皮肤的黑色素瘤	C43	1	0.14	0.30	0.22	0.00	0.05	0	0.00	0.00	0.00	0.00	0.00
其他的皮肤	C44	2	0.27	0.60	0.48	0.03	0.09	3	0.72	0.92	0.53	0.06	0.06
间皮瘤	C45	0	0.00	0.00	0.00	0.00	0.00	0	0.00	0.00	0.00	0.00	0.00
卡波西肉瘤	C46	0	0.00	0.00	0.00	0.00	0.00	0	0.00	0.00	0.00	0.00	0.00
周围神经、其他结缔组织、软组织	C47;C49	0	0.00	0.00	0.00	0.00	0.00	1	0.24	0.31	0.18	0.02	0.02
乳房	C50	0	0.00	0.00	0.00	0.00	0.00	55	13.22	16.90	9.17	0.48	0.96
外阴	C51	0	0.00	0.00	0.00	0.00	0.00	1	0.24	0.31	0.28	0.03	0.03
阴道	C52	0	0.00	0.00	0.00	0.00	0.00	0	0.00	0.00	0.00	0.00	0.00
子宫颈	C53	0	0.00	0.00	0.00	0.00	0.00	20	4.81	6.15	3.30	0.11	0.41
子宫体	C54	0	0.00	0.00	0.00	0.00	0.00	10	2.40	3.07	1.51	0.04	0.18
子宫，部位不明	C55	0	0.00	0.00	0.00	0.00	0.00	0	0.00	0.00	0.00	0.00	0.00
卵巢	C56	0	0.00	0.00	0.00	0.00	0.00	13	3.13	4.00	2.44	0.16	0.30
女性其他的生殖器	C57	0	0.00	0.00	0.00	0.00	0.00	0	0.00	0.00	0.00	0.00	0.00
胎盘	C58	0	0.00	0.00	0.00	0.00	0.00	0	0.00	0.00	0.00	0.00	0.00
阴茎	C60	1	0.14	0.30	0.12	0.00	0.00	0	0.00	0.00	0.00	0.00	0.00
前列腺	C61	15	2.03	4.47	2.84	0.07	0.07	0	0.00	0.00	0.00	0.00	0.00
睾丸	C62	1	0.14	0.30	0.20	0.00	0.03	0	0.00	0.00	0.00	0.00	0.00
男性其他的生殖器	C63	0	0.00	0.00	0.00	0.00	0.00	0	0.00	0.00	0.00	0.00	0.00
肾	C64	5	0.68	1.49	0.96	0.02	0.08	1	0.24	0.31	0.13	0.00	0.00
肾盂	C65	2	0.27	0.60	0.38	0.00	0.03	0	0.00	0.00	0.00	0.00	0.00
输尿管	C66	2	0.27	0.60	0.39	0.00	0.05	0	0.00	0.00	0.00	0.00	0.00
膀胱	C67	5	0.68	1.49	0.98	0.03	0.03	2	0.48	0.61	0.27	0.02	0.02
其他的泌尿器官	C68	0	0.00	0.00	0.00	0.00	0.00	0	0.00	0.00	0.00	0.00	0.00
眼	C69	0	0.00	0.00	0.00	0.00	0.00	0	0.00	0.00	0.00	0.00	0.00
脑、神经系统	C70–C72	20	2.71	5.96	4.12	0.16	0.39	6	1.44	1.84	1.00	0.03	0.12
甲状腺	C73	7	0.95	2.09	1.17	0.04	0.09	4	0.96	1.23	0.62	0.02	0.06
肾上腺	C74	2	0.27	0.60	0.32	0.00	0.00	0	0.00	0.00	0.00	0.00	0.00
其他的内分泌腺	C75	0	0.00	0.00	0.00	0.00	0.00	1	0.24	0.31	0.19	0.02	0.02
霍奇金病	C81	5	0.68	1.49	1.05	0.05	0.14	0	0.00	0.00	0.00	0.00	0.00
非霍奇金淋巴瘤	C82–C85;C96	4	0.54	1.19	0.70	0.00	0.03	1	0.24	0.31	0.13	0.00	0.00
免疫增生性疾病	C88	0	0.00	0.00	0.00	0.00	0.00	0	0.00	0.00	0.00	0.00	0.00
多发性骨髓瘤	C90	3	0.41	0.89	0.57	0.04	0.07	3	0.72	0.92	0.65	0.06	0.09
淋巴样白血病	C91	7	0.95	2.09	1.52	0.06	0.12	7	1.68	2.15	1.53	0.05	0.12
髓样白血病	C92–C94	7	0.95	2.09	1.49	0.05	0.17	4	0.96	1.23	0.50	0.00	0.03
白血病，未特指	C95	11	1.49	3.28	2.45	0.13	0.25	7	1.68	2.15	1.36	0.06	0.10
其他的或未指明部位	O&U	1	0.14	0.30	0.26	0.03	0.03	1	0.24	0.31	0.32	0.03	0.03
骨髓增殖性疾病	MPD	0	0.00	0.00	0.00	0.00	0.00	0	0.00	0.00	0.00	0.00	0.00
骨髓增生异常综合征	MDS	0	0.00	0.00	0.00	0.00	0.00	0	0.00	0.00	0.00	0.00	0.00
合计	ALL	738	100.00	220.01	144.91	6.08	14.72	416	100.00	127.84	68.99	2.94	7.14
C44 以外的部位	ALL but C44	736	99.73	219.41	144.43	6.05	14.63	413	99.28	126.92	68.46	2.88	7.08

表 6-63　2020 年河南省浚县恶性肿瘤发病主要指标

部位	ICD-10	男性						女性					
		病例数	构成 (%)	粗率 ($1/10^5$)	世标率 ($1/10^5$)	累积率 (%) 0~64	累积率 (%) 0~74	病例数	构成 (%)	粗率 ($1/10^5$)	世标率 ($1/10^5$)	累积率 (%) 0~64	累积率 (%) 0~74
唇	C00	1	0.12	0.28	0.19	0.00	0.00	0	0.00	0.00	0.00	0.00	0.00
舌	C01–C02	1	0.12	0.28	0.24	0.02	0.02	1	0.12	0.31	0.17	0.00	0.04
口	C03–C06	5	0.58	1.42	0.91	0.01	0.14	7	0.83	2.14	1.40	0.05	0.11
唾液腺	C07–C08	6	0.69	1.70	1.35	0.09	0.09	5	0.60	1.53	0.85	0.02	0.17
扁桃体	C09	0	0.00	0.00	0.00	0.00	0.00	0	0.00	0.00	0.00	0.00	0.00
其他的口咽	C10	0	0.00	0.00	0.00	0.00	0.00	0	0.00	0.00	0.00	0.00	0.00
鼻咽	C11	4	0.46	1.14	0.92	0.09	0.12	2	0.24	0.61	0.34	0.01	0.06
喉咽	C12–C13	3	0.35	0.85	0.55	0.00	0.14	0	0.00	0.00	0.00	0.00	0.00
咽，部位不明	C14	5	0.58	1.42	1.05	0.08	0.16	3	0.36	0.92	0.64	0.04	0.07
食管	C15	228	26.27	64.77	48.57	1.52	6.40	175	20.83	53.53	32.53	1.20	3.90
胃	C16	113	13.02	32.10	23.77	0.65	2.95	51	6.07	15.60	10.03	0.54	1.30
小肠	C17	9	1.04	2.56	1.90	0.13	0.24	4	0.48	1.22	0.85	0.04	0.10
结肠	C18	19	2.19	5.40	4.49	0.34	0.45	24	2.86	7.34	4.84	0.25	0.50
直肠	C19–C20	27	3.11	7.67	5.97	0.37	0.67	21	2.50	6.42	4.21	0.21	0.45
肛门	C21	2	0.23	0.57	0.53	0.00	0.05	3	0.36	0.92	0.47	0.00	0.04
肝脏	C22	90	10.37	25.57	20.10	1.39	2.34	43	5.12	13.15	8.29	0.46	0.85
胆囊及其他	C23–C24	9	1.04	2.56	2.30	0.15	0.26	16	1.90	4.89	2.99	0.10	0.41
胰腺	C25	17	1.96	4.83	3.83	0.17	0.44	17	2.02	5.20	3.63	0.21	0.36
鼻、鼻窦及其他	C30–C31	0	0.00	0.00	0.00	0.00	0.00	0	0.00	0.00	0.00	0.00	0.00
喉	C32	2	0.23	0.57	0.38	0.00	0.03	1	0.12	0.31	0.17	0.00	0.00
气管、支气管、肺	C33–C34	190	21.89	53.98	41.32	2.24	5.14	117	13.93	35.79	22.12	1.04	2.67
其他的胸腔器官	C37–C38	2	0.23	0.57	0.52	0.06	0.06	8	0.95	2.45	1.86	0.13	0.19
骨	C40–C41	4	0.46	1.14	1.04	0.05	0.09	10	1.19	3.06	2.10	0.12	0.26
皮肤的黑色素瘤	C43	0	0.00	0.00	0.00	0.00	0.00	0	0.00	0.00	0.00	0.00	0.00
其他的皮肤	C44	5	0.58	1.42	1.11	0.03	0.07	3	0.36	0.92	0.65	0.03	0.06
间皮瘤	C45	0	0.00	0.00	0.00	0.00	0.00	1	0.12	0.31	0.14	0.00	0.00
卡波西肉瘤	C46	0	0.00	0.00	0.00	0.00	0.00	0	0.00	0.00	0.00	0.00	0.00
周围神经、其他结缔组织、软组织	C47;C49	1	0.12	0.28	0.20	0.00	0.03	2	0.24	0.61	0.57	0.02	0.05
乳房	C50	3	0.35	0.85	0.64	0.05	0.08	127	15.12	38.85	28.49	2.38	2.91
外阴	C51	0	0.00	0.00	0.00	0.00	0.00	2	0.24	0.61	0.46	0.04	0.08
阴道	C52	0	0.00	0.00	0.00	0.00	0.00	0	0.00	0.00	0.00	0.00	0.00
子宫颈	C53	0	0.00	0.00	0.00	0.00	0.00	41	4.88	12.54	9.22	0.81	0.93
子宫体	C54	0	0.00	0.00	0.00	0.00	0.00	37	4.40	11.32	7.51	0.67	0.80
子宫，部位不明	C55	0	0.00	0.00	0.00	0.00	0.00	1	0.12	0.31	0.17	0.02	0.02
卵巢	C56	0	0.00	0.00	0.00	0.00	0.00	22	2.62	6.73	4.73	0.29	0.53
女性其他的生殖器	C57	0	0.00	0.00	0.00	0.00	0.00	1	0.12	0.31	0.17	0.02	0.02
胎盘	C58	0	0.00	0.00	0.00	0.00	0.00	0	0.00	0.00	0.00	0.00	0.00
阴茎	C60	2	0.23	0.57	0.42	0.02	0.02	0	0.00	0.00	0.00	0.00	0.00
前列腺	C61	17	1.96	4.83	3.58	0.11	0.49	0	0.00	0.00	0.00	0.00	0.00
睾丸	C62	0	0.00	0.00	0.00	0.00	0.00	0	0.00	0.00	0.00	0.00	0.00
男性其他的生殖器	C63	0	0.00	0.00	0.00	0.00	0.00	0	0.00	0.00	0.00	0.00	0.00
肾	C64	12	1.38	3.41	2.65	0.22	0.22	5	0.60	1.53	0.99	0.05	0.16
肾盂	C65	0	0.00	0.00	0.00	0.00	0.00	2	0.24	0.61	0.33	0.00	0.04
输尿管	C66	0	0.00	0.00	0.00	0.00	0.00	0	0.00	0.00	0.00	0.00	0.00
膀胱	C67	21	2.42	5.97	4.89	0.38	0.67	4	0.48	1.22	0.81	0.06	0.10
其他的泌尿器官	C68	1	0.12	0.28	0.18	0.02	0.02	0	0.00	0.00	0.00	0.00	0.00
眼	C69	3	0.35	0.85	1.62	0.07	0.12	0	0.00	0.00	0.00	0.00	0.00
脑、神经系统	C70–C72	20	2.30	5.68	4.79	0.40	0.47	12	1.43	3.67	2.67	0.16	0.25
甲状腺	C73	16	1.84	4.55	3.92	0.31	0.39	47	5.60	14.38	10.85	0.90	1.08
肾上腺	C74	3	0.35	0.85	0.67	0.04	0.09	2	0.24	0.61	0.34	0.01	0.01
其他的内分泌腺	C75	1	0.12	0.28	0.18	0.00	0.05	1	0.12	0.31	0.30	0.04	0.04
霍奇金病	C81	0	0.00	0.00	0.00	0.00	0.00	0	0.00	0.00	0.00	0.00	0.00
非霍奇金淋巴瘤	C82–C85;C96	6	0.69	1.70	2.45	0.09	0.12	1	0.12	0.31	0.14	0.00	0.00
免疫增生性疾病	C88	1	0.12	0.28	0.31	0.03	0.03	0	0.00	0.00	0.00	0.00	0.00
多发性骨髓瘤	C90	1	0.12	0.28	0.19	0.00	0.00	1	0.12	0.31	0.17	0.00	0.04
淋巴样白血病	C91	0	0.00	0.00	0.00	0.00	0.00	0	0.00	0.00	0.00	0.00	0.00
髓样白血病	C92–C94	2	0.23	0.57	0.42	0.02	0.07	1	0.12	0.31	0.18	0.00	0.03
白血病，未特指	C95	1	0.12	0.28	0.18	0.02	0.02	2	0.24	0.61	0.59	0.02	0.06
其他的或未指明部位	O&U	15	1.73	4.26	3.08	0.04	0.43	17	2.02	5.20	3.40	0.28	0.38
骨髓增殖性疾病	MPD	0	0.00	0.00	0.00	0.00	0.00	0	0.00	0.00	0.00	0.00	0.00
骨髓增生异常综合征	MDS	0	0.00	0.00	0.00	0.00	0.00	0	0.00	0.00	0.00	0.00	0.00
合计	ALL	868	100.00	246.58	191.38	9.20	23.17	840	100.00	256.96	170.38	10.22	19.05
C44 以外的部位	ALL but C44	863	99.42	245.16	190.27	9.18	23.10	837	99.64	256.04	169.73	10.19	18.99

表 6-64 2020 年河南省浚县恶性肿瘤死亡主要指标

部位	ICD-10	男性						女性					
		病例数	构成 (%)	粗率 ($1/10^5$)	世标率 ($1/10^5$)	累积率 (%) 0～64	累积率 (%) 0～74	病例数	构成 (%)	粗率 ($1/10^5$)	世标率 ($1/10^5$)	累积率 (%) 0～64	累积率 (%) 0～74
唇	C00	2	0.33	0.57	0.53	0.00	0.00	2	0.51	0.61	0.42	0.04	0.04
舌	C01–C02	2	0.33	0.57	0.38	0.00	0.03	3	0.76	0.92	0.67	0.03	0.03
口	C03–C06	4	0.66	1.14	0.73	0.02	0.06	1	0.25	0.31	0.17	0.00	0.04
唾液腺	C07–C08	1	0.17	0.28	0.19	0.00	0.00	2	0.51	0.61	0.34	0.02	0.06
扁桃体	C09	0	0.00	0.00	0.00	0.00	0.00	0	0.00	0.00	0.00	0.00	0.00
其他的口咽	C10	0	0.00	0.00	0.00	0.00	0.00	1	0.25	0.31	0.19	0.02	0.02
鼻咽	C11	3	0.50	0.85	0.72	0.09	0.09	0	0.00	0.00	0.00	0.00	0.00
喉咽	C12–C13	2	0.33	0.57	0.36	0.02	0.06	0	0.00	0.00	0.00	0.00	0.00
咽，部位不明	C14	7	1.16	1.99	1.69	0.09	0.17	4	1.01	1.22	0.66	0.00	0.08
食管	C15	160	26.49	45.45	33.52	0.67	3.75	112	28.35	34.26	19.17	0.29	1.77
胃	C16	99	16.39	28.12	20.86	0.42	2.40	43	10.89	13.15	8.13	0.31	0.77
小肠	C17	3	0.50	0.85	0.69	0.06	0.09	0	0.00	0.00	0.00	0.00	0.00
结肠	C18	9	1.49	2.56	1.74	0.02	0.10	8	2.03	2.45	1.77	0.09	0.13
直肠	C19–C20	13	2.15	3.69	2.86	0.10	0.31	4	1.01	1.22	0.64	0.04	0.04
肛门	C21	4	0.66	1.14	0.92	0.03	0.03	10	2.53	3.06	1.64	0.04	0.17
肝脏	C22	64	10.60	18.18	13.77	0.69	1.56	27	6.84	8.26	5.26	0.29	0.48
胆囊及其他	C23–C24	6	0.99	1.70	1.58	0.04	0.14	8	2.03	2.45	1.46	0.04	0.17
胰腺	C25	14	2.32	3.98	2.91	0.07	0.34	10	2.53	3.06	1.86	0.08	0.15
鼻、鼻窦及其他	C30–C31	0	0.00	0.00	0.00	0.00	0.00	1	0.25	0.31	0.17	0.00	0.04
喉	C32	3	0.50	0.85	0.84	0.04	0.09	1	0.25	0.31	0.17	0.00	0.00
气管、支气管、肺	C33–C34	131	21.69	37.21	27.85	0.99	2.85	59	14.94	18.05	10.30	0.23	0.99
其他的胸腔器官	C37–C38	2	0.33	0.57	0.52	0.06	0.06	3	0.76	0.92	0.48	0.00	0.03
骨	C40–C41	6	0.99	1.70	1.51	0.12	0.16	5	1.27	1.53	1.13	0.06	0.10
皮肤的黑色素瘤	C43	1	0.17	0.28	0.18	0.02	0.02	0	0.00	0.00	0.00	0.00	0.00
其他的皮肤	C44	2	0.33	0.57	0.53	0.00	0.00	2	0.51	0.61	0.34	0.01	0.06
间皮瘤	C45	0	0.00	0.00	0.00	0.00	0.00	0	0.00	0.00	0.00	0.00	0.00
卡波西肉瘤	C46	0	0.00	0.00	0.00	0.00	0.00	0	0.00	0.00	0.00	0.00	0.00
周围神经、其他结缔组织、软组织	C47;C49	1	0.17	0.28	0.24	0.02	0.02	1	0.25	0.31	0.30	0.04	0.04
乳房	C50	0	0.00	0.00	0.00	0.00	0.00	26	6.58	7.95	5.31	0.40	0.50
外阴	C51	0	0.00	0.00	0.00	0.00	0.00	0	0.00	0.00	0.00	0.00	0.00
阴道	C52	0	0.00	0.00	0.00	0.00	0.00	0	0.00	0.00	0.00	0.00	0.00
子宫颈	C53	0	0.00	0.00	0.00	0.00	0.00	12	3.04	3.67	2.57	0.20	0.28
子宫体	C54	0	0.00	0.00	0.00	0.00	0.00	5	1.27	1.53	0.99	0.08	0.08
子宫，部位不明	C55	0	0.00	0.00	0.00	0.00	0.00	1	0.25	0.31	0.30	0.04	0.04
卵巢	C56	0	0.00	0.00	0.00	0.00	0.00	10	2.53	3.06	1.69	0.05	0.20
女性其他的生殖器	C57	0	0.00	0.00	0.00	0.00	0.00	1	0.25	0.31	0.14	0.00	0.00
胎盘	C58	0	0.00	0.00	0.00	0.00	0.00	0	0.00	0.00	0.00	0.00	0.00
阴茎	C60	0	0.00	0.00	0.00	0.00	0.00	0	0.00	0.00	0.00	0.00	0.00
前列腺	C61	7	1.16	1.99	1.75	0.04	0.12	0	0.00	0.00	0.00	0.00	0.00
睾丸	C62	0	0.00	0.00	0.00	0.00	0.00	0	0.00	0.00	0.00	0.00	0.00
男性其他的生殖器	C63	1	0.17	0.28	0.34	0.00	0.00	0	0.00	0.00	0.00	0.00	0.00
肾	C64	2	0.33	0.57	0.36	0.02	0.02	0	0.00	0.00	0.00	0.00	0.00
肾盂	C65	0	0.00	0.00	0.00	0.00	0.00	0	0.00	0.00	0.00	0.00	0.00
输尿管	C66	0	0.00	0.00	0.00	0.00	0.00	0	0.00	0.00	0.00	0.00	0.00
膀胱	C67	5	0.83	1.42	1.21	0.06	0.14	1	0.25	0.31	0.19	0.02	0.02
其他的泌尿器官	C68	1	0.17	0.28	0.20	0.00	0.03	0	0.00	0.00	0.00	0.00	0.00
眼	C69	3	0.50	0.85	0.71	0.00	0.05	1	0.25	0.31	0.30	0.04	0.04
脑、神经系统	C70–C72	16	2.65	4.55	3.84	0.21	0.39	9	2.28	2.75	2.06	0.10	0.19
甲状腺	C73	0	0.00	0.00	0.00	0.00	0.00	1	0.25	0.31	0.17	0.00	0.04
肾上腺	C74	3	0.50	0.85	0.68	0.03	0.12	0	0.00	0.00	0.00	0.00	0.00
其他的内分泌腺	C75	1	0.17	0.28	0.18	0.00	0.05	1	0.25	0.31	0.30	0.04	0.04
霍奇金病	C81	0	0.00	0.00	0.00	0.00	0.00	0	0.00	0.00	0.00	0.00	0.00
非霍奇金淋巴瘤	C82–C85;C96	0	0.00	0.00	0.00	0.00	0.00	0	0.00	0.00	0.00	0.00	0.00
免疫增生性疾病	C88	0	0.00	0.00	0.00	0.00	0.00	0	0.00	0.00	0.00	0.00	0.00
多发性骨髓瘤	C90	2	0.33	0.57	0.37	0.00	0.05	1	0.25	0.31	0.24	0.02	0.02
淋巴样白血病	C91	1	0.17	0.28	0.19	0.00	0.00	0	0.00	0.00	0.00	0.00	0.00
髓样白血病	C92–C94	1	0.17	0.28	0.24	0.02	0.02	1	0.25	0.31	0.19	0.02	0.02
白血病，未特指	C95	1	0.17	0.28	0.19	0.00	0.00	0	0.00	0.00	0.00	0.00	0.00
其他的或未指明部位	O&U	21	3.48	5.97	5.27	0.18	0.66	17	4.30	5.20	3.61	0.20	0.31
骨髓增殖性疾病	MPD	0	0.00	0.00	0.00	0.00	0.00	0	0.00	0.00	0.00	0.00	0.00
骨髓增生异常综合征	MDS	0	0.00	0.00	0.00	0.00	0.00	1	0.25	0.31	0.30	0.04	0.04
合计	ALL	604	100.00	171.58	130.64	4.13	13.95	395	100.00	120.83	73.60	2.88	7.01
C44 以外的部位	ALL but C44	602	99.67	171.02	130.11	4.13	13.95	393	99.49	120.22	73.26	2.86	6.95

表 6-65　2020 年河南省淇县恶性肿瘤发病主要指标

部位	ICD-10	男性						女性					
		病例数	构成 (%)	粗率 (1/10^5)	世标率 (1/10^5)	累积率 (%)		病例数	构成 (%)	粗率 (1/10^5)	世标率 (1/10^5)	累积率 (%)	
						0～64	0～74					0～64	0～74
唇	C00	0	0.00	0.00	0.00	0.00	0.00	1	0.23	0.76	0.31	0.00	0.00
舌	C01–C02	2	0.41	1.42	0.80	0.08	0.08	0	0.00	0.00	0.00	0.00	0.00
口	C03–C06	2	0.41	1.42	0.88	0.00	0.08	2	0.46	1.53	0.66	0.00	0.09
唾液腺	C07–C08	2	0.41	1.42	0.87	0.00	0.18	0	0.00	0.00	0.00	0.00	0.00
扁桃体	C09	0	0.00	0.00	0.00	0.00	0.00	0	0.00	0.00	0.00	0.00	0.00
其他的口咽	C10	0	0.00	0.00	0.00	0.00	0.00	0	0.00	0.00	0.00	0.00	0.00
鼻咽	C11	0	0.00	0.00	0.00	0.00	0.00	0	0.00	0.00	0.00	0.00	0.00
喉咽	C12–C13	1	0.21	0.71	0.45	0.00	0.08	1	0.23	0.76	0.32	0.00	0.00
咽，部位不明	C14	0	0.00	0.00	0.00	0.00	0.00	0	0.00	0.00	0.00	0.00	0.00
食管	C15	165	34.16	116.87	81.73	3.34	11.01	129	29.86	98.59	51.80	1.58	6.54
胃	C16	80	16.56	56.66	41.40	2.31	5.01	52	12.04	39.74	22.68	1.18	2.87
小肠	C17	3	0.62	2.12	1.88	0.15	0.15	4	0.93	3.06	1.90	0.18	0.27
结肠	C18	11	2.28	7.79	5.23	0.28	0.49	13	3.01	9.94	5.23	0.36	0.62
直肠	C19–C20	19	3.93	13.46	8.77	0.62	1.30	15	3.47	11.46	7.67	0.68	0.75
肛门	C21	0	0.00	0.00	0.00	0.00	0.00	0	0.00	0.00	0.00	0.00	0.00
肝脏	C22	66	13.66	46.75	33.12	2.01	3.54	17	3.94	12.99	6.33	0.18	0.86
胆囊及其他	C23–C24	3	0.62	2.12	1.28	0.05	0.12	5	1.16	3.82	2.47	0.15	0.24
胰腺	C25	2	0.41	1.42	0.85	0.00	0.10	9	2.08	6.88	3.87	0.24	0.62
鼻、鼻窦及其他	C30–C31	1	0.21	0.71	0.42	0.00	0.10	0	0.00	0.00	0.00	0.00	0.00
喉	C32	2	0.41	1.42	1.23	0.10	0.17	1	0.23	0.76	0.73	0.06	0.06
气管、支气管、肺	C33–C34	67	13.87	47.46	36.37	2.30	4.41	37	8.56	28.28	15.43	0.85	1.83
其他的胸腔器官	C37–C38	1	0.21	0.71	0.39	0.05	0.05	0	0.00	0.00	0.00	0.00	0.00
骨	C40–C41	2	0.41	1.42	1.20	0.10	0.20	6	1.39	4.59	3.18	0.26	0.34
皮肤的黑色素瘤	C43	0	0.00	0.00	0.00	0.00	0.00	1	0.23	0.76	0.74	0.09	0.09
其他的皮肤	C44	6	1.24	4.25	3.76	0.25	0.43	3	0.69	2.29	1.45	0.14	0.14
间皮瘤	C45	0	0.00	0.00	0.00	0.00	0.00	0	0.00	0.00	0.00	0.00	0.00
卡波西肉瘤	C46	0	0.00	0.00	0.00	0.00	0.00	0	0.00	0.00	0.00	0.00	0.00
周围神经、其他结缔组织、软组织	C47;C49	0	0.00	0.00	0.00	0.00	0.00	0	0.00	0.00	0.00	0.00	0.00
乳房	C50	2	0.41	1.42	0.88	0.08	0.08	40	9.26	30.57	21.21	1.70	2.26
外阴	C51	0	0.00	0.00	0.00	0.00	0.00	0	0.00	0.00	0.00	0.00	0.00
阴道	C52	0	0.00	0.00	0.00	0.00	0.00	0	0.00	0.00	0.00	0.00	0.00
子宫颈	C53	0	0.00	0.00	0.00	0.00	0.00	23	5.32	17.58	13.53	1.24	1.32
子宫体	C54	0	0.00	0.00	0.00	0.00	0.00	8	1.85	6.11	4.78	0.50	0.50
子宫，部位不明	C55	0	0.00	0.00	0.00	0.00	0.00	2	0.46	1.53	1.15	0.06	0.13
卵巢	C56	0	0.00	0.00	0.00	0.00	0.00	6	1.39	4.59	3.39	0.26	0.33
女性其他的生殖器	C57	0	0.00	0.00	0.00	0.00	0.00	2	0.46	1.53	0.77	0.10	0.10
胎盘	C58	0	0.00	0.00	0.00	0.00	0.00	0	0.00	0.00	0.00	0.00	0.00
阴茎	C60	1	0.21	0.71	0.39	0.05	0.05	0	0.00	0.00	0.00	0.00	0.00
前列腺	C61	6	1.24	4.25	3.32	0.19	0.27	0	0.00	0.00	0.00	0.00	0.00
睾丸	C62	1	0.21	0.71	0.45	0.00	0.08	0	0.00	0.00	0.00	0.00	0.00
男性其他的生殖器	C63	0	0.00	0.00	0.00	0.00	0.00	0	0.00	0.00	0.00	0.00	0.00
肾	C64	7	1.45	4.96	3.39	0.14	0.47	6	1.39	4.59	3.16	0.36	0.36
肾盂	C65	0	0.00	0.00	0.00	0.00	0.00	0	0.00	0.00	0.00	0.00	0.00
输尿管	C66	0	0.00	0.00	0.00	0.00	0.00	2	0.46	1.53	1.17	0.09	0.16
膀胱	C67	3	0.62	2.12	1.65	0.10	0.10	1	0.23	0.76	0.74	0.09	0.09
其他的泌尿器官	C68	0	0.00	0.00	0.00	0.00	0.00	1	0.23	0.76	0.42	0.00	0.07
眼	C69	0	0.00	0.00	0.00	0.00	0.00	0	0.00	0.00	0.00	0.00	0.00
脑、神经系统	C70–C72	10	2.07	7.08	5.71	0.38	0.45	10	2.31	7.64	5.65	0.45	0.54
甲状腺	C73	6	1.24	4.25	3.60	0.26	0.34	23	5.32	17.58	12.12	1.13	1.29
肾上腺	C74	0	0.00	0.00	0.00	0.00	0.00	0	0.00	0.00	0.00	0.00	0.00
其他的内分泌腺	C75	0	0.00	0.00	0.00	0.00	0.00	1	0.23	0.76	0.31	0.00	0.00
霍奇金病	C81	0	0.00	0.00	0.00	0.00	0.00	0	0.00	0.00	0.00	0.00	0.00
非霍奇金淋巴瘤	C82–C85;C96	1	0.21	0.71	0.42	0.00	0.10	0	0.00	0.00	0.00	0.00	0.00
免疫增生性疾病	C88	0	0.00	0.00	0.00	0.00	0.00	1	0.23	0.76	0.74	0.09	0.09
多发性骨髓瘤	C90	1	0.21	0.71	0.78	0.10	0.10	0	0.00	0.00	0.00	0.00	0.00
淋巴样白血病	C91	0	0.00	0.00	0.00	0.00	0.00	0	0.00	0.00	0.00	0.00	0.00
髓样白血病	C92–C94	0	0.00	0.00	0.00	0.00	0.00	1	0.23	0.76	0.38	0.05	0.05
白血病，未特指	C95	2	0.41	1.42	0.80	0.08	0.08	2	0.46	1.53	1.40	0.15	0.15
其他的或未指明部位	O&U	8	1.66	5.67	4.61	0.36	0.61	7	1.62	5.35	3.53	0.24	0.31
骨髓增殖性疾病	MPD	0	0.00	0.00	0.00	0.00	0.00	0	0.00	0.00	0.00	0.00	0.00
骨髓增生异常综合征	MDS	0	0.00	0.00	0.00	0.00	0.00	0	0.00	0.00	0.00	0.00	0.00
合计	ALL	483	100.00	342.11	246.65	13.37	30.22	432	100.00	330.16	199.25	12.47	23.08
C44 以外的部位	ALL but C44	477	98.76	337.86	242.89	13.12	29.79	429	99.31	327.86	197.80	12.33	22.94

表 6-66 2020 年河南省淇县恶性肿瘤死亡主要指标

部位	ICD-10	男性						女性					
		病例数	构成(%)	粗率($1/10^5$)	世标率($1/10^5$)	累积率(%) 0~64	累积率(%) 0~74	病例数	构成(%)	粗率($1/10^5$)	世标率($1/10^5$)	累积率(%) 0~64	累积率(%) 0~74
唇	C00	0	0.00	0.00	0.00	0.00	0.00	0	0.00	0.00	0.00	0.00	0.00
舌	C01–C02	1	0.37	0.71	0.44	0.00	0.00	0	0.00	0.00	0.00	0.00	0.00
口	C03–C06	0	0.00	0.00	0.00	0.00	0.00	0	0.00	0.00	0.00	0.00	0.00
唾液腺	C07–C08	0	0.00	0.00	0.00	0.00	0.00	0	0.00	0.00	0.00	0.00	0.00
扁桃体	C09	0	0.00	0.00	0.00	0.00	0.00	0	0.00	0.00	0.00	0.00	0.00
其他的口咽	C10	0	0.00	0.00	0.00	0.00	0.00	0	0.00	0.00	0.00	0.00	0.00
鼻咽	C11	1	0.37	0.71	0.44	0.00	0.00	0	0.00	0.00	0.00	0.00	0.00
喉咽	C12–C13	1	0.37	0.71	0.42	0.00	0.10	0	0.00	0.00	0.00	0.00	0.00
咽，部位不明	C14	0	0.00	0.00	0.00	0.00	0.00	0	0.00	0.00	0.00	0.00	0.00
食管	C15	95	35.06	67.29	44.38	1.00	5.37	48	34.04	36.68	17.82	0.28	1.73
胃	C16	49	18.08	34.71	24.64	1.11	3.13	21	14.89	16.05	8.38	0.27	1.35
小肠	C17	0	0.00	0.00	0.00	0.00	0.00	1	0.71	0.76	0.38	0.05	0.05
结肠	C18	3	1.11	2.12	1.47	0.14	0.14	6	4.26	4.59	3.09	0.21	0.37
直肠	C19–C20	8	2.95	5.67	3.70	0.24	0.42	2	1.42	1.53	0.78	0.04	0.13
肛门	C21	1	0.37	0.71	0.43	0.00	0.00	0	0.00	0.00	0.00	0.00	0.00
肝脏	C22	38	14.02	26.92	18.65	1.28	2.07	10	7.09	7.64	3.64	0.04	0.53
胆囊及其他	C23–C24	3	1.11	2.12	1.58	0.06	0.06	1	0.71	0.76	0.32	0.00	0.00
胰腺	C25	4	1.48	2.83	2.04	0.14	0.24	3	2.13	2.29	0.99	0.00	0.09
鼻、鼻窦及其他	C30–C31	0	0.00	0.00	0.00	0.00	0.00	0	0.00	0.00	0.00	0.00	0.00
喉	C32	0	0.00	0.00	0.00	0.00	0.00	1	0.71	0.76	0.73	0.06	0.06
气管、支气管、肺	C33–C34	44	16.24	31.17	22.28	1.14	2.72	11	7.80	8.41	4.73	0.23	0.54
其他的胸腔器官	C37–C38	0	0.00	0.00	0.00	0.00	0.00	1	0.71	0.76	0.74	0.09	0.09
骨	C40–C41	5	1.85	3.54	2.34	0.15	0.33	4	2.84	3.06	1.37	0.00	0.26
皮肤的黑色素瘤	C43	0	0.00	0.00	0.00	0.00	0.00	0	0.00	0.00	0.00	0.00	0.00
其他的皮肤	C44	1	0.37	0.71	0.40	0.04	0.04	0	0.00	0.00	0.00	0.00	0.00
间皮瘤	C45	0	0.00	0.00	0.00	0.00	0.00	0	0.00	0.00	0.00	0.00	0.00
卡波西肉瘤	C46	0	0.00	0.00	0.00	0.00	0.00	0	0.00	0.00	0.00	0.00	0.00
周围神经、其他结缔组织、软组织	C47;C49	2	0.74	1.42	0.87	0.00	0.18	0	0.00	0.00	0.00	0.00	0.00
乳房	C50	0	0.00	0.00	0.00	0.00	0.00	7	4.96	5.35	3.17	0.27	0.34
外阴	C51	0	0.00	0.00	0.00	0.00	0.00	0	0.00	0.00	0.00	0.00	0.00
阴道	C52	0	0.00	0.00	0.00	0.00	0.00	0	0.00	0.00	0.00	0.00	0.00
子宫颈	C53	0	0.00	0.00	0.00	0.00	0.00	0	0.00	0.00	0.00	0.00	0.00
子宫体	C54	0	0.00	0.00	0.00	0.00	0.00	2	1.42	1.53	1.06	0.09	0.09
子宫，部位不明	C55	0	0.00	0.00	0.00	0.00	0.00	0	0.00	0.00	0.00	0.00	0.00
卵巢	C56	0	0.00	0.00	0.00	0.00	0.00	1	0.71	0.76	0.32	0.00	0.00
女性其他的生殖器	C57	0	0.00	0.00	0.00	0.00	0.00	0	0.00	0.00	0.00	0.00	0.00
胎盘	C58	0	0.00	0.00	0.00	0.00	0.00	0	0.00	0.00	0.00	0.00	0.00
阴茎	C60	0	0.00	0.00	0.00	0.00	0.00	0	0.00	0.00	0.00	0.00	0.00
前列腺	C61	2	0.74	1.42	1.09	0.00	0.10	0	0.00	0.00	0.00	0.00	0.00
睾丸	C62	0	0.00	0.00	0.00	0.00	0.00	0	0.00	0.00	0.00	0.00	0.00
男性其他的生殖器	C63	0	0.00	0.00	0.00	0.00	0.00	0	0.00	0.00	0.00	0.00	0.00
肾	C64	2	0.74	1.42	1.45	0.10	0.10	0	0.00	0.00	0.00	0.00	0.00
肾盂	C65	0	0.00	0.00	0.00	0.00	0.00	0	0.00	0.00	0.00	0.00	0.00
输尿管	C66	0	0.00	0.00	0.00	0.00	0.00	0	0.00	0.00	0.00	0.00	0.00
膀胱	C67	0	0.00	0.00	0.00	0.00	0.00	0	0.00	0.00	0.00	0.00	0.00
其他的泌尿器官	C68	0	0.00	0.00	0.00	0.00	0.00	0	0.00	0.00	0.00	0.00	0.00
眼	C69	0	0.00	0.00	0.00	0.00	0.00	0	0.00	0.00	0.00	0.00	0.00
脑、神经系统	C70–C72	1	0.37	0.71	0.78	0.10	0.10	8	5.67	6.11	4.93	0.39	0.47
甲状腺	C73	0	0.00	0.00	0.00	0.00	0.00	1	0.71	0.76	0.32	0.00	0.00
肾上腺	C74	1	0.37	0.71	0.44	0.00	0.00	0	0.00	0.00	0.00	0.00	0.00
其他的内分泌腺	C75	1	0.37	0.71	0.39	0.05	0.05	0	0.00	0.00	0.00	0.00	0.00
霍奇金病	C81	0	0.00	0.00	0.00	0.00	0.00	0	0.00	0.00	0.00	0.00	0.00
非霍奇金淋巴瘤	C82–C85;C96	0	0.00	0.00	0.00	0.00	0.00	2	1.42	1.53	0.85	0.04	0.11
免疫增生性疾病	C88	0	0.00	0.00	0.00	0.00	0.00	0	0.00	0.00	0.00	0.00	0.00
多发性骨髓瘤	C90	0	0.00	0.00	0.00	0.00	0.00	0	0.00	0.00	0.00	0.00	0.00
淋巴样白血病	C91	0	0.00	0.00	0.00	0.00	0.00	0	0.00	0.00	0.00	0.00	0.00
髓样白血病	C92–C94	0	0.00	0.00	0.00	0.00	0.00	0	0.00	0.00	0.00	0.00	0.00
白血病，未特指	C95	1	0.37	0.71	0.40	0.04	0.04	1	0.71	0.76	0.43	0.04	0.04
其他的或未指明部位	O&U	7	2.58	4.96	3.52	0.16	0.52	10	7.09	7.64	4.00	0.10	0.42
骨髓增殖性疾病	MPD	0	0.00	0.00	0.00	0.00	0.00	0	0.00	0.00	0.00	0.00	0.00
骨髓增生异常综合征	MDS	0	0.00	0.00	0.00	0.00	0.00	0	0.00	0.00	0.00	0.00	0.00
合计	ALL	271	100.00	191.95	132.14	5.72	15.72	141	100.00	107.76	58.07	2.21	6.68
C44 以外的部位	ALL but C44	270	99.63	191.24	131.74	5.68	15.68	141	100.00	107.76	58.07	2.21	6.68

表 6-67　2020 年河南省辉县市恶性肿瘤发病主要指标

部位	ICD-10	男性						女性					
		病例数	构成 (%)	粗率 (1/10⁵)	世标率 (1/10⁵)	累积率 (%) 0~64	累积率 (%) 0~74	病例数	构成 (%)	粗率 (1/10⁵)	世标率 (1/10⁵)	累积率 (%) 0~64	累积率 (%) 0~74
唇	C00	0	0.00	0.00	0.00	0.00	0.00	1	0.09	0.22	0.14	0.00	0.02
舌	C01–C02	3	0.26	0.65	0.44	0.03	0.06	3	0.28	0.67	0.45	0.02	0.07
口	C03–C06	5	0.43	1.08	0.68	0.02	0.08	6	0.56	1.34	0.96	0.05	0.08
唾液腺	C07–C08	4	0.34	0.86	0.49	0.00	0.00	1	0.09	0.22	0.14	0.01	0.01
扁桃体	C09	1	0.09	0.22	0.19	0.00	0.00	0	0.00	0.00	0.00	0.00	0.00
其他的口咽	C10	3	0.26	0.65	0.39	0.01	0.01	0	0.00	0.00	0.00	0.00	0.00
鼻咽	C11	3	0.26	0.65	0.48	0.03	0.07	0	0.00	0.00	0.00	0.00	0.00
喉咽	C12–C13	3	0.26	0.65	0.45	0.01	0.08	0	0.00	0.00	0.00	0.00	0.00
咽，部位不明	C14	1	0.09	0.22	0.16	0.00	0.04	0	0.00	0.00	0.00	0.00	0.00
食管	C15	272	23.43	58.78	39.60	1.32	5.22	175	16.39	38.94	21.88	0.46	2.90
胃	C16	226	19.47	48.84	32.86	1.52	4.33	77	7.21	17.14	10.02	0.50	1.25
小肠	C17	7	0.60	1.51	1.19	0.06	0.13	5	0.47	1.11	0.66	0.05	0.10
结肠	C18	51	4.39	11.02	7.67	0.34	0.92	47	4.40	10.46	6.81	0.37	0.75
直肠	C19–C20	45	3.88	9.72	6.86	0.31	0.86	31	2.90	6.90	4.22	0.22	0.53
肛门	C21	1	0.09	0.22	0.16	0.00	0.04	0	0.00	0.00	0.00	0.00	0.00
肝脏	C22	120	10.34	25.93	18.54	1.31	2.37	47	4.40	10.46	6.13	0.32	0.78
胆囊及其他	C23–C24	13	1.12	2.81	1.92	0.09	0.22	16	1.50	3.56	2.05	0.08	0.23
胰腺	C25	24	2.07	5.19	3.80	0.16	0.43	18	1.69	4.01	2.29	0.09	0.25
鼻、鼻窦及其他	C30–C31	1	0.09	0.22	0.10	0.00	0.00	0	0.00	0.00	0.00	0.00	0.00
喉	C32	8	0.69	1.73	1.20	0.07	0.13	0	0.00	0.00	0.00	0.00	0.00
气管、支气管、肺	C33–C34	189	16.28	40.84	27.88	1.40	3.71	129	12.08	28.71	17.35	0.92	1.94
其他的胸腔器官	C37–C38	3	0.26	0.65	0.42	0.01	0.06	1	0.09	0.22	0.34	0.01	0.01
骨	C40–C41	4	0.34	0.86	0.64	0.05	0.09	3	0.28	0.67	0.54	0.05	0.05
皮肤的黑色素瘤	C43	2	0.17	0.43	0.28	0.00	0.05	2	0.19	0.45	0.25	0.00	0.00
其他的皮肤	C44	2	0.17	0.43	0.28	0.00	0.04	7	0.66	1.56	1.09	0.03	0.13
间皮瘤	C45	0	0.00	0.00	0.00	0.00	0.00	1	0.09	0.22	0.13	0.02	0.02
卡波西肉瘤	C46	0	0.00	0.00	0.00	0.00	0.00	0	0.00	0.00	0.00	0.00	0.00
周围神经、其他结缔组织、软组织	C47;C49	2	0.17	0.43	0.40	0.03	0.03	4	0.37	0.89	0.59	0.06	0.06
乳房	C50	0	0.00	0.00	0.00	0.00	0.00	153	14.33	34.05	23.70	1.92	2.62
外阴	C51	0	0.00	0.00	0.00	0.00	0.00	1	0.09	0.22	0.12	0.00	0.00
阴道	C52	0	0.00	0.00	0.00	0.00	0.00	2	0.19	0.45	0.36	0.02	0.04
子宫颈	C53	0	0.00	0.00	0.00	0.00	0.00	70	6.55	15.58	11.30	0.98	1.20
子宫体	C54	0	0.00	0.00	0.00	0.00	0.00	56	5.24	12.46	8.26	0.72	0.97
子宫，部位不明	C55	0	0.00	0.00	0.00	0.00	0.00	5	0.47	1.11	0.63	0.02	0.04
卵巢	C56	0	0.00	0.00	0.00	0.00	0.00	23	2.15	5.12	3.24	0.27	0.36
女性其他的生殖器	C57	0	0.00	0.00	0.00	0.00	0.00	3	0.28	0.67	0.63	0.05	0.05
胎盘	C58	0	0.00	0.00	0.00	0.00	0.00	0	0.00	0.00	0.00	0.00	0.00
阴茎	C60	4	0.34	0.86	0.63	0.03	0.06	0	0.00	0.00	0.00	0.00	0.00
前列腺	C61	20	1.72	4.32	2.77	0.07	0.27	0	0.00	0.00	0.00	0.00	0.00
睾丸	C62	0	0.00	0.00	0.00	0.00	0.00	0	0.00	0.00	0.00	0.00	0.00
男性其他的生殖器	C63	0	0.00	0.00	0.00	0.00	0.00	0	0.00	0.00	0.00	0.00	0.00
肾	C64	16	1.38	3.46	2.40	0.16	0.28	14	1.31	3.12	1.99	0.17	0.22
肾盂	C65	0	0.00	0.00	0.00	0.00	0.00	0	0.00	0.00	0.00	0.00	0.00
输尿管	C66	2	0.17	0.43	0.32	0.02	0.06	0	0.00	0.00	0.00	0.00	0.00
膀胱	C67	23	1.98	4.97	3.45	0.23	0.36	4	0.37	0.89	0.52	0.01	0.07
其他的泌尿器官	C68	1	0.09	0.22	0.14	0.02	0.02	1	0.09	0.22	0.14	0.00	0.02
眼	C69	0	0.00	0.00	0.00	0.00	0.00	1	0.09	0.22	0.13	0.00	0.03
脑、神经系统	C70–C72	23	1.98	4.97	3.89	0.20	0.36	22	2.06	4.90	3.66	0.22	0.39
甲状腺	C73	26	2.24	5.62	4.55	0.37	0.42	95	8.90	21.14	16.80	1.41	1.62
肾上腺	C74	0	0.00	0.00	0.00	0.00	0.00	0	0.00	0.00	0.00	0.00	0.00
其他的内分泌腺	C75	1	0.09	0.22	0.16	0.02	0.02	1	0.09	0.22	0.12	0.00	0.00
霍奇金病	C81	2	0.17	0.43	0.30	0.02	0.06	7	0.66	1.56	1.25	0.09	0.09
非霍奇金淋巴瘤	C82–C85;C96	13	1.12	2.81	2.08	0.14	0.19	13	1.22	2.89	2.32	0.10	0.18
免疫增生性疾病	C88	0	0.00	0.00	0.00	0.00	0.00	0	0.00	0.00	0.00	0.00	0.00
多发性骨髓瘤	C90	6	0.52	1.30	0.87	0.07	0.12	1	0.09	0.22	0.13	0.02	0.02
淋巴样白血病	C91	0	0.00	0.00	0.00	0.00	0.00	2	0.19	0.45	0.37	0.02	0.02
髓样白血病	C92–C94	5	0.43	1.08	1.06	0.08	0.08	3	0.28	0.67	0.40	0.02	0.04
白血病，未特指	C95	7	0.60	1.51	1.40	0.09	0.13	8	0.75	1.78	1.45	0.09	0.14
其他的或未指明部位	O&U	18	1.55	3.89	2.88	0.15	0.34	9	0.84	2.00	1.26	0.06	0.06
骨髓增殖性疾病	MPD	1	0.09	0.22	0.14	0.01	0.01	0	0.00	0.00	0.00	0.00	0.00
骨髓增生异常综合征	MDS	0	0.00	0.00	0.00	0.00	0.00	0	0.00	0.00	0.00	0.00	0.00
合计	ALL	1 161	100.00	250.88	174.15	8.50	21.75	1 068	100.00	237.67	154.76	9.45	17.37
C44 以外的部位	ALL but C44	1 159	99.83	250.45	173.86	8.50	21.71	1 061	99.34	236.11	153.67	9.42	17.24

表 6-68　2020 年河南省辉县市恶性肿瘤死亡主要指标

部位	ICD-10	男性						女性					
		病例数	构成(%)	粗率(1/10^5)	世标率(1/10^5)	累积率(%)		病例数	构成(%)	粗率(1/10^5)	世标率(1/10^5)	累积率(%)	
						0~64	0~74					0~64	0~74
唇	C00	0	0.00	0.00	0.00	0.00	0.00	1	0.18	0.22	0.13	0.02	0.02
舌	C01-C02	2	0.23	0.43	0.30	0.03	0.03	2	0.36	0.45	0.26	0.00	0.06
口	C03-C06	0	0.00	0.00	0.00	0.00	0.00	4	0.72	0.89	0.52	0.02	0.10
唾液腺	C07-C08	4	0.45	0.86	0.63	0.01	0.04	0	0.00	0.00	0.00	0.00	0.00
扁桃体	C09	0	0.00	0.00	0.00	0.00	0.00	0	0.00	0.00	0.00	0.00	0.00
其他的口咽	C10	0	0.00	0.00	0.00	0.00	0.00	0	0.00	0.00	0.00	0.00	0.00
鼻咽	C11	4	0.45	0.86	0.55	0.02	0.08	1	0.18	0.22	0.14	0.01	0.01
喉咽	C12-C13	1	0.11	0.22	0.12	0.00	0.00	0	0.00	0.00	0.00	0.00	0.00
咽，部位不明	C14	1	0.11	0.22	0.12	0.00	0.00	0	0.00	0.00	0.00	0.00	0.00
食管	C15	269	30.43	58.13	38.63	0.59	4.19	153	27.52	34.05	18.16	0.30	1.54
胃	C16	159	17.99	34.36	22.88	0.66	2.48	70	12.59	15.58	8.63	0.30	0.90
小肠	C17	4	0.45	0.86	0.65	0.03	0.08	3	0.54	0.67	0.33	0.00	0.03
结肠	C18	19	2.15	4.11	2.76	0.08	0.27	16	2.88	3.56	2.00	0.05	0.18
直肠	C19-C20	24	2.71	5.19	3.32	0.07	0.37	17	3.06	3.78	2.02	0.03	0.15
肛门	C21	1	0.11	0.22	0.16	0.00	0.04	0	0.00	0.00	0.00	0.00	0.00
肝脏	C22	114	12.90	24.63	17.49	1.01	2.15	34	6.12	7.57	4.53	0.15	0.50
胆囊及其他	C23-C24	8	0.90	1.73	1.15	0.04	0.12	6	1.08	1.34	0.65	0.02	0.02
胰腺	C25	23	2.60	4.97	3.47	0.12	0.45	20	3.60	4.45	2.70	0.17	0.24
鼻、鼻窦及其他	C30-C31	1	0.11	0.22	0.12	0.00	0.00	1	0.18	0.22	0.12	0.00	0.00
喉	C32	5	0.57	1.08	0.65	0.03	0.03	0	0.00	0.00	0.00	0.00	0.00
气管、支气管、肺	C33-C34	131	14.82	28.31	19.09	0.66	2.18	74	13.31	16.47	9.11	0.42	0.94
其他的胸腔器官	C37-C38	2	0.23	0.43	0.28	0.01	0.04	2	0.36	0.45	0.27	0.03	0.03
骨	C40-C41	9	1.02	1.94	1.73	0.07	0.17	0	0.00	0.00	0.00	0.00	0.00
皮肤的黑色素瘤	C43	3	0.34	0.65	0.50	0.03	0.07	1	0.18	0.22	0.12	0.00	0.00
其他的皮肤	C44	2	0.23	0.43	0.20	0.00	0.00	2	0.36	0.45	0.20	0.00	0.00
间皮瘤	C45	0	0.00	0.00	0.00	0.00	0.00	0	0.00	0.00	0.00	0.00	0.00
卡波西肉瘤	C46	0	0.00	0.00	0.00	0.00	0.00	0	0.00	0.00	0.00	0.00	0.00
周围神经、其他结缔组织、软组织	C47;C49	1	0.11	0.22	0.14	0.02	0.02	0	0.00	0.00	0.00	0.00	0.00
乳房	C50	2	0.23	0.43	0.22	0.00	0.00	42	7.55	9.35	5.64	0.32	0.76
外阴	C51	0	0.00	0.00	0.00	0.00	0.00	1	0.18	0.22	0.13	0.02	0.02
阴道	C52	0	0.00	0.00	0.00	0.00	0.00	2	0.36	0.45	0.21	0.02	0.02
子宫颈	C53	0	0.00	0.00	0.00	0.00	0.00	21	3.78	4.67	3.01	0.18	0.36
子宫体	C54	0	0.00	0.00	0.00	0.00	0.00	7	1.26	1.56	0.91	0.08	0.11
子宫，部位不明	C55	0	0.00	0.00	0.00	0.00	0.00	5	0.90	1.11	0.65	0.04	0.04
卵巢	C56	0	0.00	0.00	0.00	0.00	0.00	17	3.06	3.78	2.35	0.20	0.28
女性其他的生殖器	C57	0	0.00	0.00	0.00	0.00	0.00	0	0.00	0.00	0.00	0.00	0.00
胎盘	C58	0	0.00	0.00	0.00	0.00	0.00	0	0.00	0.00	0.00	0.00	0.00
阴茎	C60	1	0.11	0.22	0.10	0.00	0.00	0	0.00	0.00	0.00	0.00	0.00
前列腺	C61	18	2.04	3.89	2.45	0.03	0.27	0	0.00	0.00	0.00	0.00	0.00
睾丸	C62	0	0.00	0.00	0.00	0.00	0.00	0	0.00	0.00	0.00	0.00	0.00
男性其他的生殖器	C63	0	0.00	0.00	0.00	0.00	0.00	0	0.00	0.00	0.00	0.00	0.00
肾	C64	6	0.68	1.30	0.87	0.00	0.11	4	0.72	0.89	0.51	0.01	0.05
肾盂	C65	1	0.11	0.22	0.14	0.02	0.02	0	0.00	0.00	0.00	0.00	0.00
输尿管	C66	4	0.45	0.86	0.46	0.00	0.04	1	0.18	0.22	0.13	0.02	0.02
膀胱	C67	7	0.79	1.51	1.04	0.01	0.01	4	0.72	0.89	0.40	0.00	0.00
其他的泌尿器官	C68	0	0.00	0.00	0.00	0.00	0.00	0	0.00	0.00	0.00	0.00	0.00
眼	C69	0	0.00	0.00	0.00	0.00	0.00	0	0.00	0.00	0.00	0.00	0.00
脑、神经系统	C70-C72	23	2.60	4.97	3.65	0.25	0.44	19	3.42	4.23	2.69	0.13	0.34
甲状腺	C73	1	0.11	0.22	0.12	0.00	0.00	2	0.36	0.45	0.26	0.02	0.04
肾上腺	C74	0	0.00	0.00	0.00	0.00	0.00	0	0.00	0.00	0.00	0.00	0.00
其他的内分泌腺	C75	0	0.00	0.00	0.00	0.00	0.00	1	0.18	0.22	0.12	0.00	0.00
霍奇金病	C81	0	0.00	0.00	0.00	0.00	0.00	3	0.54	0.67	0.39	0.03	0.03
非霍奇金淋巴瘤	C82-C85;C96	7	0.79	1.51	1.14	0.04	0.15	9	1.62	2.00	1.18	0.03	0.16
免疫增生性疾病	C88	1	0.11	0.22	0.14	0.00	0.02	0	0.00	0.00	0.00	0.00	0.00
多发性骨髓瘤	C90	5	0.57	1.08	0.78	0.08	0.10	0	0.00	0.00	0.00	0.00	0.00
淋巴样白血病	C91	1	0.11	0.22	0.14	0.01	0.01	1	0.18	0.22	0.24	0.02	0.02
髓样白血病	C92-C94	3	0.34	0.65	0.40	0.02	0.06	3	0.54	0.67	0.44	0.03	0.05
白血病，未特指	C95	2	0.23	0.43	0.28	0.02	0.04	2	0.36	0.45	0.42	0.01	0.01
其他的或未指明部位	O&U	12	1.36	2.59	2.04	0.05	0.18	4	0.72	0.89	0.53	0.01	0.07
骨髓增殖性疾病	MPD	0	0.00	0.00	0.00	0.00	0.00	0	0.00	0.00	0.00	0.00	0.00
骨髓增生异常综合征	MDS	3	0.34	0.65	0.58	0.02	0.06	1	0.18	0.22	0.13	0.02	0.02
合计	ALL	884	100.00	191.03	129.51	4.06	14.35	556	100.00	123.73	70.22	2.69	7.13
C44 以外的部位	ALL but C44	882	99.77	190.59	129.31	4.06	14.35	554	99.64	123.29	70.02	2.69	7.13

表 6-69　2020 年河南省焦作市城区恶性肿瘤发病主要指标

部位	ICD-10	男性						女性					
		病例数	构成(%)	粗率 $(1/10^5)$	世标率 $(1/10^5)$	累积率(%)		病例数	构成(%)	粗率 $(1/10^5)$	世标率 $(1/10^5)$	累积率(%)	
						0~64	0~74					0~64	0~74
唇	C00	1	0.12	0.30	0.09	0.00	0.00	0	0.00	0.00	0.00	0.00	0.00
舌	C01–C02	3	0.35	0.91	0.66	0.07	0.07	1	0.12	0.30	0.15	0.02	0.02
口	C03–C06	8	0.94	2.43	1.28	0.08	0.15	2	0.23	0.60	0.35	0.00	0.09
唾液腺	C07–C08	1	0.12	0.30	0.14	0.00	0.00	0	0.00	0.00	0.00	0.00	0.00
扁桃体	C09	1	0.12	0.30	0.14	0.02	0.02	0	0.00	0.00	0.00	0.00	0.00
其他的口咽	C10	2	0.24	0.61	0.38	0.02	0.06	1	0.12	0.30	0.15	0.02	0.02
鼻咽	C11	4	0.47	1.22	0.71	0.03	0.11	0	0.00	0.00	0.00	0.00	0.00
喉咽	C12–C13	4	0.47	1.22	0.63	0.00	0.06	0	0.00	0.00	0.00	0.00	0.00
咽，部位不明	C14	7	0.83	2.13	1.18	0.09	0.14	0	0.00	0.00	0.00	0.00	0.00
食管	C15	48	5.66	14.59	7.78	0.43	0.93	27	3.14	8.10	3.56	0.11	0.38
胃	C16	102	12.03	31.01	16.88	0.60	2.19	45	5.23	13.49	6.90	0.37	0.72
小肠	C17	6	0.71	1.82	1.04	0.05	0.17	5	0.58	1.50	0.66	0.02	0.06
结肠	C18	46	5.42	13.99	7.88	0.38	1.02	41	4.77	12.29	6.15	0.28	0.77
直肠	C19–C20	35	4.13	10.64	5.91	0.26	0.83	35	4.07	10.49	5.69	0.37	0.57
肛门	C21	0	0.00	0.00	0.00	0.00	0.00	1	0.12	0.30	0.19	0.02	0.02
肝脏	C22	95	11.20	28.88	16.10	1.09	1.92	39	4.53	11.69	5.92	0.32	0.82
胆囊及其他	C23–C24	16	1.89	4.86	2.43	0.11	0.33	19	2.21	5.70	2.43	0.09	0.20
胰腺	C25	14	1.65	4.26	2.10	0.09	0.24	12	1.40	3.60	1.56	0.04	0.18
鼻、鼻窦及其他	C30–C31	0	0.00	0.00	0.00	0.00	0.00	2	0.23	0.60	0.23	0.00	0.03
喉	C32	10	1.18	3.04	1.62	0.06	0.18	0	0.00	0.00	0.00	0.00	0.00
气管、支气管、肺	C33–C34	206	24.29	62.63	33.95	1.68	4.12	132	15.35	39.58	20.71	1.33	2.48
其他的胸腔器官	C37–C38	5	0.59	1.52	0.83	0.08	0.08	2	0.23	0.60	0.27	0.02	0.02
骨	C40–C41	4	0.47	1.22	1.47	0.08	0.08	2	0.23	0.60	0.35	0.02	0.04
皮肤的黑色素瘤	C43	2	0.24	0.61	0.34	0.03	0.03	1	0.12	0.30	0.17	0.00	0.04
其他的皮肤	C44	6	0.71	1.82	0.86	0.00	0.06	5	0.58	1.50	0.70	0.04	0.07
间皮瘤	C45	1	0.12	0.30	0.09	0.00	0.00	0	0.00	0.00	0.00	0.00	0.00
卡波西肉瘤	C46	0	0.00	0.00	0.00	0.00	0.00	0	0.00	0.00	0.00	0.00	0.00
周围神经、其他结缔组织、软组织	C47;C49	3	0.35	0.91	0.53	0.04	0.07	5	0.58	1.50	0.77	0.06	0.06
乳房	C50	0	0.00	0.00	0.00	0.00	0.00	140	16.28	41.98	25.64	1.90	2.88
外阴	C51	0	0.00	0.00	0.00	0.00	0.00	0	0.00	0.00	0.00	0.00	0.00
阴道	C52	0	0.00	0.00	0.00	0.00	0.00	1	0.12	0.30	0.16	0.00	0.03
子宫颈	C53	0	0.00	0.00	0.00	0.00	0.00	51	5.93	15.29	9.94	0.78	1.08
子宫体	C54	0	0.00	0.00	0.00	0.00	0.00	26	3.02	7.80	4.42	0.32	0.55
子宫，部位不明	C55	0	0.00	0.00	0.00	0.00	0.00	1	0.12	0.30	0.15	0.02	0.02
卵巢	C56	0	0.00	0.00	0.00	0.00	0.00	22	2.56	6.60	5.16	0.40	0.44
女性其他的生殖器	C57	0	0.00	0.00	0.00	0.00	0.00	1	0.12	0.30	0.10	0.00	0.00
胎盘	C58	0	0.00	0.00	0.00	0.00	0.00	0	0.00	0.00	0.00	0.00	0.00
阴茎	C60	2	0.24	0.61	0.41	0.03	0.03	0	0.00	0.00	0.00	0.00	0.00
前列腺	C61	39	4.60	11.86	5.76	0.06	0.66	0	0.00	0.00	0.00	0.00	0.00
睾丸	C62	1	0.12	0.30	0.32	0.03	0.03	0	0.00	0.00	0.00	0.00	0.00
男性其他的生殖器	C63	1	0.12	0.30	0.20	0.03	0.03	0	0.00	0.00	0.00	0.00	0.00
肾	C64	25	2.95	7.60	4.04	0.15	0.57	10	1.16	3.00	1.67	0.13	0.21
肾盂	C65	1	0.12	0.30	0.17	0.00	0.03	4	0.47	1.20	0.51	0.00	0.07
输尿管	C66	4	0.47	1.22	0.55	0.04	0.06	3	0.35	0.90	0.24	0.00	0.00
膀胱	C67	36	4.25	10.94	5.83	0.31	0.72	8	0.93	2.40	1.28	0.10	0.12
其他的泌尿器官	C68	0	0.00	0.00	0.00	0.00	0.00	0	0.00	0.00	0.00	0.00	0.00
眼	C69	0	0.00	0.00	0.00	0.00	0.00	0	0.00	0.00	0.00	0.00	0.00
脑、神经系统	C70–C72	21	2.48	6.38	4.43	0.33	0.43	26	3.02	7.80	4.74	0.33	0.48
甲状腺	C73	26	3.07	7.90	6.19	0.52	0.55	126	14.65	37.78	25.73	2.28	2.56
肾上腺	C74	0	0.00	0.00	0.00	0.00	0.00	0	0.00	0.00	0.00	0.00	0.00
其他的内分泌腺	C75	1	0.12	0.30	0.14	0.02	0.02	0	0.00	0.00	0.00	0.00	0.00
霍奇金病	C81	0	0.00	0.00	0.00	0.00	0.00	0	0.00	0.00	0.00	0.00	0.00
非霍奇金淋巴瘤	C82–C85;C96	23	2.71	6.99	4.29	0.24	0.58	20	2.33	6.00	3.37	0.20	0.48
免疫增生性疾病	C88	0	0.00	0.00	0.00	0.00	0.00	0	0.00	0.00	0.00	0.00	0.00
多发性骨髓瘤	C90	4	0.47	1.22	0.71	0.05	0.08	5	0.58	1.50	0.77	0.06	0.06
淋巴样白血病	C91	7	0.83	2.13	2.07	0.07	0.19	5	0.58	1.50	2.07	0.11	0.15
髓样白血病	C92–C94	13	1.53	3.95	1.96	0.07	0.18	16	1.86	4.80	3.00	0.20	0.22
白血病，未特指	C95	0	0.00	0.00	0.00	0.00	0.00	3	0.35	0.90	1.02	0.04	0.09
其他的或未指明部位	O&U	12	1.42	3.65	1.87	0.09	0.16	14	1.63	4.20	2.07	0.10	0.19
骨髓增殖性疾病	MPD	2	0.24	0.61	0.59	0.04	0.04	1	0.12	0.30	0.16	0.02	0.02
骨髓增生异常综合征	MDS	0	0.00	0.00	0.00	0.00	0.00	0	0.00	0.00	0.00	0.00	0.00
合计	ALL	848	100.00	257.82	144.58	7.35	17.19	860	100.00	257.87	149.12	10.09	16.22
C44 以外的部位	ALL but C44	842	99.29	255.99	143.72	7.35	17.13	855	99.42	256.37	148.42	10.05	16.15

表 6-70　2020 年河南省焦作市城区恶性肿瘤死亡主要指标

部位	ICD-10	男性						女性					
		病例数	构成 (%)	粗率 ($1/10^5$)	世标率 ($1/10^5$)	累积率 (%)		病例数	构成 (%)	粗率 ($1/10^5$)	世标率 ($1/10^5$)	累积率 (%)	
						0~64	0~74					0~64	0~74
唇	C00	0	0.00	0.00	0.00	0.00	0.00	0	0.00	0.00	0.00	0.00	0.00
舌	C01–C02	1	0.18	0.30	0.20	0.02	0.02	1	0.25	0.30	0.10	0.00	0.00
口	C03–C06	2	0.35	0.61	0.29	0.02	0.02	1	0.25	0.30	0.07	0.00	0.00
唾液腺	C07–C08	2	0.35	0.61	0.33	0.00	0.05	0	0.00	0.00	0.00	0.00	0.00
扁桃体	C09	1	0.18	0.30	0.20	0.03	0.03	0	0.00	0.00	0.00	0.00	0.00
其他的口咽	C10	1	0.18	0.30	0.19	0.00	0.05	0	0.00	0.00	0.00	0.00	0.00
鼻咽	C11	2	0.35	0.61	0.35	0.04	0.04	0	0.00	0.00	0.00	0.00	0.00
喉咽	C12–C13	3	0.53	0.91	0.47	0.02	0.06	0	0.00	0.00	0.00	0.00	0.00
咽，部位不明	C14	1	0.18	0.30	0.09	0.00	0.00	0	0.00	0.00	0.00	0.00	0.00
食管	C15	52	9.15	15.81	8.01	0.25	0.88	36	9.14	10.79	4.69	0.07	0.54
胃	C16	78	13.73	23.71	12.82	0.27	1.70	37	9.39	11.09	5.07	0.20	0.44
小肠	C17	2	0.35	0.61	0.26	0.00	0.03	4	1.02	1.20	0.51	0.02	0.06
结肠	C18	25	4.40	7.60	4.00	0.16	0.43	20	5.08	6.00	3.00	0.11	0.32
直肠	C19–C20	23	4.05	6.99	3.65	0.23	0.33	12	3.05	3.60	1.44	0.07	0.10
肛门	C21	0	0.00	0.00	0.00	0.00	0.00	1	0.25	0.30	0.19	0.02	0.02
肝脏	C22	87	15.32	26.45	14.62	0.96	1.73	39	9.90	11.69	5.78	0.27	0.78
胆囊及其他	C23–C24	18	3.17	5.47	2.60	0.09	0.29	18	4.57	5.40	2.45	0.12	0.24
胰腺	C25	14	2.46	4.26	2.23	0.10	0.16	15	3.81	4.50	1.98	0.09	0.20
鼻、鼻窦及其他	C30–C31	1	0.18	0.30	0.25	0.02	0.02	1	0.25	0.30	0.07	0.00	0.00
喉	C32	8	1.41	2.43	1.41	0.07	0.21	1	0.25	0.30	0.10	0.00	0.00
气管、支气管、肺	C33–C34	156	27.46	47.43	24.84	0.95	2.90	74	18.78	22.19	10.95	0.42	1.41
其他的胸腔器官	C37–C38	1	0.18	0.30	0.20	0.03	0.03	1	0.25	0.30	0.11	0.00	0.00
骨	C40–C41	0	0.00	0.00	0.00	0.00	0.00	4	1.02	1.20	0.58	0.03	0.05
皮肤的黑色素瘤	C43	0	0.00	0.00	0.00	0.00	0.00	1	0.25	0.30	0.17	0.00	0.04
其他的皮肤	C44	0	0.00	0.00	0.00	0.00	0.00	1	0.25	0.30	0.23	0.02	0.02
间皮瘤	C45	1	0.18	0.30	0.09	0.00	0.00	0	0.00	0.00	0.00	0.00	0.00
卡波西肉瘤	C46	0	0.00	0.00	0.00	0.00	0.00	0	0.00	0.00	0.00	0.00	0.00
周围神经、其他结缔组织、软组织	C47;C49	1	0.18	0.30	0.17	0.00	0.03	0	0.00	0.00	0.00	0.00	0.00
乳房	C50	1	0.18	0.30	0.19	0.00	0.05	29	7.36	8.70	4.87	0.36	0.49
外阴	C51	0	0.00	0.00	0.00	0.00	0.00	0	0.00	0.00	0.00	0.00	0.00
阴道	C52	0	0.00	0.00	0.00	0.00	0.00	3	0.76	0.90	0.43	0.02	0.06
子宫颈	C53	0	0.00	0.00	0.00	0.00	0.00	21	5.33	6.30	3.26	0.22	0.36
子宫体	C54	0	0.00	0.00	0.00	0.00	0.00	7	1.78	2.10	1.05	0.08	0.12
子宫，部位不明	C55	0	0.00	0.00	0.00	0.00	0.00	1	0.25	0.30	0.15	0.02	0.02
卵巢	C56	0	0.00	0.00	0.00	0.00	0.00	11	2.79	3.30	1.66	0.08	0.21
女性其他的生殖器	C57	0	0.00	0.00	0.00	0.00	0.00	1	0.25	0.30	0.10	0.00	0.00
胎盘	C58	0	0.00	0.00	0.00	0.00	0.00	0	0.00	0.00	0.00	0.00	0.00
阴茎	C60	0	0.00	0.00	0.00	0.00	0.00	0	0.00	0.00	0.00	0.00	0.00
前列腺	C61	13	2.29	3.95	1.82	0.05	0.09	0	0.00	0.00	0.00	0.00	0.00
睾丸	C62	0	0.00	0.00	0.00	0.00	0.00	0	0.00	0.00	0.00	0.00	0.00
男性其他的生殖器	C63	1	0.18	0.30	0.15	0.00	0.00	0	0.00	0.00	0.00	0.00	0.00
肾	C64	14	2.46	4.26	2.23	0.08	0.24	2	0.51	0.60	0.27	0.00	0.04
肾盂	C65	0	0.00	0.00	0.00	0.00	0.00	0	0.00	0.00	0.00	0.00	0.00
输尿管	C66	1	0.18	0.30	0.15	0.00	0.00	1	0.25	0.30	0.10	0.00	0.00
膀胱	C67	8	1.41	2.43	0.94	0.02	0.06	2	0.51	0.60	0.33	0.02	0.06
其他的泌尿器官	C68	0	0.00	0.00	0.00	0.00	0.00	0	0.00	0.00	0.00	0.00	0.00
眼	C69	0	0.00	0.00	0.00	0.00	0.00	0	0.00	0.00	0.00	0.00	0.00
脑、神经系统	C70–C72	8	1.41	2.43	1.58	0.11	0.14	9	2.28	2.70	1.25	0.03	0.17
甲状腺	C73	1	0.18	0.30	0.20	0.03	0.03	2	0.51	0.60	0.27	0.00	0.03
肾上腺	C74	0	0.00	0.00	0.00	0.00	0.00	0	0.00	0.00	0.00	0.00	0.00
其他的内分泌腺	C75	1	0.18	0.30	0.14	0.02	0.02	0	0.00	0.00	0.00	0.00	0.00
霍奇金病	C81	0	0.00	0.00	0.00	0.00	0.00	1	0.25	0.30	0.16	0.00	0.03
非霍奇金淋巴瘤	C82–C85;C96	10	1.76	3.04	1.76	0.09	0.24	7	1.78	2.10	1.18	0.04	0.14
免疫增生性疾病	C88	0	0.00	0.00	0.00	0.00	0.00	0	0.00	0.00	0.00	0.00	0.00
多发性骨髓瘤	C90	4	0.70	1.22	0.67	0.02	0.12	4	1.02	1.20	0.52	0.03	0.03
淋巴样白血病	C91	1	0.18	0.30	0.20	0.03	0.03	1	0.25	0.30	0.16	0.02	0.02
髓样白血病	C92–C94	6	1.06	1.82	0.97	0.03	0.07	5	1.27	1.50	0.78	0.05	0.08
白血病，未特指	C95	0	0.00	0.00	0.00	0.00	0.00	3	0.76	0.90	0.43	0.02	0.06
其他的或未指明部位	O&U	15	2.64	4.56	2.54	0.15	0.28	12	3.05	3.60	1.82	0.10	0.19
骨髓增殖性疾病	MPD	0	0.00	0.00	0.00	0.00	0.00	0	0.00	0.00	0.00	0.00	0.00
骨髓增生异常综合征	MDS	4	0.70	1.22	0.65	0.00	0.08	5	1.27	1.50	0.80	0.03	0.13
合计	ALL	568	100.00	172.69	91.48	3.84	10.44	394	100.00	118.14	57.10	2.55	6.45
C44 以外的部位	ALL but C44	568	100.00	172.69	91.48	3.84	10.44	393	99.75	117.84	56.87	2.53	6.43

表 6–71　2020 年河南省范县恶性肿瘤发病主要指标

部位	ICD-10	男性						女性					
		病例数	构成 (%)	粗率 ($1/10^5$)	世标率 ($1/10^5$)	累积率 (%) 0～64	累积率 (%) 0～74	病例数	构成 (%)	粗率 ($1/10^5$)	世标率 ($1/10^5$)	累积率 (%) 0～64	累积率 (%) 0～74
唇	C00	0	0.00	0.00	0.00	0.00	0.00	0	0.00	0.00	0.00	0.00	0.00
舌	C01–C02	0	0.00	0.00	0.00	0.00	0.00	0	0.00	0.00	0.00	0.00	0.00
口	C03–C06	4	0.48	1.33	1.23	0.12	0.12	3	0.38	1.05	0.89	0.06	0.06
唾液腺	C07–C08	2	0.24	0.66	0.62	0.04	0.12	4	0.50	1.39	1.22	0.09	0.15
扁桃体	C09	1	0.12	0.33	0.36	0.02	0.02	1	0.13	0.35	0.23	0.00	0.00
其他的口咽	C10	10	1.21	3.31	3.16	0.21	0.33	4	0.50	1.39	1.06	0.08	0.08
鼻咽	C11	9	1.09	2.98	2.67	0.15	0.40	5	0.63	1.74	1.43	0.08	0.21
喉咽	C12–C13	5	0.61	1.66	1.47	0.03	0.16	1	0.13	0.35	0.29	0.00	0.05
咽，部位不明	C14	3	0.36	0.99	0.95	0.03	0.19	2	0.25	0.70	0.59	0.03	0.08
食管	C15	71	8.60	23.52	20.01	0.52	2.58	29	3.66	10.11	7.27	0.24	1.08
胃	C16	86	10.41	28.49	25.12	0.88	2.72	47	5.93	16.38	11.64	0.62	1.01
小肠	C17	5	0.61	1.66	1.47	0.06	0.20	5	0.63	1.74	1.16	0.02	0.02
结肠	C18	18	2.18	5.96	5.29	0.26	0.67	14	1.77	4.88	3.61	0.14	0.35
直肠	C19–C20	43	5.21	14.24	12.62	0.58	1.49	32	4.04	11.15	7.77	0.36	0.75
肛门	C21	3	0.36	0.99	0.91	0.08	0.08	1	0.13	0.35	0.26	0.02	0.02
肝脏	C22	94	11.38	31.14	27.79	1.60	3.39	32	4.04	11.15	8.91	0.52	1.04
胆囊及其他	C23–C24	1	0.12	0.33	0.29	0.00	0.05	3	0.38	1.05	0.78	0.00	0.11
胰腺	C25	21	2.54	6.96	5.85	0.27	0.74	25	3.15	8.71	6.33	0.39	0.65
鼻、鼻窦及其他	C30–C31	2	0.24	0.66	0.64	0.07	0.07	0	0.00	0.00	0.00	0.00	0.00
喉	C32	15	1.82	4.97	4.46	0.11	0.62	1	0.13	0.35	0.29	0.00	0.05
气管、支气管、肺	C33–C34	259	31.36	85.79	75.92	3.11	8.85	123	15.51	42.86	30.51	1.40	3.52
其他的胸腔器官	C37–C38	3	0.36	0.99	1.04	0.09	0.09	3	0.38	1.05	0.78	0.00	0.11
骨	C40–C41	9	1.09	2.98	2.67	0.18	0.30	13	1.64	4.53	3.98	0.23	0.44
皮肤的黑色素瘤	C43	0	0.00	0.00	0.00	0.00	0.00	0	0.00	0.00	0.00	0.00	0.00
其他的皮肤	C44	4	0.48	1.33	1.32	0.06	0.11	4	0.50	1.39	0.90	0.04	0.09
间皮瘤	C45	0	0.00	0.00	0.00	0.00	0.00	0	0.00	0.00	0.00	0.00	0.00
卡波西肉瘤	C46	0	0.00	0.00	0.00	0.00	0.00	0	0.00	0.00	0.00	0.00	0.00
周围神经、其他结缔组织、软组织	C47;C49	3	0.36	0.99	0.94	0.10	0.10	1	0.13	0.35	0.32	0.04	0.04
乳房	C50	2	0.24	0.66	0.61	0.03	0.08	131	16.52	45.65	38.34	3.21	4.11
外阴	C51	0	0.00	0.00	0.00	0.00	0.00	0	0.00	0.00	0.00	0.00	0.00
阴道	C52	0	0.00	0.00	0.00	0.00	0.00	1	0.13	0.35	0.34	0.04	0.04
子宫颈	C53	0	0.00	0.00	0.00	0.00	0.00	54	6.81	18.82	15.73	1.31	1.79
子宫体	C54	0	0.00	0.00	0.00	0.00	0.00	46	5.80	16.03	12.57	1.01	1.22
子宫，部位不明	C55	0	0.00	0.00	0.00	0.00	0.00	16	2.02	5.58	4.61	0.35	0.57
卵巢	C56	0	0.00	0.00	0.00	0.00	0.00	24	3.03	8.36	7.01	0.49	0.59
女性其他的生殖器	C57	0	0.00	0.00	0.00	0.00	0.00	3	0.38	1.05	1.01	0.05	0.05
胎盘	C58	0	0.00	0.00	0.00	0.00	0.00	0	0.00	0.00	0.00	0.00	0.00
阴茎	C60	2	0.24	0.66	0.58	0.04	0.04	0	0.00	0.00	0.00	0.00	0.00
前列腺	C61	10	1.21	3.31	2.68	0.16	0.28	0	0.00	0.00	0.00	0.00	0.00
睾丸	C62	4	0.48	1.33	1.23	0.06	0.22	0	0.00	0.00	0.00	0.00	0.00
男性其他的生殖器	C63	0	0.00	0.00	0.00	0.00	0.00	0	0.00	0.00	0.00	0.00	0.00
肾	C64	14	1.69	4.64	4.06	0.24	0.47	14	1.77	4.88	3.78	0.18	0.41
肾盂	C65	1	0.12	0.33	0.25	0.02	0.02	1	0.13	0.35	0.29	0.00	0.05
输尿管	C66	2	0.24	0.66	0.61	0.04	0.09	0	0.00	0.00	0.00	0.00	0.00
膀胱	C67	15	1.82	4.97	4.21	0.07	0.36	5	0.63	1.74	1.16	0.08	0.08
其他的泌尿器官	C68	0	0.00	0.00	0.00	0.00	0.00	0	0.00	0.00	0.00	0.00	0.00
眼	C69	0	0.00	0.00	0.00	0.00	0.00	0	0.00	0.00	0.00	0.00	0.00
脑、神经系统	C70–C72	30	3.63	9.94	9.56	0.59	0.79	23	2.90	8.01	6.80	0.45	0.75
甲状腺	C73	29	3.51	9.61	8.86	0.74	1.01	96	12.11	33.45	28.08	2.41	3.10
肾上腺	C74	2	0.24	0.66	0.56	0.02	0.10	1	0.13	0.35	0.26	0.02	0.02
其他的内分泌腺	C75	0	0.00	0.00	0.00	0.00	0.00	1	0.13	0.35	0.34	0.04	0.04
霍奇金病	C81	0	0.00	0.00	0.00	0.00	0.00	0	0.00	0.00	0.00	0.00	0.00
非霍奇金淋巴瘤	C82–C85;C96	2	0.24	0.66	0.63	0.03	0.11	3	0.38	1.05	0.85	0.07	0.07
免疫增生性疾病	C88	0	0.00	0.00	0.00	0.00	0.00	0	0.00	0.00	0.00	0.00	0.00
多发性骨髓瘤	C90	0	0.00	0.00	0.00	0.00	0.00	1	0.13	0.35	0.34	0.03	0.03
淋巴样白血病	C91	0	0.00	0.00	0.00	0.00	0.00	1	0.13	0.35	0.34	0.04	0.04
髓样白血病	C92–C94	1	0.12	0.33	0.31	0.00	0.08	0	0.00	0.00	0.00	0.00	0.00
白血病，未特指	C95	3	0.36	0.99	0.89	0.06	0.11	2	0.25	0.70	0.58	0.04	0.10
其他的或未指明部位	O&U	38	4.60	12.59	11.61	0.74	1.04	17	2.14	5.92	5.06	0.34	0.54
骨髓增殖性疾病	MPD	0	0.00	0.00	0.00	0.00	0.00	0	0.00	0.00	0.00	0.00	0.00
骨髓增生异常综合征	MDS	0	0.00	0.00	0.00	0.00	0.00	0	0.00	0.00	0.00	0.00	0.00
合计	ALL	826	100.00	273.61	243.42	11.42	28.20	793	100.00	276.33	217.68	14.51	23.53
C44 以外的部位	ALL but C44	822	99.52	272.29	242.10	11.36	28.08	789	99.50	274.94	216.78	14.46	23.44

表 6-72 2020 年河南省范县恶性肿瘤死亡主要指标

部位	ICD-10	男性						女性					
		病例数	构成(%)	粗率(1/10^5)	世标率(1/10^5)	累积率(%)		病例数	构成(%)	粗率(1/10^5)	世标率(1/10^5)	累积率(%)	
						0~64	0~74					0~64	0~74
唇	C00	0	0.00	0.00	0.00	0.00	0.00	1	0.31	0.35	0.14	0.00	0.00
舌	C01-C02	0	0.00	0.00	0.00	0.00	0.00	0	0.00	0.00	0.00	0.00	0.00
口	C03-C06	1	0.18	0.33	0.32	0.03	0.03	1	0.31	0.35	0.13	0.00	0.00
唾液腺	C07-C08	2	0.36	0.66	0.67	0.04	0.04	0	0.00	0.00	0.00	0.00	0.00
扁桃体	C09	0	0.00	0.00	0.00	0.00	0.00	0	0.00	0.00	0.00	0.00	0.00
其他的口咽	C10	3	0.54	0.99	0.95	0.04	0.09	0	0.00	0.00	0.00	0.00	0.00
鼻咽	C11	3	0.54	0.99	0.91	0.04	0.12	2	0.61	0.70	0.52	0.00	0.13
喉咽	C12-C13	1	0.18	0.33	0.31	0.00	0.08	0	0.00	0.00	0.00	0.00	0.00
咽，部位不明	C14	1	0.18	0.33	0.32	0.03	0.03	0	0.00	0.00	0.00	0.00	0.00
食管	C15	71	12.75	23.52	19.78	0.37	2.48	21	6.42	7.32	5.24	0.12	0.80
胃	C16	57	10.23	18.88	16.89	0.40	1.81	31	9.48	10.80	7.02	0.33	0.48
小肠	C17	2	0.36	0.66	0.59	0.04	0.09	2	0.61	0.70	0.38	0.00	0.00
结肠	C18	7	1.26	2.32	2.17	0.10	0.25	7	2.14	2.44	1.56	0.04	0.14
直肠	C19-C20	19	3.41	6.29	5.84	0.34	0.75	17	5.20	5.92	3.79	0.12	0.33
肛门	C21	1	0.18	0.33	0.31	0.00	0.08	0	0.00	0.00	0.00	0.00	0.00
肝脏	C22	72	12.93	23.85	21.58	1.12	2.78	17	5.20	5.92	4.06	0.12	0.33
胆囊及其他	C23-C24	2	0.36	0.66	0.50	0.00	0.08	2	0.61	0.70	0.52	0.00	0.05
胰腺	C25	15	2.69	4.97	4.16	0.11	0.44	13	3.98	4.53	2.77	0.08	0.13
鼻、鼻窦及其他	C30-C31	1	0.18	0.33	0.18	0.00	0.00	0	0.00	0.00	0.00	0.00	0.00
喉	C32	5	0.90	1.66	1.46	0.04	0.21	0	0.00	0.00	0.00	0.00	0.00
气管、支气管、肺	C33-C34	218	39.14	72.21	63.43	2.53	6.96	68	20.80	23.70	15.80	0.66	1.64
其他的胸腔器官	C37-C38	3	0.54	0.99	0.87	0.00	0.13	0	0.00	0.00	0.00	0.00	0.00
骨	C40-C41	1	0.18	0.33	0.27	0.00	0.00	4	1.22	1.39	0.85	0.03	0.09
皮肤的黑色素瘤	C43	0	0.00	0.00	0.00	0.00	0.00	0	0.00	0.00	0.00	0.00	0.00
其他的皮肤	C44	1	0.18	0.33	0.29	0.00	0.05	1	0.31	0.35	0.34	0.03	0.03
间皮瘤	C45	0	0.00	0.00	0.00	0.00	0.00	0	0.00	0.00	0.00	0.00	0.00
卡波西肉瘤	C46	0	0.00	0.00	0.00	0.00	0.00	0	0.00	0.00	0.00	0.00	0.00
周围神经、其他结缔组织、软组织	C47;C49	0	0.00	0.00	0.00	0.00	0.00	0	0.00	0.00	0.00	0.00	0.00
乳房	C50	0	0.00	0.00	0.00	0.00	0.00	35	10.70	12.20	9.49	0.56	1.02
外阴	C51	0	0.00	0.00	0.00	0.00	0.00	0	0.00	0.00	0.00	0.00	0.00
阴道	C52	0	0.00	0.00	0.00	0.00	0.00	1	0.31	0.35	0.34	0.04	0.04
子宫颈	C53	0	0.00	0.00	0.00	0.00	0.00	17	5.20	5.92	4.40	0.27	0.48
子宫体	C54	0	0.00	0.00	0.00	0.00	0.00	13	3.98	4.53	2.70	0.11	0.21
子宫，部位不明	C55	0	0.00	0.00	0.00	0.00	0.00	2	0.61	0.70	0.58	0.00	0.10
卵巢	C56	0	0.00	0.00	0.00	0.00	0.00	13	3.98	4.53	3.54	0.20	0.48
女性其他的生殖器	C57	0	0.00	0.00	0.00	0.00	0.00	0	0.00	0.00	0.00	0.00	0.00
胎盘	C58	0	0.00	0.00	0.00	0.00	0.00	0	0.00	0.00	0.00	0.00	0.00
阴茎	C60	1	0.18	0.33	0.29	0.00	0.05	0	0.00	0.00	0.00	0.00	0.00
前列腺	C61	1	0.18	0.33	0.31	0.00	0.08	0	0.00	0.00	0.00	0.00	0.00
睾丸	C62	1	0.18	0.33	0.29	0.02	0.02	0	0.00	0.00	0.00	0.00	0.00
男性其他的生殖器	C63	0	0.00	0.00	0.00	0.00	0.00	0	0.00	0.00	0.00	0.00	0.00
肾	C64	9	1.62	2.98	2.73	0.17	0.29	7	2.14	2.44	1.77	0.12	0.12
肾盂	C65	1	0.18	0.33	0.25	0.02	0.02	0	0.00	0.00	0.00	0.00	0.00
输尿管	C66	0	0.00	0.00	0.00	0.00	0.00	0	0.00	0.00	0.00	0.00	0.00
膀胱	C67	5	0.90	1.66	1.39	0.00	0.08	3	0.92	1.05	0.61	0.04	0.04
其他的泌尿器官	C68	0	0.00	0.00	0.00	0.00	0.00	1	0.31	0.35	0.14	0.00	0.00
眼	C69	2	0.36	0.66	0.63	0.00	0.05	0	0.00	0.00	0.00	0.00	0.00
脑、神经系统	C70-C72	24	4.31	7.95	7.29	0.51	0.51	15	4.59	5.23	4.14	0.19	0.40
甲状腺	C73	1	0.18	0.33	0.32	0.03	0.03	23	7.03	8.01	6.49	0.51	0.66
肾上腺	C74	2	0.36	0.66	0.61	0.06	0.06	0	0.00	0.00	0.00	0.00	0.00
其他的内分泌腺	C75	0	0.00	0.00	0.00	0.00	0.00	1	0.31	0.35	0.34	0.04	0.04
霍奇金病	C81	0	0.00	0.00	0.00	0.00	0.00	0	0.00	0.00	0.00	0.00	0.00
非霍奇金淋巴瘤	C82-C85;C96	1	0.18	0.33	0.31	0.00	0.08	1	0.31	0.35	0.13	0.00	0.00
免疫增生性疾病	C88	0	0.00	0.00	0.00	0.00	0.00	0	0.00	0.00	0.00	0.00	0.00
多发性骨髓瘤	C90	0	0.00	0.00	0.00	0.00	0.00	0	0.00	0.00	0.00	0.00	0.00
淋巴样白血病	C91	0	0.00	0.00	0.00	0.00	0.00	0	0.00	0.00	0.00	0.00	0.00
髓样白血病	C92-C94	0	0.00	0.00	0.00	0.00	0.00	0	0.00	0.00	0.00	0.00	0.00
白血病，未特指	C95	2	0.36	0.66	0.55	0.06	0.06	2	0.61	0.70	0.58	0.04	0.10
其他的或未指明部位	O&U	21	3.77	6.96	6.28	0.27	0.54	5	1.53	1.74	1.21	0.04	0.11
骨髓增殖性疾病	MPD	0	0.00	0.00	0.00	0.00	0.00	0	0.00	0.00	0.00	0.00	0.00
骨髓增生异常综合征	MDS	0	0.00	0.00	0.00	0.00	0.00	1	0.31	0.35	0.34	0.04	0.04
合计	ALL	557	100.00	184.51	163.07	6.38	18.36	327	100.00	113.95	79.90	3.74	8.00
C44 以外的部位	ALL but C44	556	99.82	184.18	162.79	6.38	18.31	326	99.69	113.60	79.56	3.71	7.97

表 6-73 2020 年河南省濮阳县恶性肿瘤发病主要指标

部位	ICD-10	男性						女性					
		病例数	构成 (%)	粗率 ($1/10^5$)	世标率 ($1/10^5$)	累积率 (%) 0~64	累积率 (%) 0~74	病例数	构成 (%)	粗率 ($1/10^5$)	世标率 ($1/10^5$)	累积率 (%) 0~64	累积率 (%) 0~74
唇	C00	5	0.28	0.87	0.77	0.05	0.09	2	0.11	0.35	0.36	0.01	0.01
舌	C01–C02	1	0.06	0.17	0.16	0.02	0.02	4	0.21	0.71	0.51	0.01	0.05
口	C03–C06	6	0.33	1.04	0.80	0.09	0.09	1	0.05	0.18	0.12	0.01	0.01
唾液腺	C07–C08	2	0.11	0.35	0.30	0.01	0.04	2	0.11	0.35	0.25	0.02	0.02
扁桃体	C09	1	0.06	0.17	0.25	0.01	0.01	2	0.11	0.35	0.52	0.02	0.02
其他的口咽	C10	3	0.17	0.52	0.50	0.00	0.03	0	0.00	0.00	0.00	0.00	0.00
鼻咽	C11	10	0.55	1.74	1.42	0.09	0.20	6	0.32	1.06	0.95	0.05	0.09
喉咽	C12–C13	2	0.11	0.35	0.34	0.02	0.02	0	0.00	0.00	0.00	0.00	0.00
咽，部位不明	C14	3	0.17	0.52	0.52	0.00	0.13	3	0.16	0.53	0.40	0.01	0.05
食管	C15	209	11.50	36.39	36.74	0.93	4.78	153	8.06	27.01	23.00	0.39	2.46
胃	C16	205	11.28	35.70	34.64	1.23	4.11	100	5.27	17.65	15.81	0.48	1.44
小肠	C17	7	0.39	1.22	1.22	0.06	0.06	6	0.32	1.06	0.82	0.03	0.10
结肠	C18	60	3.30	10.45	9.55	0.39	1.13	26	1.37	4.59	3.97	0.12	0.46
直肠	C19–C20	73	4.02	12.71	11.65	0.50	1.52	58	3.06	10.24	8.90	0.25	0.95
肛门	C21	1	0.06	0.17	0.16	0.02	0.02	0	0.00	0.00	0.00	0.00	0.00
肝脏	C22	219	12.05	38.13	33.47	1.90	4.09	99	5.22	17.48	15.82	0.53	1.50
胆囊及其他	C23–C24	17	0.94	2.96	3.21	0.11	0.34	27	1.42	4.77	4.01	0.09	0.38
胰腺	C25	32	1.76	5.57	5.68	0.15	0.61	19	1.00	3.35	2.73	0.05	0.30
鼻、鼻窦及其他	C30–C31	2	0.11	0.35	0.28	0.03	0.03	2	0.11	0.35	0.24	0.01	0.01
喉	C32	20	1.10	3.48	3.53	0.19	0.44	1	0.05	0.18	0.12	0.00	0.00
气管、支气管、肺	C33–C34	607	33.39	105.69	101.01	3.52	12.23	291	15.33	51.37	43.29	1.57	4.87
其他的胸腔器官	C37–C38	8	0.44	1.39	1.04	0.07	0.11	5	0.26	0.88	0.71	0.06	0.06
骨	C40–C41	16	0.88	2.79	2.53	0.14	0.17	17	0.90	3.00	2.39	0.17	0.25
皮肤的黑色素瘤	C43	0	0.00	0.00	0.00	0.00	0.00	3	0.16	0.53	0.57	0.00	0.05
其他的皮肤	C44	6	0.33	1.04	0.92	0.03	0.06	4	0.21	0.71	0.76	0.04	0.07
间皮瘤	C45	1	0.06	0.17	0.18	0.00	0.03	0	0.00	0.00	0.00	0.00	0.00
卡波西肉瘤	C46	0	0.00	0.00	0.00	0.00	0.00	0	0.00	0.00	0.00	0.00	0.00
周围神经、其他结缔组织、软组织	C47;C49	7	0.39	1.22	1.04	0.05	0.10	5	0.26	0.88	0.77	0.06	0.10
乳房	C50	3	0.17	0.52	0.47	0.01	0.09	326	17.18	57.54	43.28	3.44	4.54
外阴	C51	0	0.00	0.00	0.00	0.00	0.00	5	0.26	0.88	0.63	0.05	0.08
阴道	C52	0	0.00	0.00	0.00	0.00	0.00	4	0.21	0.71	0.63	0.02	0.08
子宫颈	C53	0	0.00	0.00	0.00	0.00	0.00	168	8.85	29.65	22.48	1.73	2.46
子宫体	C54	0	0.00	0.00	0.00	0.00	0.00	89	4.69	15.71	11.84	0.93	1.21
子宫，部位不明	C55	0	0.00	0.00	0.00	0.00	0.00	12	0.63	2.12	1.76	0.15	0.19
卵巢	C56	0	0.00	0.00	0.00	0.00	0.00	59	3.11	10.41	8.01	0.61	0.87
女性其他的生殖器	C57	0	0.00	0.00	0.00	0.00	0.00	2	0.11	0.35	0.27	0.02	0.02
胎盘	C58	0	0.00	0.00	0.00	0.00	0.00	0	0.00	0.00	0.00	0.00	0.00
阴茎	C60	4	0.22	0.70	0.63	0.03	0.11	0	0.00	0.00	0.00	0.00	0.00
前列腺	C61	40	2.20	6.97	7.46	0.11	0.96	0	0.00	0.00	0.00	0.00	0.00
睾丸	C62	3	0.17	0.52	0.37	0.02	0.02	0	0.00	0.00	0.00	0.00	0.00
男性其他的生殖器	C63	0	0.00	0.00	0.00	0.00	0.00	0	0.00	0.00	0.00	0.00	0.00
肾	C64	26	1.43	4.53	4.34	0.18	0.49	19	1.00	3.35	2.76	0.10	0.29
肾盂	C65	4	0.22	0.70	0.60	0.04	0.07	2	0.11	0.35	0.41	0.00	0.03
输尿管	C66	4	0.22	0.70	0.65	0.03	0.09	0	0.00	0.00	0.00	0.00	0.00
膀胱	C67	37	2.04	6.44	5.87	0.19	0.55	13	0.68	2.29	1.94	0.04	0.15
其他的泌尿器官	C68	1	0.06	0.17	0.17	0.00	0.04	0	0.00	0.00	0.00	0.00	0.00
眼	C69	1	0.06	0.17	0.11	0.01	0.01	1	0.05	0.18	0.12	0.01	0.01
脑、神经系统	C70–C72	45	2.48	7.84	7.25	0.28	0.84	41	2.16	7.24	7.40	0.37	0.55
甲状腺	C73	59	3.25	10.27	8.15	0.60	0.81	271	14.28	47.84	35.47	3.00	3.89
肾上腺	C74	4	0.22	0.70	0.46	0.05	0.05	2	0.11	0.35	0.25	0.03	0.03
其他的内分泌腺	C75	1	0.06	0.17	0.14	0.00	0.00	0	0.00	0.00	0.00	0.00	0.00
霍奇金病	C81	3	0.17	0.52	0.43	0.02	0.05	0	0.00	0.00	0.00	0.00	0.00
非霍奇金淋巴瘤	C82–C85;C96	9	0.50	1.57	1.65	0.08	0.19	9	0.47	1.59	1.29	0.05	0.21
免疫增生性疾病	C88	0	0.00	0.00	0.00	0.00	0.00	0	0.00	0.00	0.00	0.00	0.00
多发性骨髓瘤	C90	1	0.06	0.17	0.12	0.01	0.01	1	0.05	0.18	0.12	0.00	0.00
淋巴样白血病	C91	5	0.28	0.87	0.96	0.05	0.14	1	0.05	0.18	0.12	0.01	0.01
髓样白血病	C92–C94	2	0.11	0.35	0.30	0.01	0.04	2	0.11	0.35	0.28	0.01	0.04
白血病，未特指	C95	9	0.50	1.57	1.29	0.05	0.19	5	0.26	0.88	0.70	0.06	0.06
其他的或未指明部位	O&U	34	1.87	5.92	5.84	0.31	0.64	30	1.58	5.30	4.46	0.27	0.47
骨髓增殖性疾病	MPD	0	0.00	0.00	0.00	0.00	0.00	0	0.00	0.00	0.00	0.00	0.00
骨髓增生异常综合征	MDS	0	0.00	0.00	0.00	0.00	0.00	0	0.00	0.00	0.00	0.00	0.00
合计	ALL	1 818	100.00	316.56	299.20	11.72	35.85	1 898	100.00	335.03	271.23	14.88	28.41
C44 以外的部位	ALL but C44	1 812	99.67	315.52	298.28	11.69	35.79	1 894	99.79	334.32	270.46	14.84	28.35

表 6-74 2020 年河南省濮阳县恶性肿瘤死亡主要指标

部位	ICD-10	男性						女性					
		病例数	构成 (%)	粗率 (1/10^5)	世标率 (1/10^5)	累积率 (%)		病例数	构成 (%)	粗率 (1/10^5)	世标率 (1/10^5)	累积率 (%)	
						0~64	0~74					0~64	0~74
唇	C00	1	0.09	0.17	0.14	0.00	0.00	0	0.00	0.00	0.00	0.00	0.00
舌	C01–C02	0	0.00	0.00	0.00	0.00	0.00	0	0.00	0.00	0.00	0.00	0.00
口	C03–C06	1	0.09	0.17	0.18	0.00	0.03	0	0.00	0.00	0.00	0.00	0.00
唾液腺	C07–C08	0	0.00	0.00	0.00	0.00	0.00	0	0.00	0.00	0.00	0.00	0.00
扁桃体	C09	0	0.00	0.00	0.00	0.00	0.00	1	0.15	0.18	0.12	0.00	0.00
其他的口咽	C10	2	0.18	0.35	0.36	0.00	0.06	0	0.00	0.00	0.00	0.00	0.00
鼻咽	C11	3	0.28	0.52	0.47	0.03	0.07	2	0.29	0.35	0.38	0.01	0.01
喉咽	C12–C13	1	0.09	0.17	0.18	0.00	0.03	0	0.00	0.00	0.00	0.00	0.00
咽，部位不明	C14	0	0.00	0.00	0.00	0.00	0.00	1	0.15	0.18	0.16	0.00	0.03
食管	C15	131	12.04	22.81	23.82	0.33	2.73	130	19.09	22.95	20.29	0.36	1.82
胃	C16	125	11.49	21.77	22.56	0.46	2.64	62	9.10	10.94	10.01	0.25	1.02
小肠	C17	7	0.64	1.22	1.24	0.07	0.10	1	0.15	0.18	0.16	0.00	0.03
结肠	C18	24	2.21	4.18	4.82	0.08	0.36	13	1.91	2.29	2.08	0.02	0.16
直肠	C19–C20	28	2.57	4.88	4.82	0.08	0.81	16	2.35	2.82	2.66	0.03	0.28
肛门	C21	0	0.00	0.00	0.00	0.00	0.00	0	0.00	0.00	0.00	0.00	0.00
肝脏	C22	163	14.98	28.38	25.72	1.25	3.37	79	11.60	13.94	12.73	0.34	1.19
胆囊及其他	C23–C24	7	0.64	1.22	1.07	0.05	0.16	11	1.62	1.94	1.55	0.06	0.09
胰腺	C25	28	2.57	4.88	4.70	0.19	0.53	20	2.94	3.53	2.89	0.06	0.36
鼻、鼻窦及其他	C30–C31	1	0.09	0.17	0.41	0.00	0.00	2	0.29	0.35	0.24	0.01	0.01
喉	C32	15	1.38	2.61	3.19	0.08	0.25	1	0.15	0.18	0.12	0.00	0.00
气管、支气管、肺	C33–C34	441	40.53	76.79	78.83	1.93	8.74	176	25.84	31.07	27.35	0.53	2.47
其他的胸腔器官	C37–C38	2	0.18	0.35	0.32	0.00	0.04	0	0.00	0.00	0.00	0.00	0.00
骨	C40–C41	5	0.46	0.87	1.36	0.00	0.10	1	0.15	0.18	0.17	0.01	0.01
皮肤的黑色素瘤	C43	0	0.00	0.00	0.00	0.00	0.00	1	0.15	0.18	0.15	0.00	0.04
其他的皮肤	C44	2	0.18	0.35	0.59	0.00	0.03	2	0.29	0.35	0.23	0.01	0.01
间皮瘤	C45	1	0.09	0.17	0.18	0.00	0.03	0	0.00	0.00	0.00	0.00	0.00
卡波西肉瘤	C46	0	0.00	0.00	0.00	0.00	0.00	0	0.00	0.00	0.00	0.00	0.00
周围神经、其他结缔组织、软组织	C47;C49	1	0.09	0.17	0.41	0.00	0.00	0	0.00	0.00	0.00	0.00	0.00
乳房	C50	0	0.00	0.00	0.00	0.00	0.00	42	6.17	7.41	5.81	0.33	0.68
外阴	C51	0	0.00	0.00	0.00	0.00	0.00	1	0.15	0.18	0.24	0.00	0.00
阴道	C52	0	0.00	0.00	0.00	0.00	0.00	0	0.00	0.00	0.00	0.00	0.00
子宫颈	C53	0	0.00	0.00	0.00	0.00	0.00	22	3.23	3.88	3.05	0.19	0.41
子宫体	C54	0	0.00	0.00	0.00	0.00	0.00	13	1.91	2.29	1.94	0.06	0.14
子宫，部位不明	C55	0	0.00	0.00	0.00	0.00	0.00	5	0.73	0.88	0.81	0.04	0.08
卵巢	C56	0	0.00	0.00	0.00	0.00	0.00	18	2.64	3.18	2.42	0.15	0.28
女性其他的生殖器	C57	0	0.00	0.00	0.00	0.00	0.00	0	0.00	0.00	0.00	0.00	0.00
胎盘	C58	0	0.00	0.00	0.00	0.00	0.00	0	0.00	0.00	0.00	0.00	0.00
阴茎	C60	0	0.00	0.00	0.00	0.00	0.00	0	0.00	0.00	0.00	0.00	0.00
前列腺	C61	8	0.74	1.39	1.77	0.01	0.06	0	0.00	0.00	0.00	0.00	0.00
睾丸	C62	1	0.09	0.17	0.11	0.01	0.01	0	0.00	0.00	0.00	0.00	0.00
男性其他的生殖器	C63	0	0.00	0.00	0.00	0.00	0.00	0	0.00	0.00	0.00	0.00	0.00
肾	C64	9	0.83	1.57	1.45	0.03	0.19	6	0.88	1.06	0.89	0.01	0.13
肾盂	C65	0	0.00	0.00	0.00	0.00	0.00	1	0.15	0.18	0.24	0.00	0.00
输尿管	C66	4	0.37	0.70	0.71	0.02	0.11	0	0.00	0.00	0.00	0.00	0.00
膀胱	C67	15	1.38	2.61	3.04	0.04	0.28	4	0.59	0.71	0.64	0.00	0.03
其他的泌尿器官	C68	0	0.00	0.00	0.00	0.00	0.00	0	0.00	0.00	0.00	0.00	0.00
眼	C69	0	0.00	0.00	0.00	0.00	0.00	0	0.00	0.00	0.00	0.00	0.00
脑、神经系统	C70–C72	24	2.21	4.18	3.73	0.19	0.37	25	3.67	4.41	4.57	0.13	0.33
甲状腺	C73	5	0.46	0.87	0.82	0.01	0.17	8	1.17	1.41	1.14	0.06	0.13
肾上腺	C74	0	0.00	0.00	0.00	0.00	0.00	0	0.00	0.00	0.00	0.00	0.00
其他的内分泌腺	C75	1	0.09	0.17	0.14	0.00	0.00	0	0.00	0.00	0.00	0.00	0.00
霍奇金病	C81	0	0.00	0.00	0.00	0.00	0.00	1	0.15	0.18	0.11	0.01	0.01
非霍奇金淋巴瘤	C82–C85;C96	4	0.37	0.70	0.60	0.01	0.04	4	0.59	0.71	0.55	0.02	0.05
免疫增生性疾病	C88	0	0.00	0.00	0.00	0.00	0.00	0	0.00	0.00	0.00	0.00	0.00
多发性骨髓瘤	C90	1	0.09	0.17	0.16	0.02	0.02	0	0.00	0.00	0.00	0.00	0.00
淋巴样白血病	C91	3	0.28	0.52	0.75	0.05	0.05	0	0.00	0.00	0.00	0.00	0.00
髓样白血病	C92–C94	1	0.09	0.17	0.11	0.01	0.01	1	0.15	0.18	0.16	0.00	0.03
白血病，未特指	C95	10	0.92	1.74	1.57	0.09	0.20	2	0.29	0.35	0.30	0.00	0.08
其他的或未指明部位	O&U	13	1.19	2.26	2.32	0.08	0.33	9	1.32	1.59	1.57	0.05	0.13
骨髓增殖性疾病	MPD	0	0.00	0.00	0.00	0.00	0.00	0	0.00	0.00	0.00	0.00	0.00
骨髓增生异常综合征	MDS	0	0.00	0.00	0.00	0.00	0.00	0	0.00	0.00	0.00	0.00	0.00
合计	ALL	1 088	100.00	189.45	192.66	5.12	21.94	681	100.00	120.21	105.75	2.75	10.02
C44 以外的部位	ALL but C44	1 086	99.82	189.10	192.06	5.12	21.91	679	99.71	119.85	105.51	2.74	10.01

表 6-75　2020 年河南省许昌市城区恶性肿瘤发病主要指标

部位	ICD-10	男性						女性					
		病例数	构成 (%)	粗率 (1/10^5)	世标率 (1/10^5)	累积率 (%) 0~64	累积率 (%) 0~74	病例数	构成 (%)	粗率 (1/10^5)	世标率 (1/10^5)	累积率 (%) 0~64	累积率 (%) 0~74
唇	C00	0	0.00	0.00	0.00	0.00	0.00	1	0.15	0.60	0.33	0.00	0.05
舌	C01–C02	2	0.35	1.25	0.88	0.10	0.10	0	0.00	0.00	0.00	0.00	0.00
口	C03–C06	5	0.87	3.12	1.95	0.14	0.26	0	0.00	0.00	0.00	0.00	0.00
唾液腺	C07–C08	2	0.35	1.25	0.70	0.05	0.12	1	0.15	0.60	0.25	0.00	0.06
扁桃体	C09	1	0.17	0.62	0.41	0.05	0.05	0	0.00	0.00	0.00	0.00	0.00
其他的口咽	C10	0	0.00	0.00	0.00	0.00	0.00	0	0.00	0.00	0.00	0.00	0.00
鼻咽	C11	4	0.69	2.50	1.64	0.15	0.21	2	0.30	1.20	0.77	0.08	0.08
喉咽	C12–C13	3	0.52	1.87	0.69	0.00	0.06	0	0.00	0.00	0.00	0.00	0.00
咽，部位不明	C14	1	0.17	0.62	0.37	0.00	0.06	1	0.15	0.60	1.20	0.07	0.07
食管	C15	35	6.07	21.87	11.06	0.67	1.35	12	1.82	7.20	3.51	0.09	0.55
胃	C16	30	5.20	18.75	10.12	0.59	1.40	13	1.97	7.80	4.03	0.28	0.57
小肠	C17	2	0.35	1.25	0.58	0.03	0.03	2	0.30	1.20	0.72	0.04	0.09
结肠	C18	33	5.72	20.62	10.50	0.63	1.29	26	3.93	15.59	7.48	0.31	0.93
直肠	C19–C20	43	7.45	26.87	13.79	0.86	1.61	16	2.42	9.60	4.48	0.26	0.48
肛门	C21	1	0.17	0.62	0.38	0.03	0.03	1	0.15	0.60	0.25	0.00	0.06
肝脏	C22	50	8.67	31.24	18.99	1.49	2.21	28	4.24	16.79	9.00	0.52	1.09
胆囊及其他	C23–C24	8	1.39	5.00	1.79	0.05	0.12	22	3.33	13.20	5.39	0.18	0.71
胰腺	C25	13	2.25	8.12	4.14	0.26	0.39	14	2.12	8.40	4.46	0.32	0.38
鼻、鼻窦及其他	C30–C31	0	0.00	0.00	0.00	0.00	0.00	1	0.15	0.60	0.40	0.05	0.05
喉	C32	10	1.73	6.25	3.10	0.14	0.41	1	0.15	0.60	0.25	0.00	0.06
气管、支气管、肺	C33–C34	179	31.02	111.85	56.38	2.81	7.35	94	14.22	56.38	27.15	1.67	3.19
其他的胸腔器官	C37–C38	0	0.00	0.00	0.00	0.00	0.00	1	0.15	0.60	0.25	0.00	0.06
骨	C40–C41	3	0.52	1.87	1.09	0.05	0.19	1	0.15	0.60	0.25	0.00	0.06
皮肤的黑色素瘤	C43	0	0.00	0.00	0.00	0.00	0.00	1	0.15	0.60	0.25	0.00	0.06
其他的皮肤	C44	3	0.52	1.87	0.96	0.09	0.09	2	0.30	1.20	1.43	0.06	0.06
间皮瘤	C45	0	0.00	0.00	0.00	0.00	0.00	0	0.00	0.00	0.00	0.00	0.00
卡波西肉瘤	C46	0	0.00	0.00	0.00	0.00	0.00	0	0.00	0.00	0.00	0.00	0.00
周围神经、其他结缔组织、软组织	C47;C49	2	0.35	1.25	0.57	0.05	0.05	1	0.15	0.60	0.16	0.00	0.00
乳房	C50	2	0.35	1.25	0.87	0.09	0.09	174	26.32	104.37	64.52	5.49	7.04
外阴	C51	0	0.00	0.00	0.00	0.00	0.00	1	0.15	0.60	0.11	0.00	0.00
阴道	C52	0	0.00	0.00	0.00	0.00	0.00	0	0.00	0.00	0.00	0.00	0.00
子宫颈	C53	0	0.00	0.00	0.00	0.00	0.00	36	5.45	21.59	12.66	1.12	1.35
子宫体	C54	0	0.00	0.00	0.00	0.00	0.00	18	2.72	10.80	6.50	0.54	0.70
子宫，部位不明	C55	0	0.00	0.00	0.00	0.00	0.00	7	1.06	4.20	2.28	0.15	0.26
卵巢	C56	0	0.00	0.00	0.00	0.00	0.00	21	3.18	12.60	7.18	0.63	0.82
女性其他的生殖器	C57	0	0.00	0.00	0.00	0.00	0.00	1	0.15	0.60	0.11	0.00	0.00
胎盘	C58	0	0.00	0.00	0.00	0.00	0.00	0	0.00	0.00	0.00	0.00	0.00
阴茎	C60	1	0.17	0.62	0.38	0.03	0.03	0	0.00	0.00	0.00	0.00	0.00
前列腺	C61	27	4.68	16.87	6.97	0.22	0.69	0	0.00	0.00	0.00	0.00	0.00
睾丸	C62	0	0.00	0.00	0.00	0.00	0.00	0	0.00	0.00	0.00	0.00	0.00
男性其他的生殖器	C63	0	0.00	0.00	0.00	0.00	0.00	0	0.00	0.00	0.00	0.00	0.00
肾	C64	10	1.73	6.25	3.28	0.27	0.34	3	0.45	1.80	0.69	0.03	0.03
肾盂	C65	1	0.17	0.62	0.19	0.00	0.00	0	0.00	0.00	0.00	0.00	0.00
输尿管	C66	1	0.17	0.62	0.41	0.05	0.05	0	0.00	0.00	0.00	0.00	0.00
膀胱	C67	21	3.64	13.12	5.92	0.16	0.92	6	0.91	3.60	1.86	0.12	0.24
其他的泌尿器官	C68	0	0.00	0.00	0.00	0.00	0.00	0	0.00	0.00	0.00	0.00	0.00
眼	C69	0	0.00	0.00	0.00	0.00	0.00	0	0.00	0.00	0.00	0.00	0.00
脑、神经系统	C70–C72	8	1.39	5.00	2.90	0.19	0.39	2	0.30	1.20	0.31	0.00	0.00
甲状腺	C73	37	6.41	23.12	18.00	1.61	1.75	116	17.55	69.58	46.81	4.26	4.80
肾上腺	C74	1	0.17	0.62	0.73	0.06	0.06	4	0.61	2.40	1.39	0.09	0.09
其他的内分泌腺	C75	0	0.00	0.00	0.00	0.00	0.00	0	0.00	0.00	0.00	0.00	0.00
霍奇金病	C81	1	0.17	0.62	0.91	0.06	0.06	1	0.15	0.60	0.42	0.04	0.04
非霍奇金淋巴瘤	C82–C85;C96	6	1.04	3.75	2.07	0.09	0.27	3	0.45	1.80	0.87	0.04	0.09
免疫增生性疾病	C88	0	0.00	0.00	0.00	0.00	0.00	0	0.00	0.00	0.00	0.00	0.00
多发性骨髓瘤	C90	5	0.87	3.12	1.93	0.15	0.28	2	0.30	1.20	0.27	0.00	0.00
淋巴样白血病	C91	3	0.52	1.87	2.77	0.12	0.12	2	0.30	1.20	1.42	0.11	0.11
髓样白血病	C92–C94	6	1.04	3.75	1.91	0.10	0.23	5	0.76	3.00	1.77	0.12	0.23
白血病，未特指	C95	2	0.35	1.25	1.60	0.06	0.06	2	0.30	1.20	0.78	0.06	0.06
其他的或未指明部位	O&U	10	1.73	6.25	3.83	0.10	0.57	13	1.97	7.80	4.28	0.28	0.45
骨髓增殖性疾病	MPD	5	0.87	3.12	1.89	0.11	0.30	3	0.45	1.80	0.87	0.04	0.10
骨髓增生异常综合征	MDS	0	0.00	0.00	0.00	0.00	0.00	0	0.00	0.00	0.00	0.00	0.00
合计	ALL	577	100.00	360.53	196.64	11.71	23.59	661	100.00	396.47	227.09	17.06	25.08
C44 以外的部位	ALL but C44	574	99.48	358.66	195.67	11.62	23.50	659	99.70	395.27	225.65	16.99	25.02

表 6-76 2020 年河南省许昌市城区恶性肿瘤死亡主要指标

部位	ICD-10	男性						女性					
		病例数	构成 (%)	粗率 ($1/10^5$)	世标率 ($1/10^5$)	累积率 (%)		病例数	构成 (%)	粗率 ($1/10^5$)	世标率 ($1/10^5$)	累积率 (%)	
						0~64	0~74					0~64	0~74
唇	C00	0	0.00	0.00	0.00	0.00	0.00	0	0.00	0.00	0.00	0.00	0.00
舌	C01–C02	1	0.35	0.62	0.37	0.00	0.06	0	0.00	0.00	0.00	0.00	0.00
口	C03–C06	1	0.35	0.62	0.14	0.00	0.00	1	0.49	0.60	0.11	0.00	0.00
唾液腺	C07–C08	0	0.00	0.00	0.00	0.00	0.00	0	0.00	0.00	0.00	0.00	0.00
扁桃体	C09	0	0.00	0.00	0.00	0.00	0.00	0	0.00	0.00	0.00	0.00	0.00
其他的口咽	C10	0	0.00	0.00	0.00	0.00	0.00	0	0.00	0.00	0.00	0.00	0.00
鼻咽	C11	4	1.38	2.50	1.55	0.15	0.15	0	0.00	0.00	0.00	0.00	0.00
喉咽	C12–C13	1	0.35	0.62	0.25	0.00	0.00	0	0.00	0.00	0.00	0.00	0.00
咽，部位不明	C14	1	0.35	0.62	0.29	0.00	0.07	1	0.49	0.60	1.20	0.07	0.07
食管	C15	25	8.65	15.62	7.75	0.34	1.01	11	5.34	6.60	2.39	0.04	0.14
胃	C16	14	4.84	8.75	4.38	0.21	0.55	8	3.88	4.80	1.85	0.10	0.10
小肠	C17	1	0.35	0.62	0.45	0.04	0.04	2	0.97	1.20	0.51	0.00	0.05
结肠	C18	10	3.46	6.25	2.95	0.11	0.38	17	8.25	10.20	3.97	0.18	0.36
直肠	C19–C20	8	2.77	5.00	1.78	0.00	0.06	5	2.43	3.00	1.11	0.03	0.09
肛门	C21	0	0.00	0.00	0.00	0.00	0.00	0	0.00	0.00	0.00	0.00	0.00
肝脏	C22	31	10.73	19.37	11.10	0.76	1.36	11	5.34	6.60	3.19	0.10	0.35
胆囊及其他	C23–C24	7	2.42	4.37	1.50	0.05	0.05	13	6.31	7.80	2.55	0.05	0.23
胰腺	C25	15	5.19	9.37	4.62	0.30	0.57	15	7.28	9.00	4.01	0.31	0.36
鼻、鼻窦及其他	C30–C31	1	0.35	0.62	0.19	0.00	0.00	0	0.00	0.00	0.00	0.00	0.00
喉	C32	2	0.69	1.25	0.28	0.00	0.00	0	0.00	0.00	0.00	0.00	0.00
气管、支气管、肺	C33–C34	110	38.06	68.73	31.60	1.11	3.84	44	21.36	26.39	10.02	0.21	1.03
其他的胸腔器官	C37–C38	3	1.04	1.87	1.22	0.09	0.15	0	0.00	0.00	0.00	0.00	0.00
骨	C40–C41	1	0.35	0.62	0.43	0.05	0.05	0	0.00	0.00	0.00	0.00	0.00
皮肤的黑色素瘤	C43	0	0.00	0.00	0.00	0.00	0.00	0	0.00	0.00	0.00	0.00	0.00
其他的皮肤	C44	1	0.35	0.62	0.14	0.00	0.00	0	0.00	0.00	0.00	0.00	0.00
间皮瘤	C45	0	0.00	0.00	0.00	0.00	0.00	0	0.00	0.00	0.00	0.00	0.00
卡波西肉瘤	C46	0	0.00	0.00	0.00	0.00	0.00	0	0.00	0.00	0.00	0.00	0.00
周围神经、其他结缔组织、软组织	C47;C49	1	0.35	0.62	0.43	0.05	0.05	0	0.00	0.00	0.00	0.00	0.00
乳房	C50	1	0.35	0.62	0.41	0.05	0.05	24	11.65	14.40	7.42	0.62	0.74
外阴	C51	0	0.00	0.00	0.00	0.00	0.00	1	0.49	0.60	0.18	0.00	0.00
阴道	C52	0	0.00	0.00	0.00	0.00	0.00	0	0.00	0.00	0.00	0.00	0.00
子宫颈	C53	0	0.00	0.00	0.00	0.00	0.00	11	5.34	6.60	3.77	0.33	0.44
子宫体	C54	0	0.00	0.00	0.00	0.00	0.00	1	0.49	0.60	0.40	0.05	0.05
子宫，部位不明	C55	0	0.00	0.00	0.00	0.00	0.00	0	0.00	0.00	0.00	0.00	0.00
卵巢	C56	0	0.00	0.00	0.00	0.00	0.00	12	5.83	7.20	3.58	0.26	0.38
女性其他的生殖器	C57	0	0.00	0.00	0.00	0.00	0.00	0	0.00	0.00	0.00	0.00	0.00
胎盘	C58	0	0.00	0.00	0.00	0.00	0.00	0	0.00	0.00	0.00	0.00	0.00
阴茎	C60	0	0.00	0.00	0.00	0.00	0.00	0	0.00	0.00	0.00	0.00	0.00
前列腺	C61	5	1.73	3.12	1.02	0.00	0.00	0	0.00	0.00	0.00	0.00	0.00
睾丸	C62	1	0.35	0.62	0.39	0.03	0.03	0	0.00	0.00	0.00	0.00	0.00
男性其他的生殖器	C63	0	0.00	0.00	0.00	0.00	0.00	0	0.00	0.00	0.00	0.00	0.00
肾	C64	1	0.35	0.62	0.19	0.00	0.00	0	0.00	0.00	0.00	0.00	0.00
肾盂	C65	0	0.00	0.00	0.00	0.00	0.00	0	0.00	0.00	0.00	0.00	0.00
输尿管	C66	1	0.35	0.62	0.37	0.00	0.06	0	0.00	0.00	0.00	0.00	0.00
膀胱	C67	6	2.08	3.75	1.36	0.00	0.07	2	0.97	1.20	0.22	0.00	0.00
其他的泌尿器官	C68	0	0.00	0.00	0.00	0.00	0.00	0	0.00	0.00	0.00	0.00	0.00
眼	C69	0	0.00	0.00	0.00	0.00	0.00	0	0.00	0.00	0.00	0.00	0.00
脑、神经系统	C70–C72	3	1.04	1.87	0.84	0.05	0.12	2	0.97	1.20	0.31	0.00	0.00
甲状腺	C73	2	0.69	1.25	0.54	0.00	0.07	3	1.46	1.80	0.38	0.00	0.00
肾上腺	C74	0	0.00	0.00	0.00	0.00	0.00	1	0.49	0.60	0.18	0.00	0.00
其他的内分泌腺	C75	0	0.00	0.00	0.00	0.00	0.00	0	0.00	0.00	0.00	0.00	0.00
霍奇金病	C81	0	0.00	0.00	0.00	0.00	0.00	0	0.00	0.00	0.00	0.00	0.00
非霍奇金淋巴瘤	C82–C85;C96	5	1.73	3.12	1.41	0.03	0.16	3	1.46	1.80	0.88	0.03	0.16
免疫增生性疾病	C88	0	0.00	0.00	0.00	0.00	0.00	0	0.00	0.00	0.00	0.00	0.00
多发性骨髓瘤	C90	4	1.38	2.50	1.27	0.05	0.19	1	0.49	0.60	0.11	0.00	0.00
淋巴样白血病	C91	2	0.69	1.25	0.69	0.04	0.04	0	0.00	0.00	0.00	0.00	0.00
髓样白血病	C92–C94	3	1.04	1.87	0.84	0.05	0.12	1	0.49	0.60	0.33	0.00	0.05
白血病，未特指	C95	2	0.69	1.25	1.86	0.09	0.09	1	0.49	0.60	0.38	0.03	0.03
其他的或未指明部位	O&U	13	4.50	8.12	4.96	0.21	0.67	12	5.83	7.20	2.85	0.13	0.31
骨髓增殖性疾病	MPD	0	0.00	0.00	0.00	0.00	0.00	2	0.97	1.20	0.51	0.00	0.05
骨髓增生异常综合征	MDS	2	0.69	1.25	0.78	0.05	0.11	1	0.49	0.60	0.16	0.00	0.00
合计	ALL	289	100.00	180.58	88.34	3.94	10.21	206	100.00	123.56	52.57	2.52	5.00
C44 以外的部位	ALL but C44	288	99.65	179.95	88.20	3.94	10.21	206	100.00	123.56	52.57	2.52	5.00

表 6-77　2020 年河南省禹州市恶性肿瘤发病主要指标

部位	ICD-10	男性						女性					
		病例数	构成 (%)	粗率 ($1/10^5$)	世标率 ($1/10^5$)	累积率 (%) 0~64	累积率 (%) 0~74	病例数	构成 (%)	粗率 ($1/10^5$)	世标率 ($1/10^5$)	累积率 (%) 0~64	累积率 (%) 0~74
唇	C00	0	0.00	0.00	0.00	0.00	0.00	0	0.00	0.00	0.00	0.00	0.00
舌	C01–C02	4	0.21	0.57	0.48	0.02	0.05	0	0.00	0.00	0.00	0.00	0.00
口	C03–C06	3	0.16	0.43	0.41	0.03	0.03	3	0.18	0.47	0.28	0.00	0.00
唾液腺	C07–C08	2	0.10	0.29	0.29	0.03	0.03	4	0.24	0.63	0.55	0.06	0.06
扁桃体	C09	0	0.00	0.00	0.00	0.00	0.00	0	0.00	0.00	0.00	0.00	0.00
其他的口咽	C10	0	0.00	0.00	0.00	0.00	0.00	0	0.00	0.00	0.00	0.00	0.00
鼻咽	C11	3	0.16	0.43	0.36	0.02	0.02	1	0.06	0.16	0.19	0.02	0.02
喉咽	C12–C13	1	0.05	0.14	0.14	0.00	0.03	0	0.00	0.00	0.00	0.00	0.00
咽，部位不明	C14	3	0.16	0.43	0.45	0.04	0.06	0	0.00	0.00	0.00	0.00	0.00
食管	C15	133	6.90	19.01	21.27	0.45	1.89	57	3.48	8.95	6.83	0.13	0.63
胃	C16	177	9.18	25.30	28.24	0.70	2.42	115	7.03	18.06	14.00	0.31	1.32
小肠	C17	5	0.26	0.71	0.64	0.03	0.03	4	0.24	0.63	0.61	0.06	0.06
结肠	C18	53	2.75	7.57	7.12	0.38	0.88	43	2.63	6.75	5.88	0.28	0.67
直肠	C19–C20	73	3.79	10.43	10.98	0.38	1.25	52	3.18	8.16	6.95	0.29	0.90
肛门	C21	1	0.05	0.14	0.12	0.01	0.01	3	0.18	0.47	0.40	0.00	0.03
肝脏	C22	281	14.57	40.16	42.06	1.94	4.80	168	10.27	26.38	22.26	0.85	2.56
胆囊及其他	C23–C24	13	0.67	1.86	2.02	0.07	0.20	27	1.65	4.24	3.53	0.11	0.40
胰腺	C25	22	1.14	3.14	3.58	0.15	0.41	20	1.22	3.14	2.91	0.13	0.40
鼻、鼻窦及其他	C30–C31	1	0.05	0.14	0.15	0.02	0.02	2	0.12	0.31	0.33	0.04	0.04
喉	C32	17	0.88	2.43	2.32	0.10	0.33	1	0.06	0.16	0.19	0.02	0.02
气管、支气管、肺	C33–C34	783	40.61	111.90	119.46	3.67	12.67	318	19.44	49.93	41.94	1.94	4.51
其他的胸腔器官	C37–C38	4	0.21	0.57	0.54	0.02	0.02	2	0.12	0.31	0.28	0.00	0.06
骨	C40–C41	27	1.40	3.86	4.39	0.24	0.45	21	1.28	3.30	2.53	0.12	0.26
皮肤的黑色素瘤	C43	1	0.05	0.14	0.17	0.02	0.02	0	0.00	0.00	0.00	0.00	0.00
其他的皮肤	C44	21	1.09	3.00	2.98	0.07	0.31	15	0.92	2.36	1.80	0.05	0.15
间皮瘤	C45	0	0.00	0.00	0.00	0.00	0.00	0	0.00	0.00	0.00	0.00	0.00
卡波西肉瘤	C46	0	0.00	0.00	0.00	0.00	0.00	0	0.00	0.00	0.00	0.00	0.00
周围神经、其他结缔组织、软组织	C47;C49	1	0.05	0.14	0.12	0.00	0.00	1	0.06	0.16	0.13	0.00	0.00
乳房	C50	8	0.41	1.14	1.11	0.07	0.14	294	17.97	46.16	42.78	3.48	4.71
外阴	C51	0	0.00	0.00	0.00	0.00	0.00	3	0.18	0.47	0.41	0.01	0.07
阴道	C52	0	0.00	0.00	0.00	0.00	0.00	3	0.18	0.47	0.41	0.02	0.05
子宫颈	C53	0	0.00	0.00	0.00	0.00	0.00	138	8.44	21.67	19.73	1.47	2.15
子宫体	C54	0	0.00	0.00	0.00	0.00	0.00	54	3.30	8.48	8.14	0.68	1.03
子宫，部位不明	C55	0	0.00	0.00	0.00	0.00	0.00	15	0.92	2.36	2.26	0.17	0.23
卵巢	C56	0	0.00	0.00	0.00	0.00	0.00	29	1.77	4.55	4.17	0.36	0.47
女性其他的生殖器	C57	0	0.00	0.00	0.00	0.00	0.00	2	0.12	0.31	0.37	0.04	0.04
胎盘	C58	0	0.00	0.00	0.00	0.00	0.00	0	0.00	0.00	0.00	0.00	0.00
阴茎	C60	4	0.21	0.57	0.54	0.03	0.03	0	0.00	0.00	0.00	0.00	0.00
前列腺	C61	59	3.06	8.43	9.50	0.09	0.72	0	0.00	0.00	0.00	0.00	0.00
睾丸	C62	0	0.00	0.00	0.00	0.00	0.00	0	0.00	0.00	0.00	0.00	0.00
男性其他的生殖器	C63	0	0.00	0.00	0.00	0.00	0.00	0	0.00	0.00	0.00	0.00	0.00
肾	C64	19	0.99	2.72	2.49	0.13	0.29	11	0.67	1.73	1.47	0.07	0.19
肾盂	C65	1	0.05	0.14	0.14	0.00	0.02	1	0.06	0.16	0.09	0.00	0.00
输尿管	C66	1	0.05	0.14	0.14	0.00	0.03	2	0.12	0.31	0.27	0.02	0.02
膀胱	C67	69	3.58	9.86	10.18	0.33	1.18	14	0.86	2.20	1.90	0.08	0.24
其他的泌尿器官	C68	0	0.00	0.00	0.00	0.00	0.00	0	0.00	0.00	0.00	0.00	0.00
眼	C69	0	0.00	0.00	0.00	0.00	0.00	0	0.00	0.00	0.00	0.00	0.00
脑、神经系统	C70–C72	43	2.23	6.15	6.02	0.30	0.81	41	2.51	6.44	5.77	0.26	0.64
甲状腺	C73	30	1.56	4.29	4.03	0.24	0.45	113	6.91	17.74	15.92	1.36	1.64
肾上腺	C74	2	0.10	0.29	0.25	0.00	0.02	1	0.06	0.16	0.13	0.00	0.03
其他的内分泌腺	C75	0	0.00	0.00	0.00	0.00	0.00	0	0.00	0.00	0.00	0.00	0.00
霍奇金病	C81	2	0.10	0.29	0.24	0.02	0.02	0	0.00	0.00	0.00	0.00	0.00
非霍奇金淋巴瘤	C82–C85;C96	11	0.57	1.57	1.45	0.05	0.20	5	0.31	0.79	0.83	0.08	0.08
免疫增生性疾病	C88	0	0.00	0.00	0.00	0.00	0.00	0	0.00	0.00	0.00	0.00	0.00
多发性骨髓瘤	C90	3	0.16	0.43	0.37	0.00	0.03	1	0.06	0.16	0.14	0.01	0.01
淋巴样白血病	C91	1	0.05	0.14	0.20	0.01	0.01	2	0.12	0.31	0.49	0.02	0.02
髓样白血病	C92–C94	1	0.05	0.14	0.17	0.02	0.02	2	0.12	0.31	0.44	0.02	0.02
白血病，未特指	C95	9	0.47	1.29	1.35	0.07	0.16	7	0.43	1.10	0.86	0.03	0.08
其他的或未指明部位	O&U	35	1.82	5.00	4.85	0.28	0.50	39	2.38	6.12	5.19	0.23	0.58
骨髓增殖性疾病	MPD	1	0.05	0.14	0.15	0.02	0.02	2	0.12	0.31	0.32	0.02	0.02
骨髓增生异常综合征	MDS	0	0.00	0.00	0.00	0.00	0.00	0	0.00	0.00	0.00	0.00	0.00
合计	ALL	1 928	100.00	275.54	291.46	10.10	30.63	1 636	100.00	256.88	223.66	12.86	24.45
C44 以外的部位	ALL but C44	1 907	98.91	272.54	288.48	10.02	30.33	1 621	99.08	254.53	221.86	12.81	24.30

表 6-78 2020 年河南省禹州市恶性肿瘤死亡主要指标

部位	ICD-10	男性						女性					
		病例数	构成(%)	粗率(1/10^5)	世标率(1/10^5)	累积率(%)		病例数	构成(%)	粗率(1/10^5)	世标率(1/10^5)	累积率(%)	
						0~64	0~74					0~64	0~74
唇	C00	1	0.07	0.14	0.17	0.02	0.02	0	0.00	0.00	0.00	0.00	0.00
舌	C01–C02	1	0.07	0.14	0.13	0.00	0.00	0	0.00	0.00	0.00	0.00	0.00
口	C03–C06	0	0.00	0.00	0.00	0.00	0.00	1	0.12	0.16	0.08	0.00	0.00
唾液腺	C07–C08	0	0.00	0.00	0.00	0.00	0.00	0	0.00	0.00	0.00	0.00	0.00
扁桃体	C09	0	0.00	0.00	0.00	0.00	0.00	0	0.00	0.00	0.00	0.00	0.00
其他的口咽	C10	0	0.00	0.00	0.00	0.00	0.00	0	0.00	0.00	0.00	0.00	0.00
鼻咽	C11	2	0.14	0.29	0.25	0.00	0.00	1	0.12	0.16	0.08	0.00	0.00
喉咽	C12–C13	2	0.14	0.29	0.25	0.00	0.03	0	0.00	0.00	0.00	0.00	0.00
咽，部位不明	C14	1	0.07	0.14	0.08	0.01	0.01	1	0.12	0.16	0.09	0.00	0.00
食管	C15	108	7.54	15.43	18.13	0.31	1.38	39	4.57	6.12	4.69	0.12	0.29
胃	C16	128	8.93	18.29	20.81	0.38	1.60	86	10.08	13.50	9.94	0.14	0.79
小肠	C17	5	0.35	0.71	0.69	0.05	0.05	4	0.47	0.63	0.59	0.04	0.10
结肠	C18	19	1.33	2.72	2.59	0.06	0.30	22	2.58	3.45	2.54	0.05	0.23
直肠	C19–C20	27	1.88	3.86	4.26	0.13	0.44	27	3.17	4.24	3.34	0.12	0.35
肛门	C21	1	0.07	0.14	0.12	0.01	0.01	1	0.12	0.16	0.13	0.00	0.03
肝脏	C22	249	17.38	35.59	38.33	1.38	3.83	155	18.17	24.34	19.78	0.58	1.97
胆囊及其他	C23–C24	10	0.70	1.43	1.60	0.04	0.18	19	2.23	2.98	2.39	0.06	0.31
胰腺	C25	20	1.40	2.86	3.34	0.16	0.38	13	1.52	2.04	1.81	0.07	0.26
鼻、鼻窦及其他	C30–C31	3	0.21	0.43	0.40	0.04	0.04	1	0.12	0.16	0.18	0.02	0.02
喉	C32	1	0.07	0.14	0.12	0.00	0.00	0	0.00	0.00	0.00	0.00	0.00
气管、支气管、肺	C33–C34	671	46.82	95.90	103.88	2.66	10.48	242	28.37	38.00	30.62	1.02	3.21
其他的胸腔器官	C37–C38	2	0.14	0.29	0.33	0.03	0.03	2	0.23	0.31	0.28	0.00	0.06
骨	C40–C41	19	1.33	2.72	2.72	0.15	0.23	13	1.52	2.04	1.64	0.07	0.19
皮肤的黑色素瘤	C43	1	0.07	0.14	0.12	0.01	0.01	0	0.00	0.00	0.00	0.00	0.00
其他的皮肤	C44	9	0.63	1.29	1.35	0.00	0.06	8	0.94	1.26	1.03	0.06	0.06
间皮瘤	C45	0	0.00	0.00	0.00	0.00	0.00	0	0.00	0.00	0.00	0.00	0.00
卡波西肉瘤	C46	0	0.00	0.00	0.00	0.00	0.00	0	0.00	0.00	0.00	0.00	0.00
周围神经、其他结缔组织、软组织	C47;C49	0	0.00	0.00	0.00	0.00	0.00	0	0.00	0.00	0.00	0.00	0.00
乳房	C50	3	0.21	0.43	0.45	0.04	0.07	49	5.74	7.69	6.80	0.43	0.92
外阴	C51	0	0.00	0.00	0.00	0.00	0.00	1	0.12	0.16	0.13	0.00	0.03
阴道	C52	0	0.00	0.00	0.00	0.00	0.00	2	0.23	0.31	0.16	0.00	0.00
子宫颈	C53	0	0.00	0.00	0.00	0.00	0.00	44	5.16	6.91	5.67	0.31	0.63
子宫体	C54	0	0.00	0.00	0.00	0.00	0.00	27	3.17	4.24	3.63	0.22	0.39
子宫，部位不明	C55	0	0.00	0.00	0.00	0.00	0.00	4	0.47	0.63	0.48	0.02	0.02
卵巢	C56	0	0.00	0.00	0.00	0.00	0.00	10	1.17	1.57	1.51	0.12	0.19
女性其他的生殖器	C57	0	0.00	0.00	0.00	0.00	0.00	0	0.00	0.00	0.00	0.00	0.00
胎盘	C58	0	0.00	0.00	0.00	0.00	0.00	0	0.00	0.00	0.00	0.00	0.00
阴茎	C60	1	0.07	0.14	0.13	0.00	0.00	0	0.00	0.00	0.00	0.00	0.00
前列腺	C61	23	1.61	3.29	3.67	0.00	0.24	0	0.00	0.00	0.00	0.00	0.00
睾丸	C62	0	0.00	0.00	0.00	0.00	0.00	0	0.00	0.00	0.00	0.00	0.00
男性其他的生殖器	C63	0	0.00	0.00	0.00	0.00	0.00	0	0.00	0.00	0.00	0.00	0.00
肾	C64	9	0.63	1.29	1.19	0.06	0.12	9	1.06	1.41	1.14	0.03	0.16
肾盂	C65	3	0.21	0.43	0.47	0.04	0.06	0	0.00	0.00	0.00	0.00	0.00
输尿管	C66	2	0.14	0.29	0.28	0.00	0.07	1	0.12	0.16	0.09	0.00	0.00
膀胱	C67	32	2.23	4.57	4.90	0.11	0.34	4	0.47	0.63	0.54	0.02	0.06
其他的泌尿器官	C68	0	0.00	0.00	0.00	0.00	0.00	0	0.00	0.00	0.00	0.00	0.00
眼	C69	0	0.00	0.00	0.00	0.00	0.00	0	0.00	0.00	0.00	0.00	0.00
脑、神经系统	C70–C72	33	2.30	4.72	4.51	0.21	0.72	33	3.87	5.18	4.81	0.26	0.51
甲状腺	C73	1	0.07	0.14	0.14	0.00	0.03	4	0.47	0.63	0.59	0.05	0.08
肾上腺	C74	1	0.07	0.14	0.12	0.00	0.00	2	0.23	0.31	0.22	0.01	0.01
其他的内分泌腺	C75	0	0.00	0.00	0.00	0.00	0.00	0	0.00	0.00	0.00	0.00	0.00
霍奇金病	C81	1	0.07	0.14	0.12	0.01	0.01	0	0.00	0.00	0.00	0.00	0.00
非霍奇金淋巴瘤	C82–C85;C96	8	0.56	1.14	1.04	0.03	0.12	6	0.70	0.94	0.69	0.01	0.04
免疫增生性疾病	C88	0	0.00	0.00	0.00	0.00	0.00	0	0.00	0.00	0.00	0.00	0.00
多发性骨髓瘤	C90	4	0.28	0.57	0.49	0.00	0.03	0	0.00	0.00	0.00	0.00	0.00
淋巴样白血病	C91	0	0.00	0.00	0.00	0.00	0.00	1	0.12	0.16	0.19	0.02	0.02
髓样白血病	C92–C94	1	0.07	0.14	0.17	0.02	0.02	1	0.12	0.16	0.21	0.01	0.01
白血病，未特指	C95	4	0.28	0.57	0.61	0.01	0.08	3	0.35	0.47	0.36	0.00	0.05
其他的或未指明部位	O&U	26	1.81	3.72	3.52	0.17	0.40	15	1.76	2.36	1.91	0.09	0.18
骨髓增殖性疾病	MPD	0	0.00	0.00	0.00	0.00	0.00	1	0.12	0.16	0.13	0.00	0.00
骨髓增生异常综合征	MDS	1	0.07	0.14	0.15	0.02	0.02	1	0.12	0.16	0.15	0.01	0.01
合计	ALL	1 433	100.00	204.80	221.62	6.18	21.44	853	100.00	133.94	108.62	3.98	11.19
C44 以外的部位	ALL but C44	1 424	99.37	203.51	220.28	6.18	21.38	845	99.06	132.68	107.59	3.92	11.13

表 6-79　2020 年河南省漯河市城区恶性肿瘤发病主要指标

部位	ICD-10	男性						女性					
		病例数	构成 (%)	粗率 (1/10^5)	世标率 (1/10^5)	累积率 (%)		病例数	构成 (%)	粗率 (1/10^5)	世标率 (1/10^5)	累积率 (%)	
						0~64	0~74					0~64	0~74
唇	C00	5	0.23	0.71	0.60	0.00	0.09	2	0.10	0.30	0.25	0.02	0.05
舌	C01–C02	10	0.47	1.42	1.20	0.07	0.16	7	0.36	1.04	0.76	0.05	0.08
口	C03–C06	11	0.51	1.56	1.50	0.09	0.17	5	0.26	0.74	0.50	0.02	0.08
唾液腺	C07–C08	4	0.19	0.57	0.40	0.04	0.04	4	0.20	0.60	0.44	0.04	0.04
扁桃体	C09	1	0.05	0.14	0.16	0.00	0.03	0	0.00	0.00	0.00	0.00	0.00
其他的口咽	C10	1	0.05	0.14	0.09	0.01	0.01	0	0.00	0.00	0.00	0.00	0.00
鼻咽	C11	7	0.33	0.99	0.92	0.05	0.12	5	0.26	0.74	0.58	0.04	0.07
喉咽	C12–C13	6	0.28	0.85	0.83	0.04	0.12	0	0.00	0.00	0.00	0.00	0.00
咽，部位不明	C14	2	0.09	0.28	0.19	0.01	0.01	0	0.00	0.00	0.00	0.00	0.00
食管	C15	181	8.45	25.69	21.94	0.63	2.90	79	4.05	11.75	8.08	0.24	1.16
胃	C16	200	9.34	28.38	24.92	1.07	3.32	91	4.66	13.54	9.58	0.52	1.15
小肠	C17	7	0.33	0.99	0.88	0.05	0.11	7	0.36	1.04	0.85	0.04	0.12
结肠	C18	91	4.25	12.91	11.24	0.46	1.45	82	4.20	12.20	8.99	0.39	1.14
直肠	C19–C20	114	5.32	16.18	14.11	0.70	1.87	90	4.61	13.39	9.43	0.50	1.25
肛门	C21	2	0.09	0.28	0.23	0.00	0.03	3	0.15	0.45	0.33	0.02	0.05
肝脏	C22	302	14.11	42.86	36.87	2.12	4.71	124	6.35	18.45	13.32	0.56	1.84
胆囊及其他	C23–C24	37	1.73	5.25	4.74	0.20	0.57	39	2.00	5.80	3.81	0.11	0.44
胰腺	C25	40	1.87	5.68	4.88	0.26	0.61	25	1.28	3.72	2.84	0.10	0.46
鼻、鼻窦及其他	C30–C31	4	0.19	0.57	0.59	0.03	0.03	0	0.00	0.00	0.00	0.00	0.00
喉	C32	18	0.84	2.55	2.16	0.14	0.29	2	0.10	0.30	0.17	0.00	0.03
气管、支气管、肺	C33–C34	591	27.60	83.87	73.72	3.05	9.85	260	13.32	38.68	26.98	1.36	2.96
其他的胸腔器官	C37–C38	6	0.28	0.85	0.77	0.05	0.10	6	0.31	0.89	0.67	0.02	0.11
骨	C40–C41	25	1.17	3.55	3.22	0.23	0.30	5	0.26	0.74	0.57	0.04	0.06
皮肤的黑色素瘤	C43	3	0.14	0.43	0.30	0.02	0.02	2	0.10	0.30	0.19	0.01	0.01
其他的皮肤	C44	12	0.56	1.70	1.43	0.04	0.16	19	0.97	2.83	1.79	0.05	0.22
间皮瘤	C45	0	0.00	0.00	0.00	0.00	0.00	0	0.00	0.00	0.00	0.00	0.00
卡波西肉瘤	C46	0	0.00	0.00	0.00	0.00	0.00	0	0.00	0.00	0.00	0.00	0.00
周围神经、其他结缔组织、软组织	C47;C49	8	0.37	1.14	1.10	0.06	0.12	5	0.26	0.74	0.57	0.02	0.07
乳房	C50	3	0.14	0.43	0.40	0.02	0.05	417	21.36	62.03	48.69	3.98	5.52
外阴	C51	0	0.00	0.00	0.00	0.00	0.00	2	0.10	0.30	0.17	0.01	0.01
阴道	C52	0	0.00	0.00	0.00	0.00	0.00	3	0.15	0.45	0.39	0.02	0.05
子宫颈	C53	0	0.00	0.00	0.00	0.00	0.00	163	8.35	24.25	18.98	1.48	2.23
子宫体	C54	0	0.00	0.00	0.00	0.00	0.00	61	3.13	9.07	7.32	0.53	0.90
子宫，部位不明	C55	0	0.00	0.00	0.00	0.00	0.00	9	0.46	1.34	1.03	0.11	0.11
卵巢	C56	0	0.00	0.00	0.00	0.00	0.00	58	2.97	8.63	6.40	0.43	0.68
女性其他的生殖器	C57	0	0.00	0.00	0.00	0.00	0.00	5	0.26	0.74	0.51	0.02	0.05
胎盘	C58	0	0.00	0.00	0.00	0.00	0.00	0	0.00	0.00	0.00	0.00	0.00
阴茎	C60	9	0.42	1.28	1.14	0.03	0.16	0	0.00	0.00	0.00	0.00	0.00
前列腺	C61	82	3.83	11.64	10.61	0.11	1.23	0	0.00	0.00	0.00	0.00	0.00
睾丸	C62	1	0.05	0.14	0.11	0.01	0.01	0	0.00	0.00	0.00	0.00	0.00
男性其他的生殖器	C63	0	0.00	0.00	0.00	0.00	0.00	0	0.00	0.00	0.00	0.00	0.00
肾	C64	29	1.35	4.12	3.65	0.24	0.46	21	1.08	3.12	2.71	0.16	0.36
肾盂	C65	1	0.05	0.14	0.16	0.00	0.03	2	0.10	0.30	0.25	0.02	0.05
输尿管	C66	4	0.19	0.57	0.58	0.03	0.09	2	0.10	0.30	0.23	0.01	0.04
膀胱	C67	49	2.29	6.95	6.14	0.19	0.66	13	0.67	1.93	1.36	0.05	0.17
其他的泌尿器官	C68	2	0.09	0.28	0.29	0.01	0.04	2	0.10	0.30	0.21	0.00	0.02
眼	C69	3	0.14	0.43	0.62	0.02	0.06	0	0.00	0.00	0.00	0.00	0.00
脑、神经系统	C70–C72	50	2.34	7.10	6.24	0.38	0.70	45	2.31	6.69	6.16	0.39	0.65
甲状腺	C73	41	1.91	5.82	4.66	0.35	0.46	165	8.45	24.54	19.30	1.61	1.96
肾上腺	C74	5	0.23	0.71	0.64	0.03	0.06	3	0.15	0.45	0.53	0.03	0.03
其他的内分泌腺	C75	3	0.14	0.43	0.31	0.03	0.03	1	0.05	0.15	0.09	0.01	0.01
霍奇金病	C81	5	0.23	0.71	0.71	0.01	0.12	2	0.10	0.30	0.16	0.00	0.00
非霍奇金淋巴瘤	C82–C85;C96	39	1.82	5.53	5.04	0.31	0.72	31	1.59	4.61	3.58	0.20	0.46
免疫增生性疾病	C88	0	0.00	0.00	0.00	0.00	0.00	0	0.00	0.00	0.00	0.00	0.00
多发性骨髓瘤	C90	22	1.03	3.12	2.93	0.11	0.29	11	0.56	1.64	1.32	0.09	0.17
淋巴样白血病	C91	8	0.37	1.14	1.24	0.02	0.11	11	0.56	1.64	1.51	0.09	0.15
髓样白血病	C92–C94	22	1.03	3.12	2.90	0.13	0.34	14	0.72	2.08	1.76	0.12	0.20
白血病，未特指	C95	9	0.42	1.28	1.72	0.09	0.09	11	0.56	1.64	1.71	0.09	0.16
其他的或未指明部位	O&U	62	2.90	8.80	8.08	0.37	0.89	35	1.79	5.21	3.58	0.23	0.40
骨髓增殖性疾病	MPD	4	0.19	0.57	0.47	0.03	0.05	3	0.15	0.45	0.31	0.02	0.02
骨髓增生异常综合征	MDS	0	0.00	0.00	0.00	0.00	0.00	0	0.00	0.00	0.00	0.00	0.00
合计	ALL	2 141	100.00	303.84	267.60	11.95	33.80	1 952	100.00	290.37	218.98	13.84	25.77
C44 以外的部位	ALL but C44	2 129	99.44	302.14	266.18	11.90	33.64	1 933	99.03	287.55	217.19	13.79	25.55

表 6-80 2020 年河南省漯河市城区恶性肿瘤死亡主要指标

部位	ICD-10	男性						女性					
		病例数	构成(%)	粗率($1/10^5$)	世标率($1/10^5$)	累积率(%)		病例数	构成(%)	粗率($1/10^5$)	世标率($1/10^5$)	累积率(%)	
						0~64	0~74					0~64	0~74
唇	C00	1	0.07	0.14	0.16	0.00	0.00	0	0.00	0.00	0.00	0.00	0.00
舌	C01–C02	3	0.21	0.43	0.36	0.04	0.04	3	0.32	0.45	0.33	0.03	0.03
口	C03–C06	3	0.21	0.43	0.33	0.03	0.03	5	0.53	0.74	0.47	0.00	0.06
唾液腺	C07–C08	2	0.14	0.28	0.26	0.01	0.01	0	0.00	0.00	0.00	0.00	0.00
扁桃体	C09	1	0.07	0.14	0.16	0.00	0.03	0	0.00	0.00	0.00	0.00	0.00
其他的口咽	C10	0	0.00	0.00	0.00	0.00	0.00	0	0.00	0.00	0.00	0.00	0.00
鼻咽	C11	4	0.27	0.57	0.54	0.02	0.07	3	0.32	0.45	0.30	0.03	0.03
喉咽	C12–C13	1	0.07	0.14	0.09	0.01	0.01	0	0.00	0.00	0.00	0.00	0.00
咽，部位不明	C14	3	0.21	0.43	0.30	0.00	0.03	0	0.00	0.00	0.00	0.00	0.00
食管	C15	139	9.55	19.73	17.47	0.40	2.30	59	6.27	8.78	5.62	0.07	0.61
胃	C16	151	10.37	21.43	17.86	0.53	1.98	58	6.16	8.63	5.51	0.14	0.56
小肠	C17	8	0.55	1.14	0.88	0.01	0.11	4	0.43	0.60	0.32	0.01	0.01
结肠	C18	34	2.34	4.83	4.46	0.19	0.44	40	4.25	5.95	4.04	0.11	0.45
直肠	C19–C20	46	3.16	6.53	5.72	0.23	0.77	30	3.19	4.46	3.01	0.08	0.33
肛门	C21	1	0.07	0.14	0.09	0.00	0.00	2	0.21	0.30	0.22	0.01	0.01
肝脏	C22	260	17.86	36.90	32.08	1.49	3.84	109	11.58	16.21	11.78	0.52	1.56
胆囊及其他	C23–C24	30	2.06	4.26	3.87	0.15	0.43	39	4.14	5.80	3.68	0.07	0.45
胰腺	C25	31	2.13	4.40	3.72	0.17	0.47	22	2.34	3.27	2.37	0.06	0.36
鼻、鼻窦及其他	C30–C31	0	0.00	0.00	0.00	0.00	0.00	2	0.21	0.30	0.17	0.01	0.01
喉	C32	7	0.48	0.99	0.84	0.05	0.10	0	0.00	0.00	0.00	0.00	0.00
气管、支气管、肺	C33–C34	492	33.79	69.82	60.42	1.81	7.22	197	20.94	29.31	19.31	0.67	2.02
其他的胸腔器官	C37–C38	5	0.34	0.71	0.69	0.07	0.07	1	0.11	0.15	0.12	0.00	0.03
骨	C40–C41	11	0.76	1.56	1.33	0.04	0.20	6	0.64	0.89	0.54	0.01	0.03
皮肤的黑色素瘤	C43	1	0.07	0.14	0.14	0.00	0.03	1	0.11	0.15	0.13	0.01	0.01
其他的皮肤	C44	4	0.27	0.57	0.61	0.00	0.09	8	0.85	1.19	0.79	0.01	0.10
间皮瘤	C45	0	0.00	0.00	0.00	0.00	0.00	2	0.21	0.30	0.26	0.00	0.05
卡波西肉瘤	C46	0	0.00	0.00	0.00	0.00	0.00	0	0.00	0.00	0.00	0.00	0.00
周围神经、其他结缔组织、软组织	C47;C49	2	0.14	0.28	0.36	0.03	0.03	2	0.21	0.30	0.42	0.02	0.05
乳房	C50	1	0.07	0.14	0.10	0.01	0.01	113	12.01	16.81	12.74	0.82	1.50
外阴	C51	0	0.00	0.00	0.00	0.00	0.00	0	0.00	0.00	0.00	0.00	0.00
阴道	C52	0	0.00	0.00	0.00	0.00	0.00	1	0.11	0.15	0.14	0.00	0.02
子宫颈	C53	0	0.00	0.00	0.00	0.00	0.00	45	4.78	6.69	5.14	0.31	0.71
子宫体	C54	0	0.00	0.00	0.00	0.00	0.00	17	1.81	2.53	1.86	0.12	0.25
子宫，部位不明	C55	0	0.00	0.00	0.00	0.00	0.00	5	0.53	0.74	0.57	0.06	0.06
卵巢	C56	0	0.00	0.00	0.00	0.00	0.00	36	3.83	5.36	4.00	0.23	0.47
女性其他的生殖器	C57	0	0.00	0.00	0.00	0.00	0.00	1	0.11	0.15	0.09	0.01	0.01
胎盘	C58	0	0.00	0.00	0.00	0.00	0.00	0	0.00	0.00	0.00	0.00	0.00
阴茎	C60	5	0.34	0.71	0.60	0.00	0.09	0	0.00	0.00	0.00	0.00	0.00
前列腺	C61	29	1.99	4.12	3.71	0.01	0.25	0	0.00	0.00	0.00	0.00	0.00
睾丸	C62	0	0.00	0.00	0.00	0.00	0.00	0	0.00	0.00	0.00	0.00	0.00
男性其他的生殖器	C63	0	0.00	0.00	0.00	0.00	0.00	0	0.00	0.00	0.00	0.00	0.00
肾	C64	18	1.24	2.55	2.33	0.07	0.37	6	0.64	0.89	0.63	0.06	0.06
肾盂	C65	1	0.07	0.14	0.12	0.01	0.01	0	0.00	0.00	0.00	0.00	0.00
输尿管	C66	3	0.21	0.43	0.29	0.03	0.03	1	0.11	0.15	0.11	0.01	0.01
膀胱	C67	18	1.24	2.55	2.14	0.06	0.22	6	0.64	0.89	0.67	0.03	0.07
其他的泌尿器官	C68	0	0.00	0.00	0.00	0.00	0.00	1	0.11	0.15	0.14	0.00	0.02
眼	C69	0	0.00	0.00	0.00	0.00	0.00	1	0.11	0.15	0.12	0.00	0.03
脑、神经系统	C70–C72	32	2.20	4.54	4.26	0.25	0.53	28	2.98	4.17	3.47	0.16	0.44
甲状腺	C73	5	0.34	0.71	0.47	0.01	0.05	11	1.17	1.64	1.30	0.07	0.17
肾上腺	C74	1	0.07	0.14	0.16	0.00	0.00	0	0.00	0.00	0.00	0.00	0.00
其他的内分泌腺	C75	0	0.00	0.00	0.00	0.00	0.00	1	0.11	0.15	0.12	0.00	0.03
霍奇金病	C81	2	0.14	0.28	0.27	0.01	0.05	2	0.21	0.30	0.16	0.00	0.00
非霍奇金淋巴瘤	C82–C85;C96	16	1.10	2.27	1.93	0.13	0.25	4	0.43	0.60	0.43	0.01	0.07
免疫增生性疾病	C88	0	0.00	0.00	0.00	0.00	0.00	0	0.00	0.00	0.00	0.00	0.00
多发性骨髓瘤	C90	10	0.69	1.42	1.12	0.04	0.11	6	0.64	0.89	0.52	0.04	0.04
淋巴样白血病	C91	9	0.62	1.28	1.41	0.06	0.12	4	0.43	0.60	0.34	0.01	0.01
髓样白血病	C92–C94	20	1.37	2.84	2.53	0.09	0.38	14	1.49	2.08	1.82	0.10	0.23
白血病，未特指	C95	9	0.62	1.28	1.17	0.07	0.07	10	1.06	1.49	1.21	0.06	0.17
其他的或未指明部位	O&U	33	2.27	4.68	3.94	0.16	0.52	29	3.08	4.31	3.21	0.13	0.34
骨髓增殖性疾病	MPD	1	0.07	0.14	0.13	0.01	0.01	1	0.11	0.15	0.08	0.00	0.00
骨髓增生异常综合征	MDS	3	0.21	0.43	0.34	0.00	0.00	5	0.53	0.74	0.62	0.03	0.07
合计	ALL	1 456	100.00	206.63	179.76	6.30	21.35	941	100.00	139.98	98.89	4.12	11.55
C44 以外的部位	ALL but C44	1 452	99.73	206.06	179.14	6.30	21.26	933	99.15	138.79	98.10	4.11	11.45

表 6-81　2020 年河南省舞阳县恶性肿瘤发病主要指标

部位	ICD-10	男性						女性					
		病例数	构成 (%)	粗率 (1/10^5)	世标率 (1/10^5)	累积率 (%) 0~64	累积率 (%) 0~74	病例数	构成 (%)	粗率 (1/10^5)	世标率 (1/10^5)	累积率 (%) 0~64	累积率 (%) 0~74
唇	C00	0	0.00	0.00	0.00	0.00	0.00	0	0.00	0.00	0.00	0.00	0.00
舌	C01–C02	5	0.58	1.62	1.36	0.12	0.12	2	0.22	0.70	0.57	0.05	0.05
口	C03–C06	6	0.69	1.94	1.13	0.09	0.13	2	0.22	0.70	0.33	0.02	0.02
唾液腺	C07–C08	2	0.23	0.65	0.34	0.02	0.06	2	0.22	0.70	0.60	0.06	0.06
扁桃体	C09	1	0.12	0.32	0.21	0.00	0.03	0	0.00	0.00	0.00	0.00	0.00
其他的口咽	C10	3	0.35	0.97	0.63	0.05	0.05	0	0.00	0.00	0.00	0.00	0.00
鼻咽	C11	3	0.35	0.97	0.63	0.06	0.06	3	0.34	1.05	0.81	0.02	0.10
喉咽	C12–C13	0	0.00	0.00	0.00	0.00	0.00	0	0.00	0.00	0.00	0.00	0.00
咽，部位不明	C14	1	0.12	0.32	0.33	0.02	0.02	1	0.11	0.35	0.06	0.00	0.00
食管	C15	72	8.30	23.28	10.82	0.35	1.51	57	6.38	19.91	9.48	0.24	1.32
胃	C16	108	12.46	34.92	18.16	0.69	2.85	43	4.82	15.02	7.94	0.40	1.12
小肠	C17	1	0.12	0.32	0.27	0.03	0.03	5	0.56	1.75	1.07	0.08	0.14
结肠	C18	28	3.23	9.05	5.04	0.28	0.56	26	2.91	9.08	5.35	0.35	0.56
直肠	C19–C20	39	4.50	12.61	6.96	0.28	1.01	42	4.70	14.67	8.68	0.54	1.20
肛门	C21	0	0.00	0.00	0.00	0.00	0.00	1	0.11	0.35	0.07	0.00	0.00
肝脏	C22	115	13.26	37.18	23.18	1.41	3.03	48	5.38	16.77	8.91	0.33	1.32
胆囊及其他	C23–C24	19	2.19	6.14	3.04	0.15	0.39	18	2.02	6.29	3.74	0.18	0.48
胰腺	C25	20	2.31	6.47	3.76	0.18	0.54	19	2.13	6.64	3.24	0.20	0.32
鼻、鼻窦及其他	C30–C31	1	0.12	0.32	0.21	0.00	0.03	1	0.11	0.35	0.19	0.02	0.02
喉	C32	12	1.38	3.88	2.35	0.13	0.36	0	0.00	0.00	0.00	0.00	0.00
气管、支气管、肺	C33–C34	245	28.26	79.21	42.19	1.86	5.75	123	13.77	42.96	24.49	1.52	3.24
其他的胸腔器官	C37–C38	1	0.12	0.32	0.21	0.00	0.03	1	0.11	0.35	0.25	0.03	0.03
骨	C40–C41	5	0.58	1.62	0.88	0.00	0.15	3	0.34	1.05	0.57	0.02	0.06
皮肤的黑色素瘤	C43	0	0.00	0.00	0.00	0.00	0.00	0	0.00	0.00	0.00	0.00	0.00
其他的皮肤	C44	4	0.46	1.29	0.55	0.00	0.08	6	0.67	2.10	0.66	0.02	0.08
间皮瘤	C45	0	0.00	0.00	0.00	0.00	0.00	1	0.11	0.35	0.24	0.00	0.04
卡波西肉瘤	C46	0	0.00	0.00	0.00	0.00	0.00	0	0.00	0.00	0.00	0.00	0.00
周围神经、其他结缔组织、软组织	C47;C49	3	0.35	0.97	0.80	0.06	0.06	3	0.34	1.05	1.04	0.06	0.10
乳房	C50	3	0.35	0.97	0.53	0.05	0.05	143	16.01	49.95	36.74	3.10	3.93
外阴	C51	0	0.00	0.00	0.00	0.00	0.00	0	0.00	0.00	0.00	0.00	0.00
阴道	C52	0	0.00	0.00	0.00	0.00	0.00	0	0.00	0.00	0.00	0.00	0.00
子宫颈	C53	0	0.00	0.00	0.00	0.00	0.00	135	15.12	47.15	34.78	2.91	3.68
子宫体	C54	0	0.00	0.00	0.00	0.00	0.00	22	2.46	7.68	5.36	0.44	0.67
子宫，部位不明	C55	0	0.00	0.00	0.00	0.00	0.00	5	0.56	1.75	1.12	0.09	0.09
卵巢	C56	0	0.00	0.00	0.00	0.00	0.00	31	3.47	10.83	7.94	0.52	0.89
女性其他的生殖器	C57	0	0.00	0.00	0.00	0.00	0.00	2	0.22	0.70	0.44	0.06	0.06
胎盘	C58	0	0.00	0.00	0.00	0.00	0.00	0	0.00	0.00	0.00	0.00	0.00
阴茎	C60	4	0.46	1.29	0.71	0.04	0.12	0	0.00	0.00	0.00	0.00	0.00
前列腺	C61	28	3.23	9.05	4.35	0.11	0.58	0	0.00	0.00	0.00	0.00	0.00
睾丸	C62	0	0.00	0.00	0.00	0.00	0.00	0	0.00	0.00	0.00	0.00	0.00
男性其他的生殖器	C63	0	0.00	0.00	0.00	0.00	0.00	0	0.00	0.00	0.00	0.00	0.00
肾	C64	12	1.38	3.88	2.48	0.15	0.35	8	0.90	2.79	1.95	0.08	0.24
肾盂	C65	1	0.12	0.32	0.27	0.02	0.02	0	0.00	0.00	0.00	0.00	0.00
输尿管	C66	1	0.12	0.32	0.21	0.00	0.03	2	0.22	0.70	0.46	0.03	0.08
膀胱	C67	19	2.19	6.14	2.96	0.10	0.38	5	0.56	1.75	0.84	0.00	0.13
其他的泌尿器官	C68	0	0.00	0.00	0.00	0.00	0.00	0	0.00	0.00	0.00	0.00	0.00
眼	C69	2	0.23	0.65	0.25	0.00	0.04	0	0.00	0.00	0.00	0.00	0.00
脑、神经系统	C70–C72	17	1.96	5.50	4.58	0.30	0.37	15	1.68	5.24	3.07	0.19	0.36
甲状腺	C73	21	2.42	6.79	5.62	0.44	0.56	72	8.06	25.15	21.22	1.86	1.99
肾上腺	C74	2	0.23	0.65	0.38	0.03	0.07	1	0.11	0.35	0.25	0.03	0.03
其他的内分泌腺	C75	0	0.00	0.00	0.00	0.00	0.00	0	0.00	0.00	0.00	0.00	0.00
霍奇金病	C81	1	0.12	0.32	0.51	0.03	0.03	0	0.00	0.00	0.00	0.00	0.00
非霍奇金淋巴瘤	C82–C85;C96	7	0.81	2.26	1.88	0.14	0.18	8	0.90	2.79	1.82	0.06	0.23
免疫增生性疾病	C88	0	0.00	0.00	0.00	0.00	0.00	0	0.00	0.00	0.00	0.00	0.00
多发性骨髓瘤	C90	8	0.92	2.59	1.61	0.07	0.26	7	0.78	2.44	1.46	0.06	0.23
淋巴样白血病	C91	3	0.35	0.97	0.46	0.05	0.05	1	0.11	0.35	0.19	0.02	0.02
髓样白血病	C92–C94	17	1.96	5.50	3.67	0.23	0.47	5	0.56	1.75	0.77	0.07	0.07
白血病，未特指	C95	4	0.46	1.29	1.46	0.08	0.12	3	0.34	1.05	1.15	0.08	0.08
其他的或未指明部位	O&U	23	2.65	7.44	5.58	0.39	0.67	19	2.13	6.64	4.83	0.31	0.53
骨髓增殖性疾病	MPD	0	0.00	0.00	0.00	0.00	0.00	1	0.11	0.35	0.26	0.02	0.02
骨髓增生异常综合征	MDS	0	0.00	0.00	0.00	0.00	0.00	1	0.11	0.35	0.10	0.00	0.00
合计	ALL	867	100.00	280.31	160.54	8.01	21.19	893	100.00	311.91	203.05	14.11	23.62
C44 以外的部位	ALL but C44	863	99.54	279.02	159.99	8.01	21.11	887	99.33	309.81	202.39	14.09	23.54

表 6-82 2020 年河南省舞阳县恶性肿瘤死亡主要指标

部位	ICD-10	男性						女性					
		病例数	构成 (%)	粗率 ($1/10^5$)	世标率 ($1/10^5$)	累积率 (%) 0~64	累积率 (%) 0~74	病例数	构成 (%)	粗率 ($1/10^5$)	世标率 ($1/10^5$)	累积率 (%) 0~64	累积率 (%) 0~74
唇	C00	0	0.00	0.00	0.00	0.00	0.00	0	0.00	0.00	0.00	0.00	0.00
舌	C01–C02	2	0.29	0.65	0.56	0.06	0.06	1	0.26	0.35	0.24	0.00	0.04
口	C03–C06	2	0.29	0.65	0.34	0.02	0.06	0	0.00	0.00	0.00	0.00	0.00
唾液腺	C07–C08	0	0.00	0.00	0.00	0.00	0.00	3	0.77	1.05	0.58	0.03	0.08
扁桃体	C09	0	0.00	0.00	0.00	0.00	0.00	0	0.00	0.00	0.00	0.00	0.00
其他的口咽	C10	0	0.00	0.00	0.00	0.00	0.00	0	0.00	0.00	0.00	0.00	0.00
鼻咽	C11	5	0.73	1.62	0.86	0.00	0.15	2	0.52	0.70	0.54	0.03	0.07
喉咽	C12–C13	0	0.00	0.00	0.00	0.00	0.00	0	0.00	0.00	0.00	0.00	0.00
咽，部位不明	C14	1	0.15	0.32	0.09	0.00	0.00	0	0.00	0.00	0.00	0.00	0.00
食管	C15	71	10.33	22.96	10.04	0.21	1.31	45	11.60	15.72	5.39	0.09	0.53
胃	C16	83	12.08	26.83	13.27	0.45	1.89	41	10.57	14.32	5.86	0.30	0.54
小肠	C17	1	0.15	0.32	0.17	0.02	0.02	0	0.00	0.00	0.00	0.00	0.00
结肠	C18	28	4.08	9.05	4.07	0.17	0.48	16	4.12	5.59	3.13	0.20	0.37
直肠	C19–C20	13	1.89	4.20	2.01	0.08	0.20	14	3.61	4.89	2.09	0.14	0.23
肛门	C21	0	0.00	0.00	0.00	0.00	0.00	2	0.52	0.70	0.31	0.00	0.04
肝脏	C22	111	16.16	35.89	21.43	1.19	2.80	44	11.34	15.37	6.96	0.21	0.91
胆囊及其他	C23–C24	9	1.31	2.91	1.11	0.06	0.11	9	2.32	3.14	1.67	0.09	0.22
胰腺	C25	8	1.16	2.59	1.24	0.03	0.19	12	3.09	4.19	2.15	0.20	0.25
鼻、鼻窦及其他	C30–C31	2	0.29	0.65	0.41	0.00	0.07	0	0.00	0.00	0.00	0.00	0.00
喉	C32	1	0.15	0.32	0.21	0.00	0.03	0	0.00	0.00	0.00	0.00	0.00
气管、支气管、肺	C33–C34	237	34.50	76.62	36.56	1.21	4.92	91	23.45	31.78	15.47	0.59	2.01
其他的胸腔器官	C37–C38	1	0.15	0.32	0.06	0.00	0.00	2	0.52	0.70	0.54	0.03	0.07
骨	C40–C41	10	1.46	3.23	1.70	0.03	0.30	3	0.77	1.05	0.40	0.00	0.04
皮肤的黑色素瘤	C43	0	0.00	0.00	0.00	0.00	0.00	0	0.00	0.00	0.00	0.00	0.00
其他的皮肤	C44	5	0.73	1.62	0.52	0.00	0.04	2	0.52	0.70	0.32	0.03	0.03
间皮瘤	C45	0	0.00	0.00	0.00	0.00	0.00	1	0.26	0.35	0.24	0.00	0.04
卡波西肉瘤	C46	0	0.00	0.00	0.00	0.00	0.00	0	0.00	0.00	0.00	0.00	0.00
周围神经、其他结缔组织、软组织	C47;C49	2	0.29	0.65	0.73	0.05	0.05	1	0.26	0.35	0.26	0.02	0.02
乳房	C50	0	0.00	0.00	0.00	0.00	0.00	26	6.70	9.08	5.31	0.35	0.64
外阴	C51	0	0.00	0.00	0.00	0.00	0.00	2	0.52	0.70	0.14	0.00	0.00
阴道	C52	0	0.00	0.00	0.00	0.00	0.00	0	0.00	0.00	0.00	0.00	0.00
子宫颈	C53	0	0.00	0.00	0.00	0.00	0.00	15	3.87	5.24	3.34	0.19	0.40
子宫体	C54	0	0.00	0.00	0.00	0.00	0.00	2	0.52	0.70	0.57	0.05	0.05
子宫，部位不明	C55	0	0.00	0.00	0.00	0.00	0.00	2	0.52	0.70	0.27	0.00	0.05
卵巢	C56	0	0.00	0.00	0.00	0.00	0.00	6	1.55	2.10	1.12	0.07	0.12
女性其他的生殖器	C57	0	0.00	0.00	0.00	0.00	0.00	0	0.00	0.00	0.00	0.00	0.00
胎盘	C58	0	0.00	0.00	0.00	0.00	0.00	0	0.00	0.00	0.00	0.00	0.00
阴茎	C60	0	0.00	0.00	0.00	0.00	0.00	0	0.00	0.00	0.00	0.00	0.00
前列腺	C61	15	2.18	4.85	1.86	0.02	0.26	0	0.00	0.00	0.00	0.00	0.00
睾丸	C62	0	0.00	0.00	0.00	0.00	0.00	0	0.00	0.00	0.00	0.00	0.00
男性其他的生殖器	C63	0	0.00	0.00	0.00	0.00	0.00	0	0.00	0.00	0.00	0.00	0.00
肾	C64	6	0.87	1.94	0.81	0.02	0.10	0	0.00	0.00	0.00	0.00	0.00
肾盂	C65	0	0.00	0.00	0.00	0.00	0.00	0	0.00	0.00	0.00	0.00	0.00
输尿管	C66	0	0.00	0.00	0.00	0.00	0.00	0	0.00	0.00	0.00	0.00	0.00
膀胱	C67	9	1.31	2.91	0.99	0.02	0.11	3	0.77	1.05	0.47	0.03	0.03
其他的泌尿器官	C68	0	0.00	0.00	0.00	0.00	0.00	1	0.26	0.35	0.21	0.00	0.05
眼	C69	0	0.00	0.00	0.00	0.00	0.00	2	0.52	0.70	0.17	0.00	0.00
脑、神经系统	C70–C72	17	2.47	5.50	3.72	0.25	0.37	14	3.61	4.89	2.54	0.12	0.32
甲状腺	C73	0	0.00	0.00	0.00	0.00	0.00	2	0.52	0.70	0.14	0.00	0.00
肾上腺	C74	5	0.73	1.62	0.84	0.03	0.15	0	0.00	0.00	0.00	0.00	0.00
其他的内分泌腺	C75	0	0.00	0.00	0.00	0.00	0.00	0	0.00	0.00	0.00	0.00	0.00
霍奇金病	C81	1	0.15	0.32	0.17	0.00	0.04	1	0.26	0.35	0.24	0.00	0.04
非霍奇金淋巴瘤	C82–C85;C96	4	0.58	1.29	0.76	0.03	0.15	3	0.77	1.05	0.61	0.03	0.08
免疫增生性疾病	C88	0	0.00	0.00	0.00	0.00	0.00	0	0.00	0.00	0.00	0.00	0.00
多发性骨髓瘤	C90	9	1.31	2.91	1.66	0.07	0.26	0	0.00	0.00	0.00	0.00	0.00
淋巴样白血病	C91	3	0.44	0.97	0.51	0.04	0.04	2	0.52	0.70	0.30	0.00	0.05
髓样白血病	C92–C94	4	0.58	1.29	0.88	0.06	0.10	2	0.52	0.70	0.44	0.06	0.06
白血病，未特指	C95	3	0.44	0.97	0.94	0.03	0.10	3	0.77	1.05	0.56	0.05	0.05
其他的或未指明部位	O&U	18	2.62	5.82	3.30	0.21	0.37	11	2.84	3.84	2.52	0.16	0.27
骨髓增殖性疾病	MPD	0	0.00	0.00	0.00	0.00	0.00	1	0.26	0.35	0.25	0.03	0.03
骨髓增生异常综合征	MDS	1	0.15	0.32	0.09	0.00	0.00	1	0.26	0.35	0.06	0.00	0.00
合计	ALL	687	100.00	222.12	111.93	4.37	14.73	388	100.00	135.52	65.39	3.09	7.73
C44 以外的部位	ALL but C44	682	99.27	220.50	111.41	4.37	14.69	386	99.48	134.82	65.07	3.06	7.70

表 6-83　2020 年河南省临颍县恶性肿瘤发病主要指标

部位	ICD-10	男性						女性					
		病例数	构成 (%)	粗率 (1/10^5)	世标率 (1/10^5)	累积率 (%)		病例数	构成 (%)	粗率 (1/10^5)	世标率 (1/10^5)	累积率 (%)	
						0~64	0~74					0~64	0~74
唇	C00	0	0.00	0.00	0.00	0.00	0.00	2	0.20	0.68	0.29	0.00	0.02
舌	C01–C02	3	0.29	1.01	0.68	0.03	0.08	1	0.10	0.34	0.26	0.03	0.03
口	C03–C06	4	0.38	1.35	0.69	0.02	0.09	3	0.30	1.02	0.49	0.00	0.09
唾液腺	C07–C08	1	0.10	0.34	0.28	0.03	0.03	3	0.30	1.02	0.70	0.05	0.10
扁桃体	C09	0	0.00	0.00	0.00	0.00	0.00	0	0.00	0.00	0.00	0.00	0.00
其他的口咽	C10	0	0.00	0.00	0.00	0.00	0.00	0	0.00	0.00	0.00	0.00	0.00
鼻咽	C11	2	0.19	0.68	0.43	0.02	0.05	5	0.49	1.70	0.96	0.07	0.10
喉咽	C12–C13	0	0.00	0.00	0.00	0.00	0.00	0	0.00	0.00	0.00	0.00	0.00
咽，部位不明	C14	2	0.19	0.68	0.50	0.05	0.05	1	0.10	0.34	0.15	0.00	0.02
食管	C15	73	7.00	24.69	13.04	0.38	1.60	51	5.04	17.34	7.15	0.19	0.61
胃	C16	97	9.30	32.80	18.91	0.84	2.16	51	5.04	17.34	8.93	0.54	1.05
小肠	C17	2	0.19	0.68	0.43	0.03	0.06	1	0.10	0.34	0.20	0.03	0.03
结肠	C18	32	3.07	10.82	6.86	0.45	0.86	27	2.67	9.18	5.07	0.27	0.60
直肠	C19–C20	45	4.31	15.22	9.35	0.57	1.20	44	4.35	14.96	8.24	0.55	0.98
肛门	C21	3	0.29	1.01	0.53	0.00	0.05	0	0.00	0.00	0.00	0.00	0.00
肝脏	C22	175	16.78	59.18	37.72	2.58	4.29	78	7.71	26.52	13.26	0.66	1.75
胆囊及其他	C23–C24	16	1.53	5.41	3.41	0.25	0.47	20	1.98	6.80	3.57	0.25	0.43
胰腺	C25	13	1.25	4.40	2.72	0.14	0.23	16	1.58	5.44	2.94	0.17	0.41
鼻、鼻窦及其他	C30–C31	3	0.29	1.01	0.61	0.06	0.06	1	0.10	0.34	0.20	0.03	0.03
喉	C32	10	0.96	3.38	2.24	0.14	0.26	0	0.00	0.00	0.00	0.00	0.00
气管、支气管、肺	C33–C34	329	31.54	111.26	64.19	2.78	7.79	163	16.11	55.43	27.70	1.45	3.43
其他的胸腔器官	C37–C38	5	0.48	1.69	1.14	0.07	0.12	2	0.20	0.68	0.41	0.02	0.06
骨	C40–C41	23	2.21	7.78	5.38	0.35	0.60	5	0.49	1.70	0.92	0.07	0.11
皮肤的黑色素瘤	C43	0	0.00	0.00	0.00	0.00	0.00	1	0.10	0.34	0.14	0.00	0.00
其他的皮肤	C44	7	0.67	2.37	1.29	0.06	0.08	9	0.89	3.06	1.41	0.06	0.13
间皮瘤	C45	1	0.10	0.34	0.22	0.03	0.03	0	0.00	0.00	0.00	0.00	0.00
卡波西肉瘤	C46	0	0.00	0.00	0.00	0.00	0.00	0	0.00	0.00	0.00	0.00	0.00
周围神经、其他结缔组织、软组织	C47;C49	4	0.38	1.35	1.14	0.11	0.11	6	0.59	2.04	2.27	0.16	0.16
乳房	C50	1	0.10	0.34	0.23	0.02	0.02	168	16.60	57.13	40.28	3.31	4.22
外阴	C51	0	0.00	0.00	0.00	0.00	0.00	2	0.20	0.68	0.30	0.00	0.05
阴道	C52	0	0.00	0.00	0.00	0.00	0.00	2	0.20	0.68	0.46	0.05	0.05
子宫颈	C53	0	0.00	0.00	0.00	0.00	0.00	69	6.82	23.46	15.39	1.40	1.66
子宫体	C54	0	0.00	0.00	0.00	0.00	0.00	26	2.57	8.84	5.08	0.40	0.68
子宫，部位不明	C55	0	0.00	0.00	0.00	0.00	0.00	5	0.49	1.70	1.07	0.10	0.12
卵巢	C56	0	0.00	0.00	0.00	0.00	0.00	17	1.68	5.78	3.63	0.28	0.37
女性其他的生殖器	C57	0	0.00	0.00	0.00	0.00	0.00	1	0.10	0.34	0.20	0.03	0.03
胎盘	C58	0	0.00	0.00	0.00	0.00	0.00	0	0.00	0.00	0.00	0.00	0.00
阴茎	C60	0	0.00	0.00	0.00	0.00	0.00	0	0.00	0.00	0.00	0.00	0.00
前列腺	C61	25	2.40	8.45	4.33	0.10	0.38	0	0.00	0.00	0.00	0.00	0.00
睾丸	C62	2	0.19	0.68	1.04	0.06	0.06	0	0.00	0.00	0.00	0.00	0.00
男性其他的生殖器	C63	0	0.00	0.00	0.00	0.00	0.00	0	0.00	0.00	0.00	0.00	0.00
肾	C64	8	0.77	2.71	1.80	0.12	0.26	10	0.99	3.40	1.92	0.15	0.23
肾盂	C65	3	0.29	1.01	0.72	0.06	0.06	0	0.00	0.00	0.00	0.00	0.00
输尿管	C66	4	0.38	1.35	0.77	0.02	0.05	0	0.00	0.00	0.00	0.00	0.00
膀胱	C67	25	2.40	8.45	4.59	0.17	0.58	9	0.89	3.06	1.38	0.05	0.21
其他的泌尿器官	C68	0	0.00	0.00	0.00	0.00	0.00	0	0.00	0.00	0.00	0.00	0.00
眼	C69	0	0.00	0.00	0.00	0.00	0.00	1	0.10	0.34	0.26	0.02	0.02
脑、神经系统	C70–C72	18	1.73	6.09	5.13	0.32	0.58	30	2.96	10.20	5.99	0.46	0.70
甲状腺	C73	19	1.82	6.43	6.14	0.43	0.53	86	8.50	29.24	22.42	1.90	2.12
肾上腺	C74	1	0.10	0.34	0.23	0.02	0.02	1	0.10	0.34	0.20	0.03	0.03
其他的内分泌腺	C75	0	0.00	0.00	0.00	0.00	0.00	0	0.00	0.00	0.00	0.00	0.00
霍奇金病	C81	1	0.10	0.34	0.43	0.03	0.03	0	0.00	0.00	0.00	0.00	0.00
非霍奇金淋巴瘤	C82–C85;C96	3	0.29	1.01	1.06	0.09	0.09	10	0.99	3.40	2.67	0.17	0.31
免疫增生性疾病	C88	1	0.10	0.34	0.16	0.00	0.03	0	0.00	0.00	0.00	0.00	0.00
多发性骨髓瘤	C90	5	0.48	1.69	0.82	0.00	0.12	5	0.49	1.70	0.78	0.03	0.14
淋巴样白血病	C91	0	0.00	0.00	0.00	0.00	0.00	1	0.10	0.34	0.10	0.00	0.00
髓样白血病	C92–C94	7	0.67	2.37	1.70	0.13	0.18	4	0.40	1.36	0.96	0.03	0.11
白血病，未特指	C95	12	1.15	4.06	3.29	0.21	0.31	11	1.09	3.74	4.26	0.21	0.24
其他的或未指明部位	O&U	56	5.37	18.94	11.91	0.66	1.25	61	6.03	20.74	13.10	0.95	1.42
骨髓增殖性疾病	MPD	2	0.19	0.68	0.47	0.05	0.05	3	0.30	1.02	0.99	0.05	0.05
骨髓增生异常综合征	MDS	0	0.00	0.00	0.00	0.00	0.00	0	0.00	0.00	0.00	0.00	0.00
合计	ALL	1 043	100.00	352.70	216.59	11.48	24.89	1 012	100.00	344.11	206.72	14.21	22.88
C44 以外的部位	ALL but C44	1 036	99.33	350.33	215.31	11.43	24.81	1 003	99.11	341.05	205.31	14.15	22.75

表 6-84　2020 年河南省临颍县恶性肿瘤死亡主要指标

部位	ICD-10	男性						女性					
		病例数	构成(%)	粗率(1/10^5)	世标率(1/10^5)	累积率(%) 0~64	累积率(%) 0~74	病例数	构成(%)	粗率(1/10^5)	世标率(1/10^5)	累积率(%) 0~64	累积率(%) 0~74
唇	C00	0	0.00	0.00	0.00	0.00	0.00	0	0.00	0.00	0.00	0.00	0.00
舌	C01-C02	0	0.00	0.00	0.00	0.00	0.00	2	0.43	0.68	0.44	0.03	0.08
口	C03-C06	1	0.13	0.34	0.16	0.00	0.03	3	0.64	1.02	0.55	0.05	0.05
唾液腺	C07-C08	1	0.13	0.34	0.28	0.03	0.03	0	0.00	0.00	0.00	0.00	0.00
扁桃体	C09	0	0.00	0.00	0.00	0.00	0.00	0	0.00	0.00	0.00	0.00	0.00
其他的口咽	C10	0	0.00	0.00	0.00	0.00	0.00	1	0.21	0.34	0.20	0.03	0.03
鼻咽	C11	4	0.52	1.35	1.01	0.11	0.11	0	0.00	0.00	0.00	0.00	0.00
喉咽	C12-C13	1	0.13	0.34	0.28	0.03	0.03	1	0.21	0.34	0.10	0.00	0.00
咽，部位不明	C14	0	0.00	0.00	0.00	0.00	0.00	1	0.21	0.34	0.36	0.03	0.03
食管	C15	68	8.90	22.99	13.15	0.64	1.57	58	12.34	19.72	8.43	0.22	0.89
胃	C16	78	10.21	26.38	14.48	0.62	1.50	40	8.51	13.60	6.41	0.32	0.64
小肠	C17	0	0.00	0.00	0.00	0.00	0.00	1	0.21	0.34	0.15	0.00	0.02
结肠	C18	14	1.83	4.73	2.91	0.11	0.38	7	1.49	2.38	1.07	0.03	0.12
直肠	C19-C20	11	1.44	3.72	2.12	0.12	0.16	17	3.62	5.78	2.57	0.09	0.25
肛门	C21	2	0.26	0.68	0.36	0.00	0.05	0	0.00	0.00	0.00	0.00	0.00
肝脏	C22	165	21.60	55.80	35.08	2.29	4.15	67	14.26	22.78	11.17	0.48	1.55
胆囊及其他	C23-C24	11	1.44	3.72	2.21	0.09	0.30	18	3.83	6.12	2.87	0.10	0.35
胰腺	C25	12	1.57	4.06	2.05	0.03	0.23	11	2.34	3.74	1.80	0.09	0.25
鼻、鼻窦及其他	C30-C31	3	0.39	1.01	0.58	0.04	0.04	1	0.21	0.34	0.08	0.00	0.00
喉	C32	2	0.26	0.68	0.53	0.03	0.03	0	0.00	0.00	0.00	0.00	0.00
气管、支气管、肺	C33-C34	283	37.04	95.70	53.85	2.24	6.11	98	20.85	33.32	15.14	0.64	1.67
其他的胸腔器官	C37-C38	4	0.52	1.35	1.00	0.07	0.07	1	0.21	0.34	0.15	0.00	0.02
骨	C40-C41	6	0.79	2.03	1.13	0.03	0.13	2	0.43	0.68	0.30	0.00	0.05
皮肤的黑色素瘤	C43	0	0.00	0.00	0.00	0.00	0.00	0	0.00	0.00	0.00	0.00	0.00
其他的皮肤	C44	2	0.26	0.68	0.35	0.00	0.00	0	0.00	0.00	0.00	0.00	0.00
间皮瘤	C45	1	0.13	0.34	0.10	0.00	0.00	0	0.00	0.00	0.00	0.00	0.00
卡波西肉瘤	C46	0	0.00	0.00	0.00	0.00	0.00	0	0.00	0.00	0.00	0.00	0.00
周围神经、其他结缔组织、软组织	C47;C49	1	0.13	0.34	0.28	0.03	0.03	3	0.64	1.02	0.78	0.03	0.07
乳房	C50	1	0.13	0.34	0.37	0.03	0.03	28	5.96	9.52	5.77	0.45	0.64
外阴	C51	0	0.00	0.00	0.00	0.00	0.00	0	0.00	0.00	0.00	0.00	0.00
阴道	C52	0	0.00	0.00	0.00	0.00	0.00	0	0.00	0.00	0.00	0.00	0.00
子宫颈	C53	0	0.00	0.00	0.00	0.00	0.00	24	5.11	8.16	4.84	0.38	0.55
子宫体	C54	0	0.00	0.00	0.00	0.00	0.00	5	1.06	1.70	0.82	0.05	0.05
子宫，部位不明	C55	0	0.00	0.00	0.00	0.00	0.00	1	0.21	0.34	0.08	0.00	0.00
卵巢	C56	0	0.00	0.00	0.00	0.00	0.00	8	1.70	2.72	1.43	0.09	0.16
女性其他的生殖器	C57	0	0.00	0.00	0.00	0.00	0.00	0	0.00	0.00	0.00	0.00	0.00
胎盘	C58	0	0.00	0.00	0.00	0.00	0.00	0	0.00	0.00	0.00	0.00	0.00
阴茎	C60	0	0.00	0.00	0.00	0.00	0.00	0	0.00	0.00	0.00	0.00	0.00
前列腺	C61	14	1.83	4.73	2.11	0.00	0.09	0	0.00	0.00	0.00	0.00	0.00
睾丸	C62	0	0.00	0.00	0.00	0.00	0.00	0	0.00	0.00	0.00	0.00	0.00
男性其他的生殖器	C63	0	0.00	0.00	0.00	0.00	0.00	0	0.00	0.00	0.00	0.00	0.00
肾	C64	2	0.26	0.68	0.39	0.03	0.03	2	0.43	0.68	0.31	0.02	0.02
肾盂	C65	2	0.26	0.68	0.45	0.03	0.03	0	0.00	0.00	0.00	0.00	0.00
输尿管	C66	2	0.26	0.68	0.35	0.00	0.00	0	0.00	0.00	0.00	0.00	0.00
膀胱	C67	3	0.39	1.01	0.55	0.00	0.09	6	1.28	2.04	0.86	0.06	0.06
其他的泌尿器官	C68	0	0.00	0.00	0.00	0.00	0.00	0	0.00	0.00	0.00	0.00	0.00
眼	C69	0	0.00	0.00	0.00	0.00	0.00	1	0.21	0.34	0.14	0.00	0.00
脑、神经系统	C70-C72	14	1.83	4.73	3.26	0.17	0.38	13	2.77	4.42	2.56	0.09	0.37
甲状腺	C73	3	0.39	1.01	0.61	0.03	0.06	4	0.85	1.36	0.63	0.02	0.09
肾上腺	C74	1	0.13	0.34	0.35	0.03	0.03	0	0.00	0.00	0.00	0.00	0.00
其他的内分泌腺	C75	0	0.00	0.00	0.00	0.00	0.00	0	0.00	0.00	0.00	0.00	0.00
霍奇金病	C81	0	0.00	0.00	0.00	0.00	0.00	0	0.00	0.00	0.00	0.00	0.00
非霍奇金淋巴瘤	C82-C85;C96	5	0.65	1.69	1.35	0.08	0.12	2	0.43	0.68	0.35	0.03	0.05
免疫增生性疾病	C88	0	0.00	0.00	0.00	0.00	0.00	0	0.00	0.00	0.00	0.00	0.00
多发性骨髓瘤	C90	1	0.13	0.34	0.28	0.03	0.03	3	0.64	1.02	0.47	0.00	0.07
淋巴样白血病	C91	0	0.00	0.00	0.00	0.00	0.00	0	0.00	0.00	0.00	0.00	0.00
髓样白血病	C92-C94	3	0.39	1.01	0.69	0.05	0.10	0	0.00	0.00	0.00	0.00	0.00
白血病，未特指	C95	6	0.79	2.03	1.33	0.05	0.13	12	2.55	4.08	4.54	0.21	0.28
其他的或未指明部位	O&U	35	4.58	11.84	7.24	0.45	0.85	25	5.32	8.50	5.77	0.29	0.59
骨髓增殖性疾病	MPD	0	0.00	0.00	0.00	0.00	0.00	1	0.21	0.34	0.10	0.00	0.00
骨髓增生异常综合征	MDS	2	0.26	0.68	0.36	0.00	0.05	3	0.64	1.02	0.50	0.00	0.11
合计	ALL	764	100.00	258.36	151.55	7.52	16.99	470	100.00	159.82	81.73	3.82	9.10
C44 以外的部位	ALL but C44	762	99.74	257.68	151.20	7.52	16.99	470	100.00	159.82	81.73	3.82	9.10

表 6-85 2020 年河南省渑池县恶性肿瘤发病主要指标

部位	ICD-10	男性						女性					
		病例数	构成 (%)	粗率 ($1/10^5$)	世标率 ($1/10^5$)	累积率 (%)		病例数	构成 (%)	粗率 ($1/10^5$)	世标率 ($1/10^5$)	累积率 (%)	
						0~64	0~74					0~64	0~74
唇	C00	0	0.00	0.00	0.00	0.00	0.00	0	0.00	0.00	0.00	0.00	0.00
舌	C01–C02	0	0.00	0.00	0.00	0.00	0.00	1	0.24	0.58	0.41	0.05	0.05
口	C03–C06	1	0.24	0.55	0.33	0.03	0.03	2	0.49	1.15	0.70	0.08	0.08
唾液腺	C07–C08	1	0.24	0.55	0.38	0.00	0.06	1	0.24	0.58	0.35	0.03	0.03
扁桃体	C09	0	0.00	0.00	0.00	0.00	0.00	0	0.00	0.00	0.00	0.00	0.00
其他的口咽	C10	1	0.24	0.55	0.36	0.03	0.03	1	0.24	0.58	0.37	0.00	0.06
鼻咽	C11	1	0.24	0.55	0.44	0.00	0.11	1	0.24	0.58	0.35	0.04	0.04
喉咽	C12–C13	1	0.24	0.55	0.38	0.00	0.06	0	0.00	0.00	0.00	0.00	0.00
咽，部位不明	C14	2	0.47	1.10	0.81	0.00	0.17	0	0.00	0.00	0.00	0.00	0.00
食管	C15	57	13.48	31.22	21.90	0.46	3.12	39	9.49	22.44	13.52	0.40	1.50
胃	C16	87	20.57	47.65	33.27	1.19	4.54	31	7.54	17.84	10.75	0.11	1.20
小肠	C17	1	0.24	0.55	0.38	0.00	0.06	0	0.00	0.00	0.00	0.00	0.00
结肠	C18	10	2.36	5.48	3.76	0.25	0.36	9	2.19	5.18	3.30	0.30	0.42
直肠	C19–C20	12	2.84	6.57	4.68	0.16	0.63	15	3.65	8.63	5.81	0.36	0.85
肛门	C21	0	0.00	0.00	0.00	0.00	0.00	1	0.24	0.58	0.31	0.00	0.00
肝脏	C22	26	6.15	14.24	9.94	0.60	1.26	20	4.87	11.51	7.12	0.26	0.79
胆囊及其他	C23–C24	5	1.18	2.74	1.76	0.14	0.20	11	2.68	6.33	3.79	0.17	0.49
胰腺	C25	5	1.18	2.74	1.97	0.08	0.32	10	2.43	5.75	3.32	0.12	0.31
鼻、鼻窦及其他	C30–C31	0	0.00	0.00	0.00	0.00	0.00	0	0.00	0.00	0.00	0.00	0.00
喉	C32	6	1.42	3.29	2.10	0.06	0.25	1	0.24	0.58	0.37	0.00	0.06
气管、支气管、肺	C33–C34	127	30.02	69.56	47.53	2.29	6.36	58	14.11	33.37	21.11	1.16	2.52
其他的胸腔器官	C37–C38	2	0.47	1.10	0.83	0.00	0.06	1	0.24	0.58	0.35	0.03	0.03
骨	C40–C41	1	0.24	0.55	0.35	0.00	0.00	3	0.73	1.73	1.05	0.00	0.12
皮肤的黑色素瘤	C43	1	0.24	0.55	0.44	0.00	0.11	0	0.00	0.00	0.00	0.00	0.00
其他的皮肤	C44	5	1.18	2.74	2.60	0.10	0.21	2	0.49	1.15	0.72	0.00	0.10
间皮瘤	C45	0	0.00	0.00	0.00	0.00	0.00	0	0.00	0.00	0.00	0.00	0.00
卡波西肉瘤	C46	0	0.00	0.00	0.00	0.00	0.00	0	0.00	0.00	0.00	0.00	0.00
周围神经、其他结缔组织、软组织	C47;C49	1	0.24	0.55	0.44	0.00	0.11	0	0.00	0.00	0.00	0.00	0.00
乳房	C50	2	0.47	1.10	0.61	0.03	0.03	58	14.11	33.37	22.73	1.86	2.43
外阴	C51	0	0.00	0.00	0.00	0.00	0.00	1	0.24	0.58	0.31	0.00	0.00
阴道	C52	0	0.00	0.00	0.00	0.00	0.00	1	0.24	0.58	0.35	0.04	0.04
子宫颈	C53	0	0.00	0.00	0.00	0.00	0.00	42	10.22	24.17	16.30	1.27	1.78
子宫体	C54	0	0.00	0.00	0.00	0.00	0.00	21	5.11	12.08	8.00	0.60	0.99
子宫，部位不明	C55	0	0.00	0.00	0.00	0.00	0.00	4	0.97	2.30	1.57	0.18	0.18
卵巢	C56	0	0.00	0.00	0.00	0.00	0.00	10	2.43	5.75	3.95	0.35	0.46
女性其他的生殖器	C57	0	0.00	0.00	0.00	0.00	0.00	1	0.24	0.58	0.39	0.03	0.03
胎盘	C58	0	0.00	0.00	0.00	0.00	0.00	0	0.00	0.00	0.00	0.00	0.00
阴茎	C60	2	0.47	1.10	0.74	0.03	0.09	0	0.00	0.00	0.00	0.00	0.00
前列腺	C61	13	3.07	7.12	4.90	0.04	0.62	0	0.00	0.00	0.00	0.00	0.00
睾丸	C62	0	0.00	0.00	0.00	0.00	0.00	0	0.00	0.00	0.00	0.00	0.00
男性其他的生殖器	C63	0	0.00	0.00	0.00	0.00	0.00	0	0.00	0.00	0.00	0.00	0.00
肾	C64	3	0.71	1.64	1.07	0.04	0.11	4	0.97	2.30	1.45	0.08	0.08
肾盂	C65	2	0.47	1.10	0.76	0.00	0.13	0	0.00	0.00	0.00	0.00	0.00
输尿管	C66	0	0.00	0.00	0.00	0.00	0.00	0	0.00	0.00	0.00	0.00	0.00
膀胱	C67	10	2.36	5.48	4.02	0.28	0.51	2	0.49	1.15	0.76	0.03	0.09
其他的泌尿器官	C68	0	0.00	0.00	0.00	0.00	0.00	0	0.00	0.00	0.00	0.00	0.00
眼	C69	0	0.00	0.00	0.00	0.00	0.00	0	0.00	0.00	0.00	0.00	0.00
脑、神经系统	C70–C72	13	3.07	7.12	5.51	0.39	0.50	11	2.68	6.33	4.02	0.24	0.46
甲状腺	C73	5	1.18	2.74	2.21	0.14	0.20	34	8.27	19.56	13.38	1.17	1.29
肾上腺	C74	0	0.00	0.00	0.00	0.00	0.00	0	0.00	0.00	0.00	0.00	0.00
其他的内分泌腺	C75	0	0.00	0.00	0.00	0.00	0.00	0	0.00	0.00	0.00	0.00	0.00
霍奇金病	C81	0	0.00	0.00	0.00	0.00	0.00	0	0.00	0.00	0.00	0.00	0.00
非霍奇金淋巴瘤	C82–C85;C96	1	0.24	0.55	0.42	0.05	0.05	3	0.73	1.73	0.99	0.04	0.15
免疫增生性疾病	C88	0	0.00	0.00	0.00	0.00	0.00	0	0.00	0.00	0.00	0.00	0.00
多发性骨髓瘤	C90	0	0.00	0.00	0.00	0.00	0.00	3	0.73	1.73	1.65	0.10	0.20
淋巴样白血病	C91	0	0.00	0.00	0.00	0.00	0.00	0	0.00	0.00	0.00	0.00	0.00
髓样白血病	C92–C94	2	0.47	1.10	0.71	0.03	0.10	2	0.49	1.15	0.78	0.05	0.11
白血病，未特指	C95	2	0.47	1.10	0.71	0.03	0.10	3	0.73	1.73	1.79	0.12	0.12
其他的或未指明部位	O&U	15	3.55	8.22	5.61	0.38	0.68	4	0.97	2.30	1.56	0.05	0.28
骨髓增殖性疾病	MPD	0	0.00	0.00	0.00	0.00	0.00	0	0.00	0.00	0.00	0.00	0.00
骨髓增生异常综合征	MDS	0	0.00	0.00	0.00	0.00	0.00	0	0.00	0.00	0.00	0.00	0.00
合计	ALL	423	100.00	231.68	161.91	6.85	21.18	411	100.00	236.50	153.69	9.34	17.38
C44 以外的部位	ALL but C44	418	98.82	228.94	159.31	6.75	20.97	409	99.51	235.35	152.97	9.34	17.28

表 6-86 2020 年河南省渑池县恶性肿瘤死亡主要指标

部位	ICD-10	男性						女性					
		病例数	构成 (%)	粗率 (1/10^5)	世标率 (1/10^5)	累积率 (%)		病例数	构成 (%)	粗率 (1/10^5)	世标率 (1/10^5)	累积率 (%)	
						0~64	0~74					0~64	0~74
唇	C00	1	0.30	0.55	0.45	0.00	0.00	0	0.00	0.00	0.00	0.00	0.00
舌	C01-C02	0	0.00	0.00	0.00	0.00	0.00	0	0.00	0.00	0.00	0.00	0.00
口	C03-C06	1	0.30	0.55	0.38	0.00	0.06	2	1.00	1.15	0.70	0.08	0.08
唾液腺	C07-C08	0	0.00	0.00	0.00	0.00	0.00	0	0.00	0.00	0.00	0.00	0.00
扁桃体	C09	0	0.00	0.00	0.00	0.00	0.00	0	0.00	0.00	0.00	0.00	0.00
其他的口咽	C10	0	0.00	0.00	0.00	0.00	0.00	0	0.00	0.00	0.00	0.00	0.00
鼻咽	C11	1	0.30	0.55	0.42	0.05	0.05	0	0.00	0.00	0.00	0.00	0.00
喉咽	C12-C13	0	0.00	0.00	0.00	0.00	0.00	0	0.00	0.00	0.00	0.00	0.00
咽，部位不明	C14	1	0.30	0.55	0.35	0.00	0.00	0	0.00	0.00	0.00	0.00	0.00
食管	C15	55	16.27	30.12	20.91	0.66	2.60	28	13.93	16.11	9.81	0.10	1.23
胃	C16	79	23.37	43.27	29.86	1.07	4.06	29	14.43	16.69	10.28	0.35	1.10
小肠	C17	0	0.00	0.00	0.00	0.00	0.00	1	0.50	0.58	0.37	0.00	0.06
结肠	C18	8	2.37	4.38	2.94	0.00	0.19	6	2.99	3.45	2.17	0.19	0.29
直肠	C19-C20	7	2.07	3.83	2.60	0.00	0.34	10	4.98	5.75	3.57	0.17	0.33
肛门	C21	0	0.00	0.00	0.00	0.00	0.00	0	0.00	0.00	0.00	0.00	0.00
肝脏	C22	36	10.65	19.72	13.75	0.73	1.76	22	10.95	12.66	7.64	0.17	0.87
胆囊及其他	C23-C24	4	1.18	2.19	1.67	0.08	0.19	12	5.97	6.91	4.35	0.09	0.68
胰腺	C25	8	2.37	4.38	3.07	0.09	0.43	9	4.48	5.18	2.81	0.08	0.26
鼻、鼻窦及其他	C30-C31	0	0.00	0.00	0.00	0.00	0.00	0	0.00	0.00	0.00	0.00	0.00
喉	C32	1	0.30	0.55	0.38	0.00	0.06	0	0.00	0.00	0.00	0.00	0.00
气管、支气管、肺	C33-C34	101	29.88	55.32	38.67	1.00	5.05	34	16.92	19.56	11.13	0.31	1.13
其他的胸腔器官	C37-C38	0	0.00	0.00	0.00	0.00	0.00	0	0.00	0.00	0.00	0.00	0.00
骨	C40-C41	4	1.18	2.19	1.56	0.08	0.19	4	1.99	2.30	1.41	0.12	0.12
皮肤的黑色素瘤	C43	1	0.30	0.55	0.44	0.00	0.11	0	0.00	0.00	0.00	0.00	0.00
其他的皮肤	C44	2	0.59	1.10	0.87	0.05	0.05	0	0.00	0.00	0.00	0.00	0.00
间皮瘤	C45	0	0.00	0.00	0.00	0.00	0.00	0	0.00	0.00	0.00	0.00	0.00
卡波西肉瘤	C46	0	0.00	0.00	0.00	0.00	0.00	0	0.00	0.00	0.00	0.00	0.00
周围神经、其他结缔组织、软组织	C47;C49	0	0.00	0.00	0.00	0.00	0.00	0	0.00	0.00	0.00	0.00	0.00
乳房	C50	0	0.00	0.00	0.00	0.00	0.00	8	3.98	4.60	3.03	0.21	0.43
外阴	C51	0	0.00	0.00	0.00	0.00	0.00	0	0.00	0.00	0.00	0.00	0.00
阴道	C52	0	0.00	0.00	0.00	0.00	0.00	0	0.00	0.00	0.00	0.00	0.00
子宫颈	C53	0	0.00	0.00	0.00	0.00	0.00	9	4.48	5.18	3.28	0.03	0.51
子宫体	C54	0	0.00	0.00	0.00	0.00	0.00	3	1.49	1.73	1.03	0.03	0.10
子宫，部位不明	C55	0	0.00	0.00	0.00	0.00	0.00	1	0.50	0.58	0.41	0.05	0.05
卵巢	C56	0	0.00	0.00	0.00	0.00	0.00	3	1.49	1.73	1.05	0.07	0.07
女性其他的生殖器	C57	0	0.00	0.00	0.00	0.00	0.00	0	0.00	0.00	0.00	0.00	0.00
胎盘	C58	0	0.00	0.00	0.00	0.00	0.00	0	0.00	0.00	0.00	0.00	0.00
阴茎	C60	0	0.00	0.00	0.00	0.00	0.00	0	0.00	0.00	0.00	0.00	0.00
前列腺	C61	2	0.59	1.10	0.62	0.00	0.00	0	0.00	0.00	0.00	0.00	0.00
睾丸	C62	0	0.00	0.00	0.00	0.00	0.00	0	0.00	0.00	0.00	0.00	0.00
男性其他的生殖器	C63	0	0.00	0.00	0.00	0.00	0.00	0	0.00	0.00	0.00	0.00	0.00
肾	C64	1	0.30	0.55	0.44	0.00	0.11	3	1.49	1.73	0.93	0.00	0.00
肾盂	C65	0	0.00	0.00	0.00	0.00	0.00	0	0.00	0.00	0.00	0.00	0.00
输尿管	C66	0	0.00	0.00	0.00	0.00	0.00	0	0.00	0.00	0.00	0.00	0.00
膀胱	C67	2	0.59	1.10	0.83	0.00	0.06	1	0.50	0.58	0.37	0.00	0.06
其他的泌尿器官	C68	0	0.00	0.00	0.00	0.00	0.00	0	0.00	0.00	0.00	0.00	0.00
眼	C69	0	0.00	0.00	0.00	0.00	0.00	0	0.00	0.00	0.00	0.00	0.00
脑、神经系统	C70-C72	9	2.66	4.93	4.02	0.20	0.32	6	2.99	3.45	2.21	0.11	0.27
甲状腺	C73	0	0.00	0.00	0.00	0.00	0.00	1	0.50	0.58	0.41	0.05	0.05
肾上腺	C74	0	0.00	0.00	0.00	0.00	0.00	0	0.00	0.00	0.00	0.00	0.00
其他的内分泌腺	C75	0	0.00	0.00	0.00	0.00	0.00	0	0.00	0.00	0.00	0.00	0.00
霍奇金病	C81	1	0.30	0.55	0.44	0.00	0.11	0	0.00	0.00	0.00	0.00	0.00
非霍奇金淋巴瘤	C82-C85;C96	2	0.59	1.10	0.87	0.00	0.22	2	1.00	1.15	0.66	0.03	0.03
免疫增生性疾病	C88	0	0.00	0.00	0.00	0.00	0.00	0	0.00	0.00	0.00	0.00	0.00
多发性骨髓瘤	C90	0	0.00	0.00	0.00	0.00	0.00	0	0.00	0.00	0.00	0.00	0.00
淋巴样白血病	C91	0	0.00	0.00	0.00	0.00	0.00	0	0.00	0.00	0.00	0.00	0.00
髓样白血病	C92-C94	1	0.30	0.55	0.33	0.03	0.03	2	1.00	1.15	0.72	0.03	0.10
白血病，未特指	C95	1	0.30	0.55	0.33	0.03	0.03	1	0.50	0.58	0.31	0.00	0.00
其他的或未指明部位	O&U	9	2.66	4.93	3.54	0.16	0.56	4	1.99	2.30	1.36	0.00	0.12
骨髓增殖性疾病	MPD	0	0.00	0.00	0.00	0.00	0.00	0	0.00	0.00	0.00	0.00	0.00
骨髓增生异常综合征	MDS	0	0.00	0.00	0.00	0.00	0.00	0	0.00	0.00	0.00	0.00	0.00
合计	ALL	338	100.00	185.13	129.72	4.22	16.60	201	100.00	115.66	70.02	2.28	7.95
C44 以外的部位	ALL but C44	336	99.41	184.03	128.85	4.17	16.55	201	100.00	115.66	70.02	2.28	7.95

表 6-87　2020 年河南省三门峡市陕州区恶性肿瘤发病主要指标

部位	ICD-10	男性						女性					
		病例数	构成 (%)	粗率 ($1/10^5$)	世标率 ($1/10^5$)	累积率 (%) 0~64	累积率 (%) 0~74	病例数	构成 (%)	粗率 ($1/10^5$)	世标率 ($1/10^5$)	累积率 (%) 0~64	累积率 (%) 0~74
唇	C00	0	0.00	0.00	0.00	0.00	0.00	0	0.00	0.00	0.00	0.00	0.00
舌	C01–C02	1	0.26	0.54	0.25	0.00	0.00	2	0.49	1.20	0.69	0.04	0.04
口	C03–C06	1	0.26	0.54	0.65	0.04	0.04	0	0.00	0.00	0.00	0.00	0.00
唾液腺	C07–C08	1	0.26	0.54	0.36	0.00	0.06	1	0.24	0.60	0.23	0.00	0.00
扁桃体	C09	0	0.00	0.00	0.00	0.00	0.00	0	0.00	0.00	0.00	0.00	0.00
其他的口咽	C10	1	0.26	0.54	0.35	0.04	0.04	0	0.00	0.00	0.00	0.00	0.00
鼻咽	C11	0	0.00	0.00	0.00	0.00	0.00	0	0.00	0.00	0.00	0.00	0.00
喉咽	C12–C13	0	0.00	0.00	0.00	0.00	0.00	0	0.00	0.00	0.00	0.00	0.00
咽，部位不明	C14	0	0.00	0.00	0.00	0.00	0.00	0	0.00	0.00	0.00	0.00	0.00
食管	C15	45	11.57	24.50	15.72	0.83	1.99	25	6.10	15.01	8.28	0.23	0.98
胃	C16	48	12.34	26.13	16.78	0.59	2.12	26	6.34	15.61	8.30	0.39	0.83
小肠	C17	3	0.77	1.63	1.08	0.04	0.17	1	0.24	0.60	0.63	0.04	0.04
结肠	C18	20	5.14	10.89	6.86	0.29	0.62	9	2.20	5.40	2.95	0.15	0.38
直肠	C19–C20	11	2.83	5.99	3.82	0.22	0.51	15	3.66	9.01	5.21	0.18	0.67
肛门	C21	0	0.00	0.00	0.00	0.00	0.00	0	0.00	0.00	0.00	0.00	0.00
肝脏	C22	30	7.71	16.33	10.64	0.49	0.84	22	5.37	13.21	7.65	0.27	1.02
胆囊及其他	C23–C24	7	1.80	3.81	2.60	0.07	0.24	20	4.88	12.01	7.12	0.28	1.03
胰腺	C25	13	3.34	7.08	4.07	0.14	0.41	6	1.46	3.60	2.33	0.05	0.35
鼻、鼻窦及其他	C30–C31	2	0.51	1.09	0.60	0.04	0.04	1	0.24	0.60	0.31	0.03	0.03
喉	C32	3	0.77	1.63	0.91	0.09	0.09	1	0.24	0.60	0.36	0.00	0.00
气管、支气管、肺	C33–C34	97	24.94	52.80	33.96	1.28	4.72	61	14.88	36.63	20.78	0.98	2.46
其他的胸腔器官	C37–C38	2	0.51	1.09	0.76	0.03	0.09	1	0.24	0.60	0.41	0.00	0.10
骨	C40–C41	2	0.51	1.09	0.84	0.00	0.00	0	0.00	0.00	0.00	0.00	0.00
皮肤的黑色素瘤	C43	0	0.00	0.00	0.00	0.00	0.00	0	0.00	0.00	0.00	0.00	0.00
其他的皮肤	C44	8	2.06	4.35	2.90	0.08	0.31	4	0.98	2.40	1.31	0.00	0.06
间皮瘤	C45	0	0.00	0.00	0.00	0.00	0.00	0	0.00	0.00	0.00	0.00	0.00
卡波西肉瘤	C46	0	0.00	0.00	0.00	0.00	0.00	0	0.00	0.00	0.00	0.00	0.00
周围神经、其他结缔组织、软组织	C47;C49	1	0.26	0.54	0.43	0.00	0.11	1	0.24	0.60	0.39	0.05	0.05
乳房	C50	0	0.00	0.00	0.00	0.00	0.00	59	14.39	35.43	23.25	1.95	2.44
外阴	C51	0	0.00	0.00	0.00	0.00	0.00	0	0.00	0.00	0.00	0.00	0.00
阴道	C52	0	0.00	0.00	0.00	0.00	0.00	0	0.00	0.00	0.00	0.00	0.00
子宫颈	C53	0	0.00	0.00	0.00	0.00	0.00	24	5.85	14.41	9.47	0.69	1.12
子宫体	C54	0	0.00	0.00	0.00	0.00	0.00	25	6.10	15.01	9.07	0.79	1.07
子宫，部位不明	C55	0	0.00	0.00	0.00	0.00	0.00	1	0.24	0.60	0.38	0.03	0.03
卵巢	C56	0	0.00	0.00	0.00	0.00	0.00	17	4.15	10.21	5.84	0.30	0.69
女性其他的生殖器	C57	0	0.00	0.00	0.00	0.00	0.00	0	0.00	0.00	0.00	0.00	0.00
胎盘	C58	0	0.00	0.00	0.00	0.00	0.00	0	0.00	0.00	0.00	0.00	0.00
阴茎	C60	2	0.51	1.09	0.70	0.03	0.13	0	0.00	0.00	0.00	0.00	0.00
前列腺	C61	20	5.14	10.89	7.29	0.13	0.83	0	0.00	0.00	0.00	0.00	0.00
睾丸	C62	0	0.00	0.00	0.00	0.00	0.00	0	0.00	0.00	0.00	0.00	0.00
男性其他的生殖器	C63	0	0.00	0.00	0.00	0.00	0.00	0	0.00	0.00	0.00	0.00	0.00
肾	C64	6	1.54	3.27	1.93	0.22	0.22	5	1.22	3.00	1.86	0.09	0.25
肾盂	C65	0	0.00	0.00	0.00	0.00	0.00	1	0.24	0.60	0.26	0.00	0.00
输尿管	C66	1	0.26	0.54	0.36	0.00	0.06	1	0.24	0.60	0.23	0.00	0.00
膀胱	C67	15	3.86	8.17	4.98	0.31	0.60	2	0.49	1.20	0.77	0.00	0.16
其他的泌尿器官	C68	0	0.00	0.00	0.00	0.00	0.00	1	0.24	0.60	0.36	0.00	0.06
眼	C69	0	0.00	0.00	0.00	0.00	0.00	0	0.00	0.00	0.00	0.00	0.00
脑、神经系统	C70–C72	4	1.03	2.18	1.43	0.03	0.26	9	2.20	5.40	3.26	0.22	0.34
甲状腺	C73	14	3.60	7.62	5.80	0.50	0.56	51	12.44	30.62	20.64	2.01	2.23
肾上腺	C74	0	0.00	0.00	0.00	0.00	0.00	0	0.00	0.00	0.00	0.00	0.00
其他的内分泌腺	C75	0	0.00	0.00	0.00	0.00	0.00	0	0.00	0.00	0.00	0.00	0.00
霍奇金病	C81	0	0.00	0.00	0.00	0.00	0.00	0	0.00	0.00	0.00	0.00	0.00
非霍奇金淋巴瘤	C82–C85;C96	4	1.03	2.18	1.37	0.04	0.04	6	1.46	3.60	2.15	0.14	0.14
免疫增生性疾病	C88	0	0.00	0.00	0.00	0.00	0.00	0	0.00	0.00	0.00	0.00	0.00
多发性骨髓瘤	C90	6	1.54	3.27	2.04	0.14	0.26	3	0.73	1.80	1.18	0.04	0.10
淋巴样白血病	C91	3	0.77	1.63	1.62	0.11	0.11	1	0.24	0.60	0.39	0.05	0.05
髓样白血病	C92–C94	5	1.29	2.72	2.47	0.09	0.31	1	0.24	0.60	0.38	0.03	0.03
白血病，未特指	C95	5	1.29	2.72	3.54	0.23	0.23	2	0.49	1.20	0.94	0.07	0.07
其他的或未指明部位	O&U	7	1.80	3.81	3.81	0.16	0.29	5	1.22	3.00	1.83	0.12	0.18
骨髓增殖性疾病	MPD	1	0.26	0.54	0.52	0.04	0.04	0	0.00	0.00	0.00	0.00	0.00
骨髓增生异常综合征	MDS	0	0.00	0.00	0.00	0.00	0.00	0	0.00	0.00	0.00	0.00	0.00
合计	ALL	389	100.00	211.75	141.45	6.31	16.36	410	100.00	246.20	149.19	9.23	17.01
C44 以外的部位	ALL but C44	381	97.94	207.40	138.55	6.23	16.05	406	99.02	243.80	147.88	9.23	16.95

表 6-88　2020 年河南省三门峡市陕州区恶性肿瘤死亡主要指标

部位	ICD-10	男性						女性					
		病例数	构成 (%)	粗率 ($1/10^5$)	世标率 ($1/10^5$)	累积率 (%)		病例数	构成 (%)	粗率 ($1/10^5$)	世标率 ($1/10^5$)	累积率 (%)	
						0~64	0~74					0~64	0~74
唇	C00	0	0.00	0.00	0.00	0.00	0.00	0	0.00	0.00	0.00	0.00	0.00
舌	C01-C02	2	0.66	1.09	0.88	0.03	0.03	1	0.44	0.60	0.23	0.00	0.00
口	C03-C06	0	0.00	0.00	0.00	0.00	0.00	0	0.00	0.00	0.00	0.00	0.00
唾液腺	C07-C08	0	0.00	0.00	0.00	0.00	0.00	2	0.88	1.20	0.74	0.03	0.09
扁桃体	C09	0	0.00	0.00	0.00	0.00	0.00	0	0.00	0.00	0.00	0.00	0.00
其他的口咽	C10	0	0.00	0.00	0.00	0.00	0.00	0	0.00	0.00	0.00	0.00	0.00
鼻咽	C11	0	0.00	0.00	0.00	0.00	0.00	1	0.44	0.60	0.31	0.03	0.03
喉咽	C12-C13	0	0.00	0.00	0.00	0.00	0.00	0	0.00	0.00	0.00	0.00	0.00
咽，部位不明	C14	1	0.33	0.54	0.25	0.00	0.00	0	0.00	0.00	0.00	0.00	0.00
食管	C15	31	10.26	16.87	10.69	0.35	1.14	22	9.69	13.21	6.92	0.08	0.77
胃	C16	46	15.23	25.04	15.77	0.61	2.22	15	6.61	9.01	5.17	0.26	0.57
小肠	C17	1	0.33	0.54	0.28	0.00	0.00	0	0.00	0.00	0.00	0.00	0.00
结肠	C18	8	2.65	4.35	3.02	0.09	0.31	8	3.52	4.80	2.45	0.05	0.21
直肠	C19-C20	7	2.32	3.81	2.22	0.04	0.21	5	2.20	3.00	1.67	0.06	0.06
肛门	C21	0	0.00	0.00	0.00	0.00	0.00	0	0.00	0.00	0.00	0.00	0.00
肝脏	C22	37	12.25	20.14	13.26	0.60	0.94	30	13.22	18.01	10.24	0.41	1.22
胆囊及其他	C23-C24	6	1.99	3.27	2.29	0.14	0.25	19	8.37	11.41	6.16	0.05	0.76
胰腺	C25	19	6.29	10.34	6.09	0.27	0.51	8	3.52	4.80	3.07	0.00	0.53
鼻、鼻窦及其他	C30-C31	0	0.00	0.00	0.00	0.00	0.00	0	0.00	0.00	0.00	0.00	0.00
喉	C32	2	0.66	1.09	0.78	0.04	0.15	1	0.44	0.60	0.36	0.00	0.00
气管、支气管、肺	C33-C34	94	31.13	51.17	33.87	1.02	4.60	43	18.94	25.82	14.68	0.59	1.75
其他的胸腔器官	C37-C38	1	0.33	0.54	0.25	0.00	0.00	0	0.00	0.00	0.00	0.00	0.00
骨	C40-C41	3	0.99	1.63	1.22	0.08	0.08	2	0.88	1.20	1.09	0.09	0.09
皮肤的黑色素瘤	C43	0	0.00	0.00	0.00	0.00	0.00	0	0.00	0.00	0.00	0.00	0.00
其他的皮肤	C44	1	0.33	0.54	0.28	0.00	0.00	0	0.00	0.00	0.00	0.00	0.00
间皮瘤	C45	0	0.00	0.00	0.00	0.00	0.00	1	0.44	0.60	0.41	0.00	0.10
卡波西肉瘤	C46	0	0.00	0.00	0.00	0.00	0.00	0	0.00	0.00	0.00	0.00	0.00
周围神经、其他结缔组织、软组织	C47;C49	0	0.00	0.00	0.00	0.00	0.00	0	0.00	0.00	0.00	0.00	0.00
乳房	C50	0	0.00	0.00	0.00	0.00	0.00	17	7.49	10.21	5.93	0.51	0.63
外阴	C51	0	0.00	0.00	0.00	0.00	0.00	1	0.44	0.60	0.39	0.05	0.05
阴道	C52	0	0.00	0.00	0.00	0.00	0.00	0	0.00	0.00	0.00	0.00	0.00
子宫颈	C53	0	0.00	0.00	0.00	0.00	0.00	10	4.41	6.00	3.58	0.09	0.36
子宫体	C54	0	0.00	0.00	0.00	0.00	0.00	3	1.32	1.80	1.08	0.03	0.13
子宫，部位不明	C55	0	0.00	0.00	0.00	0.00	0.00	0	0.00	0.00	0.00	0.00	0.00
卵巢	C56	0	0.00	0.00	0.00	0.00	0.00	12	5.29	7.21	3.88	0.11	0.43
女性其他的生殖器	C57	0	0.00	0.00	0.00	0.00	0.00	0	0.00	0.00	0.00	0.00	0.00
胎盘	C58	0	0.00	0.00	0.00	0.00	0.00	0	0.00	0.00	0.00	0.00	0.00
阴茎	C60	1	0.33	0.54	0.27	0.03	0.03	0	0.00	0.00	0.00	0.00	0.00
前列腺	C61	11	3.64	5.99	3.85	0.13	0.19	0	0.00	0.00	0.00	0.00	0.00
睾丸	C62	0	0.00	0.00	0.00	0.00	0.00	0	0.00	0.00	0.00	0.00	0.00
男性其他的生殖器	C63	1	0.33	0.54	0.43	0.00	0.11	0	0.00	0.00	0.00	0.00	0.00
肾	C64	1	0.33	0.54	0.25	0.00	0.00	2	0.88	1.20	0.72	0.00	0.06
肾盂	C65	0	0.00	0.00	0.00	0.00	0.00	0	0.00	0.00	0.00	0.00	0.00
输尿管	C66	0	0.00	0.00	0.00	0.00	0.00	0	0.00	0.00	0.00	0.00	0.00
膀胱	C67	6	1.99	3.27	2.39	0.08	0.14	0	0.00	0.00	0.00	0.00	0.00
其他的泌尿器官	C68	0	0.00	0.00	0.00	0.00	0.00	0	0.00	0.00	0.00	0.00	0.00
眼	C69	0	0.00	0.00	0.00	0.00	0.00	0	0.00	0.00	0.00	0.00	0.00
脑、神经系统	C70-C72	6	1.99	3.27	1.97	0.07	0.23	6	2.64	3.60	1.81	0.09	0.15
甲状腺	C73	2	0.66	1.09	0.80	0.07	0.07	2	0.88	1.20	0.75	0.05	0.11
肾上腺	C74	0	0.00	0.00	0.00	0.00	0.00	0	0.00	0.00	0.00	0.00	0.00
其他的内分泌腺	C75	0	0.00	0.00	0.00	0.00	0.00	0	0.00	0.00	0.00	0.00	0.00
霍奇金病	C81	0	0.00	0.00	0.00	0.00	0.00	0	0.00	0.00	0.00	0.00	0.00
非霍奇金淋巴瘤	C82-C85;C96	2	0.66	1.09	1.08	0.04	0.04	5	2.20	3.00	1.51	0.03	0.13
免疫增生性疾病	C88	0	0.00	0.00	0.00	0.00	0.00	0	0.00	0.00	0.00	0.00	0.00
多发性骨髓瘤	C90	1	0.33	0.54	0.36	0.00	0.06	1	0.44	0.60	0.36	0.00	0.06
淋巴样白血病	C91	0	0.00	0.00	0.00	0.00	0.00	1	0.44	0.60	0.39	0.05	0.05
髓样白血病	C92-C94	2	0.66	1.09	0.88	0.03	0.09	2	0.88	1.20	0.75	0.05	0.11
白血病，未特指	C95	2	0.66	1.09	0.68	0.04	0.10	2	0.88	1.20	0.98	0.04	0.04
其他的或未指明部位	O&U	8	2.65	4.35	3.23	0.04	0.33	5	2.20	3.00	1.67	0.00	0.12
骨髓增殖性疾病	MPD	0	0.00	0.00	0.00	0.00	0.00	0	0.00	0.00	0.00	0.00	0.00
骨髓增生异常综合征	MDS	0	0.00	0.00	0.00	0.00	0.00	0	0.00	0.00	0.00	0.00	0.00
合计	ALL	302	100.00	164.39	107.37	3.83	11.85	227	100.00	136.31	77.29	2.75	8.61
C44 以外的部位	ALL but C44	301	99.67	163.85	107.08	3.83	11.85	227	100.00	136.31	77.29	2.75	8.61

表 6-89　2020 年河南省南召县恶性肿瘤发病主要指标

部位	ICD-10	男性						女性					
		病例数	构成(%)	粗率(1/10^5)	世标率(1/10^5)	累积率(%)		病例数	构成(%)	粗率(1/10^5)	世标率(1/10^5)	累积率(%)	
						0~64	0~74					0~64	0~74
唇	C00	0	0.00	0.00	0.00	0.00	0.00	0	0.00	0.00	0.00	0.00	0.00
舌	C01–C02	2	0.23	0.70	0.65	0.04	0.09	1	0.15	0.37	0.29	0.00	0.07
口	C03–C06	0	0.00	0.00	0.00	0.00	0.00	0	0.00	0.00	0.00	0.00	0.00
唾液腺	C07–C08	2	0.23	0.70	0.65	0.03	0.03	3	0.45	1.10	0.72	0.08	0.08
扁桃体	C09	0	0.00	0.00	0.00	0.00	0.00	1	0.15	0.37	0.33	0.04	0.04
其他的口咽	C10	0	0.00	0.00	0.00	0.00	0.00	0	0.00	0.00	0.00	0.00	0.00
鼻咽	C11	11	1.26	3.83	3.05	0.22	0.34	1	0.15	0.37	0.24	0.03	0.03
喉咽	C12–C13	0	0.00	0.00	0.00	0.00	0.00	2	0.30	0.73	0.39	0.03	0.03
咽，部位不明	C14	0	0.00	0.00	0.00	0.00	0.00	1	0.15	0.37	0.29	0.00	0.07
食管	C15	102	11.67	35.47	28.76	0.84	3.49	40	5.97	14.64	11.28	0.37	1.56
胃	C16	251	28.72	87.29	70.46	3.02	8.96	77	11.49	28.18	20.58	1.10	2.11
小肠	C17	5	0.57	1.74	1.31	0.15	0.15	1	0.15	0.37	0.29	0.00	0.07
结肠	C18	28	3.20	9.74	7.89	0.55	0.93	24	3.58	8.78	6.93	0.35	1.00
直肠	C19–C20	36	4.12	12.52	10.29	0.52	1.25	30	4.48	10.98	7.84	0.46	1.06
肛门	C21	1	0.11	0.35	0.20	0.00	0.00	0	0.00	0.00	0.00	0.00	0.00
肝脏	C22	90	10.30	31.30	25.30	1.52	2.88	33	4.93	12.08	9.46	0.42	1.08
胆囊及其他	C23–C24	2	0.23	0.70	0.71	0.00	0.07	4	0.60	1.46	1.27	0.06	0.18
胰腺	C25	18	2.06	6.26	5.10	0.15	0.59	9	1.34	3.29	2.42	0.15	0.26
鼻、鼻窦及其他	C30–C31	3	0.34	1.04	0.86	0.11	0.11	0	0.00	0.00	0.00	0.00	0.00
喉	C32	5	0.57	1.74	1.43	0.09	0.22	1	0.15	0.37	0.35	0.00	0.06
气管、支气管、肺	C33–C34	168	19.22	58.42	46.79	2.31	5.60	78	11.64	28.55	21.03	0.90	2.57
其他的胸腔器官	C37–C38	4	0.46	1.39	0.97	0.10	0.10	2	0.30	0.73	0.59	0.05	0.05
骨	C40–C41	4	0.46	1.39	1.12	0.08	0.15	4	0.60	1.46	1.53	0.09	0.15
皮肤的黑色素瘤	C43	0	0.00	0.00	0.00	0.00	0.00	0	0.00	0.00	0.00	0.00	0.00
其他的皮肤	C44	2	0.23	0.70	0.54	0.00	0.06	2	0.30	0.73	0.53	0.03	0.10
间皮瘤	C45	0	0.00	0.00	0.00	0.00	0.00	0	0.00	0.00	0.00	0.00	0.00
卡波西肉瘤	C46	0	0.00	0.00	0.00	0.00	0.00	0	0.00	0.00	0.00	0.00	0.00
周围神经、其他结缔组织、软组织	C47;C49	1	0.11	0.35	0.30	0.03	0.03	0	0.00	0.00	0.00	0.00	0.00
乳房	C50	6	0.69	2.09	1.92	0.09	0.15	107	15.97	39.16	30.22	2.52	3.13
外阴	C51	0	0.00	0.00	0.00	0.00	0.00	0	0.00	0.00	0.00	0.00	0.00
阴道	C52	0	0.00	0.00	0.00	0.00	0.00	2	0.30	0.73	0.51	0.04	0.04
子宫颈	C53	0	0.00	0.00	0.00	0.00	0.00	77	11.49	28.18	21.60	1.70	2.52
子宫体	C54	0	0.00	0.00	0.00	0.00	0.00	30	4.48	10.98	8.58	0.70	1.02
子宫，部位不明	C55	0	0.00	0.00	0.00	0.00	0.00	15	2.24	5.49	4.06	0.21	0.56
卵巢	C56	0	0.00	0.00	0.00	0.00	0.00	18	2.69	6.59	5.13	0.38	0.51
女性其他的生殖器	C57	0	0.00	0.00	0.00	0.00	0.00	0	0.00	0.00	0.00	0.00	0.00
胎盘	C58	0	0.00	0.00	0.00	0.00	0.00	0	0.00	0.00	0.00	0.00	0.00
阴茎	C60	4	0.46	1.39	1.09	0.07	0.14	0	0.00	0.00	0.00	0.00	0.00
前列腺	C61	23	2.63	8.00	6.62	0.11	1.01	0	0.00	0.00	0.00	0.00	0.00
睾丸	C62	1	0.11	0.35	0.23	0.02	0.02	0	0.00	0.00	0.00	0.00	0.00
男性其他的生殖器	C63	0	0.00	0.00	0.00	0.00	0.00	0	0.00	0.00	0.00	0.00	0.00
肾	C64	10	1.14	3.48	2.63	0.20	0.27	4	0.60	1.46	1.30	0.09	0.15
肾盂	C65	1	0.11	0.35	0.20	0.00	0.00	0	0.00	0.00	0.00	0.00	0.00
输尿管	C66	0	0.00	0.00	0.00	0.00	0.00	3	0.45	1.10	0.88	0.00	0.12
膀胱	C67	23	2.63	8.00	6.32	0.28	0.75	7	1.04	2.56	1.94	0.06	0.23
其他的泌尿器官	C68	0	0.00	0.00	0.00	0.00	0.00	0	0.00	0.00	0.00	0.00	0.00
眼	C69	0	0.00	0.00	0.00	0.00	0.00	0	0.00	0.00	0.00	0.00	0.00
脑、神经系统	C70–C72	22	2.52	7.65	6.39	0.44	0.66	22	3.28	8.05	6.37	0.44	0.76
甲状腺	C73	11	1.26	3.83	3.41	0.25	0.31	46	6.87	16.84	13.44	1.16	1.27
肾上腺	C74	0	0.00	0.00	0.00	0.00	0.00	0	0.00	0.00	0.00	0.00	0.00
其他的内分泌腺	C75	0	0.00	0.00	0.00	0.00	0.00	0	0.00	0.00	0.00	0.00	0.00
霍奇金病	C81	1	0.11	0.35	0.29	0.00	0.07	1	0.15	0.37	0.24	0.03	0.03
非霍奇金淋巴瘤	C82–C85;C96	12	1.37	4.17	3.42	0.15	0.55	8	1.19	2.93	2.37	0.23	0.23
免疫增生性疾病	C88	0	0.00	0.00	0.00	0.00	0.00	0	0.00	0.00	0.00	0.00	0.00
多发性骨髓瘤	C90	1	0.11	0.35	0.20	0.00	0.00	2	0.30	0.73	0.38	0.00	0.00
淋巴样白血病	C91	1	0.11	0.35	0.23	0.02	0.02	0	0.00	0.00	0.00	0.00	0.00
髓样白血病	C92–C94	5	0.57	1.74	1.46	0.08	0.21	3	0.45	1.10	0.95	0.09	0.09
白血病，未特指	C95	6	0.69	2.09	1.65	0.12	0.17	5	0.75	1.83	1.57	0.06	0.14
其他的或未指明部位	O&U	12	1.37	4.17	3.25	0.10	0.41	6	0.90	2.20	1.69	0.14	0.22
骨髓增殖性疾病	MPD	0	0.00	0.00	0.00	0.00	0.00	0	0.00	0.00	0.00	0.00	0.00
骨髓增生异常综合征	MDS	0	0.00	0.00	0.00	0.00	0.00	0	0.00	0.00	0.00	0.00	0.00
合计	ALL	874	100.00	303.93	245.70	11.68	29.80	670	100.00	245.23	187.58	12.03	21.59
C44 以外的部位	ALL but C44	872	99.77	303.24	245.16	11.68	29.74	668	99.70	244.50	187.05	12.00	21.49

表 6-90 2020 年河南省南召县恶性肿瘤死亡主要指标

部位	ICD-10	男性						女性					
		病例数	构成 (%)	粗率 ($1/10^5$)	世标率 ($1/10^5$)	累积率 (%)		病例数	构成 (%)	粗率 ($1/10^5$)	世标率 ($1/10^5$)	累积率 (%)	
						0~64	0~74					0~64	0~74
唇	C00	0	0.00	0.00	0.00	0.00	0.00	0	0.00	0.00	0.00	0.00	0.00
舌	C01–C02	2	0.31	0.70	0.65	0.04	0.09	0	0.00	0.00	0.00	0.00	0.00
口	C03–C06	0	0.00	0.00	0.00	0.00	0.00	1	0.31	0.37	0.29	0.00	0.07
唾液腺	C07–C08	0	0.00	0.00	0.00	0.00	0.00	1	0.31	0.37	0.32	0.03	0.03
扁桃体	C09	0	0.00	0.00	0.00	0.00	0.00	0	0.00	0.00	0.00	0.00	0.00
其他的口咽	C10	0	0.00	0.00	0.00	0.00	0.00	0	0.00	0.00	0.00	0.00	0.00
鼻咽	C11	3	0.47	1.04	0.84	0.10	0.10	1	0.31	0.37	0.29	0.00	0.07
喉咽	C12–C13	0	0.00	0.00	0.00	0.00	0.00	0	0.00	0.00	0.00	0.00	0.00
咽，部位不明	C14	0	0.00	0.00	0.00	0.00	0.00	1	0.31	0.37	0.29	0.00	0.07
食管	C15	77	11.98	26.78	22.52	0.49	2.29	30	9.35	10.98	7.11	0.33	0.61
胃	C16	213	33.13	74.07	57.65	1.84	6.89	62	19.31	22.69	16.56	0.76	1.67
小肠	C17	0	0.00	0.00	0.00	0.00	0.00	1	0.31	0.37	0.29	0.00	0.07
结肠	C18	9	1.40	3.13	2.64	0.11	0.39	8	2.49	2.93	2.16	0.09	0.30
直肠	C19–C20	27	4.20	9.39	7.42	0.23	0.87	19	5.92	6.95	5.10	0.36	0.63
肛门	C21	0	0.00	0.00	0.00	0.00	0.00	1	0.31	0.37	0.16	0.00	0.00
肝脏	C22	82	12.75	28.52	22.48	1.13	2.64	33	10.28	12.08	8.66	0.43	0.88
胆囊及其他	C23–C24	2	0.31	0.70	0.64	0.00	0.00	5	1.56	1.83	1.46	0.06	0.18
胰腺	C25	13	2.02	4.52	3.45	0.04	0.38	5	1.56	1.83	1.32	0.08	0.14
鼻、鼻窦及其他	C30–C31	1	0.16	0.35	0.31	0.04	0.04	0	0.00	0.00	0.00	0.00	0.00
喉	C32	5	0.78	1.74	1.18	0.03	0.08	0	0.00	0.00	0.00	0.00	0.00
气管、支气管、肺	C33–C34	136	21.15	47.29	39.38	1.73	5.12	64	19.94	23.43	16.21	0.70	1.67
其他的胸腔器官	C37–C38	4	0.62	1.39	1.08	0.05	0.10	1	0.31	0.37	0.29	0.00	0.07
骨	C40–C41	8	1.24	2.78	2.11	0.10	0.10	5	1.56	1.83	1.62	0.12	0.19
皮肤的黑色素瘤	C43	0	0.00	0.00	0.00	0.00	0.00	0	0.00	0.00	0.00	0.00	0.00
其他的皮肤	C44	4	0.62	1.39	1.23	0.07	0.20	2	0.62	0.73	0.48	0.03	0.03
间皮瘤	C45	0	0.00	0.00	0.00	0.00	0.00	0	0.00	0.00	0.00	0.00	0.00
卡波西肉瘤	C46	0	0.00	0.00	0.00	0.00	0.00	0	0.00	0.00	0.00	0.00	0.00
周围神经、其他结缔组织、软组织	C47;C49	0	0.00	0.00	0.00	0.00	0.00	2	0.62	0.73	0.38	0.00	0.00
乳房	C50	1	0.16	0.35	0.21	0.00	0.00	19	5.92	6.95	5.21	0.47	0.61
外阴	C51	0	0.00	0.00	0.00	0.00	0.00	0	0.00	0.00	0.00	0.00	0.00
阴道	C52	0	0.00	0.00	0.00	0.00	0.00	1	0.31	0.37	0.27	0.02	0.02
子宫颈	C53	0	0.00	0.00	0.00	0.00	0.00	15	4.67	5.49	3.95	0.21	0.47
子宫体	C54	0	0.00	0.00	0.00	0.00	0.00	4	1.25	1.46	1.22	0.03	0.22
子宫，部位不明	C55	0	0.00	0.00	0.00	0.00	0.00	4	1.25	1.46	1.03	0.05	0.12
卵巢	C56	0	0.00	0.00	0.00	0.00	0.00	6	1.87	2.20	1.56	0.11	0.26
女性其他的生殖器	C57	0	0.00	0.00	0.00	0.00	0.00	0	0.00	0.00	0.00	0.00	0.00
胎盘	C58	0	0.00	0.00	0.00	0.00	0.00	0	0.00	0.00	0.00	0.00	0.00
阴茎	C60	1	0.16	0.35	0.29	0.00	0.07	0	0.00	0.00	0.00	0.00	0.00
前列腺	C61	9	1.40	3.13	2.93	0.04	0.48	0	0.00	0.00	0.00	0.00	0.00
睾丸	C62	0	0.00	0.00	0.00	0.00	0.00	0	0.00	0.00	0.00	0.00	0.00
男性其他的生殖器	C63	0	0.00	0.00	0.00	0.00	0.00	0	0.00	0.00	0.00	0.00	0.00
肾	C64	7	1.09	2.43	1.85	0.08	0.21	1	0.31	0.37	0.35	0.00	0.06
肾盂	C65	0	0.00	0.00	0.00	0.00	0.00	0	0.00	0.00	0.00	0.00	0.00
输尿管	C66	1	0.16	0.35	0.31	0.04	0.04	0	0.00	0.00	0.00	0.00	0.00
膀胱	C67	7	1.09	2.43	1.78	0.06	0.12	4	1.25	1.46	0.88	0.00	0.06
其他的泌尿器官	C68	0	0.00	0.00	0.00	0.00	0.00	0	0.00	0.00	0.00	0.00	0.00
眼	C69	0	0.00	0.00	0.00	0.00	0.00	0	0.00	0.00	0.00	0.00	0.00
脑、神经系统	C70–C72	9	1.40	3.13	2.78	0.20	0.27	11	3.43	4.03	3.30	0.18	0.43
甲状腺	C73	3	0.47	1.04	0.77	0.02	0.09	2	0.62	0.73	0.58	0.03	0.03
肾上腺	C74	0	0.00	0.00	0.00	0.00	0.00	0	0.00	0.00	0.00	0.00	0.00
其他的内分泌腺	C75	0	0.00	0.00	0.00	0.00	0.00	0	0.00	0.00	0.00	0.00	0.00
霍奇金病	C81	0	0.00	0.00	0.00	0.00	0.00	0	0.00	0.00	0.00	0.00	0.00
非霍奇金淋巴瘤	C82–C85;C96	7	1.09	2.43	1.95	0.10	0.23	3	0.93	1.10	1.01	0.05	0.11
免疫增生性疾病	C88	0	0.00	0.00	0.00	0.00	0.00	0	0.00	0.00	0.00	0.00	0.00
多发性骨髓瘤	C90	0	0.00	0.00	0.00	0.00	0.00	1	0.31	0.37	0.19	0.00	0.00
淋巴样白血病	C91	0	0.00	0.00	0.00	0.00	0.00	0	0.00	0.00	0.00	0.00	0.00
髓样白血病	C92–C94	3	0.47	1.04	0.89	0.06	0.13	1	0.31	0.37	0.57	0.03	0.03
白血病，未特指	C95	1	0.16	0.35	0.39	0.02	0.02	3	0.93	1.10	0.82	0.03	0.17
其他的或未指明部位	O&U	8	1.24	2.78	2.43	0.04	0.40	4	1.25	1.46	0.96	0.05	0.12
骨髓增殖性疾病	MPD	0	0.00	0.00	0.00	0.00	0.00	0	0.00	0.00	0.00	0.00	0.00
骨髓增生异常综合征	MDS	0	0.00	0.00	0.00	0.00	0.00	0	0.00	0.00	0.00	0.00	0.00
合计	ALL	643	100.00	223.60	180.17	6.63	21.35	321	100.00	117.49	84.88	4.24	9.40
C44 以外的部位	ALL but C44	639	99.38	222.21	178.94	6.56	21.15	319	99.38	116.76	84.40	4.21	9.37

表 6-91　2020 年河南省方城县恶性肿瘤发病主要指标

部位	ICD-10	男性						女性					
		病例数	构成(%)	粗率($1/10^5$)	世标率($1/10^5$)	累积率(%)		病例数	构成(%)	粗率($1/10^5$)	世标率($1/10^5$)	累积率(%)	
						0~64	0~74					0~64	0~74
唇	C00	0	0.00	0.00	0.00	0.00	0.00	0	0.00	0.00	0.00	0.00	0.00
舌	C01−C02	3	0.17	0.50	0.36	0.02	0.04	1	0.06	0.19	0.11	0.01	0.01
口	C03−C06	2	0.11	0.33	0.20	0.00	0.00	3	0.17	0.56	0.35	0.04	0.04
唾液腺	C07−C08	3	0.17	0.50	0.36	0.04	0.04	6	0.35	1.12	0.82	0.07	0.10
扁桃体	C09	0	0.00	0.00	0.00	0.00	0.00	0	0.00	0.00	0.00	0.00	0.00
其他的口咽	C10	0	0.00	0.00	0.00	0.00	0.00	2	0.12	0.37	0.28	0.03	0.03
鼻咽	C11	7	0.39	1.17	1.04	0.06	0.13	5	0.29	0.94	0.65	0.05	0.08
喉咽	C12−C13	3	0.17	0.50	0.34	0.00	0.07	2	0.12	0.37	0.21	0.00	0.04
咽，部位不明	C14	2	0.11	0.33	0.25	0.02	0.02	1	0.06	0.19	0.08	0.00	0.00
食管	C15	213	11.99	35.63	24.04	0.98	3.00	86	5.00	16.09	10.35	0.40	1.35
胃	C16	311	17.51	52.02	35.12	1.49	4.41	124	7.21	23.21	14.72	0.63	1.60
小肠	C17	9	0.51	1.51	1.09	0.03	0.17	5	0.29	0.94	0.66	0.03	0.08
结肠	C18	42	2.36	7.03	4.93	0.19	0.67	45	2.62	8.42	5.32	0.40	0.55
直肠	C19−C20	86	4.84	14.38	10.28	0.47	1.46	56	3.26	10.48	7.07	0.37	1.00
肛门	C21	7	0.39	1.17	0.64	0.01	0.03	2	0.12	0.37	0.23	0.00	0.02
肝脏	C22	201	11.32	33.62	23.99	1.52	3.03	92	5.35	17.22	11.03	0.51	1.28
胆囊及其他	C23−C24	26	1.46	4.35	3.03	0.12	0.39	16	0.93	2.99	1.84	0.10	0.20
胰腺	C25	26	1.46	4.35	3.01	0.14	0.39	17	0.99	3.18	2.18	0.07	0.33
鼻、鼻窦及其他	C30−C31	6	0.34	1.00	0.70	0.02	0.08	5	0.29	0.94	0.95	0.06	0.08
喉	C32	13	0.73	2.17	1.54	0.08	0.22	2	0.12	0.37	0.25	0.03	0.03
气管、支气管、肺	C33−C34	427	24.04	71.42	48.86	2.01	6.06	187	10.88	35.00	22.34	1.06	2.57
其他的胸腔器官	C37−C38	13	0.73	2.17	1.47	0.06	0.15	9	0.52	1.68	1.15	0.04	0.14
骨	C40−C41	33	1.86	5.52	5.05	0.33	0.42	26	1.51	4.87	4.17	0.21	0.45
皮肤的黑色素瘤	C43	3	0.17	0.50	0.32	0.01	0.01	0	0.00	0.00	0.00	0.00	0.00
其他的皮肤	C44	17	0.96	2.84	1.82	0.04	0.20	16	0.93	2.99	1.77	0.08	0.18
间皮瘤	C45	1	0.06	0.17	0.14	0.00	0.03	0	0.00	0.00	0.00	0.00	0.00
卡波西肉瘤	C46	0	0.00	0.00	0.00	0.00	0.00	0	0.00	0.00	0.00	0.00	0.00
周围神经、其他结缔组织、软组织	C47;C49	6	0.34	1.00	0.66	0.03	0.05	3	0.17	0.56	0.57	0.03	0.07
乳房	C50	5	0.28	0.84	0.56	0.04	0.08	314	18.27	58.76	42.88	3.61	4.53
外阴	C51	0	0.00	0.00	0.00	0.00	0.00	1	0.06	0.19	0.14	0.01	0.01
阴道	C52	0	0.00	0.00	0.00	0.00	0.00	4	0.23	0.75	0.45	0.03	0.06
子宫颈	C53	0	0.00	0.00	0.00	0.00	0.00	168	9.77	31.44	23.31	1.95	2.34
子宫体	C54	0	0.00	0.00	0.00	0.00	0.00	103	5.99	19.28	13.30	1.17	1.40
子宫，部位不明	C55	0	0.00	0.00	0.00	0.00	0.00	9	0.52	1.68	1.18	0.05	0.15
卵巢	C56	0	0.00	0.00	0.00	0.00	0.00	69	4.01	12.91	10.35	0.76	1.01
女性其他的生殖器	C57	0	0.00	0.00	0.00	0.00	0.00	3	0.17	0.56	0.39	0.05	0.05
胎盘	C58	0	0.00	0.00	0.00	0.00	0.00	0	0.00	0.00	0.00	0.00	0.00
阴茎	C60	5	0.28	0.84	0.51	0.03	0.05	0	0.00	0.00	0.00	0.00	0.00
前列腺	C61	42	2.36	7.03	4.82	0.15	0.60	0	0.00	0.00	0.00	0.00	0.00
睾丸	C62	5	0.28	0.84	0.62	0.06	0.06	0	0.00	0.00	0.00	0.00	0.00
男性其他的生殖器	C63	0	0.00	0.00	0.00	0.00	0.00	0	0.00	0.00	0.00	0.00	0.00
肾	C64	21	1.18	3.51	2.74	0.12	0.41	17	0.99	3.18	2.44	0.15	0.29
肾盂	C65	4	0.23	0.67	0.43	0.04	0.04	3	0.17	0.56	0.41	0.03	0.06
输尿管	C66	1	0.06	0.17	0.11	0.01	0.01	1	0.06	0.19	0.10	0.00	0.00
膀胱	C67	44	2.48	7.36	4.75	0.23	0.51	12	0.70	2.25	1.48	0.07	0.18
其他的泌尿器官	C68	1	0.06	0.17	0.14	0.00	0.03	0	0.00	0.00	0.00	0.00	0.00
眼	C69	0	0.00	0.00	0.00	0.00	0.00	1	0.06	0.19	0.37	0.02	0.02
脑、神经系统	C70−C72	70	3.94	11.71	9.06	0.47	0.93	58	3.37	10.85	7.74	0.54	0.76
甲状腺	C73	41	2.31	6.86	5.49	0.37	0.52	177	10.30	33.12	25.28	1.92	2.60
肾上腺	C74	2	0.11	0.33	0.33	0.01	0.01	1	0.06	0.19	0.10	0.00	0.00
其他的内分泌腺	C75	0	0.00	0.00	0.00	0.00	0.00	0	0.00	0.00	0.00	0.00	0.00
霍奇金病	C81	1	0.06	0.17	0.18	0.01	0.01	2	0.12	0.37	0.34	0.01	0.05
非霍奇金淋巴瘤	C82−C85;C96	15	0.84	2.51	2.44	0.15	0.27	9	0.52	1.68	1.14	0.06	0.15
免疫增生性疾病	C88	0	0.00	0.00	0.00	0.00	0.00	0	0.00	0.00	0.00	0.00	0.00
多发性骨髓瘤	C90	3	0.17	0.50	0.34	0.01	0.03	4	0.23	0.75	0.45	0.04	0.04
淋巴样白血病	C91	4	0.23	0.67	0.70	0.04	0.07	2	0.12	0.37	0.22	0.01	0.01
髓样白血病	C92−C94	12	0.68	2.01	1.65	0.08	0.20	9	0.52	1.68	1.42	0.10	0.13
白血病，未特指	C95	7	0.39	1.17	1.01	0.06	0.10	11	0.64	2.06	1.75	0.09	0.17
其他的或未指明部位	O&U	33	1.86	5.52	4.39	0.21	0.49	30	1.75	5.61	4.03	0.19	0.42
骨髓增殖性疾病	MPD	0	0.00	0.00	0.00	0.00	0.00	0	0.00	0.00	0.00	0.00	0.00
骨髓增生异常综合征	MDS	0	0.00	0.00	0.00	0.00	0.00	0	0.00	0.00	0.00	0.00	0.00
合计	ALL	1 776	100.00	297.06	209.49	9.76	25.51	1 719	100.00	321.70	226.38	15.08	24.66
C44 以外的部位	ALL but C44	1 759	99.04	294.22	207.67	9.73	25.32	1 703	99.07	318.70	224.61	15.00	24.48

表 6-92　2020 年河南省方城县恶性肿瘤死亡主要指标

部位	ICD-10	男性						女性					
		病例数	构成(%)	粗率(1/10^5)	世标率(1/10^5)	累积率(%)		病例数	构成(%)	粗率(1/10^5)	世标率(1/10^5)	累积率(%)	
						0～64	0～74					0～64	0～74
唇	C00	1	0.07	0.17	0.13	0.01	0.01	1	0.12	0.19	0.11	0.01	0.01
舌	C01–C02	0	0.00	0.00	0.00	0.00	0.00	1	0.12	0.19	0.15	0.01	0.01
口	C03–C06	1	0.07	0.17	0.10	0.00	0.00	1	0.12	0.19	0.13	0.02	0.02
唾液腺	C07–C08	0	0.00	0.00	0.00	0.00	0.00	2	0.25	0.37	0.15	0.00	0.00
扁桃体	C09	1	0.07	0.17	0.12	0.00	0.02	0	0.00	0.00	0.00	0.00	0.00
其他的口咽	C10	0	0.00	0.00	0.00	0.00	0.00	2	0.25	0.37	0.28	0.03	0.03
鼻咽	C11	4	0.29	0.67	0.51	0.03	0.10	0	0.00	0.00	0.00	0.00	0.00
喉咽	C12–C13	3	0.21	0.50	0.35	0.00	0.03	1	0.12	0.19	0.06	0.00	0.00
咽，部位不明	C14	4	0.29	0.67	0.42	0.02	0.02	2	0.25	0.37	0.25	0.00	0.02
食管	C15	133	9.53	22.25	14.70	0.20	1.71	55	6.84	10.29	6.14	0.17	0.65
胃	C16	273	19.56	45.66	30.50	0.96	3.66	108	13.43	20.21	12.31	0.48	1.33
小肠	C17	3	0.21	0.50	0.40	0.00	0.09	5	0.62	0.94	0.64	0.00	0.10
结肠	C18	17	1.22	2.84	1.86	0.10	0.23	23	2.86	4.30	2.53	0.10	0.21
直肠	C19–C20	38	2.72	6.36	4.49	0.13	0.65	32	3.98	5.99	3.72	0.14	0.44
肛门	C21	43	3.08	7.19	4.45	0.14	0.37	15	1.87	2.81	1.57	0.04	0.17
肝脏	C22	207	14.83	34.62	24.10	1.23	2.97	86	10.70	16.09	9.91	0.32	1.18
胆囊及其他	C23–C24	6	0.43	1.00	0.65	0.01	0.03	27	3.36	5.05	2.94	0.10	0.30
胰腺	C25	31	2.22	5.19	3.49	0.12	0.46	15	1.87	2.81	1.77	0.07	0.21
鼻、鼻窦及其他	C30–C31	3	0.21	0.50	0.34	0.02	0.02	3	0.37	0.56	0.38	0.01	0.04
喉	C32	13	0.93	2.17	1.43	0.04	0.18	0	0.00	0.00	0.00	0.00	0.00
气管、支气管、肺	C33–C34	413	29.58	69.08	46.38	1.42	5.66	168	20.90	31.44	19.62	0.64	2.47
其他的胸腔器官	C37–C38	8	0.57	1.34	0.90	0.04	0.11	6	0.75	1.12	0.71	0.03	0.05
骨	C40–C41	10	0.72	1.67	1.18	0.05	0.12	11	1.37	2.06	1.36	0.09	0.18
皮肤的黑色素瘤	C43	0	0.00	0.00	0.00	0.00	0.00	0	0.00	0.00	0.00	0.00	0.00
其他的皮肤	C44	7	0.50	1.17	0.78	0.03	0.10	4	0.50	0.75	0.48	0.01	0.04
间皮瘤	C45	0	0.00	0.00	0.00	0.00	0.00	0	0.00	0.00	0.00	0.00	0.00
卡波西肉瘤	C46	0	0.00	0.00	0.00	0.00	0.00	0	0.00	0.00	0.00	0.00	0.00
周围神经、其他结缔组织、软组织	C47;C49	1	0.07	0.17	0.12	0.01	0.01	3	0.37	0.56	0.36	0.01	0.05
乳房	C50	1	0.07	0.17	0.12	0.00	0.02	46	5.72	8.61	6.06	0.32	0.82
外阴	C51	0	0.00	0.00	0.00	0.00	0.00	0	0.00	0.00	0.00	0.00	0.00
阴道	C52	0	0.00	0.00	0.00	0.00	0.00	1	0.12	0.19	0.11	0.01	0.01
子宫颈	C53	0	0.00	0.00	0.00	0.00	0.00	33	4.10	6.18	4.00	0.29	0.45
子宫体	C54	0	0.00	0.00	0.00	0.00	0.00	23	2.86	4.30	2.80	0.19	0.31
子宫，部位不明	C55	0	0.00	0.00	0.00	0.00	0.00	3	0.37	0.56	0.39	0.04	0.04
卵巢	C56	0	0.00	0.00	0.00	0.00	0.00	21	2.61	3.93	2.79	0.17	0.31
女性其他的生殖器	C57	0	0.00	0.00	0.00	0.00	0.00	1	0.12	0.19	0.11	0.01	0.01
胎盘	C58	0	0.00	0.00	0.00	0.00	0.00	0	0.00	0.00	0.00	0.00	0.00
阴茎	C60	1	0.07	0.17	0.14	0.00	0.03	0	0.00	0.00	0.00	0.00	0.00
前列腺	C61	17	1.22	2.84	2.06	0.03	0.32	0	0.00	0.00	0.00	0.00	0.00
睾丸	C62	1	0.07	0.17	0.12	0.01	0.01	0	0.00	0.00	0.00	0.00	0.00
男性其他的生殖器	C63	0	0.00	0.00	0.00	0.00	0.00	0	0.00	0.00	0.00	0.00	0.00
肾	C64	11	0.79	1.84	1.37	0.06	0.21	5	0.62	0.94	0.65	0.03	0.09
肾盂	C65	3	0.21	0.50	0.37	0.02	0.06	0	0.00	0.00	0.00	0.00	0.00
输尿管	C66	0	0.00	0.00	0.00	0.00	0.00	0	0.00	0.00	0.00	0.00	0.00
膀胱	C67	19	1.36	3.18	2.02	0.05	0.18	1	0.12	0.19	0.15	0.00	0.02
其他的泌尿器官	C68	0	0.00	0.00	0.00	0.00	0.00	1	0.12	0.19	0.15	0.00	0.02
眼	C69	0	0.00	0.00	0.00	0.00	0.00	0	0.00	0.00	0.00	0.00	0.00
脑、神经系统	C70–C72	43	3.08	7.19	5.46	0.25	0.49	27	3.36	5.05	3.55	0.16	0.34
甲状腺	C73	3	0.21	0.50	0.32	0.00	0.00	3	0.37	0.56	0.40	0.01	0.05
肾上腺	C74	3	0.21	0.50	0.35	0.02	0.02	1	0.12	0.19	0.10	0.00	0.00
其他的内分泌腺	C75	0	0.00	0.00	0.00	0.00	0.00	0	0.00	0.00	0.00	0.00	0.00
霍奇金病	C81	6	0.43	1.00	0.74	0.01	0.07	13	1.62	2.43	1.61	0.07	0.15
非霍奇金淋巴瘤	C82–C85;C96	19	1.36	3.18	2.43	0.06	0.31	9	1.12	1.68	1.01	0.03	0.12
免疫增生性疾病	C88	0	0.00	0.00	0.00	0.00	0.00	0	0.00	0.00	0.00	0.00	0.00
多发性骨髓瘤	C90	5	0.36	0.84	0.61	0.03	0.05	6	0.75	1.12	0.75	0.04	0.10
淋巴样白血病	C91	5	0.36	0.84	0.87	0.03	0.10	2	0.25	0.37	0.22	0.01	0.01
髓样白血病	C92–C94	8	0.57	1.34	1.20	0.06	0.13	5	0.62	0.94	0.69	0.04	0.12
白血病，未特指	C95	5	0.36	0.84	0.59	0.03	0.09	7	0.87	1.31	1.16	0.03	0.09
其他的或未指明部位	O&U	26	1.86	4.35	3.06	0.15	0.37	23	2.86	4.30	2.51	0.07	0.31
骨髓增殖性疾病	MPD	0	0.00	0.00	0.00	0.00	0.00	2	0.25	0.37	0.35	0.02	0.02
骨髓增生异常综合征	MDS	0	0.00	0.00	0.00	0.00	0.00	0	0.00	0.00	0.00	0.00	0.00
合计	ALL	1 396	100.00	233.50	159.21	5.39	19.04	804	100.00	150.46	95.14	3.84	10.90
C44 以外的部位	ALL but C44	1 389	99.50	232.33	158.44	5.36	18.94	800	99.50	149.71	94.66	3.83	10.86

表 6-93　2020 年河南省镇平县恶性肿瘤发病主要指标

部位	ICD-10	男性						女性					
		病例数	构成 (%)	粗率 ($1/10^5$)	世标率 ($1/10^5$)	累积率 (%)		病例数	构成 (%)	粗率 ($1/10^5$)	世标率 ($1/10^5$)	累积率 (%)	
						0～64	0～74					0～64	0～74
唇	C00	2	0.14	0.42	0.22	0.00	0.03	0	0.00	0.00	0.00	0.00	0.00
舌	C01–C02	1	0.07	0.21	0.12	0.00	0.03	0	0.00	0.00	0.00	0.00	0.00
口	C03–C06	5	0.35	1.04	0.68	0.04	0.08	2	0.18	0.46	0.25	0.01	0.03
唾液腺	C07–C08	2	0.14	0.42	0.31	0.03	0.03	0	0.00	0.00	0.00	0.00	0.00
扁桃体	C09	0	0.00	0.00	0.00	0.00	0.00	0	0.00	0.00	0.00	0.00	0.00
其他的口咽	C10	0	0.00	0.00	0.00	0.00	0.00	0	0.00	0.00	0.00	0.00	0.00
鼻咽	C11	6	0.42	1.25	0.82	0.07	0.09	4	0.36	0.92	0.44	0.03	0.03
喉咽	C12–C13	5	0.35	1.04	0.79	0.04	0.04	1	0.09	0.23	0.10	0.00	0.00
咽，部位不明	C14	0	0.00	0.00	0.00	0.00	0.00	0	0.00	0.00	0.00	0.00	0.00
食管	C15	260	18.13	54.15	34.82	1.64	4.27	118	10.77	27.01	14.56	0.73	1.71
胃	C16	283	19.74	58.94	37.63	1.85	4.59	93	8.49	21.29	11.82	0.57	1.45
小肠	C17	7	0.49	1.46	0.98	0.04	0.12	8	0.73	1.83	1.20	0.11	0.11
结肠	C18	43	3.00	8.96	5.96	0.30	0.69	44	4.01	10.07	5.54	0.34	0.58
直肠	C19–C20	69	4.81	14.37	9.43	0.53	1.15	46	4.20	10.53	6.07	0.36	0.73
肛门	C21	1	0.07	0.21	0.13	0.01	0.01	1	0.09	0.23	0.10	0.01	0.01
肝脏	C22	144	10.04	29.99	21.29	1.54	2.33	59	5.38	13.51	7.53	0.46	0.81
胆囊及其他	C23–C24	15	1.05	3.12	1.94	0.07	0.23	14	1.28	3.21	1.46	0.02	0.11
胰腺	C25	9	0.63	1.87	1.11	0.04	0.20	7	0.64	1.60	0.82	0.06	0.08
鼻、鼻窦及其他	C30–C31	4	0.28	0.83	0.80	0.07	0.07	0	0.00	0.00	0.00	0.00	0.00
喉	C32	17	1.19	3.54	2.45	0.20	0.33	1	0.09	0.23	0.10	0.00	0.00
气管、支气管、肺	C33–C34	329	22.94	68.52	46.62	2.96	5.97	141	12.86	32.28	18.35	1.13	2.08
其他的胸腔器官	C37–C38	5	0.35	1.04	1.17	0.08	0.08	2	0.18	0.46	0.21	0.00	0.02
骨	C40–C41	11	0.77	2.29	1.57	0.10	0.20	9	0.82	2.06	1.30	0.07	0.13
皮肤的黑色素瘤	C43	1	0.07	0.21	0.10	0.00	0.00	3	0.27	0.69	0.46	0.04	0.07
其他的皮肤	C44	8	0.56	1.67	1.01	0.01	0.10	7	0.64	1.60	1.10	0.05	0.16
间皮瘤	C45	1	0.07	0.21	0.12	0.00	0.03	0	0.00	0.00	0.00	0.00	0.00
卡波西肉瘤	C46	0	0.00	0.00	0.00	0.00	0.00	0	0.00	0.00	0.00	0.00	0.00
周围神经、其他结缔组织、软组织	C47;C49	2	0.14	0.42	0.25	0.01	0.04	0	0.00	0.00	0.00	0.00	0.00
乳房	C50	3	0.21	0.62	0.39	0.03	0.05	198	18.07	45.33	30.72	2.48	3.32
外阴	C51	0	0.00	0.00	0.00	0.00	0.00	2	0.18	0.46	0.74	0.04	0.07
阴道	C52	0	0.00	0.00	0.00	0.00	0.00	0	0.00	0.00	0.00	0.00	0.00
子宫颈	C53	0	0.00	0.00	0.00	0.00	0.00	67	6.11	15.34	11.72	0.92	1.16
子宫体	C54	0	0.00	0.00	0.00	0.00	0.00	85	7.76	19.46	12.04	1.03	1.35
子宫，部位不明	C55	0	0.00	0.00	0.00	0.00	0.00	3	0.27	0.69	0.44	0.03	0.06
卵巢	C56	0	0.00	0.00	0.00	0.00	0.00	22	2.01	5.04	3.46	0.26	0.34
女性其他的生殖器	C57	0	0.00	0.00	0.00	0.00	0.00	1	0.09	0.23	0.12	0.00	0.02
胎盘	C58	0	0.00	0.00	0.00	0.00	0.00	0	0.00	0.00	0.00	0.00	0.00
阴茎	C60	3	0.21	0.62	0.35	0.00	0.05	0	0.00	0.00	0.00	0.00	0.00
前列腺	C61	30	2.09	6.25	3.90	0.13	0.39	0	0.00	0.00	0.00	0.00	0.00
睾丸	C62	1	0.07	0.21	0.19	0.02	0.02	0	0.00	0.00	0.00	0.00	0.00
男性其他的生殖器	C63	0	0.00	0.00	0.00	0.00	0.00	0	0.00	0.00	0.00	0.00	0.00
肾	C64	9	0.63	1.87	1.48	0.13	0.15	7	0.64	1.60	0.87	0.05	0.11
肾盂	C65	1	0.07	0.21	0.10	0.00	0.00	0	0.00	0.00	0.00	0.00	0.00
输尿管	C66	1	0.07	0.21	0.13	0.01	0.01	2	0.18	0.46	0.23	0.00	0.03
膀胱	C67	25	1.74	5.21	3.45	0.15	0.44	7	0.64	1.60	0.79	0.03	0.08
其他的泌尿器官	C68	1	0.07	0.21	0.13	0.00	0.02	0	0.00	0.00	0.00	0.00	0.00
眼	C69	0	0.00	0.00	0.00	0.00	0.00	0	0.00	0.00	0.00	0.00	0.00
脑、神经系统	C70–C72	29	2.02	6.04	5.01	0.37	0.50	32	2.92	7.33	4.76	0.39	0.57
甲状腺	C73	20	1.39	4.17	3.06	0.27	0.31	60	5.47	13.74	10.65	0.92	1.00
肾上腺	C74	1	0.07	0.21	0.13	0.00	0.02	1	0.09	0.23	0.10	0.01	0.01
其他的内分泌腺	C75	1	0.07	0.21	0.10	0.00	0.00	0	0.00	0.00	0.00	0.00	0.00
霍奇金病	C81	0	0.00	0.00	0.00	0.00	0.00	1	0.09	0.23	0.13	0.00	0.03
非霍奇金淋巴瘤	C82–C85;C96	16	1.12	3.33	3.34	0.25	0.33	11	1.00	2.52	1.50	0.10	0.12
免疫增生性疾病	C88	0	0.00	0.00	0.00	0.00	0.00	0	0.00	0.00	0.00	0.00	0.00
多发性骨髓瘤	C90	1	0.07	0.21	0.12	0.00	0.03	1	0.09	0.23	0.20	0.03	0.03
淋巴样白血病	C91	2	0.14	0.42	0.32	0.02	0.04	1	0.09	0.23	0.10	0.01	0.01
髓样白血病	C92–C94	7	0.49	1.46	0.94	0.07	0.12	3	0.27	0.69	0.44	0.03	0.05
白血病，未特指	C95	6	0.42	1.25	1.84	0.12	0.14	6	0.55	1.37	0.92	0.06	0.08
其他的或未指明部位	O&U	44	3.07	9.16	6.60	0.41	0.67	25	2.28	5.72	4.42	0.21	0.41
骨髓增殖性疾病	MPD	3	0.21	0.62	0.48	0.04	0.04	1	0.09	0.23	0.20	0.03	0.03
骨髓增生异常综合征	MDS	0	0.00	0.00	0.00	0.00	0.00	0	0.00	0.00	0.00	0.00	0.00
合计	ALL	1 434	100.00	298.65	202.36	11.63	24.05	1 096	100.00	250.92	155.94	10.60	16.98
C44 以外的部位	ALL but C44	1 426	99.44	296.99	201.35	11.62	23.95	1 089	99.36	249.31	154.84	10.55	16.82

表 6-94　2020 年河南省镇平县恶性肿瘤死亡主要指标

部位	ICD-10	男性						女性					
		病例数	构成(%)	粗率($1/10^5$)	世标率($1/10^5$)	累积率(%) 0~64	累积率(%) 0~74	病例数	构成(%)	粗率($1/10^5$)	世标率($1/10^5$)	累积率(%) 0~64	累积率(%) 0~74
唇	C00	1	0.09	0.21	0.19	0.02	0.02	0	0.00	0.00	0.00	0.00	0.00
舌	C01–C02	1	0.09	0.21	0.13	0.00	0.02	0	0.00	0.00	0.00	0.00	0.00
口	C03–C06	2	0.18	0.42	0.20	0.00	0.00	1	0.17	0.23	0.12	0.00	0.02
唾液腺	C07–C08	2	0.18	0.42	0.40	0.04	0.04	0	0.00	0.00	0.00	0.00	0.00
扁桃体	C09	2	0.18	0.42	0.26	0.01	0.03	0	0.00	0.00	0.00	0.00	0.00
其他的口咽	C10	0	0.00	0.00	0.00	0.00	0.00	0	0.00	0.00	0.00	0.00	0.00
鼻咽	C11	3	0.26	0.62	0.44	0.04	0.04	4	0.66	0.92	0.51	0.04	0.04
喉咽	C12–C13	3	0.26	0.62	0.40	0.01	0.01	0	0.00	0.00	0.00	0.00	0.00
咽，部位不明	C14	0	0.00	0.00	0.00	0.00	0.00	0	0.00	0.00	0.00	0.00	0.00
食管	C15	191	16.78	39.78	24.59	0.85	2.97	92	15.28	21.06	10.90	0.50	1.18
胃	C16	280	24.60	58.31	36.80	1.64	4.22	99	16.45	22.66	12.05	0.60	1.32
小肠	C17	4	0.35	0.83	0.46	0.03	0.05	2	0.33	0.46	0.30	0.04	0.04
结肠	C18	18	1.58	3.75	2.20	0.12	0.29	23	3.82	5.27	2.69	0.11	0.35
直肠	C19–C20	30	2.64	6.25	4.09	0.17	0.40	16	2.66	3.66	1.88	0.06	0.21
肛门	C21	1	0.09	0.21	0.12	0.01	0.01	1	0.17	0.23	0.10	0.01	0.01
肝脏	C22	155	13.62	32.28	21.46	1.23	2.36	78	12.96	17.86	9.29	0.35	1.06
胆囊及其他	C23–C24	13	1.14	2.71	1.54	0.03	0.18	8	1.33	1.83	1.04	0.04	0.12
胰腺	C25	8	0.70	1.67	0.93	0.04	0.11	9	1.50	2.06	1.23	0.08	0.16
鼻、鼻窦及其他	C30–C31	1	0.09	0.21	0.13	0.01	0.01	1	0.17	0.23	0.10	0.00	0.00
喉	C32	2	0.18	0.42	0.26	0.00	0.00	1	0.17	0.23	0.12	0.00	0.02
气管、支气管、肺	C33–C34	287	25.22	59.77	38.97	2.09	4.84	108	17.94	24.73	13.97	0.74	1.39
其他的胸腔器官	C37–C38	4	0.35	0.83	0.61	0.05	0.05	4	0.66	0.92	0.38	0.01	0.03
骨	C40–C41	13	1.14	2.71	1.65	0.05	0.23	3	0.50	0.69	0.30	0.00	0.02
皮肤的黑色素瘤	C43	1	0.09	0.21	0.12	0.01	0.01	0	0.00	0.00	0.00	0.00	0.00
其他的皮肤	C44	4	0.35	0.83	0.55	0.01	0.06	1	0.17	0.23	0.07	0.00	0.00
间皮瘤	C45	0	0.00	0.00	0.00	0.00	0.00	0	0.00	0.00	0.00	0.00	0.00
卡波西肉瘤	C46	0	0.00	0.00	0.00	0.00	0.00	0	0.00	0.00	0.00	0.00	0.00
周围神经、其他结缔组织、软组织	C47;C49	1	0.09	0.21	0.17	0.01	0.01	1	0.17	0.23	0.13	0.01	0.01
乳房	C50	0	0.00	0.00	0.00	0.00	0.00	63	10.47	14.42	9.15	0.80	1.04
外阴	C51	0	0.00	0.00	0.00	0.00	0.00	0	0.00	0.00	0.00	0.00	0.00
阴道	C52	0	0.00	0.00	0.00	0.00	0.00	0	0.00	0.00	0.00	0.00	0.00
子宫颈	C53	0	0.00	0.00	0.00	0.00	0.00	21	3.49	4.81	3.06	0.24	0.39
子宫体	C54	0	0.00	0.00	0.00	0.00	0.00	6	1.00	1.37	0.67	0.04	0.08
子宫，部位不明	C55	0	0.00	0.00	0.00	0.00	0.00	7	1.16	1.60	0.91	0.05	0.14
卵巢	C56	0	0.00	0.00	0.00	0.00	0.00	8	1.33	1.83	1.12	0.11	0.11
女性其他的生殖器	C57	0	0.00	0.00	0.00	0.00	0.00	0	0.00	0.00	0.00	0.00	0.00
胎盘	C58	0	0.00	0.00	0.00	0.00	0.00	0	0.00	0.00	0.00	0.00	0.00
阴茎	C60	0	0.00	0.00	0.00	0.00	0.00	0	0.00	0.00	0.00	0.00	0.00
前列腺	C61	9	0.79	1.87	1.16	0.00	0.08	0	0.00	0.00	0.00	0.00	0.00
睾丸	C62	0	0.00	0.00	0.00	0.00	0.00	0	0.00	0.00	0.00	0.00	0.00
男性其他的生殖器	C63	0	0.00	0.00	0.00	0.00	0.00	0	0.00	0.00	0.00	0.00	0.00
肾	C64	2	0.18	0.42	0.34	0.03	0.05	1	0.17	0.23	0.12	0.00	0.02
肾盂	C65	0	0.00	0.00	0.00	0.00	0.00	1	0.17	0.23	0.09	0.00	0.00
输尿管	C66	0	0.00	0.00	0.00	0.00	0.00	0	0.00	0.00	0.00	0.00	0.00
膀胱	C67	9	0.79	1.87	1.16	0.03	0.14	3	0.50	0.69	0.28	0.00	0.00
其他的泌尿器官	C68	0	0.00	0.00	0.00	0.00	0.00	0	0.00	0.00	0.00	0.00	0.00
眼	C69	0	0.00	0.00	0.00	0.00	0.00	1	0.17	0.23	0.20	0.03	0.03
脑、神经系统	C70–C72	26	2.28	5.41	4.17	0.29	0.42	9	1.50	2.06	0.97	0.01	0.12
甲状腺	C73	2	0.18	0.42	0.25	0.01	0.04	2	0.33	0.46	0.20	0.01	0.01
肾上腺	C74	1	0.09	0.21	0.13	0.00	0.02	0	0.00	0.00	0.00	0.00	0.00
其他的内分泌腺	C75	0	0.00	0.00	0.00	0.00	0.00	0	0.00	0.00	0.00	0.00	0.00
霍奇金病	C81	0	0.00	0.00	0.00	0.00	0.00	1	0.17	0.23	0.13	0.00	0.03
非霍奇金淋巴瘤	C82–C85;C96	9	0.79	1.87	1.24	0.08	0.19	4	0.66	0.92	0.56	0.02	0.08
免疫增生性疾病	C88	0	0.00	0.00	0.00	0.00	0.00	0	0.00	0.00	0.00	0.00	0.00
多发性骨髓瘤	C90	1	0.09	0.21	0.12	0.00	0.03	0	0.00	0.00	0.00	0.00	0.00
淋巴样白血病	C91	2	0.18	0.42	0.25	0.00	0.04	0	0.00	0.00	0.00	0.00	0.00
髓样白血病	C92–C94	0	0.00	0.00	0.00	0.00	0.00	1	0.17	0.23	0.12	0.00	0.02
白血病，未特指	C95	8	0.70	1.67	1.62	0.10	0.14	2	0.33	0.46	0.31	0.02	0.02
其他的或未指明部位	O&U	41	3.60	8.54	5.47	0.30	0.55	19	3.16	4.35	2.50	0.14	0.31
骨髓增殖性疾病	MPD	1	0.09	0.21	0.28	0.02	0.02	0	0.00	0.00	0.00	0.00	0.00
骨髓增生异常综合征	MDS	0	0.00	0.00	0.00	0.00	0.00	1	0.17	0.23	0.10	0.01	0.01
合计	ALL	1 138	100.00	237.01	152.85	7.35	17.69	602	100.00	137.82	75.67	4.08	8.38
C44 以外的部位	ALL but C44	1 134	99.65	236.17	152.29	7.34	17.63	601	99.83	137.59	75.60	4.08	8.38

表 6-95　2020 年河南省内乡县恶性肿瘤发病主要指标

部位	ICD-10	男性						女性					
		病例数	构成(%)	粗率(1/10^5)	世标率(1/10^5)	累积率(%) 0~64	累积率(%) 0~74	病例数	构成(%)	粗率(1/10^5)	世标率(1/10^5)	累积率(%) 0~64	累积率(%) 0~74
唇	C00	1	0.08	0.27	0.16	0.02	0.02	1	0.11	0.28	0.17	0.00	0.03
舌	C01–C02	4	0.34	1.08	0.88	0.07	0.07	1	0.11	0.28	0.14	0.00	0.00
口	C03–C06	5	0.42	1.35	0.91	0.04	0.14	1	0.11	0.28	0.28	0.02	0.02
唾液腺	C07–C08	3	0.25	0.81	0.62	0.06	0.06	0	0.00	0.00	0.00	0.00	0.00
扁桃体	C09	1	0.08	0.27	0.18	0.00	0.00	0	0.00	0.00	0.00	0.00	0.00
其他的口咽	C10	2	0.17	0.54	0.42	0.00	0.00	1	0.11	0.28	0.25	0.03	0.03
鼻咽	C11	5	0.42	1.35	0.92	0.05	0.11	3	0.34	0.85	0.51	0.06	0.06
喉咽	C12–C13	4	0.34	1.08	0.68	0.02	0.02	1	0.11	0.28	0.11	0.00	0.00
咽，部位不明	C14	3	0.25	0.81	0.52	0.02	0.05	1	0.11	0.28	0.27	0.02	0.02
食管	C15	247	20.91	66.60	47.05	1.93	5.75	131	14.77	37.09	21.34	0.88	2.40
胃	C16	276	23.37	74.42	51.58	2.64	6.61	88	9.92	24.91	15.15	0.78	1.76
小肠	C17	6	0.51	1.62	1.09	0.08	0.16	3	0.34	0.85	0.55	0.05	0.05
结肠	C18	43	3.64	11.60	8.12	0.44	1.00	30	3.38	8.49	5.12	0.31	0.50
直肠	C19–C20	42	3.56	11.33	8.28	0.57	0.82	34	3.83	9.63	6.57	0.44	0.72
肛门	C21	4	0.34	1.08	0.70	0.00	0.09	1	0.11	0.28	0.12	0.00	0.00
肝脏	C22	87	7.37	23.46	17.35	1.13	2.11	41	4.62	11.61	7.29	0.39	0.95
胆囊及其他	C23–C24	8	0.68	2.16	1.41	0.05	0.05	8	0.90	2.26	1.48	0.10	0.20
胰腺	C25	10	0.85	2.70	1.77	0.09	0.20	15	1.69	4.25	2.91	0.23	0.34
鼻、鼻窦及其他	C30–C31	4	0.34	1.08	0.77	0.03	0.11	0	0.00	0.00	0.00	0.00	0.00
喉	C32	11	0.93	2.97	2.05	0.15	0.18	5	0.56	1.42	0.84	0.02	0.04
气管、支气管、肺	C33–C34	256	21.68	69.03	49.05	2.72	6.28	119	13.42	33.69	22.82	1.49	2.62
其他的胸腔器官	C37–C38	6	0.51	1.62	1.22	0.08	0.13	6	0.68	1.70	1.17	0.11	0.11
骨	C40–C41	5	0.42	1.35	1.13	0.10	0.10	6	0.68	1.70	1.18	0.07	0.10
皮肤的黑色素瘤	C43	2	0.17	0.54	0.43	0.00	0.05	3	0.34	0.85	0.56	0.03	0.06
其他的皮肤	C44	6	0.51	1.62	1.13	0.02	0.17	4	0.45	1.13	0.55	0.00	0.03
间皮瘤	C45	9	0.76	2.43	1.64	0.14	0.17	4	0.45	1.13	0.82	0.09	0.09
卡波西肉瘤	C46	0	0.00	0.00	0.00	0.00	0.00	0	0.00	0.00	0.00	0.00	0.00
周围神经、其他结缔组织、软组织	C47;C49	3	0.25	0.81	0.58	0.00	0.00	2	0.23	0.57	0.65	0.04	0.04
乳房	C50	1	0.08	0.27	0.16	0.02	0.02	140	15.78	39.63	30.47	2.52	3.35
外阴	C51	0	0.00	0.00	0.00	0.00	0.00	4	0.45	1.13	0.80	0.04	0.11
阴道	C52	0	0.00	0.00	0.00	0.00	0.00	2	0.23	0.57	0.36	0.03	0.03
子宫颈	C53	0	0.00	0.00	0.00	0.00	0.00	44	4.96	12.46	9.84	0.80	0.99
子宫体	C54	0	0.00	0.00	0.00	0.00	0.00	28	3.16	7.93	5.19	0.41	0.68
子宫，部位不明	C55	0	0.00	0.00	0.00	0.00	0.00	5	0.56	1.42	0.96	0.10	0.10
卵巢	C56	0	0.00	0.00	0.00	0.00	0.00	17	1.92	4.81	3.56	0.33	0.41
女性其他的生殖器	C57	0	0.00	0.00	0.00	0.00	0.00	0	0.00	0.00	0.00	0.00	0.00
胎盘	C58	0	0.00	0.00	0.00	0.00	0.00	1	0.11	0.28	0.16	0.02	0.02
阴茎	C60	2	0.17	0.54	0.41	0.04	0.04	0	0.00	0.00	0.00	0.00	0.00
前列腺	C61	13	1.10	3.51	2.43	0.11	0.21	0	0.00	0.00	0.00	0.00	0.00
睾丸	C62	0	0.00	0.00	0.00	0.00	0.00	0	0.00	0.00	0.00	0.00	0.00
男性其他的生殖器	C63	1	0.08	0.27	0.24	0.00	0.00	0	0.00	0.00	0.00	0.00	0.00
肾	C64	7	0.59	1.89	1.42	0.06	0.20	5	0.56	1.42	1.03	0.09	0.09
肾盂	C65	3	0.25	0.81	0.57	0.04	0.04	2	0.23	0.57	0.34	0.00	0.06
输尿管	C66	2	0.17	0.54	0.34	0.02	0.05	1	0.11	0.28	0.16	0.02	0.02
膀胱	C67	14	1.19	3.78	2.88	0.18	0.26	3	0.34	0.85	0.48	0.02	0.05
其他的泌尿器官	C68	0	0.00	0.00	0.00	0.00	0.00	1	0.11	0.28	0.17	0.00	0.03
眼	C69	1	0.08	0.27	0.21	0.02	0.02	1	0.11	0.28	0.17	0.00	0.03
脑、神经系统	C70–C72	19	1.61	5.12	4.06	0.31	0.46	25	2.82	7.08	5.17	0.36	0.53
甲状腺	C73	12	1.02	3.24	2.82	0.24	0.29	54	6.09	15.29	11.53	1.02	1.10
肾上腺	C74	0	0.00	0.00	0.00	0.00	0.00	0	0.00	0.00	0.00	0.00	0.00
其他的内分泌腺	C75	0	0.00	0.00	0.00	0.00	0.00	1	0.11	0.28	0.43	0.02	0.02
霍奇金病	C81	3	0.25	0.81	0.72	0.06	0.06	3	0.34	0.85	0.48	0.04	0.04
非霍奇金淋巴瘤	C82–C85;C96	17	1.44	4.58	3.48	0.23	0.34	10	1.13	2.83	2.05	0.11	0.32
免疫增生性疾病	C88	0	0.00	0.00	0.00	0.00	0.00	0	0.00	0.00	0.00	0.00	0.00
多发性骨髓瘤	C90	7	0.59	1.89	1.28	0.07	0.15	4	0.45	1.13	0.69	0.02	0.11
淋巴样白血病	C91	3	0.25	0.81	0.67	0.04	0.09	8	0.90	2.26	2.35	0.10	0.20
髓样白血病	C92–C94	10	0.85	2.70	2.12	0.15	0.18	6	0.68	1.70	1.72	0.12	0.12
白血病，未特指	C95	7	0.59	1.89	1.54	0.08	0.15	3	0.34	0.85	0.51	0.02	0.07
其他的或未指明部位	O&U	3	0.25	0.81	0.57	0.02	0.02	8	0.90	2.26	1.39	0.03	0.24
骨髓增殖性疾病	MPD	3	0.25	0.81	0.61	0.04	0.09	2	0.23	0.57	0.34	0.02	0.05
骨髓增生异常综合征	MDS	0	0.00	0.00	0.00	0.00	0.00	0	0.00	0.00	0.00	0.00	0.00
合计	ALL	1 181	100.00	318.46	227.17	12.21	27.12	887	100.00	251.11	171.19	11.41	18.96
C44 以外的部位	ALL but C44	1 175	99.49	316.84	226.04	12.19	26.94	883	99.55	249.98	170.64	11.41	18.93

表 6-96 2020 年河南省内乡县恶性肿瘤死亡主要指标

部位	ICD-10	男性						女性					
		病例数	构成 (%)	粗率 ($1/10^5$)	世标率 ($1/10^5$)	累积率 (%)		病例数	构成 (%)	粗率 ($1/10^5$)	世标率 ($1/10^5$)	累积率 (%)	
						0~64	0~74					0~64	0~74
唇	C00	0	0.00	0.00	0.00	0.00	0.00	0	0.00	0.00	0.00	0.00	0.00
舌	C01–C02	2	0.25	0.54	0.53	0.05	0.05	1	0.21	0.28	0.14	0.00	0.00
口	C03–C06	3	0.38	0.81	0.50	0.02	0.05	0	0.00	0.00	0.00	0.00	0.00
唾液腺	C07–C08	3	0.38	0.81	0.53	0.02	0.06	0	0.00	0.00	0.00	0.00	0.00
扁桃体	C09	0	0.00	0.00	0.00	0.00	0.00	0	0.00	0.00	0.00	0.00	0.00
其他的口咽	C10	3	0.38	0.81	0.60	0.00	0.00	0	0.00	0.00	0.00	0.00	0.00
鼻咽	C11	3	0.38	0.81	0.61	0.02	0.10	2	0.42	0.57	0.42	0.03	0.06
喉咽	C12–C13	4	0.50	1.08	0.69	0.04	0.04	0	0.00	0.00	0.00	0.00	0.00
咽，部位不明	C14	1	0.13	0.27	0.24	0.00	0.00	0	0.00	0.00	0.00	0.00	0.00
食管	C15	185	23.15	49.89	34.95	1.15	3.93	106	22.36	30.01	16.70	0.40	1.91
胃	C16	189	23.65	50.96	35.15	1.22	4.59	73	15.40	20.67	12.45	0.44	1.35
小肠	C17	3	0.38	0.81	0.58	0.04	0.07	2	0.42	0.57	0.26	0.00	0.00
结肠	C18	14	1.75	3.78	2.65	0.06	0.17	16	3.38	4.53	2.80	0.17	0.28
直肠	C19–C20	23	2.88	6.20	4.20	0.13	0.50	14	2.95	3.96	2.27	0.12	0.22
肛门	C21	2	0.25	0.54	0.36	0.00	0.08	1	0.21	0.28	0.14	0.00	0.00
肝脏	C22	69	8.64	18.61	13.86	0.81	1.67	33	6.96	9.34	4.95	0.13	0.44
胆囊及其他	C23–C24	5	0.63	1.35	0.85	0.03	0.09	8	1.69	2.26	1.27	0.05	0.12
胰腺	C25	14	1.75	3.78	2.68	0.11	0.32	9	1.90	2.55	1.56	0.04	0.19
鼻、鼻窦及其他	C30–C31	1	0.13	0.27	0.17	0.00	0.03	1	0.21	0.28	0.16	0.02	0.02
喉	C32	7	0.88	1.89	1.26	0.04	0.07	3	0.63	0.85	0.43	0.00	0.03
气管、支气管、肺	C33–C34	179	22.40	48.27	33.64	1.33	4.06	64	13.50	18.12	10.55	0.40	1.15
其他的胸腔器官	C37–C38	3	0.38	0.81	0.53	0.00	0.08	3	0.63	0.85	0.48	0.00	0.08
骨	C40–C41	4	0.50	1.08	1.08	0.05	0.05	4	0.84	1.13	0.65	0.02	0.09
皮肤的黑色素瘤	C43	2	0.25	0.54	0.40	0.00	0.00	3	0.63	0.85	0.51	0.03	0.03
其他的皮肤	C44	4	0.50	1.08	0.85	0.04	0.09	1	0.21	0.28	0.17	0.02	0.02
间皮瘤	C45	8	1.00	2.16	1.57	0.15	0.20	2	0.42	0.57	0.44	0.04	0.04
卡波西肉瘤	C46	0	0.00	0.00	0.00	0.00	0.00	0	0.00	0.00	0.00	0.00	0.00
周围神经、其他结缔组织、软组织	C47;C49	1	0.13	0.27	0.16	0.00	0.00	2	0.42	0.57	0.36	0.00	0.08
乳房	C50	0	0.00	0.00	0.00	0.00	0.00	30	6.33	8.49	6.44	0.56	0.80
外阴	C51	0	0.00	0.00	0.00	0.00	0.00	0	0.00	0.00	0.00	0.00	0.00
阴道	C52	0	0.00	0.00	0.00	0.00	0.00	2	0.42	0.57	0.28	0.02	0.02
子宫颈	C53	0	0.00	0.00	0.00	0.00	0.00	8	1.69	2.26	1.52	0.11	0.16
子宫体	C54	0	0.00	0.00	0.00	0.00	0.00	11	2.32	3.11	1.87	0.13	0.22
子宫，部位不明	C55	0	0.00	0.00	0.00	0.00	0.00	2	0.42	0.57	0.34	0.00	0.06
卵巢	C56	0	0.00	0.00	0.00	0.00	0.00	9	1.90	2.55	1.58	0.09	0.15
女性其他的生殖器	C57	0	0.00	0.00	0.00	0.00	0.00	0	0.00	0.00	0.00	0.00	0.00
胎盘	C58	0	0.00	0.00	0.00	0.00	0.00	0	0.00	0.00	0.00	0.00	0.00
阴茎	C60	0	0.00	0.00	0.00	0.00	0.00	0	0.00	0.00	0.00	0.00	0.00
前列腺	C61	2	0.25	0.54	0.36	0.00	0.00	0	0.00	0.00	0.00	0.00	0.00
睾丸	C62	0	0.00	0.00	0.00	0.00	0.00	0	0.00	0.00	0.00	0.00	0.00
男性其他的生殖器	C63	0	0.00	0.00	0.00	0.00	0.00	0	0.00	0.00	0.00	0.00	0.00
肾	C64	4	0.50	1.08	0.77	0.05	0.13	4	0.84	1.13	0.70	0.00	0.14
肾盂	C65	1	0.13	0.27	0.24	0.03	0.03	0	0.00	0.00	0.00	0.00	0.00
输尿管	C66	1	0.13	0.27	0.24	0.00	0.00	1	0.21	0.28	0.14	0.00	0.00
膀胱	C67	2	0.25	0.54	0.48	0.00	0.00	2	0.42	0.57	0.26	0.00	0.00
其他的泌尿器官	C68	0	0.00	0.00	0.00	0.00	0.00	1	0.21	0.28	0.12	0.00	0.00
眼	C69	1	0.13	0.27	0.16	0.02	0.02	0	0.00	0.00	0.00	0.00	0.00
脑、神经系统	C70–C72	17	2.13	4.58	3.13	0.11	0.25	16	3.38	4.53	2.78	0.11	0.24
甲状腺	C73	4	0.50	1.08	0.68	0.03	0.08	9	1.90	2.55	1.71	0.08	0.21
肾上腺	C74	0	0.00	0.00	0.00	0.00	0.00	0	0.00	0.00	0.00	0.00	0.00
其他的内分泌腺	C75	0	0.00	0.00	0.00	0.00	0.00	0	0.00	0.00	0.00	0.00	0.00
霍奇金病	C81	2	0.25	0.54	0.34	0.02	0.05	2	0.42	0.57	0.33	0.00	0.05
非霍奇金淋巴瘤	C82–C85;C96	8	1.00	2.16	1.44	0.07	0.21	11	2.32	3.11	2.40	0.18	0.35
免疫增生性疾病	C88	0	0.00	0.00	0.00	0.00	0.00	0	0.00	0.00	0.00	0.00	0.00
多发性骨髓瘤	C90	5	0.63	1.35	1.00	0.07	0.13	5	1.05	1.42	0.87	0.02	0.15
淋巴样白血病	C91	3	0.38	0.81	0.53	0.02	0.09	5	1.05	1.42	1.34	0.08	0.08
髓样白血病	C92–C94	7	0.88	1.89	1.89	0.14	0.14	4	0.84	1.13	0.95	0.08	0.13
白血病，未特指	C95	5	0.63	1.35	1.04	0.08	0.11	2	0.42	0.57	0.34	0.02	0.05
其他的或未指明部位	O&U	2	0.25	0.54	0.35	0.00	0.05	1	0.21	0.28	0.11	0.00	0.00
骨髓增殖性疾病	MPD	0	0.00	0.00	0.00	0.00	0.00	1	0.21	0.28	0.17	0.00	0.03
骨髓增生异常综合征	MDS	3	0.38	0.81	0.55	0.04	0.07	0	0.00	0.00	0.00	0.00	0.00
合计	ALL	799	100.00	215.45	151.83	5.98	17.61	474	100.00	134.19	80.97	3.41	8.93
C44 以外的部位	ALL but C44	795	99.50	214.37	150.98	5.94	17.53	473	99.79	133.91	80.79	3.39	8.91

表 6-97 2020 年河南省新野县恶性肿瘤发病主要指标

部位	ICD-10	男性						女性					
		病例数	构成(%)	粗率(1/10^5)	世标率(1/10^5)	累积率(%)		病例数	构成(%)	粗率(1/10^5)	世标率(1/10^5)	累积率(%)	
						0~64	0~74					0~64	0~74
唇	C00	4	0.28	1.15	0.56	0.00	0.12	1	0.10	0.29	0.16	0.02	0.02
舌	C01–C02	2	0.14	0.58	0.29	0.00	0.02	3	0.30	0.86	0.66	0.05	0.05
口	C03–C06	7	0.50	2.01	0.84	0.02	0.08	3	0.30	0.86	0.62	0.04	0.04
唾液腺	C07–C08	0	0.00	0.00	0.00	0.00	0.00	1	0.10	0.29	0.14	0.00	0.02
扁桃体	C09	0	0.00	0.00	0.00	0.00	0.00	0	0.00	0.00	0.00	0.00	0.00
其他的口咽	C10	0	0.00	0.00	0.00	0.00	0.00	0	0.00	0.00	0.00	0.00	0.00
鼻咽	C11	9	0.64	2.59	2.79	0.21	0.23	3	0.30	0.86	0.43	0.02	0.06
喉咽	C12–C13	2	0.14	0.58	0.45	0.02	0.02	0	0.00	0.00	0.00	0.00	0.00
咽，部位不明	C14	5	0.36	1.44	1.00	0.10	0.10	0	0.00	0.00	0.00	0.00	0.00
食管	C15	206	14.64	59.26	31.08	1.62	3.74	109	10.79	31.20	16.08	0.62	1.71
胃	C16	271	19.26	77.96	40.68	1.95	5.20	117	11.58	33.49	17.53	0.58	1.78
小肠	C17	4	0.28	1.15	0.82	0.07	0.11	1	0.10	0.29	0.22	0.03	0.03
结肠	C18	34	2.42	9.78	6.62	0.36	0.79	32	3.17	9.16	5.41	0.36	0.65
直肠	C19–C20	50	3.55	14.38	7.68	0.35	0.89	49	4.85	14.03	8.10	0.56	0.84
肛门	C21	2	0.14	0.58	0.68	0.07	0.07	1	0.10	0.29	0.16	0.02	0.02
肝脏	C22	166	11.80	47.76	31.64	2.08	3.33	65	6.44	18.61	11.23	0.58	1.14
胆囊及其他	C23–C24	20	1.42	5.75	3.92	0.22	0.50	13	1.29	3.72	2.03	0.12	0.21
胰腺	C25	17	1.21	4.89	2.27	0.07	0.29	9	0.89	2.58	1.33	0.04	0.04
鼻、鼻窦及其他	C30–C31	1	0.07	0.29	0.16	0.02	0.02	1	0.10	0.29	0.17	0.02	0.02
喉	C32	11	0.78	3.16	2.11	0.18	0.24	0	0.00	0.00	0.00	0.00	0.00
气管、支气管、肺	C33–C34	376	26.72	108.17	61.31	3.64	7.62	139	13.76	39.79	22.34	1.17	2.19
其他的胸腔器官	C37–C38	4	0.28	1.15	0.66	0.07	0.07	6	0.59	1.72	1.07	0.11	0.11
骨	C40–C41	8	0.57	2.30	1.79	0.12	0.16	7	0.69	2.00	1.05	0.03	0.19
皮肤的黑色素瘤	C43	0	0.00	0.00	0.00	0.00	0.00	0	0.00	0.00	0.00	0.00	0.00
其他的皮肤	C44	7	0.50	2.01	0.97	0.05	0.07	1	0.10	0.29	0.11	0.00	0.00
间皮瘤	C45	2	0.14	0.58	0.31	0.02	0.04	0	0.00	0.00	0.00	0.00	0.00
卡波西肉瘤	C46	0	0.00	0.00	0.00	0.00	0.00	0	0.00	0.00	0.00	0.00	0.00
周围神经、其他结缔组织、软组织	C47;C49	5	0.36	1.44	1.01	0.07	0.13	0	0.00	0.00	0.00	0.00	0.00
乳房	C50	0	0.00	0.00	0.00	0.00	0.00	183	18.12	52.39	35.75	3.09	3.92
外阴	C51	0	0.00	0.00	0.00	0.00	0.00	1	0.10	0.29	0.14	0.00	0.03
阴道	C52	0	0.00	0.00	0.00	0.00	0.00	0	0.00	0.00	0.00	0.00	0.00
子宫颈	C53	0	0.00	0.00	0.00	0.00	0.00	62	6.14	17.75	12.50	1.03	1.31
子宫体	C54	0	0.00	0.00	0.00	0.00	0.00	38	3.76	10.88	6.69	0.52	0.79
子宫，部位不明	C55	0	0.00	0.00	0.00	0.00	0.00	5	0.50	1.43	0.91	0.09	0.09
卵巢	C56	0	0.00	0.00	0.00	0.00	0.00	30	2.97	8.59	6.17	0.48	0.64
女性其他的生殖器	C57	0	0.00	0.00	0.00	0.00	0.00	0	0.00	0.00	0.00	0.00	0.00
胎盘	C58	0	0.00	0.00	0.00	0.00	0.00	0	0.00	0.00	0.00	0.00	0.00
阴茎	C60	2	0.14	0.58	0.24	0.00	0.02	0	0.00	0.00	0.00	0.00	0.00
前列腺	C61	28	1.99	8.06	3.66	0.08	0.39	0	0.00	0.00	0.00	0.00	0.00
睾丸	C62	0	0.00	0.00	0.00	0.00	0.00	0	0.00	0.00	0.00	0.00	0.00
男性其他的生殖器	C63	0	0.00	0.00	0.00	0.00	0.00	0	0.00	0.00	0.00	0.00	0.00
肾	C64	12	0.85	3.45	1.96	0.13	0.29	4	0.40	1.15	0.66	0.06	0.06
肾盂	C65	3	0.21	0.86	0.62	0.06	0.06	3	0.30	0.86	0.39	0.00	0.05
输尿管	C66	6	0.43	1.73	0.71	0.00	0.10	2	0.20	0.57	0.27	0.00	0.05
膀胱	C67	21	1.49	6.04	3.48	0.17	0.38	4	0.40	1.15	0.54	0.00	0.02
其他的泌尿器官	C68	2	0.14	0.58	0.26	0.02	0.02	0	0.00	0.00	0.00	0.00	0.00
眼	C69	0	0.00	0.00	0.00	0.00	0.00	1	0.10	0.29	0.16	0.02	0.02
脑、神经系统	C70–C72	36	2.56	10.36	6.23	0.41	0.79	37	3.66	10.59	8.19	0.55	0.77
甲状腺	C73	12	0.85	3.45	4.35	0.33	0.33	30	2.97	8.59	7.38	0.56	0.60
肾上腺	C74	0	0.00	0.00	0.00	0.00	0.00	1	0.10	0.29	0.33	0.03	0.03
其他的内分泌腺	C75	0	0.00	0.00	0.00	0.00	0.00	0	0.00	0.00	0.00	0.00	0.00
霍奇金病	C81	1	0.07	0.29	0.15	0.00	0.04	0	0.00	0.00	0.00	0.00	0.00
非霍奇金淋巴瘤	C82–C85;C96	26	1.85	7.48	6.43	0.43	0.66	15	1.49	4.29	2.99	0.17	0.29
免疫增生性疾病	C88	0	0.00	0.00	0.00	0.00	0.00	0	0.00	0.00	0.00	0.00	0.00
多发性骨髓瘤	C90	0	0.00	0.00	0.00	0.00	0.00	0	0.00	0.00	0.00	0.00	0.00
淋巴样白血病	C91	8	0.57	2.30	1.47	0.07	0.15	5	0.50	1.43	1.32	0.09	0.16
髓样白血病	C92–C94	5	0.36	1.44	0.88	0.04	0.11	0	0.00	0.00	0.00	0.00	0.00
白血病，未特指	C95	4	0.28	1.15	1.14	0.11	0.11	6	0.59	1.72	1.92	0.13	0.15
其他的或未指明部位	O&U	28	1.99	8.06	5.39	0.34	0.57	22	2.18	6.30	3.83	0.24	0.39
骨髓增殖性疾病	MPD	0	0.00	0.00	0.00	0.00	0.00	0	0.00	0.00	0.00	0.00	0.00
骨髓增生异常综合征	MDS	0	0.00	0.00	0.00	0.00	0.00	0	0.00	0.00	0.00	0.00	0.00
合计	ALL	1 407	100.00	404.77	236.58	13.48	27.85	1 010	100.00	289.14	178.98	11.41	18.48
C44 以外的部位	ALL but C44	1 400	99.50	402.76	235.61	13.44	27.78	1 009	99.90	288.85	178.88	11.41	18.48

表 6-98　2020 年河南省新野县恶性肿瘤死亡主要指标

部位	ICD-10	男性						女性					
		病例数	构成 (%)	粗率 ($1/10^5$)	世标率 ($1/10^5$)	累积率 (%)		病例数	构成 (%)	粗率 ($1/10^5$)	世标率 ($1/10^5$)	累积率 (%)	
						0～64	0～74					0～64	0～74
唇	C00	3	0.27	0.86	0.43	0.00	0.10	2	0.34	0.57	0.23	0.00	0.00
舌	C01–C02	1	0.09	0.29	0.13	0.00	0.02	1	0.17	0.29	0.30	0.03	0.03
口	C03–C06	3	0.27	0.86	0.32	0.00	0.00	1	0.17	0.29	0.12	0.00	0.00
唾液腺	C07–C08	0	0.00	0.00	0.00	0.00	0.00	0	0.00	0.00	0.00	0.00	0.00
扁桃体	C09	0	0.00	0.00	0.00	0.00	0.00	0	0.00	0.00	0.00	0.00	0.00
其他的口咽	C10	2	0.18	0.58	0.35	0.04	0.04	0	0.00	0.00	0.00	0.00	0.00
鼻咽	C11	1	0.09	0.29	0.16	0.02	0.02	3	0.52	0.86	0.59	0.03	0.06
喉咽	C12–C13	3	0.27	0.86	0.58	0.03	0.03	1	0.17	0.29	0.11	0.00	0.00
咽，部位不明	C14	5	0.44	1.44	0.97	0.08	0.10	0	0.00	0.00	0.00	0.00	0.00
食管	C15	163	14.44	46.89	22.77	0.75	2.58	65	11.19	18.61	9.75	0.31	1.13
胃	C16	233	20.64	67.03	33.12	1.09	4.11	109	18.76	31.20	15.83	0.32	1.36
小肠	C17	4	0.35	1.15	0.75	0.05	0.09	0	0.00	0.00	0.00	0.00	0.00
结肠	C18	21	1.86	6.04	3.16	0.13	0.26	19	3.27	5.44	2.63	0.06	0.27
直肠	C19–C20	30	2.66	8.63	5.02	0.26	0.53	23	3.96	6.58	3.59	0.12	0.44
肛门	C21	2	0.18	0.58	0.63	0.05	0.05	1	0.17	0.29	0.12	0.00	0.00
肝脏	C22	171	15.15	49.19	29.02	1.73	3.03	68	11.70	19.47	11.05	0.58	1.11
胆囊及其他	C23–C24	18	1.59	5.18	2.92	0.15	0.39	10	1.72	2.86	1.43	0.05	0.13
胰腺	C25	21	1.86	6.04	3.33	0.20	0.43	12	2.07	3.44	2.04	0.11	0.11
鼻、鼻窦及其他	C30–C31	1	0.09	0.29	0.18	0.02	0.02	1	0.17	0.29	0.22	0.03	0.03
喉	C32	6	0.53	1.73	1.05	0.10	0.10	1	0.17	0.29	0.16	0.00	0.00
气管、支气管、肺	C33–C34	295	26.13	84.87	44.16	2.24	5.62	105	18.07	30.06	15.54	0.64	1.75
其他的胸腔器官	C37–C38	7	0.62	2.01	0.84	0.00	0.10	3	0.52	0.86	0.63	0.05	0.05
骨	C40–C41	7	0.62	2.01	1.17	0.05	0.09	4	0.69	1.15	0.60	0.01	0.08
皮肤的黑色素瘤	C43	0	0.00	0.00	0.00	0.00	0.00	0	0.00	0.00	0.00	0.00	0.00
其他的皮肤	C44	3	0.27	0.86	0.28	0.00	0.00	4	0.69	1.15	0.54	0.00	0.06
间皮瘤	C45	0	0.00	0.00	0.00	0.00	0.00	0	0.00	0.00	0.00	0.00	0.00
卡波西肉瘤	C46	0	0.00	0.00	0.00	0.00	0.00	0	0.00	0.00	0.00	0.00	0.00
周围神经、其他结缔组织、软组织	C47;C49	3	0.27	0.86	0.76	0.05	0.07	0	0.00	0.00	0.00	0.00	0.00
乳房	C50	0	0.00	0.00	0.00	0.00	0.00	34	5.85	9.73	5.69	0.45	0.70
外阴	C51	0	0.00	0.00	0.00	0.00	0.00	0	0.00	0.00	0.00	0.00	0.00
阴道	C52	0	0.00	0.00	0.00	0.00	0.00	0	0.00	0.00	0.00	0.00	0.00
子宫颈	C53	0	0.00	0.00	0.00	0.00	0.00	24	4.13	6.87	4.40	0.37	0.47
子宫体	C54	0	0.00	0.00	0.00	0.00	0.00	5	0.86	1.43	0.69	0.02	0.10
子宫，部位不明	C55	0	0.00	0.00	0.00	0.00	0.00	7	1.20	2.00	1.03	0.04	0.07
卵巢	C56	0	0.00	0.00	0.00	0.00	0.00	7	1.20	2.00	1.44	0.10	0.15
女性其他的生殖器	C57	0	0.00	0.00	0.00	0.00	0.00	0	0.00	0.00	0.00	0.00	0.00
胎盘	C58	0	0.00	0.00	0.00	0.00	0.00	0	0.00	0.00	0.00	0.00	0.00
阴茎	C60	0	0.00	0.00	0.00	0.00	0.00	0	0.00	0.00	0.00	0.00	0.00
前列腺	C61	17	1.51	4.89	2.74	0.12	0.30	0	0.00	0.00	0.00	0.00	0.00
睾丸	C62	0	0.00	0.00	0.00	0.00	0.00	0	0.00	0.00	0.00	0.00	0.00
男性其他的生殖器	C63	0	0.00	0.00	0.00	0.00	0.00	0	0.00	0.00	0.00	0.00	0.00
肾	C64	8	0.71	2.30	1.48	0.08	0.22	2	0.34	0.57	0.22	0.00	0.00
肾盂	C65	2	0.18	0.58	0.43	0.02	0.06	2	0.34	0.57	0.26	0.00	0.03
输尿管	C66	4	0.35	1.15	0.77	0.02	0.02	0	0.00	0.00	0.00	0.00	0.00
膀胱	C67	12	1.06	3.45	2.49	0.18	0.24	5	0.86	1.43	0.62	0.00	0.00
其他的泌尿器官	C68	0	0.00	0.00	0.00	0.00	0.00	0	0.00	0.00	0.00	0.00	0.00
眼	C69	0	0.00	0.00	0.00	0.00	0.00	0	0.00	0.00	0.00	0.00	0.00
脑、神经系统	C70–C72	28	2.48	8.06	4.53	0.22	0.51	23	3.96	6.58	4.64	0.26	0.42
甲状腺	C73	0	0.00	0.00	0.00	0.00	0.00	2	0.34	0.57	0.22	0.00	0.00
肾上腺	C74	0	0.00	0.00	0.00	0.00	0.00	0	0.00	0.00	0.00	0.00	0.00
其他的内分泌腺	C75	0	0.00	0.00	0.00	0.00	0.00	0	0.00	0.00	0.00	0.00	0.00
霍奇金病	C81	5	0.44	1.44	0.89	0.05	0.11	0	0.00	0.00	0.00	0.00	0.00
非霍奇金淋巴瘤	C82–C85;C96	20	1.77	5.75	3.65	0.23	0.41	5	0.86	1.43	0.73	0.06	0.06
免疫增生性疾病	C88	0	0.00	0.00	0.00	0.00	0.00	0	0.00	0.00	0.00	0.00	0.00
多发性骨髓瘤	C90	1	0.09	0.29	0.23	0.03	0.03	0	0.00	0.00	0.00	0.00	0.00
淋巴样白血病	C91	4	0.35	1.15	0.70	0.06	0.06	3	0.52	0.86	0.55	0.06	0.06
髓样白血病	C92–C94	0	0.00	0.00	0.00	0.00	0.00	1	0.17	0.29	0.14	0.00	0.02
白血病，未特指	C95	4	0.35	1.15	0.62	0.05	0.07	5	0.86	1.43	1.76	0.11	0.14
其他的或未指明部位	O&U	20	1.77	5.75	3.46	0.20	0.44	22	3.79	6.30	3.72	0.25	0.43
骨髓增殖性疾病	MPD	0	0.00	0.00	0.00	0.00	0.00	1	0.17	0.29	0.14	0.00	0.02
骨髓增生异常综合征	MDS	1	0.09	0.29	0.31	0.03	0.03	0	0.00	0.00	0.00	0.00	0.00
合计	ALL	1 129	100.00	324.79	174.39	8.32	20.27	581	100.00	166.33	91.70	4.05	9.26
C44 以外的部位	ALL but C44	1 126	99.73	323.93	174.11	8.32	20.27	577	99.31	165.18	91.16	4.05	9.20

表 6-99　2020 年河南省桐柏县恶性肿瘤发病主要指标

部位	ICD-10	男性						女性					
		病例数	构成 (%)	粗率 ($1/10^5$)	世标率 ($1/10^5$)	累积率 (%)		病例数	构成 (%)	粗率 ($1/10^5$)	世标率 ($1/10^5$)	累积率 (%)	
						0～64	0～74					0～64	0～74
唇	C00	0	0.00	0.00	0.00	0.00	0.00	0	0.00	0.00	0.00	0.00	0.00
舌	C01–C02	2	0.36	1.05	0.92	0.12	0.12	0	0.00	0.00	0.00	0.00	0.00
口	C03–C06	0	0.00	0.00	0.00	0.00	0.00	1	0.20	0.49	0.91	0.00	0.00
唾液腺	C07–C08	1	0.18	0.52	0.36	0.04	0.04	2	0.40	0.98	0.92	0.06	0.06
扁桃体	C09	1	0.18	0.52	0.56	0.07	0.07	1	0.20	0.49	0.35	0.04	0.04
其他的口咽	C10	0	0.00	0.00	0.00	0.00	0.00	0	0.00	0.00	0.00	0.00	0.00
鼻咽	C11	7	1.27	3.67	3.04	0.10	0.31	2	0.40	0.98	0.94	0.10	0.10
喉咽	C12–C13	0	0.00	0.00	0.00	0.00	0.00	0	0.00	0.00	0.00	0.00	0.00
咽，部位不明	C14	0	0.00	0.00	0.00	0.00	0.00	1	0.20	0.49	0.47	0.05	0.05
食管	C15	46	8.35	24.10	21.46	0.82	2.99	9	1.82	4.43	3.56	0.15	0.51
胃	C16	83	15.06	43.49	38.10	1.35	5.38	31	6.28	15.26	13.87	0.78	1.29
小肠	C17	6	1.09	3.14	2.72	0.09	0.47	3	0.61	1.48	1.19	0.00	0.15
结肠	C18	20	3.63	10.48	9.52	0.54	1.49	14	2.83	6.89	5.98	0.47	0.77
直肠	C19–C20	25	4.54	13.10	11.00	0.47	1.47	21	4.25	10.34	8.51	0.42	1.01
肛门	C21	1	0.18	0.52	0.50	0.00	0.08	0	0.00	0.00	0.00	0.00	0.00
肝脏	C22	71	12.89	37.20	33.09	1.67	3.92	25	5.06	12.31	10.77	0.34	1.22
胆囊及其他	C23–C24	4	0.73	2.10	2.06	0.07	0.36	6	1.21	2.95	3.41	0.07	0.26
胰腺	C25	6	1.09	3.14	2.99	0.00	0.62	11	2.23	5.42	4.68	0.11	0.81
鼻、鼻窦及其他	C30–C31	0	0.00	0.00	0.00	0.00	0.00	1	0.20	0.49	0.47	0.05	0.05
喉	C32	2	0.36	1.05	0.92	0.12	0.12	0	0.00	0.00	0.00	0.00	0.00
气管、支气管、肺	C33–C34	112	20.33	58.69	49.43	2.16	5.82	57	11.54	28.06	22.91	1.24	2.85
其他的胸腔器官	C37–C38	1	0.18	0.52	0.35	0.03	0.03	3	0.61	1.48	1.06	0.12	0.12
骨	C40–C41	2	0.36	1.05	1.07	0.03	0.03	2	0.40	0.98	1.44	0.11	0.11
皮肤的黑色素瘤	C43	1	0.18	0.52	0.34	0.00	0.00	1	0.20	0.49	0.44	0.00	0.07
其他的皮肤	C44	10	1.81	5.24	4.85	0.37	0.66	2	0.40	0.98	0.86	0.03	0.03
间皮瘤	C45	0	0.00	0.00	0.00	0.00	0.00	0	0.00	0.00	0.00	0.00	0.00
卡波西肉瘤	C46	0	0.00	0.00	0.00	0.00	0.00	0	0.00	0.00	0.00	0.00	0.00
周围神经、其他结缔组织、软组织	C47;C49	3	0.54	1.57	1.57	0.08	0.21	3	0.61	1.48	1.45	0.08	0.19
乳房	C50	6	1.09	3.14	2.54	0.18	0.43	90	18.22	44.31	37.41	3.08	3.82
外阴	C51	0	0.00	0.00	0.00	0.00	0.00	0	0.00	0.00	0.00	0.00	0.00
阴道	C52	0	0.00	0.00	0.00	0.00	0.00	0	0.00	0.00	0.00	0.00	0.00
子宫颈	C53	0	0.00	0.00	0.00	0.00	0.00	33	6.68	16.25	14.34	1.06	1.43
子宫体	C54	0	0.00	0.00	0.00	0.00	0.00	17	3.44	8.37	6.92	0.51	0.91
子宫，部位不明	C55	0	0.00	0.00	0.00	0.00	0.00	9	1.82	4.43	3.40	0.31	0.31
卵巢	C56	0	0.00	0.00	0.00	0.00	0.00	17	3.44	8.37	6.70	0.55	0.73
女性其他的生殖器	C57	0	0.00	0.00	0.00	0.00	0.00	7	1.42	3.45	2.78	0.18	0.25
胎盘	C58	0	0.00	0.00	0.00	0.00	0.00	0	0.00	0.00	0.00	0.00	0.00
阴茎	C60	2	0.36	1.05	1.06	0.07	0.15	0	0.00	0.00	0.00	0.00	0.00
前列腺	C61	23	4.17	12.05	10.25	0.09	0.88	0	0.00	0.00	0.00	0.00	0.00
睾丸	C62	1	0.18	0.52	0.49	0.03	0.03	0	0.00	0.00	0.00	0.00	0.00
男性其他的生殖器	C63	0	0.00	0.00	0.00	0.00	0.00	0	0.00	0.00	0.00	0.00	0.00
肾	C64	7	1.27	3.67	2.84	0.17	0.29	7	1.42	3.45	3.12	0.19	0.48
肾盂	C65	2	0.36	1.05	0.84	0.00	0.08	0	0.00	0.00	0.00	0.00	0.00
输尿管	C66	0	0.00	0.00	0.00	0.00	0.00	2	0.40	0.98	0.88	0.00	0.18
膀胱	C67	19	3.45	9.96	8.57	0.37	1.08	6	1.21	2.95	2.46	0.11	0.26
其他的泌尿器官	C68	0	0.00	0.00	0.00	0.00	0.00	1	0.20	0.49	0.35	0.04	0.04
眼	C69	0	0.00	0.00	0.00	0.00	0.00	2	0.40	0.98	0.65	0.07	0.07
脑、神经系统	C70–C72	18	3.27	9.43	8.66	0.65	0.82	26	5.26	12.80	11.65	0.92	1.39
甲状腺	C73	17	3.09	8.91	7.76	0.63	0.76	42	8.50	20.68	18.52	1.56	1.85
肾上腺	C74	2	0.36	1.05	0.79	0.07	0.07	1	0.20	0.49	0.31	0.00	0.00
其他的内分泌腺	C75	0	0.00	0.00	0.00	0.00	0.00	0	0.00	0.00	0.00	0.00	0.00
霍奇金病	C81	0	0.00	0.00	0.00	0.00	0.00	0	0.00	0.00	0.00	0.00	0.00
非霍奇金淋巴瘤	C82–C85;C96	7	1.27	3.67	3.41	0.27	0.27	5	1.01	2.46	2.16	0.10	0.36
免疫增生性疾病	C88	0	0.00	0.00	0.00	0.00	0.00	0	0.00	0.00	0.00	0.00	0.00
多发性骨髓瘤	C90	4	0.73	2.10	1.79	0.14	0.22	2	0.40	0.98	0.91	0.05	0.12
淋巴样白血病	C91	1	0.18	0.52	0.86	0.05	0.05	1	0.20	0.49	0.77	0.04	0.04
髓样白血病	C92–C94	1	0.18	0.52	0.50	0.00	0.12	4	0.81	1.97	2.16	0.14	0.21
白血病，未特指	C95	3	0.54	1.57	1.40	0.00	0.21	3	0.61	1.48	1.40	0.11	0.22
其他的或未指明部位	O&U	34	6.17	17.82	16.00	0.83	1.45	23	4.66	11.32	9.83	0.65	1.09
骨髓增殖性疾病	MPD	0	0.00	0.00	0.00	0.00	0.00	0	0.00	0.00	0.00	0.00	0.00
骨髓增生异常综合征	MDS	0	0.00	0.00	0.00	0.00	0.00	0	0.00	0.00	0.00	0.00	0.00
合计	ALL	551	100.00	288.73	252.63	11.69	31.10	494	100.00	243.23	210.92	13.90	23.47
C44 以外的部位	ALL but C44	541	98.19	283.49	247.78	11.31	30.44	492	99.60	242.24	210.05	13.88	23.44

表 6-100 2020 年河南省桐柏县恶性肿瘤死亡主要指标

部位	ICD-10	男性						女性					
		病例数	构成(%)	粗率(1/10⁵)	世标率(1/10⁵)	累积率(%)		病例数	构成(%)	粗率(1/10⁵)	世标率(1/10⁵)	累积率(%)	
						0~64	0~74					0~64	0~74
唇	C00	0	0.00	0.00	0.00	0.00	0.00	0	0.00	0.00	0.00	0.00	0.00
舌	C01–C02	0	0.00	0.00	0.00	0.00	0.00	0	0.00	0.00	0.00	0.00	0.00
口	C03–C06	0	0.00	0.00	0.00	0.00	0.00	0	0.00	0.00	0.00	0.00	0.00
唾液腺	C07–C08	0	0.00	0.00	0.00	0.00	0.00	0	0.00	0.00	0.00	0.00	0.00
扁桃体	C09	0	0.00	0.00	0.00	0.00	0.00	0	0.00	0.00	0.00	0.00	0.00
其他的口咽	C10	0	0.00	0.00	0.00	0.00	0.00	0	0.00	0.00	0.00	0.00	0.00
鼻咽	C11	2	0.50	1.05	0.94	0.03	0.03	2	1.05	0.98	0.92	0.08	0.08
喉咽	C12–C13	0	0.00	0.00	0.00	0.00	0.00	0	0.00	0.00	0.00	0.00	0.00
咽，部位不明	C14	0	0.00	0.00	0.00	0.00	0.00	0	0.00	0.00	0.00	0.00	0.00
食管	C15	28	7.02	14.67	12.84	0.36	1.48	6	3.14	2.95	2.20	0.10	0.18
胃	C16	74	18.55	38.78	34.78	1.43	5.09	21	10.99	10.34	9.09	0.32	1.05
小肠	C17	3	0.75	1.57	1.34	0.00	0.25	3	1.57	1.48	1.10	0.04	0.12
结肠	C18	7	1.75	3.67	3.49	0.00	0.67	4	2.09	1.97	1.66	0.03	0.21
直肠	C19–C20	18	4.51	9.43	8.31	0.27	1.06	7	3.66	3.45	2.72	0.05	0.34
肛门	C21	0	0.00	0.00	0.00	0.00	0.00	1	0.52	0.49	0.44	0.00	0.07
肝脏	C22	80	20.05	41.92	36.95	1.50	4.07	27	14.14	13.29	13.22	0.15	1.18
胆囊及其他	C23–C24	3	0.75	1.57	1.21	0.09	0.21	2	1.05	0.98	1.25	0.04	0.04
胰腺	C25	9	2.26	4.72	4.12	0.12	0.57	9	4.71	4.43	3.60	0.16	0.53
鼻、鼻窦及其他	C30–C31	0	0.00	0.00	0.00	0.00	0.00	0	0.00	0.00	0.00	0.00	0.00
喉	C32	0	0.00	0.00	0.00	0.00	0.00	0	0.00	0.00	0.00	0.00	0.00
气管、支气管、肺	C33–C34	90	22.56	47.16	41.51	2.02	5.31	43	22.51	21.17	20.10	0.43	1.90
其他的胸腔器官	C37–C38	1	0.25	0.52	0.47	0.05	0.05	0	0.00	0.00	0.00	0.00	0.00
骨	C40–C41	1	0.25	0.52	0.36	0.04	0.04	0	0.00	0.00	0.00	0.00	0.00
皮肤的黑色素瘤	C43	0	0.00	0.00	0.00	0.00	0.00	0	0.00	0.00	0.00	0.00	0.00
其他的皮肤	C44	4	1.00	2.10	1.93	0.12	0.20	0	0.00	0.00	0.00	0.00	0.00
间皮瘤	C45	0	0.00	0.00	0.00	0.00	0.00	0	0.00	0.00	0.00	0.00	0.00
卡波西肉瘤	C46	0	0.00	0.00	0.00	0.00	0.00	0	0.00	0.00	0.00	0.00	0.00
周围神经、其他结缔组织、软组织	C47;C49	1	0.25	0.52	0.50	0.00	0.12	0	0.00	0.00	0.00	0.00	0.00
乳房	C50	7	1.75	3.67	3.02	0.14	0.43	24	12.57	11.82	10.39	0.51	1.02
外阴	C51	0	0.00	0.00	0.00	0.00	0.00	0	0.00	0.00	0.00	0.00	0.00
阴道	C52	0	0.00	0.00	0.00	0.00	0.00	1	0.52	0.49	0.31	0.00	0.00
子宫颈	C53	0	0.00	0.00	0.00	0.00	0.00	5	2.62	2.46	1.93	0.10	0.10
子宫体	C54	0	0.00	0.00	0.00	0.00	0.00	1	0.52	0.49	0.47	0.05	0.05
子宫，部位不明	C55	1	0.25	0.52	0.47	0.05	0.05	1	0.52	0.49	0.45	0.00	0.00
卵巢	C56	0	0.00	0.00	0.00	0.00	0.00	4	2.09	1.97	1.61	0.07	0.18
女性其他的生殖器	C57	0	0.00	0.00	0.00	0.00	0.00	0	0.00	0.00	0.00	0.00	0.00
胎盘	C58	0	0.00	0.00	0.00	0.00	0.00	0	0.00	0.00	0.00	0.00	0.00
阴茎	C60	1	0.25	0.52	0.50	0.00	0.08	0	0.00	0.00	0.00	0.00	0.00
前列腺	C61	6	1.50	3.14	2.76	0.12	0.37	0	0.00	0.00	0.00	0.00	0.00
睾丸	C62	0	0.00	0.00	0.00	0.00	0.00	0	0.00	0.00	0.00	0.00	0.00
男性其他的生殖器	C63	0	0.00	0.00	0.00	0.00	0.00	0	0.00	0.00	0.00	0.00	0.00
肾	C64	5	1.25	2.62	2.04	0.08	0.21	2	1.05	0.98	0.80	0.06	0.06
肾盂	C65	0	0.00	0.00	0.00	0.00	0.00	0	0.00	0.00	0.00	0.00	0.00
输尿管	C66	0	0.00	0.00	0.00	0.00	0.00	1	0.52	0.49	0.35	0.04	0.04
膀胱	C67	9	2.26	4.72	3.89	0.20	0.45	1	0.52	0.49	0.30	0.03	0.03
其他的泌尿器官	C68	0	0.00	0.00	0.00	0.00	0.00	0	0.00	0.00	0.00	0.00	0.00
眼	C69	0	0.00	0.00	0.00	0.00	0.00	0	0.00	0.00	0.00	0.00	0.00
脑、神经系统	C70–C72	15	3.76	7.86	7.22	0.30	0.79	10	5.24	4.92	5.12	0.24	0.57
甲状腺	C73	0	0.00	0.00	0.00	0.00	0.00	0	0.00	0.00	0.00	0.00	0.00
肾上腺	C74	2	0.50	1.05	0.72	0.08	0.08	0	0.00	0.00	0.00	0.00	0.00
其他的内分泌腺	C75	0	0.00	0.00	0.00	0.00	0.00	0	0.00	0.00	0.00	0.00	0.00
霍奇金病	C81	0	0.00	0.00	0.00	0.00	0.00	0	0.00	0.00	0.00	0.00	0.00
非霍奇金淋巴瘤	C82–C85;C96	3	0.75	1.57	1.70	0.05	0.13	2	1.05	0.98	0.91	0.05	0.12
免疫增生性疾病	C88	0	0.00	0.00	0.00	0.00	0.00	0	0.00	0.00	0.00	0.00	0.00
多发性骨髓瘤	C90	1	0.25	0.52	0.57	0.00	0.00	2	1.05	0.98	0.79	0.04	0.12
淋巴样白血病	C91	0	0.00	0.00	0.00	0.00	0.00	0	0.00	0.00	0.00	0.00	0.00
髓样白血病	C92–C94	2	0.50	1.05	1.00	0.00	0.21	0	0.00	0.00	0.00	0.00	0.00
白血病，未特指	C95	5	1.25	2.62	1.96	0.09	0.21	1	0.52	0.49	0.44	0.00	0.11
其他的或未指明部位	O&U	21	5.26	11.00	9.44	0.38	1.00	11	5.76	5.42	5.19	0.32	0.58
骨髓增殖性疾病	MPD	0	0.00	0.00	0.00	0.00	0.00	0	0.00	0.00	0.00	0.00	0.00
骨髓增生异常综合征	MDS	0	0.00	0.00	0.00	0.00	0.00	0	0.00	0.00	0.00	0.00	0.00
合计	ALL	399	100.00	209.08	184.04	7.50	23.17	191	100.00	94.04	85.38	2.94	8.69
C44 以外的部位	ALL but C44	395	99.00	206.98	182.11	7.38	22.97	191	100.00	94.04	85.38	2.94	8.69

表 6-101　2020 年河南省睢县恶性肿瘤发病主要指标

部位	ICD-10	男性						女性					
		病例数	构成(%)	粗率(1/10^5)	世标率(1/10^5)	累积率(%) 0~64	累积率(%) 0~74	病例数	构成(%)	粗率(1/10^5)	世标率(1/10^5)	累积率(%) 0~64	累积率(%) 0~74
唇	C00	0	0.00	0.00	0.00	0.00	0.00	0	0.00	0.00	0.00	0.00	0.00
舌	C01–C02	5	0.46	1.10	1.05	0.08	0.08	1	0.10	0.24	0.23	0.02	0.02
口	C03–C06	4	0.37	0.88	0.71	0.03	0.11	1	0.10	0.24	0.23	0.03	0.03
唾液腺	C07–C08	2	0.19	0.44	0.41	0.04	0.04	4	0.42	0.97	0.75	0.05	0.08
扁桃体	C09	1	0.09	0.22	0.18	0.02	0.02	0	0.00	0.00	0.00	0.00	0.00
其他的口咽	C10	1	0.09	0.22	0.23	0.03	0.03	0	0.00	0.00	0.00	0.00	0.00
鼻咽	C11	3	0.28	0.66	0.66	0.06	0.06	0	0.00	0.00	0.00	0.00	0.00
喉咽	C12–C13	0	0.00	0.00	0.00	0.00	0.00	0	0.00	0.00	0.00	0.00	0.00
咽，部位不明	C14	3	0.28	0.66	0.56	0.02	0.09	2	0.21	0.49	0.42	0.03	0.06
食管	C15	49	4.54	10.76	8.78	0.43	1.10	26	2.73	6.33	4.44	0.19	0.55
胃	C16	92	8.52	20.21	15.38	0.61	1.76	46	4.83	11.21	7.48	0.25	0.90
小肠	C17	5	0.46	1.10	0.86	0.05	0.09	3	0.31	0.73	0.49	0.02	0.05
结肠	C18	20	1.85	4.39	3.97	0.24	0.59	22	2.31	5.36	3.92	0.21	0.62
直肠	C19–C20	54	5.00	11.86	9.81	0.65	1.18	34	3.57	8.28	5.62	0.22	0.72
肛门	C21	0	0.00	0.00	0.00	0.00	0.00	1	0.10	0.24	0.07	0.00	0.00
肝脏	C22	241	22.31	52.93	44.17	2.85	5.73	110	11.54	26.79	19.05	1.07	2.13
胆囊及其他	C23–C24	15	1.39	3.29	2.56	0.09	0.34	12	1.26	2.92	1.82	0.13	0.20
胰腺	C25	28	2.59	6.15	5.16	0.23	0.75	28	2.94	6.82	4.00	0.14	0.37
鼻、鼻窦及其他	C30–C31	2	0.19	0.44	0.35	0.02	0.05	2	0.21	0.49	0.26	0.00	0.00
喉	C32	10	0.93	2.20	1.73	0.06	0.25	1	0.10	0.24	0.10	0.00	0.00
气管、支气管、肺	C33–C34	347	32.13	76.21	60.08	2.78	7.86	162	17.00	39.46	28.51	1.56	3.36
其他的胸腔器官	C37–C38	2	0.19	0.44	0.35	0.01	0.06	0	0.00	0.00	0.00	0.00	0.00
骨	C40–C41	10	0.93	2.20	1.89	0.12	0.24	10	1.05	2.44	1.77	0.15	0.22
皮肤的黑色素瘤	C43	0	0.00	0.00	0.00	0.00	0.00	1	0.10	0.24	0.07	0.00	0.00
其他的皮肤	C44	8	0.74	1.76	1.53	0.10	0.14	8	0.84	1.95	1.35	0.02	0.16
间皮瘤	C45	0	0.00	0.00	0.00	0.00	0.00	0	0.00	0.00	0.00	0.00	0.00
卡波西肉瘤	C46	0	0.00	0.00	0.00	0.00	0.00	0	0.00	0.00	0.00	0.00	0.00
周围神经、其他结缔组织、软组织	C47;C49	3	0.28	0.66	0.54	0.02	0.06	5	0.52	1.22	0.73	0.04	0.04
乳房	C50	7	0.65	1.54	1.33	0.09	0.12	185	19.41	45.06	37.94	2.74	4.10
外阴	C51	0	0.00	0.00	0.00	0.00	0.00	1	0.10	0.24	0.10	0.00	0.00
阴道	C52	0	0.00	0.00	0.00	0.00	0.00	0	0.00	0.00	0.00	0.00	0.00
子宫颈	C53	1	0.09	0.22	0.20	0.00	0.03	54	5.67	13.15	10.81	0.82	1.16
子宫体	C54	0	0.00	0.00	0.00	0.00	0.00	23	2.41	5.60	4.63	0.37	0.55
子宫，部位不明	C55	0	0.00	0.00	0.00	0.00	0.00	29	3.04	7.06	6.14	0.58	0.62
卵巢	C56	0	0.00	0.00	0.00	0.00	0.00	31	3.25	7.55	5.96	0.51	0.77
女性其他的生殖器	C57	0	0.00	0.00	0.00	0.00	0.00	1	0.10	0.24	0.23	0.03	0.03
胎盘	C58	0	0.00	0.00	0.00	0.00	0.00	0	0.00	0.00	0.00	0.00	0.00
阴茎	C60	1	0.09	0.22	0.11	0.00	0.00	0	0.00	0.00	0.00	0.00	0.00
前列腺	C61	12	1.11	2.64	1.94	0.00	0.24	0	0.00	0.00	0.00	0.00	0.00
睾丸	C62	1	0.09	0.22	0.23	0.03	0.03	1	0.10	0.24	0.10	0.00	0.00
男性其他的生殖器	C63	0	0.00	0.00	0.00	0.00	0.00	0	0.00	0.00	0.00	0.00	0.00
肾	C64	38	3.52	8.35	7.11	0.45	0.81	11	1.15	2.68	2.00	0.09	0.19
肾盂	C65	1	0.09	0.22	0.20	0.00	0.00	0	0.00	0.00	0.00	0.00	0.00
输尿管	C66	2	0.19	0.44	0.41	0.04	0.04	2	0.21	0.49	0.33	0.03	0.03
膀胱	C67	16	1.48	3.51	2.71	0.14	0.38	5	0.52	1.22	1.04	0.09	0.12
其他的泌尿器官	C68	0	0.00	0.00	0.00	0.00	0.00	0	0.00	0.00	0.00	0.00	0.00
眼	C69	0	0.00	0.00	0.00	0.00	0.00	1	0.10	0.24	0.23	0.03	0.03
脑、神经系统	C70–C72	31	2.87	6.81	5.65	0.32	0.60	29	3.04	7.06	5.26	0.28	0.53
甲状腺	C73	21	1.94	4.61	4.15	0.36	0.40	56	5.88	13.64	11.38	0.92	1.13
肾上腺	C74	0	0.00	0.00	0.00	0.00	0.00	0	0.00	0.00	0.00	0.00	0.00
其他的内分泌腺	C75	0	0.00	0.00	0.00	0.00	0.00	0	0.00	0.00	0.00	0.00	0.00
霍奇金病	C81	0	0.00	0.00	0.00	0.00	0.00	0	0.00	0.00	0.00	0.00	0.00
非霍奇金淋巴瘤	C82–C85;C96	2	0.19	0.44	0.36	0.03	0.03	2	0.21	0.49	0.36	0.02	0.05
免疫增生性疾病	C88	0	0.00	0.00	0.00	0.00	0.00	0	0.00	0.00	0.00	0.00	0.00
多发性骨髓瘤	C90	1	0.09	0.22	0.23	0.03	0.03	0	0.00	0.00	0.00	0.00	0.00
淋巴样白血病	C91	1	0.09	0.22	0.15	0.02	0.02	1	0.10	0.24	0.23	0.02	0.02
髓样白血病	C92–C94	0	0.00	0.00	0.00	0.00	0.00	1	0.10	0.24	0.23	0.02	0.02
白血病，未特指	C95	11	1.02	2.42	1.99	0.06	0.20	9	0.94	2.19	2.15	0.12	0.16
其他的或未指明部位	O&U	29	2.69	6.37	5.21	0.22	0.57	32	3.36	7.79	6.06	0.38	0.64
骨髓增殖性疾病	MPD	0	0.00	0.00	0.00	0.00	0.00	0	0.00	0.00	0.00	0.00	0.00
骨髓增生异常综合征	MDS	0	0.00	0.00	0.00	0.00	0.00	0	0.00	0.00	0.00	0.00	0.00
合计	ALL	1 080	100.00	237.20	192.92	10.34	24.12	953	100.00	232.14	176.50	11.19	19.67
C44 以外的部位	ALL but C44	1 072	99.26	235.44	191.39	10.24	23.97	945	99.16	230.19	175.15	11.16	19.51

表 6-102 2020 年河南省睢县恶性肿瘤死亡主要指标

部位	ICD-10	男性						女性					
		病例数	构成 (%)	粗率 ($1/10^5$)	世标率 ($1/10^5$)	累积率 (%)		病例数	构成 (%)	粗率 ($1/10^5$)	世标率 ($1/10^5$)	累积率 (%)	
						0~64	0~74					0~64	0~74
唇	C00	0	0.00	0.00	0.00	0.00	0.00	0	0.00	0.00	0.00	0.00	0.00
舌	C01–C02	0	0.00	0.00	0.00	0.00	0.00	0	0.00	0.00	0.00	0.00	0.00
口	C03–C06	3	0.41	0.66	0.51	0.00	0.07	0	0.00	0.00	0.00	0.00	0.00
唾液腺	C07–C08	1	0.14	0.22	0.15	0.02	0.02	0	0.00	0.00	0.00	0.00	0.00
扁桃体	C09	0	0.00	0.00	0.00	0.00	0.00	0	0.00	0.00	0.00	0.00	0.00
其他的口咽	C10	0	0.00	0.00	0.00	0.00	0.00	0	0.00	0.00	0.00	0.00	0.00
鼻咽	C11	1	0.14	0.22	0.20	0.00	0.00	0	0.00	0.00	0.00	0.00	0.00
喉咽	C12–C13	0	0.00	0.00	0.00	0.00	0.00	0	0.00	0.00	0.00	0.00	0.00
咽，部位不明	C14	2	0.28	0.44	0.43	0.03	0.06	2	0.42	0.49	0.42	0.03	0.06
食管	C15	28	3.85	6.15	4.54	0.15	0.42	15	3.14	3.65	2.16	0.06	0.19
胃	C16	67	9.22	14.72	11.55	0.56	1.35	38	7.97	9.26	5.98	0.20	0.59
小肠	C17	1	0.14	0.22	0.20	0.00	0.03	1	0.21	0.24	0.19	0.00	0.03
结肠	C18	11	1.51	2.42	2.17	0.11	0.29	2	0.42	0.49	0.33	0.02	0.02
直肠	C19–C20	19	2.61	4.17	3.12	0.12	0.27	13	2.73	3.17	1.91	0.04	0.25
肛门	C21	0	0.00	0.00	0.00	0.00	0.00	0	0.00	0.00	0.00	0.00	0.00
肝脏	C22	204	28.06	44.80	37.26	2.24	4.87	82	17.19	19.97	14.51	0.81	1.60
胆囊及其他	C23–C24	10	1.38	2.20	1.85	0.06	0.19	9	1.89	2.19	1.25	0.05	0.09
胰腺	C25	18	2.48	3.95	3.18	0.08	0.52	18	3.77	4.38	2.78	0.11	0.25
鼻、鼻窦及其他	C30–C31	1	0.14	0.22	0.20	0.00	0.03	2	0.42	0.49	0.23	0.00	0.00
喉	C32	5	0.69	1.10	1.00	0.00	0.13	0	0.00	0.00	0.00	0.00	0.00
气管、支气管、肺	C33–C34	257	35.35	56.44	44.09	1.72	5.88	109	22.85	26.55	18.13	0.81	1.99
其他的胸腔器官	C37–C38	0	0.00	0.00	0.00	0.00	0.00	1	0.21	0.24	0.19	0.02	0.02
骨	C40–C41	2	0.28	0.44	0.39	0.05	0.05	4	0.84	0.97	0.62	0.04	0.08
皮肤的黑色素瘤	C43	0	0.00	0.00	0.00	0.00	0.00	0	0.00	0.00	0.00	0.00	0.00
其他的皮肤	C44	0	0.00	0.00	0.00	0.00	0.00	4	0.84	0.97	0.77	0.02	0.09
间皮瘤	C45	0	0.00	0.00	0.00	0.00	0.00	0	0.00	0.00	0.00	0.00	0.00
卡波西肉瘤	C46	0	0.00	0.00	0.00	0.00	0.00	0	0.00	0.00	0.00	0.00	0.00
周围神经、其他结缔组织、软组织	C47;C49	0	0.00	0.00	0.00	0.00	0.00	1	0.21	0.24	0.16	0.00	0.00
乳房	C50	0	0.00	0.00	0.00	0.00	0.00	43	9.01	10.47	8.62	0.70	0.97
外阴	C51	0	0.00	0.00	0.00	0.00	0.00	1	0.21	0.24	0.23	0.02	0.02
阴道	C52	0	0.00	0.00	0.00	0.00	0.00	1	0.21	0.24	0.17	0.02	0.02
子宫颈	C53	1	0.14	0.22	0.20	0.00	0.03	37	7.76	9.01	7.31	0.51	0.83
子宫体	C54	0	0.00	0.00	0.00	0.00	0.00	13	2.73	3.17	2.54	0.16	0.34
子宫，部位不明	C55	0	0.00	0.00	0.00	0.00	0.00	7	1.47	1.71	1.30	0.08	0.18
卵巢	C56	0	0.00	0.00	0.00	0.00	0.00	13	2.73	3.17	2.43	0.18	0.29
女性其他的生殖器	C57	0	0.00	0.00	0.00	0.00	0.00	3	0.63	0.73	0.62	0.05	0.05
胎盘	C58	0	0.00	0.00	0.00	0.00	0.00	0	0.00	0.00	0.00	0.00	0.00
阴茎	C60	2	0.28	0.44	0.32	0.02	0.02	0	0.00	0.00	0.00	0.00	0.00
前列腺	C61	5	0.69	1.10	0.73	0.00	0.13	0	0.00	0.00	0.00	0.00	0.00
睾丸	C62	1	0.14	0.22	0.23	0.03	0.03	1	0.21	0.24	0.10	0.00	0.00
男性其他的生殖器	C63	0	0.00	0.00	0.00	0.00	0.00	0	0.00	0.00	0.00	0.00	0.00
肾	C64	27	3.71	5.93	4.98	0.35	0.55	10	2.10	2.44	1.74	0.06	0.17
肾盂	C65	0	0.00	0.00	0.00	0.00	0.00	0	0.00	0.00	0.00	0.00	0.00
输尿管	C66	0	0.00	0.00	0.00	0.00	0.00	0	0.00	0.00	0.00	0.00	0.00
膀胱	C67	9	1.24	1.98	1.58	0.06	0.16	2	0.42	0.49	0.42	0.02	0.05
其他的泌尿器官	C68	0	0.00	0.00	0.00	0.00	0.00	0	0.00	0.00	0.00	0.00	0.00
眼	C69	0	0.00	0.00	0.00	0.00	0.00	0	0.00	0.00	0.00	0.00	0.00
脑、神经系统	C70–C72	22	3.03	4.83	3.62	0.22	0.43	18	3.77	4.38	3.37	0.14	0.31
甲状腺	C73	0	0.00	0.00	0.00	0.00	0.00	0	0.00	0.00	0.00	0.00	0.00
肾上腺	C74	0	0.00	0.00	0.00	0.00	0.00	0	0.00	0.00	0.00	0.00	0.00
其他的内分泌腺	C75	0	0.00	0.00	0.00	0.00	0.00	0	0.00	0.00	0.00	0.00	0.00
霍奇金病	C81	0	0.00	0.00	0.00	0.00	0.00	0	0.00	0.00	0.00	0.00	0.00
非霍奇金淋巴瘤	C82–C85;C96	2	0.28	0.44	0.26	0.02	0.02	1	0.21	0.24	0.10	0.00	0.00
免疫增生性疾病	C88	0	0.00	0.00	0.00	0.00	0.00	0	0.00	0.00	0.00	0.00	0.00
多发性骨髓瘤	C90	0	0.00	0.00	0.00	0.00	0.00	0	0.00	0.00	0.00	0.00	0.00
淋巴样白血病	C91	1	0.14	0.22	0.15	0.02	0.02	1	0.21	0.24	0.23	0.02	0.02
髓样白血病	C92–C94	0	0.00	0.00	0.00	0.00	0.00	1	0.21	0.24	0.17	0.02	0.02
白血病，未特指	C95	9	1.24	1.98	1.75	0.08	0.15	8	1.68	1.95	2.14	0.13	0.17
其他的或未指明部位	O&U	18	2.48	3.95	2.97	0.10	0.24	16	3.35	3.90	3.00	0.13	0.24
骨髓增殖性疾病	MPD	0	0.00	0.00	0.00	0.00	0.00	0	0.00	0.00	0.00	0.00	0.00
骨髓增生异常综合征	MDS	0	0.00	0.00	0.00	0.00	0.00	0	0.00	0.00	0.00	0.00	0.00
合计	ALL	727	100.00	159.67	127.63	6.02	15.94	477	100.00	116.19	84.11	4.47	8.93
C44 以外的部位	ALL but C44	727	100.00	159.67	127.63	6.02	15.94	473	99.16	115.22	83.34	4.45	8.84

表 6-103 2020 年河南省虞城县恶性肿瘤发病主要指标

部位	ICD-10	男性						女性					
		病例数	构成 (%)	粗率 (1/10^5)	世标率 (1/10^5)	累积率 (%) 0~64	累积率 (%) 0~74	病例数	构成 (%)	粗率 (1/10^5)	世标率 (1/10^5)	累积率 (%) 0~64	累积率 (%) 0~74
唇	C00	0	0.00	0.00	0.00	0.00	0.00	0	0.00	0.00	0.00	0.00	0.00
舌	C01–C02	2	0.15	0.34	0.30	0.00	0.07	1	0.06	0.18	0.14	0.01	0.01
口	C03–C06	0	0.00	0.00	0.00	0.00	0.00	2	0.12	0.36	0.25	0.02	0.02
唾液腺	C07–C08	8	0.58	1.34	1.26	0.10	0.10	8	0.50	1.44	1.37	0.09	0.18
扁桃体	C09	0	0.00	0.00	0.00	0.00	0.00	1	0.06	0.18	0.06	0.00	0.00
其他的口咽	C10	2	0.15	0.34	0.32	0.02	0.05	1	0.06	0.18	0.14	0.01	0.01
鼻咽	C11	7	0.51	1.17	1.11	0.09	0.12	7	0.43	1.26	1.06	0.09	0.13
喉咽	C12–C13	0	0.00	0.00	0.00	0.00	0.00	0	0.00	0.00	0.00	0.00	0.00
咽，部位不明	C14	0	0.00	0.00	0.00	0.00	0.00	0	0.00	0.00	0.00	0.00	0.00
食管	C15	188	13.69	31.56	28.39	0.90	3.43	87	5.39	15.70	12.07	0.66	1.40
胃	C16	191	13.91	32.06	28.61	1.40	3.43	94	5.82	16.96	13.51	0.83	1.58
小肠	C17	22	1.60	3.69	3.33	0.07	0.48	6	0.37	1.08	0.82	0.04	0.11
结肠	C18	43	3.13	7.22	6.33	0.37	0.77	49	3.04	8.84	7.36	0.44	0.85
直肠	C19–C20	75	5.46	12.59	11.34	0.58	1.33	66	4.09	11.91	9.96	0.66	1.07
肛门	C21	2	0.15	0.34	0.32	0.00	0.07	1	0.06	0.18	0.14	0.00	0.04
肝脏	C22	202	14.71	33.91	31.36	2.09	3.99	82	5.08	14.80	11.53	0.54	1.44
胆囊及其他	C23–C24	23	1.68	3.86	3.48	0.15	0.43	19	1.18	3.43	2.70	0.10	0.36
胰腺	C25	26	1.89	4.36	4.11	0.21	0.53	22	1.36	3.97	3.06	0.19	0.35
鼻、鼻窦及其他	C30–C31	0	0.00	0.00	0.00	0.00	0.00	0	0.00	0.00	0.00	0.00	0.00
喉	C32	6	0.44	1.01	0.92	0.08	0.11	4	0.25	0.72	0.57	0.02	0.09
气管、支气管、肺	C33–C34	353	25.71	59.25	52.61	2.32	6.50	178	11.03	32.12	24.52	1.24	3.01
其他的胸腔器官	C37–C38	1	0.07	0.17	0.17	0.02	0.02	1	0.06	0.18	0.17	0.02	0.02
骨	C40–C41	8	0.58	1.34	1.34	0.09	0.12	5	0.31	0.90	0.60	0.01	0.05
皮肤的黑色素瘤	C43	0	0.00	0.00	0.00	0.00	0.00	0	0.00	0.00	0.00	0.00	0.00
其他的皮肤	C44	3	0.22	0.50	0.51	0.04	0.04	5	0.31	0.90	0.74	0.03	0.07
间皮瘤	C45	0	0.00	0.00	0.00	0.00	0.00	0	0.00	0.00	0.00	0.00	0.00
卡波西肉瘤	C46	0	0.00	0.00	0.00	0.00	0.00	0	0.00	0.00	0.00	0.00	0.00
周围神经、其他结缔组织、软组织	C47;C49	0	0.00	0.00	0.00	0.00	0.00	0	0.00	0.00	0.00	0.00	0.00
乳房	C50	4	0.29	0.67	0.57	0.04	0.07	394	24.41	71.10	59.57	3.77	6.74
外阴	C51	0	0.00	0.00	0.00	0.00	0.00	1	0.06	0.18	0.15	0.02	0.02
阴道	C52	0	0.00	0.00	0.00	0.00	0.00	3	0.19	0.54	0.35	0.03	0.03
子宫颈	C53	0	0.00	0.00	0.00	0.00	0.00	163	10.10	29.42	24.67	1.89	2.67
子宫体	C54	0	0.00	0.00	0.00	0.00	0.00	112	6.94	20.21	16.93	1.37	1.81
子宫，部位不明	C55	0	0.00	0.00	0.00	0.00	0.00	0	0.00	0.00	0.00	0.00	0.00
卵巢	C56	0	0.00	0.00	0.00	0.00	0.00	76	4.71	13.71	11.43	0.84	1.14
女性其他的生殖器	C57	0	0.00	0.00	0.00	0.00	0.00	0	0.00	0.00	0.00	0.00	0.00
胎盘	C58	0	0.00	0.00	0.00	0.00	0.00	0	0.00	0.00	0.00	0.00	0.00
阴茎	C60	3	0.22	0.50	0.40	0.01	0.01	0	0.00	0.00	0.00	0.00	0.00
前列腺	C61	34	2.48	5.71	4.96	0.09	0.54	0	0.00	0.00	0.00	0.00	0.00
睾丸	C62	4	0.29	0.67	0.63	0.04	0.10	0	0.00	0.00	0.00	0.00	0.00
男性其他的生殖器	C63	0	0.00	0.00	0.00	0.00	0.00	0	0.00	0.00	0.00	0.00	0.00
肾	C64	29	2.11	4.87	4.44	0.25	0.55	19	1.18	3.43	3.05	0.25	0.34
肾盂	C65	3	0.22	0.50	0.44	0.02	0.09	0	0.00	0.00	0.00	0.00	0.00
输尿管	C66	2	0.15	0.34	0.28	0.03	0.03	3	0.19	0.54	0.45	0.02	0.05
膀胱	C67	37	2.69	6.21	5.37	0.20	0.54	14	0.87	2.53	1.98	0.14	0.21
其他的泌尿器官	C68	0	0.00	0.00	0.00	0.00	0.00	1	0.06	0.18	0.19	0.02	0.02
眼	C69	0	0.00	0.00	0.00	0.00	0.00	0	0.00	0.00	0.00	0.00	0.00
脑、神经系统	C70–C72	34	2.48	5.71	5.26	0.28	0.63	47	2.91	8.48	7.02	0.47	0.73
甲状腺	C73	17	1.24	2.85	2.52	0.22	0.24	116	7.19	20.93	18.46	1.59	1.77
肾上腺	C74	5	0.36	0.84	0.66	0.01	0.12	0	0.00	0.00	0.00	0.00	0.00
其他的内分泌腺	C75	0	0.00	0.00	0.00	0.00	0.00	0	0.00	0.00	0.00	0.00	0.00
霍奇金病	C81	0	0.00	0.00	0.00	0.00	0.00	1	0.06	0.18	0.14	0.01	0.01
非霍奇金淋巴瘤	C82–C85;C96	3	0.22	0.50	0.45	0.03	0.06	2	0.12	0.36	0.30	0.03	0.03
免疫增生性疾病	C88	0	0.00	0.00	0.00	0.00	0.00	0	0.00	0.00	0.00	0.00	0.00
多发性骨髓瘤	C90	10	0.73	1.68	1.54	0.09	0.23	5	0.31	0.90	0.81	0.08	0.11
淋巴样白血病	C91	5	0.36	0.84	0.81	0.06	0.12	5	0.31	0.90	0.64	0.03	0.07
髓样白血病	C92–C94	8	0.58	1.34	1.24	0.04	0.16	3	0.19	0.54	0.47	0.04	0.04
白血病，未特指	C95	3	0.22	0.50	0.38	0.03	0.03	2	0.12	0.36	0.35	0.02	0.02
其他的或未指明部位	O&U	10	0.73	1.68	1.75	0.08	0.19	8	0.50	1.44	1.24	0.06	0.19
骨髓增殖性疾病	MPD	0	0.00	0.00	0.00	0.00	0.00	0	0.00	0.00	0.00	0.00	0.00
骨髓增生异常综合征	MDS	0	0.00	0.00	0.00	0.00	0.00	0	0.00	0.00	0.00	0.00	0.00
合计	ALL	1 373	100.00	230.47	207.48	10.01	25.30	1 614	100.00	291.26	238.99	15.68	26.78
C44 以外的部位	ALL but C44	1 370	99.78	229.96	206.97	9.97	25.27	1 609	99.69	290.36	238.25	15.65	26.71

表 6-104 2020 年河南省虞城县恶性肿瘤死亡主要指标

部位	ICD-10	男性						女性					
		病例数	构成(%)	粗率(1/10^5)	世标率(1/10^5)	累积率(%) 0~64	累积率(%) 0~74	病例数	构成(%)	粗率(1/10^5)	世标率(1/10^5)	累积率(%) 0~64	累积率(%) 0~74
唇	C00	2	0.20	0.34	0.31	0.02	0.05	0	0.00	0.00	0.00	0.00	0.00
舌	C01–C02	1	0.10	0.17	0.13	0.00	0.00	1	0.12	0.18	0.18	0.00	0.03
口	C03–C06	1	0.10	0.17	0.17	0.00	0.03	1	0.12	0.18	0.17	0.02	0.02
唾液腺	C07–C08	5	0.50	0.84	0.73	0.02	0.07	0	0.00	0.00	0.00	0.00	0.00
扁桃体	C09	0	0.00	0.00	0.00	0.00	0.00	2	0.24	0.36	0.23	0.02	0.02
其他的口咽	C10	0	0.00	0.00	0.00	0.00	0.00	1	0.12	0.18	0.14	0.00	0.04
鼻咽	C11	3	0.30	0.50	0.45	0.02	0.05	4	0.48	0.72	0.60	0.06	0.06
喉咽	C12–C13	0	0.00	0.00	0.00	0.00	0.00	0	0.00	0.00	0.00	0.00	0.00
咽，部位不明	C14	1	0.10	0.17	0.17	0.00	0.03	0	0.00	0.00	0.00	0.00	0.00
食管	C15	159	15.84	26.69	23.48	0.52	2.56	78	9.27	14.08	9.67	0.27	1.13
胃	C16	154	15.34	25.85	22.80	0.64	2.92	69	8.20	12.45	9.33	0.33	1.17
小肠	C17	19	1.89	3.19	2.91	0.09	0.36	4	0.48	0.72	0.56	0.04	0.07
结肠	C18	29	2.89	4.87	4.34	0.16	0.52	32	3.80	5.77	4.07	0.18	0.45
直肠	C19–C20	49	4.88	8.22	7.39	0.23	0.70	36	4.28	6.50	4.67	0.17	0.58
肛门	C21	4	0.40	0.67	0.60	0.00	0.10	0	0.00	0.00	0.00	0.00	0.00
肝脏	C22	147	14.64	24.67	22.18	0.91	2.83	76	9.04	13.71	9.89	0.36	1.10
胆囊及其他	C23–C24	27	2.69	4.53	3.86	0.09	0.38	17	2.02	3.07	2.25	0.02	0.31
胰腺	C25	17	1.69	2.85	2.63	0.17	0.37	11	1.31	1.99	1.76	0.04	0.30
鼻、鼻窦及其他	C30–C31	1	0.10	0.17	0.17	0.00	0.03	0	0.00	0.00	0.00	0.00	0.00
喉	C32	3	0.30	0.50	0.46	0.00	0.00	1	0.12	0.18	0.18	0.00	0.03
气管、支气管、肺	C33–C34	217	21.61	36.42	31.60	0.53	3.24	109	12.96	19.67	13.63	0.40	1.55
其他的胸腔器官	C37–C38	1	0.10	0.17	0.13	0.01	0.01	5	0.59	0.90	0.58	0.04	0.07
骨	C40–C41	9	0.90	1.51	1.35	0.03	0.17	5	0.59	0.90	0.60	0.02	0.05
皮肤的黑色素瘤	C43	0	0.00	0.00	0.00	0.00	0.00	0	0.00	0.00	0.00	0.00	0.00
其他的皮肤	C44	4	0.40	0.67	0.71	0.00	0.07	4	0.48	0.72	0.42	0.02	0.02
间皮瘤	C45	0	0.00	0.00	0.00	0.00	0.00	0	0.00	0.00	0.00	0.00	0.00
卡波西肉瘤	C46	0	0.00	0.00	0.00	0.00	0.00	0	0.00	0.00	0.00	0.00	0.00
周围神经、其他结缔组织、软组织	C47;C49	1	0.10	0.17	0.17	0.00	0.03	0	0.00	0.00	0.00	0.00	0.00
乳房	C50	3	0.30	0.50	0.48	0.02	0.09	158	18.79	28.51	21.68	0.50	3.08
外阴	C51	0	0.00	0.00	0.00	0.00	0.00	1	0.12	0.18	0.11	0.00	0.00
阴道	C52	0	0.00	0.00	0.00	0.00	0.00	3	0.36	0.54	0.37	0.04	0.04
子宫颈	C53	0	0.00	0.00	0.00	0.00	0.00	63	7.49	11.37	8.78	0.45	1.05
子宫体	C54	0	0.00	0.00	0.00	0.00	0.00	42	4.99	7.58	6.28	0.39	0.74
子宫，部位不明	C55	0	0.00	0.00	0.00	0.00	0.00	4	0.48	0.72	0.60	0.06	0.06
卵巢	C56	0	0.00	0.00	0.00	0.00	0.00	16	1.90	2.89	2.07	0.07	0.24
女性其他的生殖器	C57	0	0.00	0.00	0.00	0.00	0.00	1	0.12	0.18	0.18	0.00	0.03
胎盘	C58	0	0.00	0.00	0.00	0.00	0.00	0	0.00	0.00	0.00	0.00	0.00
阴茎	C60	2	0.20	0.34	0.28	0.02	0.02	0	0.00	0.00	0.00	0.00	0.00
前列腺	C61	26	2.59	4.36	3.72	0.02	0.24	0	0.00	0.00	0.00	0.00	0.00
睾丸	C62	3	0.30	0.50	0.38	0.00	0.07	0	0.00	0.00	0.00	0.00	0.00
男性其他的生殖器	C63	0	0.00	0.00	0.00	0.00	0.00	0	0.00	0.00	0.00	0.00	0.00
肾	C64	15	1.49	2.52	2.31	0.06	0.29	9	1.07	1.62	1.40	0.10	0.20
肾盂	C65	6	0.60	1.01	0.89	0.04	0.15	1	0.12	0.18	0.18	0.00	0.03
输尿管	C66	0	0.00	0.00	0.00	0.00	0.00	2	0.24	0.36	0.17	0.00	0.00
膀胱	C67	23	2.29	3.86	3.25	0.04	0.32	6	0.71	1.08	0.64	0.00	0.07
其他的泌尿器官	C68	0	0.00	0.00	0.00	0.00	0.00	0	0.00	0.00	0.00	0.00	0.00
眼	C69	0	0.00	0.00	0.00	0.00	0.00	0	0.00	0.00	0.00	0.00	0.00
脑、神经系统	C70–C72	22	2.19	3.69	3.36	0.09	0.42	24	2.85	4.33	3.24	0.08	0.41
甲状腺	C73	6	0.60	1.01	0.87	0.06	0.11	22	2.62	3.97	3.41	0.09	0.47
肾上腺	C74	6	0.60	1.01	0.80	0.02	0.13	1	0.12	0.18	0.14	0.00	0.04
其他的内分泌腺	C75	1	0.10	0.17	0.09	0.00	0.00	0	0.00	0.00	0.00	0.00	0.00
霍奇金病	C81	0	0.00	0.00	0.00	0.00	0.00	1	0.12	0.18	0.14	0.01	0.01
非霍奇金淋巴瘤	C82–C85;C96	3	0.30	0.50	0.49	0.02	0.08	3	0.36	0.54	0.43	0.02	0.05
免疫增生性疾病	C88	0	0.00	0.00	0.00	0.00	0.00	0	0.00	0.00	0.00	0.00	0.00
多发性骨髓瘤	C90	3	0.30	0.50	0.45	0.02	0.05	8	0.95	1.44	1.06	0.00	0.17
淋巴样白血病	C91	1	0.10	0.17	0.16	0.02	0.02	2	0.24	0.36	0.19	0.00	0.00
髓样白血病	C92–C94	5	0.50	0.84	0.76	0.03	0.12	3	0.36	0.54	0.36	0.02	0.02
白血病，未特指	C95	8	0.80	1.34	1.25	0.08	0.13	1	0.12	0.18	0.11	0.00	0.00
其他的或未指明部位	O&U	17	1.69	2.85	2.72	0.05	0.32	14	1.66	2.53	1.99	0.09	0.21
骨髓增殖性疾病	MPD	0	0.00	0.00	0.00	0.00	0.00	0	0.00	0.00	0.00	0.00	0.00
骨髓增生异常综合征	MDS	0	0.00	0.00	0.00	0.00	0.00	0	0.00	0.00	0.00	0.00	0.00
合计	ALL	1 004	100.00	168.53	148.95	4.01	17.07	841	100.00	151.77	112.47	3.89	13.91
C44 以外的部位	ALL but C44	1 000	99.60	167.86	148.24	4.01	17.01	837	99.52	151.05	112.05	3.87	13.89

表 6-105　2020 年河南省罗山县恶性肿瘤发病主要指标

部位	ICD-10	男性						女性					
		病例数	构成(%)	粗率($1/10^5$)	世标率($1/10^5$)	累积率(%)		病例数	构成(%)	粗率($1/10^5$)	世标率($1/10^5$)	累积率(%)	
						0~64	0~74					0~64	0~74
唇	C00	0	0.00	0.00	0.00	0.00	0.00	0	0.00	0.00	0.00	0.00	0.00
舌	C01–C02	4	0.35	1.00	0.76	0.06	0.06	0	0.00	0.00	0.00	0.00	0.00
口	C03–C06	6	0.52	1.50	1.03	0.06	0.15	0	0.00	0.00	0.00	0.00	0.00
唾液腺	C07–C08	0	0.00	0.00	0.00	0.00	0.00	0	0.00	0.00	0.00	0.00	0.00
扁桃体	C09	0	0.00	0.00	0.00	0.00	0.00	1	0.12	0.27	0.14	0.02	0.02
其他的口咽	C10	1	0.09	0.25	0.16	0.01	0.01	0	0.00	0.00	0.00	0.00	0.00
鼻咽	C11	17	1.47	4.24	3.05	0.23	0.34	8	0.97	2.20	1.48	0.09	0.15
喉咽	C12–C13	1	0.09	0.25	0.17	0.00	0.03	0	0.00	0.00	0.00	0.00	0.00
咽，部位不明	C14	2	0.17	0.50	0.30	0.03	0.03	2	0.24	0.55	0.38	0.00	0.05
食管	C15	69	5.95	17.21	12.64	0.42	1.30	15	1.82	4.12	2.63	0.03	0.33
胃	C16	230	19.84	57.38	41.97	1.48	5.68	94	11.38	25.80	16.01	0.69	1.92
小肠	C17	2	0.17	0.50	0.33	0.02	0.04	1	0.12	0.27	0.22	0.00	0.05
结肠	C18	86	7.42	21.46	15.10	0.82	1.87	51	6.17	14.00	9.11	0.50	1.05
直肠	C19–C20	38	3.28	9.48	6.59	0.21	1.01	20	2.42	5.49	3.45	0.15	0.45
肛门	C21	6	0.52	1.50	1.03	0.05	0.14	2	0.24	0.55	0.34	0.02	0.04
肝脏	C22	177	15.27	44.16	31.46	1.69	4.00	91	11.02	24.98	15.85	0.49	1.83
胆囊及其他	C23–C24	7	0.60	1.75	1.20	0.06	0.14	15	1.82	4.12	2.35	0.15	0.18
胰腺	C25	21	1.81	5.24	3.59	0.11	0.39	25	3.03	6.86	4.22	0.26	0.54
鼻、鼻窦及其他	C30–C31	9	0.78	2.25	1.47	0.11	0.16	2	0.24	0.55	0.29	0.02	0.02
喉	C32	4	0.35	1.00	0.66	0.02	0.10	1	0.12	0.27	0.14	0.02	0.02
气管、支气管、肺	C33–C34	318	27.44	79.34	56.33	2.17	7.13	119	14.41	32.66	20.14	0.90	2.36
其他的胸腔器官	C37–C38	0	0.00	0.00	0.00	0.00	0.00	0	0.00	0.00	0.00	0.00	0.00
骨	C40–C41	12	1.04	2.99	2.01	0.14	0.22	6	0.73	1.65	1.16	0.04	0.13
皮肤的黑色素瘤	C43	0	0.00	0.00	0.00	0.00	0.00	0	0.00	0.00	0.00	0.00	0.00
其他的皮肤	C44	3	0.26	0.75	0.52	0.05	0.05	2	0.24	0.55	0.38	0.00	0.00
间皮瘤	C45	0	0.00	0.00	0.00	0.00	0.00	0	0.00	0.00	0.00	0.00	0.00
卡波西肉瘤	C46	0	0.00	0.00	0.00	0.00	0.00	0	0.00	0.00	0.00	0.00	0.00
周围神经、其他结缔组织、软组织	C47;C49	0	0.00	0.00	0.00	0.00	0.00	1	0.12	0.27	0.53	0.03	0.03
乳房	C50	3	0.26	0.75	0.51	0.02	0.02	113	13.68	31.02	19.22	1.51	1.97
外阴	C51	0	0.00	0.00	0.00	0.00	0.00	0	0.00	0.00	0.00	0.00	0.00
阴道	C52	0	0.00	0.00	0.00	0.00	0.00	0	0.00	0.00	0.00	0.00	0.00
子宫颈	C53	0	0.00	0.00	0.00	0.00	0.00	75	9.08	20.59	13.33	0.95	1.45
子宫体	C54	0	0.00	0.00	0.00	0.00	0.00	33	4.00	9.06	5.67	0.48	0.67
子宫，部位不明	C55	0	0.00	0.00	0.00	0.00	0.00	2	0.24	0.55	0.34	0.02	0.04
卵巢	C56	0	0.00	0.00	0.00	0.00	0.00	29	3.51	7.96	5.12	0.39	0.64
女性其他的生殖器	C57	0	0.00	0.00	0.00	0.00	0.00	0	0.00	0.00	0.00	0.00	0.00
胎盘	C58	0	0.00	0.00	0.00	0.00	0.00	0	0.00	0.00	0.00	0.00	0.00
阴茎	C60	2	0.17	0.50	0.37	0.00	0.05	0	0.00	0.00	0.00	0.00	0.00
前列腺	C61	24	2.07	5.99	4.17	0.08	0.38	0	0.00	0.00	0.00	0.00	0.00
睾丸	C62	2	0.17	0.50	0.33	0.03	0.03	0	0.00	0.00	0.00	0.00	0.00
男性其他的生殖器	C63	0	0.00	0.00	0.00	0.00	0.00	0	0.00	0.00	0.00	0.00	0.00
肾	C64	15	1.29	3.74	2.62	0.12	0.37	5	0.61	1.37	0.80	0.07	0.07
肾盂	C65	0	0.00	0.00	0.00	0.00	0.00	0	0.00	0.00	0.00	0.00	0.00
输尿管	C66	0	0.00	0.00	0.00	0.00	0.00	0	0.00	0.00	0.00	0.00	0.00
膀胱	C67	17	1.47	4.24	3.35	0.09	0.51	4	0.48	1.10	0.64	0.05	0.08
其他的泌尿器官	C68	0	0.00	0.00	0.00	0.00	0.00	0	0.00	0.00	0.00	0.00	0.00
眼	C69	1	0.09	0.25	0.17	0.00	0.03	0	0.00	0.00	0.00	0.00	0.00
脑、神经系统	C70–C72	20	1.73	4.99	3.86	0.18	0.45	28	3.39	7.69	5.27	0.28	0.69
甲状腺	C73	12	1.04	2.99	2.28	0.19	0.21	42	5.08	11.53	7.87	0.64	0.78
肾上腺	C74	1	0.09	0.25	0.22	0.00	0.05	0	0.00	0.00	0.00	0.00	0.00
其他的内分泌腺	C75	1	0.09	0.25	0.16	0.02	0.02	2	0.24	0.55	0.42	0.04	0.04
霍奇金病	C81	3	0.26	0.75	0.44	0.05	0.05	2	0.24	0.55	0.43	0.00	0.11
非霍奇金淋巴瘤	C82–C85;C96	2	0.17	0.50	0.35	0.01	0.01	3	0.36	0.82	0.91	0.03	0.06
免疫增生性疾病	C88	0	0.00	0.00	0.00	0.00	0.00	0	0.00	0.00	0.00	0.00	0.00
多发性骨髓瘤	C90	0	0.00	0.00	0.00	0.00	0.00	0	0.00	0.00	0.00	0.00	0.00
淋巴样白血病	C91	0	0.00	0.00	0.00	0.00	0.00	0	0.00	0.00	0.00	0.00	0.00
髓样白血病	C92–C94	2	0.17	0.50	0.31	0.02	0.02	3	0.36	0.82	0.52	0.04	0.06
白血病，未特指	C95	24	2.07	5.99	5.50	0.26	0.53	12	1.45	3.29	3.04	0.14	0.36
其他的或未指明部位	O&U	17	1.47	4.24	2.99	0.12	0.48	17	2.06	4.67	3.62	0.25	0.39
骨髓增殖性疾病	MPD	0	0.00	0.00	0.00	0.00	0.00	0	0.00	0.00	0.00	0.00	0.00
骨髓增生异常综合征	MDS	0	0.00	0.00	0.00	0.00	0.00	0	0.00	0.00	0.00	0.00	0.00
合计	ALL	1 159	100.00	289.16	208.00	8.95	26.09	826	100.00	226.72	146.02	8.30	16.57
C44 以外的部位	ALL but C44	1 156	99.74	288.41	207.49	8.89	26.04	824	99.76	226.17	145.64	8.30	16.57

表 6-106 2020 年河南省罗山县恶性肿瘤死亡主要指标

部位	ICD-10	男性						女性					
		病例数	构成(%)	粗率($1/10^5$)	世标率($1/10^5$)	累积率(%)		病例数	构成(%)	粗率($1/10^5$)	世标率($1/10^5$)	累积率(%)	
						0~64	0~74					0~64	0~74
唇	C00	1	0.13	0.25	0.16	0.02	0.02	0	0.00	0.00	0.00	0.00	0.00
舌	C01-C02	2	0.27	0.50	0.46	0.02	0.07	1	0.24	0.27	0.16	0.00	0.00
口	C03-C06	2	0.27	0.50	0.44	0.00	0.11	1	0.24	0.27	0.22	0.00	0.05
唾液腺	C07-C08	0	0.00	0.00	0.00	0.00	0.00	0	0.00	0.00	0.00	0.00	0.00
扁桃体	C09	0	0.00	0.00	0.00	0.00	0.00	0	0.00	0.00	0.00	0.00	0.00
其他的口咽	C10	0	0.00	0.00	0.00	0.00	0.00	0	0.00	0.00	0.00	0.00	0.00
鼻咽	C11	6	0.80	1.50	1.04	0.04	0.12	1	0.24	0.27	0.12	0.00	0.00
喉咽	C12-C13	0	0.00	0.00	0.00	0.00	0.00	0	0.00	0.00	0.00	0.00	0.00
咽，部位不明	C14	1	0.13	0.25	0.14	0.02	0.02	1	0.24	0.27	0.12	0.00	0.00
食管	C15	41	5.45	10.23	7.56	0.16	0.77	13	3.07	3.57	2.21	0.08	0.27
胃	C16	161	21.41	40.17	30.01	0.85	3.65	62	14.62	17.02	10.78	0.34	1.32
小肠	C17	0	0.00	0.00	0.00	0.00	0.00	1	0.24	0.27	0.22	0.00	0.05
结肠	C18	52	6.91	12.97	9.45	0.37	1.08	22	5.19	6.04	3.91	0.05	0.46
直肠	C19-C20	4	0.53	1.00	0.73	0.06	0.08	6	1.42	1.65	1.04	0.07	0.13
肛门	C21	0	0.00	0.00	0.00	0.00	0.00	0	0.00	0.00	0.00	0.00	0.00
肝脏	C22	154	20.48	38.42	27.75	1.34	3.02	80	18.87	21.96	13.72	0.41	1.37
胆囊及其他	C23-C24	2	0.27	0.50	0.39	0.00	0.05	13	3.07	3.57	2.07	0.13	0.21
胰腺	C25	17	2.26	4.24	3.15	0.06	0.39	21	4.95	5.76	3.39	0.17	0.36
鼻、鼻窦及其他	C30-C31	2	0.27	0.50	0.33	0.02	0.04	2	0.47	0.55	0.24	0.00	0.00
喉	C32	1	0.13	0.25	0.16	0.02	0.02	1	0.24	0.27	0.14	0.02	0.02
气管、支气管、肺	C33-C34	222	29.52	55.39	40.16	1.31	5.54	80	18.87	21.96	13.87	0.48	1.42
其他的胸腔器官	C37-C38	0	0.00	0.00	0.00	0.00	0.00	0	0.00	0.00	0.00	0.00	0.00
骨	C40-C41	16	2.13	3.99	2.95	0.14	0.38	6	1.42	1.65	1.49	0.10	0.13
皮肤的黑色素瘤	C43	0	0.00	0.00	0.00	0.00	0.00	0	0.00	0.00	0.00	0.00	0.00
其他的皮肤	C44	1	0.13	0.25	0.17	0.00	0.00	0	0.00	0.00	0.00	0.00	0.00
间皮瘤	C45	0	0.00	0.00	0.00	0.00	0.00	0	0.00	0.00	0.00	0.00	0.00
卡波西肉瘤	C46	0	0.00	0.00	0.00	0.00	0.00	0	0.00	0.00	0.00	0.00	0.00
周围神经、其他结缔组织、软组织	C47;C49	0	0.00	0.00	0.00	0.00	0.00	2	0.47	0.55	0.98	0.05	0.05
乳房	C50	1	0.13	0.25	0.16	0.02	0.02	24	5.66	6.59	3.97	0.21	0.40
外阴	C51	0	0.00	0.00	0.00	0.00	0.00	0	0.00	0.00	0.00	0.00	0.00
阴道	C52	0	0.00	0.00	0.00	0.00	0.00	0	0.00	0.00	0.00	0.00	0.00
子宫颈	C53	0	0.00	0.00	0.00	0.00	0.00	22	5.19	6.04	3.86	0.15	0.36
子宫体	C54	0	0.00	0.00	0.00	0.00	0.00	9	2.12	2.47	1.61	0.05	0.16
子宫，部位不明	C55	0	0.00	0.00	0.00	0.00	0.00	0	0.00	0.00	0.00	0.00	0.00
卵巢	C56	0	0.00	0.00	0.00	0.00	0.00	9	2.12	2.47	1.54	0.05	0.21
女性其他的生殖器	C57	0	0.00	0.00	0.00	0.00	0.00	0	0.00	0.00	0.00	0.00	0.00
胎盘	C58	0	0.00	0.00	0.00	0.00	0.00	0	0.00	0.00	0.00	0.00	0.00
阴茎	C60	0	0.00	0.00	0.00	0.00	0.00	0	0.00	0.00	0.00	0.00	0.00
前列腺	C61	6	0.80	1.50	1.15	0.00	0.11	0	0.00	0.00	0.00	0.00	0.00
睾丸	C62	1	0.13	0.25	0.16	0.02	0.02	0	0.00	0.00	0.00	0.00	0.00
男性其他的生殖器	C63	0	0.00	0.00	0.00	0.00	0.00	0	0.00	0.00	0.00	0.00	0.00
肾	C64	6	0.80	1.50	1.05	0.04	0.15	2	0.47	0.55	0.35	0.04	0.04
肾盂	C65	0	0.00	0.00	0.00	0.00	0.00	0	0.00	0.00	0.00	0.00	0.00
输尿管	C66	0	0.00	0.00	0.00	0.00	0.00	0	0.00	0.00	0.00	0.00	0.00
膀胱	C67	5	0.66	1.25	1.15	0.04	0.09	1	0.24	0.27	0.14	0.02	0.02
其他的泌尿器官	C68	0	0.00	0.00	0.00	0.00	0.00	0	0.00	0.00	0.00	0.00	0.00
眼	C69	0	0.00	0.00	0.00	0.00	0.00	0	0.00	0.00	0.00	0.00	0.00
脑、神经系统	C70-C72	9	1.20	2.25	1.58	0.07	0.18	20	4.72	5.49	4.07	0.20	0.50
甲状腺	C73	1	0.13	0.25	0.22	0.00	0.05	2	0.47	0.55	0.24	0.00	0.00
肾上腺	C74	1	0.13	0.25	0.22	0.00	0.05	0	0.00	0.00	0.00	0.00	0.00
其他的内分泌腺	C75	0	0.00	0.00	0.00	0.00	0.00	0	0.00	0.00	0.00	0.00	0.00
霍奇金病	C81	0	0.00	0.00	0.00	0.00	0.00	0	0.00	0.00	0.00	0.00	0.00
非霍奇金淋巴瘤	C82-C85;C96	1	0.13	0.25	0.17	0.00	0.03	2	0.47	0.55	0.34	0.00	0.00
免疫增生性疾病	C88	0	0.00	0.00	0.00	0.00	0.00	0	0.00	0.00	0.00	0.00	0.00
多发性骨髓瘤	C90	0	0.00	0.00	0.00	0.00	0.00	0	0.00	0.00	0.00	0.00	0.00
淋巴样白血病	C91	0	0.00	0.00	0.00	0.00	0.00	0	0.00	0.00	0.00	0.00	0.00
髓样白血病	C92-C94	3	0.40	0.75	0.47	0.00	0.03	0	0.00	0.00	0.00	0.00	0.00
白血病，未特指	C95	18	2.39	4.49	3.36	0.14	0.36	11	2.59	3.02	2.78	0.13	0.35
其他的或未指明部位	O&U	15	1.99	3.74	2.84	0.07	0.56	9	2.12	2.47	1.95	0.08	0.25
骨髓增殖性疾病	MPD	0	0.00	0.00	0.00	0.00	0.00	0	0.00	0.00	0.00	0.00	0.00
骨髓增生异常综合征	MDS	0	0.00	0.00	0.00	0.00	0.00	0	0.00	0.00	0.00	0.00	0.00
合计	ALL	752	100.00	187.62	137.59	4.81	17.05	424	100.00	116.38	75.54	2.82	8.12
C44 以外的部位	ALL but C44	751	99.87	187.37	137.42	4.81	17.05	424	100.00	116.38	75.54	2.82	8.12

表 6-107　2020 年河南省沈丘县恶性肿瘤发病主要指标

部位	ICD-10	男性						女性					
		病例数	构成 (%)	粗率 (1/10^5)	世标率 (1/10^5)	累积率 (%) 0~64	累积率 (%) 0~74	病例数	构成 (%)	粗率 (1/10^5)	世标率 (1/10^5)	累积率 (%) 0~64	累积率 (%) 0~74
唇	C00	1	0.06	0.16	0.14	0.00	0.02	0	0.00	0.00	0.00	0.00	0.00
舌	C01–C02	2	0.12	0.33	0.19	0.00	0.00	4	0.26	0.67	0.47	0.03	0.05
口	C03–C06	0	0.00	0.00	0.00	0.00	0.00	4	0.26	0.67	0.51	0.05	0.08
唾液腺	C07–C08	4	0.24	0.66	0.64	0.05	0.07	8	0.51	1.34	1.15	0.09	0.11
扁桃体	C09	0	0.00	0.00	0.00	0.00	0.00	1	0.06	0.17	0.12	0.00	0.02
其他的口咽	C10	1	0.06	0.16	0.13	0.00	0.00	0	0.00	0.00	0.00	0.00	0.00
鼻咽	C11	6	0.36	0.99	0.81	0.07	0.10	3	0.19	0.50	0.30	0.00	0.03
喉咽	C12–C13	1	0.06	0.16	0.15	0.02	0.02	0	0.00	0.00	0.00	0.00	0.00
咽，部位不明	C14	0	0.00	0.00	0.00	0.00	0.00	0	0.00	0.00	0.00	0.00	0.00
食管	C15	177	10.50	29.20	22.57	0.88	2.69	146	9.35	24.49	14.15	0.66	1.63
胃	C16	197	11.68	32.50	25.20	0.98	3.29	104	6.66	17.45	10.36	0.53	1.15
小肠	C17	9	0.53	1.48	1.14	0.04	0.16	5	0.32	0.84	0.60	0.01	0.11
结肠	C18	35	2.08	5.77	4.69	0.19	0.61	31	1.99	5.20	3.72	0.26	0.44
直肠	C19–C20	79	4.69	13.03	10.59	0.57	1.43	73	4.68	12.25	7.52	0.28	0.89
肛门	C21	0	0.00	0.00	0.00	0.00	0.00	0	0.00	0.00	0.00	0.00	0.00
肝脏	C22	288	17.08	47.52	38.77	2.57	4.67	147	9.42	24.66	15.81	0.87	2.00
胆囊及其他	C23–C24	14	0.83	2.31	1.79	0.05	0.20	19	1.22	3.19	1.87	0.07	0.21
胰腺	C25	19	1.13	3.13	2.48	0.15	0.25	24	1.54	4.03	2.85	0.21	0.34
鼻、鼻窦及其他	C30–C31	1	0.06	0.16	0.14	0.01	0.01	2	0.13	0.34	0.27	0.02	0.04
喉	C32	5	0.30	0.82	0.69	0.03	0.10	2	0.13	0.34	0.24	0.00	0.05
气管、支气管、肺	C33–C34	573	33.99	94.54	71.65	2.53	8.81	260	16.66	43.61	27.20	1.26	3.30
其他的胸腔器官	C37–C38	4	0.24	0.66	0.52	0.04	0.04	0	0.00	0.00	0.00	0.00	0.00
骨	C40–C41	18	1.07	2.97	2.73	0.16	0.19	18	1.15	3.02	2.40	0.18	0.20
皮肤的黑色素瘤	C43	3	0.18	0.49	0.38	0.02	0.02	1	0.06	0.17	0.13	0.01	0.01
其他的皮肤	C44	7	0.42	1.15	0.78	0.04	0.09	7	0.45	1.17	0.52	0.01	0.06
间皮瘤	C45	0	0.00	0.00	0.00	0.00	0.00	0	0.00	0.00	0.00	0.00	0.00
卡波西肉瘤	C46	0	0.00	0.00	0.00	0.00	0.00	1	0.06	0.17	0.13	0.02	0.02
周围神经、其他结缔组织、软组织	C47;C49	1	0.06	0.16	0.14	0.00	0.03	1	0.06	0.17	0.17	0.01	0.01
乳房	C50	6	0.36	0.99	0.68	0.03	0.05	271	17.36	45.46	37.39	2.99	3.95
外阴	C51	0	0.00	0.00	0.00	0.00	0.00	1	0.06	0.17	0.13	0.01	0.01
阴道	C52	0	0.00	0.00	0.00	0.00	0.00	2	0.13	0.34	0.25	0.03	0.03
子宫颈	C53	0	0.00	0.00	0.00	0.00	0.00	121	7.75	20.30	15.89	1.28	1.72
子宫体	C54	0	0.00	0.00	0.00	0.00	0.00	63	4.04	10.57	8.43	0.74	0.99
子宫，部位不明	C55	0	0.00	0.00	0.00	0.00	0.00	0	0.00	0.00	0.00	0.00	0.00
卵巢	C56	0	0.00	0.00	0.00	0.00	0.00	35	2.24	5.87	4.54	0.37	0.49
女性其他的生殖器	C57	0	0.00	0.00	0.00	0.00	0.00	2	0.13	0.34	0.26	0.02	0.02
胎盘	C58	0	0.00	0.00	0.00	0.00	0.00	0	0.00	0.00	0.00	0.00	0.00
阴茎	C60	5	0.30	0.82	0.60	0.05	0.08	0	0.00	0.00	0.00	0.00	0.00
前列腺	C61	30	1.78	4.95	3.58	0.03	0.41	0	0.00	0.00	0.00	0.00	0.00
睾丸	C62	3	0.18	0.49	0.38	0.03	0.03	0	0.00	0.00	0.00	0.00	0.00
男性其他的生殖器	C63	0	0.00	0.00	0.00	0.00	0.00	0	0.00	0.00	0.00	0.00	0.00
肾	C64	28	1.66	4.62	3.86	0.18	0.54	20	1.28	3.35	2.71	0.16	0.28
肾盂	C65	1	0.06	0.16	0.13	0.00	0.00	0	0.00	0.00	0.00	0.00	0.00
输尿管	C66	0	0.00	0.00	0.00	0.00	0.00	2	0.13	0.34	0.25	0.02	0.04
膀胱	C67	36	2.14	5.94	4.41	0.16	0.56	17	1.09	2.85	1.79	0.08	0.23
其他的泌尿器官	C68	1	0.06	0.16	0.15	0.01	0.01	0	0.00	0.00	0.00	0.00	0.00
眼	C69	2	0.12	0.33	0.41	0.01	0.05	2	0.13	0.34	0.46	0.03	0.03
脑、神经系统	C70–C72	11	0.65	1.81	1.53	0.12	0.16	23	1.47	3.86	3.30	0.23	0.37
甲状腺	C73	13	0.77	2.14	1.78	0.15	0.15	62	3.97	10.40	8.68	0.72	0.79
肾上腺	C74	2	0.12	0.33	0.27	0.03	0.03	2	0.13	0.34	0.27	0.02	0.02
其他的内分泌腺	C75	1	0.06	0.16	0.14	0.00	0.03	2	0.13	0.34	0.36	0.01	0.04
霍奇金病	C81	9	0.53	1.48	1.21	0.06	0.17	4	0.26	0.67	0.59	0.04	0.04
非霍奇金淋巴瘤	C82–C85;C96	22	1.30	3.63	3.24	0.17	0.38	12	0.77	2.01	1.71	0.12	0.14
免疫增生性疾病	C88	0	0.00	0.00	0.00	0.00	0.00	0	0.00	0.00	0.00	0.00	0.00
多发性骨髓瘤	C90	1	0.06	0.16	0.15	0.02	0.02	0	0.00	0.00	0.00	0.00	0.00
淋巴样白血病	C91	2	0.12	0.33	0.40	0.03	0.03	1	0.06	0.17	0.31	0.01	0.01
髓样白血病	C92–C94	8	0.47	1.32	1.22	0.08	0.10	7	0.45	1.17	0.96	0.05	0.10
白血病，未特指	C95	44	2.61	7.26	7.04	0.40	0.66	42	2.69	7.05	6.12	0.39	0.56
其他的或未指明部位	O&U	16	0.95	2.64	2.22	0.13	0.21	9	0.58	1.51	0.97	0.04	0.14
骨髓增殖性疾病	MPD	0	0.00	0.00	0.00	0.00	0.00	0	0.00	0.00	0.00	0.00	0.00
骨髓增生异常综合征	MDS	0	0.00	0.00	0.00	0.00	0.00	0	0.00	0.00	0.00	0.00	0.00
合计	ALL	1 686	100.00	278.17	219.72	10.08	26.49	1 561	100.00	261.86	185.86	11.96	20.76
C44 以外的部位	ALL but C44	1 679	99.58	277.02	218.94	10.04	26.40	1 554	99.55	260.68	185.34	11.95	20.70

表 6-108 2020 年河南省沈丘县恶性肿瘤死亡主要指标

部位	ICD-10	男性						女性					
		病例数	构成 (%)	粗率 ($1/10^5$)	世标率 ($1/10^5$)	累积率 (%)		病例数	构成 (%)	粗率 ($1/10^5$)	世标率 ($1/10^5$)	累积率 (%)	
						0~64	0~74					0~64	0~74
唇	C00	0	0.00	0.00	0.00	0.00	0.00	0	0.00	0.00	0.00	0.00	0.00
舌	C01–C02	1	0.08	0.16	0.13	0.00	0.00	1	0.13	0.17	0.05	0.00	0.00
口	C03–C06	2	0.17	0.33	0.29	0.02	0.05	0	0.00	0.00	0.00	0.00	0.00
唾液腺	C07–C08	1	0.08	0.16	0.14	0.00	0.03	0	0.00	0.00	0.00	0.00	0.00
扁桃体	C09	0	0.00	0.00	0.00	0.00	0.00	0	0.00	0.00	0.00	0.00	0.00
其他的口咽	C10	2	0.17	0.33	0.26	0.01	0.01	0	0.00	0.00	0.00	0.00	0.00
鼻咽	C11	3	0.25	0.49	0.38	0.02	0.04	5	0.67	0.84	0.36	0.00	0.05
喉咽	C12–C13	1	0.08	0.16	0.15	0.01	0.01	1	0.13	0.17	0.12	0.00	0.02
咽，部位不明	C14	0	0.00	0.00	0.00	0.00	0.00	1	0.13	0.17	0.03	0.00	0.00
食管	C15	143	11.92	23.59	17.29	0.40	2.01	79	10.66	13.25	7.15	0.27	0.82
胃	C16	137	11.42	22.60	16.42	0.56	1.85	78	10.53	13.08	6.90	0.31	0.75
小肠	C17	2	0.17	0.33	0.28	0.02	0.02	4	0.54	0.67	0.51	0.02	0.09
结肠	C18	17	1.42	2.80	2.36	0.13	0.29	6	0.81	1.01	0.56	0.03	0.07
直肠	C19–C20	31	2.58	5.11	3.96	0.15	0.49	32	4.32	5.37	2.67	0.06	0.24
肛门	C21	0	0.00	0.00	0.00	0.00	0.00	0	0.00	0.00	0.00	0.00	0.00
肝脏	C22	247	20.58	40.75	32.29	1.96	4.12	112	15.11	18.79	10.12	0.38	1.22
胆囊及其他	C23–C24	9	0.75	1.48	1.13	0.04	0.14	16	2.16	2.68	1.52	0.07	0.15
胰腺	C25	17	1.42	2.80	2.16	0.18	0.21	17	2.29	2.85	1.78	0.09	0.20
鼻、鼻窦及其他	C30–C31	0	0.00	0.00	0.00	0.00	0.00	1	0.13	0.17	0.15	0.02	0.02
喉	C32	8	0.67	1.32	1.08	0.05	0.17	2	0.27	0.34	0.22	0.00	0.02
气管、支气管、肺	C33–C34	442	36.83	72.93	54.56	1.31	6.69	175	23.62	29.36	16.01	0.50	1.87
其他的胸腔器官	C37–C38	3	0.25	0.49	0.35	0.00	0.00	0	0.00	0.00	0.00	0.00	0.00
骨	C40–C41	11	0.92	1.81	1.40	0.07	0.15	7	0.94	1.17	0.72	0.07	0.07
皮肤的黑色素瘤	C43	1	0.08	0.16	0.15	0.01	0.01	1	0.13	0.17	0.05	0.00	0.00
其他的皮肤	C44	7	0.58	1.15	0.81	0.03	0.09	6	0.81	1.01	0.32	0.00	0.03
间皮瘤	C45	0	0.00	0.00	0.00	0.00	0.00	0	0.00	0.00	0.00	0.00	0.00
卡波西肉瘤	C46	0	0.00	0.00	0.00	0.00	0.00	0	0.00	0.00	0.00	0.00	0.00
周围神经、其他结缔组织、软组织	C47;C49	1	0.08	0.16	0.14	0.00	0.03	1	0.13	0.17	0.11	0.00	0.03
乳房	C50	3	0.25	0.49	0.26	0.00	0.00	64	8.64	10.74	7.70	0.55	0.86
外阴	C51	0	0.00	0.00	0.00	0.00	0.00	0	0.00	0.00	0.00	0.00	0.00
阴道	C52	0	0.00	0.00	0.00	0.00	0.00	0	0.00	0.00	0.00	0.00	0.00
子宫颈	C53	0	0.00	0.00	0.00	0.00	0.00	44	5.94	7.38	5.10	0.26	0.62
子宫体	C54	0	0.00	0.00	0.00	0.00	0.00	2	0.27	0.34	0.22	0.00	0.02
子宫，部位不明	C55	0	0.00	0.00	0.00	0.00	0.00	1	0.13	0.17	0.12	0.00	0.02
卵巢	C56	0	0.00	0.00	0.00	0.00	0.00	23	3.10	3.86	2.43	0.16	0.31
女性其他的生殖器	C57	0	0.00	0.00	0.00	0.00	0.00	0	0.00	0.00	0.00	0.00	0.00
胎盘	C58	0	0.00	0.00	0.00	0.00	0.00	0	0.00	0.00	0.00	0.00	0.00
阴茎	C60	2	0.17	0.33	0.20	0.00	0.03	0	0.00	0.00	0.00	0.00	0.00
前列腺	C61	16	1.33	2.64	1.57	0.00	0.10	0	0.00	0.00	0.00	0.00	0.00
睾丸	C62	1	0.08	0.16	0.14	0.00	0.02	0	0.00	0.00	0.00	0.00	0.00
男性其他的生殖器	C63	0	0.00	0.00	0.00	0.00	0.00	0	0.00	0.00	0.00	0.00	0.00
肾	C64	16	1.33	2.64	2.12	0.13	0.26	8	1.08	1.34	0.87	0.05	0.11
肾盂	C65	0	0.00	0.00	0.00	0.00	0.00	0	0.00	0.00	0.00	0.00	0.00
输尿管	C66	0	0.00	0.00	0.00	0.00	0.00	0	0.00	0.00	0.00	0.00	0.00
膀胱	C67	6	0.50	0.99	0.63	0.03	0.03	3	0.40	0.50	0.20	0.00	0.02
其他的泌尿器官	C68	0	0.00	0.00	0.00	0.00	0.00	0	0.00	0.00	0.00	0.00	0.00
眼	C69	0	0.00	0.00	0.00	0.00	0.00	1	0.13	0.17	0.12	0.01	0.01
脑、神经系统	C70–C72	22	1.83	3.63	3.11	0.22	0.39	11	1.48	1.85	1.39	0.06	0.14
甲状腺	C73	3	0.25	0.49	0.28	0.00	0.02	4	0.54	0.67	0.23	0.00	0.02
肾上腺	C74	0	0.00	0.00	0.00	0.00	0.00	0	0.00	0.00	0.00	0.00	0.00
其他的内分泌腺	C75	0	0.00	0.00	0.00	0.00	0.00	0	0.00	0.00	0.00	0.00	0.00
霍奇金病	C81	2	0.17	0.33	0.24	0.01	0.01	1	0.13	0.17	0.16	0.01	0.01
非霍奇金淋巴瘤	C82–C85;C96	8	0.67	1.32	1.07	0.04	0.15	6	0.81	1.01	0.63	0.04	0.04
免疫增生性疾病	C88	0	0.00	0.00	0.00	0.00	0.00	0	0.00	0.00	0.00	0.00	0.00
多发性骨髓瘤	C90	3	0.25	0.49	0.42	0.02	0.08	1	0.13	0.17	0.05	0.00	0.00
淋巴样白血病	C91	1	0.08	0.16	0.13	0.02	0.02	0	0.00	0.00	0.00	0.00	0.00
髓样白血病	C92–C94	2	0.17	0.33	0.41	0.01	0.03	2	0.27	0.34	0.23	0.01	0.01
白血病，未特指	C95	13	1.08	2.14	1.91	0.12	0.17	17	2.29	2.85	2.56	0.12	0.25
其他的或未指明部位	O&U	16	1.33	2.64	1.97	0.09	0.19	8	1.08	1.34	0.80	0.01	0.12
骨髓增殖性疾病	MPD	0	0.00	0.00	0.00	0.00	0.00	0	0.00	0.00	0.00	0.00	0.00
骨髓增生异常综合征	MDS	0	0.00	0.00	0.00	0.00	0.00	0	0.00	0.00	0.00	0.00	0.00
合计	ALL	1 200	100.00	197.99	150.16	5.65	17.97	741	100.00	124.30	72.17	3.09	8.19
C44 以外的部位	ALL but C44	1 193	99.42	196.83	149.35	5.62	17.88	735	99.19	123.30	71.85	3.09	8.16

表 6-109　2020 年河南省郸城县恶性肿瘤发病主要指标

部位	ICD-10	男性						女性					
		病例数	构成 (%)	粗率 ($1/10^5$)	世标率 ($1/10^5$)	累积率 (%)		病例数	构成 (%)	粗率 ($1/10^5$)	世标率 ($1/10^5$)	累积率 (%)	
						0~64	0~74					0~64	0~74
唇	C00	4	0.21	0.55	0.61	0.01	0.10	6	0.31	0.89	0.81	0.06	0.12
舌	C01–C02	6	0.32	0.83	0.81	0.03	0.16	12	0.62	1.77	1.54	0.07	0.20
口	C03–C06	7	0.37	0.97	0.76	0.06	0.10	8	0.41	1.18	1.04	0.01	0.14
唾液腺	C07–C08	5	0.27	0.69	0.55	0.05	0.05	5	0.26	0.74	0.75	0.07	0.10
扁桃体	C09	2	0.11	0.28	0.18	0.02	0.02	3	0.15	0.44	0.32	0.01	0.04
其他的口咽	C10	3	0.16	0.42	0.35	0.04	0.04	5	0.26	0.74	0.66	0.05	0.05
鼻咽	C11	12	0.64	1.66	1.43	0.08	0.21	9	0.46	1.33	1.20	0.08	0.14
喉咽	C12–C13	2	0.11	0.28	0.27	0.00	0.00	2	0.10	0.30	0.35	0.00	0.06
咽，部位不明	C14	6	0.32	0.83	0.87	0.07	0.10	2	0.10	0.30	0.24	0.02	0.02
食管	C15	281	14.97	38.92	38.91	1.63	5.36	226	11.67	33.38	30.03	1.22	4.03
胃	C16	274	14.60	37.95	37.56	2.24	5.29	223	11.51	32.93	28.41	1.50	3.49
小肠	C17	11	0.59	1.52	1.41	0.07	0.20	8	0.41	1.18	1.12	0.05	0.14
结肠	C18	42	2.24	5.82	5.36	0.33	0.70	51	2.63	7.53	7.11	0.35	1.12
直肠	C19–C20	49	2.61	6.79	6.77	0.36	0.92	60	3.10	8.86	8.16	0.32	1.20
肛门	C21	36	1.92	4.99	4.89	0.27	0.71	29	1.50	4.28	4.18	0.24	0.71
肝脏	C22	310	16.52	42.93	41.02	2.62	5.58	201	10.38	29.68	26.89	1.58	3.61
胆囊及其他	C23–C24	12	0.64	1.66	1.60	0.12	0.21	19	0.98	2.81	2.90	0.19	0.43
胰腺	C25	21	1.12	2.91	2.80	0.12	0.47	19	0.98	2.81	2.61	0.19	0.31
鼻、鼻窦及其他	C30–C31	10	0.53	1.38	1.45	0.13	0.20	12	0.62	1.77	1.68	0.15	0.21
喉	C32	18	0.96	2.49	2.42	0.06	0.32	12	0.62	1.77	1.54	0.08	0.23
气管、支气管、肺	C33–C34	481	25.63	66.61	65.45	3.84	9.10	193	9.96	28.50	25.51	1.26	3.55
其他的胸腔器官	C37–C38	8	0.43	1.11	0.94	0.10	0.10	7	0.36	1.03	0.88	0.09	0.09
骨	C40–C41	12	0.64	1.66	2.31	0.12	0.19	10	0.52	1.48	1.33	0.08	0.14
皮肤的黑色素瘤	C43	0	0.00	0.00	0.00	0.00	0.00	0	0.00	0.00	0.00	0.00	0.00
其他的皮肤	C44	15	0.80	2.08	2.33	0.11	0.20	16	0.83	2.36	2.10	0.15	0.18
间皮瘤	C45	0	0.00	0.00	0.00	0.00	0.00	0	0.00	0.00	0.00	0.00	0.00
卡波西肉瘤	C46	0	0.00	0.00	0.00	0.00	0.00	0	0.00	0.00	0.00	0.00	0.00
周围神经、其他结缔组织、软组织	C47;C49	4	0.21	0.55	0.65	0.06	0.09	5	0.26	0.74	0.59	0.06	0.06
乳房	C50	5	0.27	0.69	0.75	0.04	0.10	418	21.58	61.73	50.81	3.32	5.51
外阴	C51	0	0.00	0.00	0.00	0.00	0.00	1	0.05	0.15	0.11	0.01	0.01
阴道	C52	0	0.00	0.00	0.00	0.00	0.00	1	0.05	0.15	0.11	0.01	0.01
子宫颈	C53	0	0.00	0.00	0.00	0.00	0.00	93	4.80	13.73	11.07	0.90	1.27
子宫体	C54	0	0.00	0.00	0.00	0.00	0.00	19	0.98	2.81	2.28	0.15	0.30
子宫，部位不明	C55	0	0.00	0.00	0.00	0.00	0.00	17	0.88	2.51	2.18	0.16	0.25
卵巢	C56	0	0.00	0.00	0.00	0.00	0.00	56	2.89	8.27	6.72	0.58	0.70
女性其他的生殖器	C57	0	0.00	0.00	0.00	0.00	0.00	7	0.36	1.03	1.12	0.07	0.10
胎盘	C58	0	0.00	0.00	0.00	0.00	0.00	1	0.05	0.15	0.10	0.01	0.01
阴茎	C60	5	0.27	0.69	0.63	0.02	0.06	0	0.00	0.00	0.00	0.00	0.00
前列腺	C61	16	0.85	2.22	2.17	0.06	0.29	0	0.00	0.00	0.00	0.00	0.00
睾丸	C62	4	0.21	0.55	0.45	0.02	0.05	0	0.00	0.00	0.00	0.00	0.00
男性其他的生殖器	C63	3	0.16	0.42	0.46	0.03	0.06	0	0.00	0.00	0.00	0.00	0.00
肾	C64	10	0.53	1.38	1.29	0.07	0.16	9	0.46	1.33	0.99	0.09	0.09
肾盂	C65	1	0.05	0.14	0.08	0.01	0.01	2	0.10	0.30	0.22	0.02	0.02
输尿管	C66	8	0.43	1.11	1.08	0.06	0.15	2	0.10	0.30	0.23	0.01	0.04
膀胱	C67	15	0.80	2.08	1.86	0.09	0.19	11	0.57	1.62	1.46	0.13	0.15
其他的泌尿器官	C68	1	0.05	0.14	0.09	0.01	0.01	3	0.15	0.44	0.32	0.03	0.03
眼	C69	2	0.11	0.28	0.19	0.02	0.02	2	0.10	0.30	0.47	0.02	0.02
脑、神经系统	C70–C72	40	2.13	5.54	5.74	0.39	0.58	41	2.12	6.05	6.17	0.36	0.64
甲状腺	C73	16	0.85	2.22	2.01	0.19	0.22	22	1.14	3.25	2.38	0.17	0.22
肾上腺	C74	0	0.00	0.00	0.00	0.00	0.00	1	0.05	0.15	0.10	0.01	0.01
其他的内分泌腺	C75	1	0.05	0.14	0.19	0.02	0.02	2	0.10	0.30	0.20	0.02	0.02
霍奇金病	C81	1	0.05	0.14	0.19	0.02	0.02	3	0.15	0.44	0.40	0.01	0.07
非霍奇金淋巴瘤	C82–C85;C96	17	0.91	2.35	2.62	0.10	0.28	9	0.46	1.33	1.31	0.06	0.12
免疫增生性疾病	C88	0	0.00	0.00	0.00	0.00	0.00	0	0.00	0.00	0.00	0.00	0.00
多发性骨髓瘤	C90	13	0.69	1.80	1.65	0.07	0.23	12	0.62	1.77	1.63	0.12	0.21
淋巴样白血病	C91	15	0.80	2.08	3.01	0.15	0.25	13	0.67	1.92	2.44	0.08	0.23
髓样白血病	C92–C94	23	1.23	3.19	3.10	0.17	0.30	15	0.77	2.22	1.78	0.14	0.20
白血病，未特指	C95	25	1.33	3.46	3.45	0.18	0.31	24	1.24	3.54	3.75	0.19	0.25
其他的或未指明部位	O&U	25	1.33	3.46	3.66	0.18	0.44	10	0.52	1.48	1.17	0.07	0.13
骨髓增殖性疾病	MPD	0	0.00	0.00	0.00	0.00	0.00	0	0.00	0.00	0.00	0.00	0.00
骨髓增生异常综合征	MDS	0	0.00	0.00	0.00	0.00	0.00	0	0.00	0.00	0.00	0.00	0.00
合计	ALL	1 877	100.00	259.94	256.35	14.46	34.16	1 937	100.00	286.05	251.47	14.65	31.02
C44 以外的部位	ALL but C44	1 862	99.20	257.87	254.02	14.35	33.96	1 921	99.17	283.69	249.37	14.50	30.84

表 6-110 2020 年河南省郸城县恶性肿瘤死亡主要指标

部位	ICD-10	男性						女性					
		病例数	构成 (%)	粗率 ($1/10^5$)	世标率 ($1/10^5$)	累积率 (%)		病例数	构成 (%)	粗率 ($1/10^5$)	世标率 ($1/10^5$)	累积率 (%)	
						0~64	0~74					0~64	0~74
唇	C00	2	0.16	0.28	0.25	0.01	0.04	2	0.21	0.30	0.35	0.00	0.06
舌	C01–C02	3	0.24	0.42	0.40	0.01	0.04	5	0.54	0.74	0.63	0.01	0.10
口	C03–C06	3	0.24	0.42	0.31	0.03	0.03	3	0.32	0.44	0.41	0.01	0.04
唾液腺	C07–C08	3	0.24	0.42	0.35	0.01	0.01	1	0.11	0.15	0.10	0.01	0.01
扁桃体	C09	2	0.16	0.28	0.29	0.01	0.04	2	0.21	0.30	0.18	0.00	0.00
其他的口咽	C10	2	0.16	0.28	0.36	0.02	0.02	2	0.21	0.30	0.24	0.01	0.05
鼻咽	C11	7	0.55	0.97	0.81	0.05	0.11	4	0.43	0.59	0.40	0.02	0.02
喉咽	C12–C13	1	0.08	0.14	0.11	0.00	0.00	1	0.11	0.15	0.13	0.00	0.03
咽，部位不明	C14	3	0.24	0.42	0.41	0.02	0.06	2	0.21	0.30	0.24	0.01	0.05
食管	C15	175	13.80	24.24	21.98	0.79	2.59	141	15.15	20.82	18.57	0.83	2.31
胃	C16	183	14.43	25.34	24.09	0.90	2.68	123	13.21	18.16	16.65	0.68	1.89
小肠	C17	8	0.63	1.11	1.02	0.05	0.14	4	0.43	0.59	0.55	0.01	0.04
结肠	C18	21	1.66	2.91	3.08	0.09	0.34	24	2.58	3.54	3.48	0.16	0.53
直肠	C19–C20	21	1.66	2.91	3.02	0.16	0.32	25	2.69	3.69	3.55	0.24	0.48
肛门	C21	19	1.50	2.63	2.55	0.18	0.28	23	2.47	3.40	3.12	0.23	0.41
肝脏	C22	256	20.19	35.45	34.58	1.64	4.59	148	15.90	21.86	18.76	1.00	2.29
胆囊及其他	C23–C24	8	0.63	1.11	1.19	0.00	0.19	14	1.50	2.07	2.04	0.10	0.29
胰腺	C25	15	1.18	2.08	2.09	0.06	0.35	14	1.50	2.07	1.90	0.08	0.23
鼻、鼻窦及其他	C30–C31	7	0.55	0.97	0.95	0.09	0.09	5	0.54	0.74	0.56	0.01	0.04
喉	C32	12	0.95	1.66	1.85	0.04	0.22	7	0.75	1.03	1.07	0.00	0.12
气管、支气管、肺	C33–C34	374	29.50	51.80	50.62	2.63	6.17	114	12.24	16.84	15.58	1.07	2.08
其他的胸腔器官	C37–C38	4	0.32	0.55	0.45	0.03	0.07	4	0.43	0.59	0.43	0.02	0.02
骨	C40–C41	6	0.47	0.83	0.90	0.04	0.04	4	0.43	0.59	0.43	0.03	0.06
皮肤的黑色素瘤	C43	0	0.00	0.00	0.00	0.00	0.00	1	0.11	0.15	0.10	0.01	0.01
其他的皮肤	C44	12	0.95	1.66	1.50	0.13	0.16	9	0.97	1.33	0.94	0.08	0.08
间皮瘤	C45	0	0.00	0.00	0.00	0.00	0.00	0	0.00	0.00	0.00	0.00	0.00
卡波西肉瘤	C46	0	0.00	0.00	0.00	0.00	0.00	0	0.00	0.00	0.00	0.00	0.00
周围神经、其他结缔组织、软组织	C47;C49	3	0.24	0.42	0.48	0.04	0.07	0	0.00	0.00	0.00	0.00	0.00
乳房	C50	1	0.08	0.14	0.09	0.00	0.00	99	10.63	14.62	13.44	1.07	1.73
外阴	C51	0	0.00	0.00	0.00	0.00	0.00	0	0.00	0.00	0.00	0.00	0.00
阴道	C52	0	0.00	0.00	0.00	0.00	0.00	1	0.11	0.15	0.09	0.00	0.00
子宫颈	C53	0	0.00	0.00	0.00	0.00	0.00	29	3.11	4.28	3.58	0.25	0.45
子宫体	C54	0	0.00	0.00	0.00	0.00	0.00	6	0.64	0.89	0.62	0.03	0.07
子宫，部位不明	C55	0	0.00	0.00	0.00	0.00	0.00	11	1.18	1.62	1.36	0.04	0.16
卵巢	C56	0	0.00	0.00	0.00	0.00	0.00	20	2.15	2.95	2.46	0.05	0.36
女性其他的生殖器	C57	0	0.00	0.00	0.00	0.00	0.00	3	0.32	0.44	0.52	0.03	0.03
胎盘	C58	0	0.00	0.00	0.00	0.00	0.00	0	0.00	0.00	0.00	0.00	0.00
阴茎	C60	3	0.24	0.42	0.29	0.01	0.01	0	0.00	0.00	0.00	0.00	0.00
前列腺	C61	8	0.63	1.11	0.96	0.02	0.16	0	0.00	0.00	0.00	0.00	0.00
睾丸	C62	3	0.24	0.42	0.29	0.01	0.01	0	0.00	0.00	0.00	0.00	0.00
男性其他的生殖器	C63	2	0.16	0.28	0.23	0.01	0.04	0	0.00	0.00	0.00	0.00	0.00
肾	C64	4	0.32	0.55	0.54	0.02	0.08	6	0.64	0.89	0.61	0.05	0.05
肾盂	C65	1	0.08	0.14	0.18	0.00	0.00	1	0.11	0.15	0.12	0.01	0.01
输尿管	C66	4	0.32	0.55	0.59	0.00	0.09	1	0.11	0.15	0.11	0.01	0.01
膀胱	C67	9	0.71	1.25	1.11	0.05	0.11	8	0.86	1.18	1.03	0.08	0.12
其他的泌尿器官	C68	0	0.00	0.00	0.00	0.00	0.00	1	0.11	0.15	0.10	0.01	0.01
眼	C69	1	0.08	0.14	0.09	0.01	0.01	1	0.11	0.15	0.12	0.01	0.01
脑、神经系统	C70–C72	25	1.97	3.46	3.27	0.17	0.36	16	1.72	2.36	2.15	0.09	0.24
甲状腺	C73	9	0.71	1.25	1.13	0.07	0.17	12	1.29	1.77	1.53	0.07	0.23
肾上腺	C74	1	0.08	0.14	0.09	0.00	0.00	0	0.00	0.00	0.00	0.00	0.00
其他的内分泌腺	C75	0	0.00	0.00	0.00	0.00	0.00	1	0.11	0.15	0.10	0.01	0.01
霍奇金病	C81	1	0.08	0.14	0.19	0.02	0.02	0	0.00	0.00	0.00	0.00	0.00
非霍奇金淋巴瘤	C82–C85;C96	8	0.63	1.11	1.25	0.05	0.18	5	0.54	0.74	0.60	0.04	0.07
免疫增生性疾病	C88	0	0.00	0.00	0.00	0.00	0.00	0	0.00	0.00	0.00	0.00	0.00
多发性骨髓瘤	C90	6	0.47	0.83	0.82	0.03	0.10	4	0.43	0.59	0.47	0.04	0.08
淋巴样白血病	C91	6	0.47	0.83	0.99	0.06	0.06	5	0.54	0.74	1.20	0.07	0.07
髓样白血病	C92–C94	11	0.87	1.52	1.47	0.07	0.10	6	0.64	0.89	0.99	0.06	0.10
白血病，未特指	C95	9	0.71	1.25	1.32	0.08	0.14	6	0.64	0.89	0.79	0.06	0.09
其他的或未指明部位	O&U	6	0.47	0.83	0.71	0.06	0.10	7	0.75	1.03	1.00	0.06	0.12
骨髓增殖性疾病	MPD	0	0.00	0.00	0.00	0.00	0.00	0	0.00	0.00	0.00	0.00	0.00
骨髓增生异常综合征	MDS	0	0.00	0.00	0.00	0.00	0.00	0	0.00	0.00	0.00	0.00	0.00
合计	ALL	1 268	100.00	175.60	169.25	7.79	20.40	931	100.00	137.49	123.40	6.74	15.22
C44 以外的部位	ALL but C44	1 256	99.05	173.94	167.75	7.66	20.24	922	99.03	136.16	122.46	6.66	15.15

表 6-111　2020 年河南省项城市恶性肿瘤发病主要指标

部位	ICD-10	男性						女性					
		病例数	构成 (%)	粗率 ($1/10^5$)	世标率 ($1/10^5$)	累积率 (%)		病例数	构成 (%)	粗率 ($1/10^5$)	世标率 ($1/10^5$)	累积率 (%)	
						0~64	0~74					0~64	0~74
唇	C00	1	0.05	0.14	0.09	0.01	0.01	0	0.00	0.00	0.00	0.00	0.00
舌	C01–C02	5	0.27	0.71	0.51	0.03	0.07	2	0.12	0.31	0.23	0.03	0.03
口	C03–C06	6	0.33	0.85	0.54	0.04	0.06	5	0.30	0.77	0.50	0.05	0.07
唾液腺	C07–C08	7	0.38	0.99	0.92	0.03	0.11	5	0.30	0.77	0.83	0.04	0.07
扁桃体	C09	1	0.05	0.14	0.09	0.01	0.01	0	0.00	0.00	0.00	0.00	0.00
其他的口咽	C10	7	0.38	0.99	0.79	0.03	0.10	1	0.06	0.15	0.10	0.00	0.02
鼻咽	C11	13	0.71	1.85	1.38	0.07	0.17	11	0.66	1.70	1.14	0.05	0.15
喉咽	C12–C13	2	0.11	0.28	0.20	0.01	0.03	0	0.00	0.00	0.00	0.00	0.00
咽，部位不明	C14	2	0.11	0.28	0.15	0.00	0.00	0	0.00	0.00	0.00	0.00	0.00
食管	C15	144	7.88	20.46	14.10	0.54	1.74	114	6.85	17.65	9.07	0.23	1.13
胃	C16	249	13.62	35.38	24.71	1.11	2.68	164	9.86	25.39	13.41	0.57	1.44
小肠	C17	7	0.38	0.99	0.73	0.04	0.07	9	0.54	1.39	0.87	0.04	0.13
结肠	C18	49	2.68	6.96	5.40	0.37	0.65	52	3.13	8.05	4.50	0.22	0.52
直肠	C19–C20	84	4.60	11.94	8.62	0.52	0.93	62	3.73	9.60	5.81	0.29	0.64
肛门	C21	1	0.05	0.14	0.09	0.00	0.02	1	0.06	0.15	0.10	0.00	0.02
肝脏	C22	307	16.79	43.62	32.73	2.22	3.85	135	8.11	20.90	11.80	0.68	1.30
胆囊及其他	C23–C24	28	1.53	3.98	3.01	0.16	0.37	21	1.26	3.25	1.80	0.08	0.18
胰腺	C25	27	1.48	3.84	2.66	0.09	0.35	18	1.08	2.79	1.45	0.05	0.17
鼻、鼻窦及其他	C30–C31	2	0.11	0.28	0.22	0.02	0.02	3	0.18	0.46	0.27	0.02	0.02
喉	C32	22	1.20	3.13	2.23	0.10	0.34	1	0.06	0.15	0.10	0.00	0.02
气管、支气管、肺	C33–C34	541	29.60	76.87	52.61	2.12	6.21	252	15.14	39.01	21.59	1.06	2.36
其他的胸腔器官	C37–C38	12	0.66	1.71	1.57	0.07	0.17	10	0.60	1.55	0.84	0.06	0.09
骨	C40–C41	12	0.66	1.71	1.29	0.08	0.14	14	0.84	2.17	1.33	0.10	0.11
皮肤的黑色素瘤	C43	1	0.05	0.14	0.14	0.01	0.01	0	0.00	0.00	0.00	0.00	0.00
其他的皮肤	C44	13	0.71	1.85	1.36	0.04	0.12	17	1.02	2.63	1.59	0.06	0.19
间皮瘤	C45	0	0.00	0.00	0.00	0.00	0.00	0	0.00	0.00	0.00	0.00	0.00
卡波西肉瘤	C46	0	0.00	0.00	0.00	0.00	0.00	0	0.00	0.00	0.00	0.00	0.00
周围神经、其他结缔组织、软组织	C47;C49	4	0.22	0.57	0.67	0.05	0.05	5	0.30	0.77	0.49	0.03	0.05
乳房	C50	3	0.16	0.43	0.25	0.02	0.02	295	17.73	45.66	34.07	2.79	3.48
外阴	C51	0	0.00	0.00	0.00	0.00	0.00	1	0.06	0.15	0.10	0.00	0.02
阴道	C52	0	0.00	0.00	0.00	0.00	0.00	3	0.18	0.46	0.48	0.02	0.02
子宫颈	C53	0	0.00	0.00	0.00	0.00	0.00	89	5.35	13.78	10.17	0.89	1.08
子宫体	C54	0	0.00	0.00	0.00	0.00	0.00	45	2.70	6.97	5.04	0.44	0.56
子宫，部位不明	C55	0	0.00	0.00	0.00	0.00	0.00	7	0.42	1.08	0.67	0.04	0.08
卵巢	C56	0	0.00	0.00	0.00	0.00	0.00	40	2.40	6.19	4.50	0.36	0.45
女性其他的生殖器	C57	0	0.00	0.00	0.00	0.00	0.00	0	0.00	0.00	0.00	0.00	0.00
胎盘	C58	0	0.00	0.00	0.00	0.00	0.00	0	0.00	0.00	0.00	0.00	0.00
阴茎	C60	4	0.22	0.57	0.37	0.03	0.05	0	0.00	0.00	0.00	0.00	0.00
前列腺	C61	22	1.20	3.13	2.01	0.08	0.23	0	0.00	0.00	0.00	0.00	0.00
睾丸	C62	2	0.11	0.28	0.20	0.01	0.03	0	0.00	0.00	0.00	0.00	0.00
男性其他的生殖器	C63	1	0.05	0.14	0.07	0.00	0.00	0	0.00	0.00	0.00	0.00	0.00
肾	C64	23	1.26	3.27	2.65	0.17	0.30	16	0.96	2.48	1.82	0.15	0.18
肾盂	C65	1	0.05	0.14	0.09	0.00	0.02	3	0.18	0.46	0.19	0.01	0.01
输尿管	C66	0	0.00	0.00	0.00	0.00	0.00	1	0.06	0.15	0.09	0.01	0.01
膀胱	C67	30	1.64	4.26	3.04	0.12	0.36	11	0.66	1.70	0.98	0.04	0.10
其他的泌尿器官	C68	1	0.05	0.14	0.09	0.00	0.02	0	0.00	0.00	0.00	0.00	0.00
眼	C69	1	0.05	0.14	0.14	0.01	0.01	0	0.00	0.00	0.00	0.00	0.00
脑、神经系统	C70–C72	74	4.05	10.52	8.56	0.51	0.93	68	4.09	10.53	7.23	0.44	0.75
甲状腺	C73	26	1.42	3.69	3.17	0.27	0.27	93	5.59	14.40	11.61	0.88	1.12
肾上腺	C74	0	0.00	0.00	0.00	0.00	0.00	1	0.06	0.15	0.09	0.01	0.01
其他的内分泌腺	C75	0	0.00	0.00	0.00	0.00	0.00	1	0.06	0.15	0.09	0.01	0.01
霍奇金病	C81	0	0.00	0.00	0.00	0.00	0.00	1	0.06	0.15	0.13	0.01	0.01
非霍奇金淋巴瘤	C82–C85;C96	19	1.04	2.70	2.15	0.13	0.26	10	0.60	1.55	1.10	0.10	0.12
免疫增生性疾病	C88	0	0.00	0.00	0.00	0.00	0.00	0	0.00	0.00	0.00	0.00	0.00
多发性骨髓瘤	C90	9	0.49	1.28	0.96	0.05	0.12	1	0.06	0.15	0.09	0.01	0.01
淋巴样白血病	C91	1	0.05	0.14	0.11	0.01	0.01	2	0.12	0.31	0.52	0.02	0.02
髓样白血病	C92–C94	11	0.60	1.56	1.51	0.08	0.11	13	0.78	2.01	1.58	0.11	0.19
白血病，未特指	C95	8	0.44	1.14	1.06	0.07	0.07	4	0.24	0.62	0.37	0.03	0.05
其他的或未指明部位	O&U	44	2.41	6.25	5.93	0.38	0.55	57	3.43	8.82	6.17	0.38	0.60
骨髓增殖性疾病	MPD	0	0.00	0.00	0.00	0.00	0.00	0	0.00	0.00	0.00	0.00	0.00
骨髓增生异常综合征	MDS	1	0.05	0.14	0.09	0.01	0.01	0	0.00	0.00	0.00	0.00	0.00
合计	ALL	1 828	100.00	259.75	189.27	9.73	21.68	1 664	100.00	257.57	164.94	10.40	17.59
C44 以外的部位	ALL but C44	1 815	99.29	257.90	187.92	9.69	21.55	1 647	98.98	254.94	163.34	10.34	17.40

表 6-112 2020 年河南省项城市恶性肿瘤死亡主要指标

部位	ICD-10	男性						女性					
		病例数	构成 (%)	粗率 (1/10^5)	世标率 (1/10^5)	累积率 (%) 0~64	累积率 (%) 0~74	病例数	构成 (%)	粗率 (1/10^5)	世标率 (1/10^5)	累积率 (%) 0~64	累积率 (%) 0~74
唇	C00	0	0.00	0.00	0.00	0.00	0.00	0	0.00	0.00	0.00	0.00	0.00
舌	C01–C02	3	0.28	0.43	0.38	0.04	0.04	2	0.27	0.31	0.19	0.01	0.03
口	C03–C06	2	0.19	0.28	0.19	0.02	0.02	1	0.13	0.15	0.05	0.00	0.00
唾液腺	C07–C08	1	0.09	0.14	0.09	0.00	0.02	0	0.00	0.00	0.00	0.00	0.00
扁桃体	C09	0	0.00	0.00	0.00	0.00	0.00	0	0.00	0.00	0.00	0.00	0.00
其他的口咽	C10	2	0.19	0.28	0.24	0.02	0.04	1	0.13	0.15	0.08	0.00	0.02
鼻咽	C11	3	0.28	0.43	0.26	0.01	0.03	3	0.40	0.46	0.33	0.04	0.04
喉咽	C12–C13	1	0.09	0.14	0.07	0.00	0.00	0	0.00	0.00	0.00	0.00	0.00
咽，部位不明	C14	0	0.00	0.00	0.00	0.00	0.00	0	0.00	0.00	0.00	0.00	0.00
食管	C15	91	8.47	12.93	8.76	0.29	0.95	72	9.64	11.14	5.38	0.12	0.53
胃	C16	184	17.13	26.15	17.15	0.53	1.72	118	15.80	18.27	8.44	0.28	0.74
小肠	C17	6	0.56	0.85	0.65	0.02	0.06	2	0.27	0.31	0.13	0.00	0.02
结肠	C18	20	1.86	2.84	1.97	0.06	0.23	20	2.68	3.10	1.33	0.03	0.10
直肠	C19–C20	37	3.45	5.26	3.39	0.11	0.35	27	3.61	4.18	2.12	0.08	0.21
肛门	C21	1	0.09	0.14	0.09	0.00	0.02	0	0.00	0.00	0.00	0.00	0.00
肝脏	C22	199	18.53	28.28	20.49	1.29	2.39	87	11.65	13.47	6.65	0.31	0.65
胆囊及其他	C23–C24	14	1.30	1.99	1.48	0.06	0.21	16	2.14	2.48	1.11	0.03	0.08
胰腺	C25	17	1.58	2.42	1.63	0.06	0.22	9	1.20	1.39	0.72	0.02	0.14
鼻、鼻窦及其他	C30–C31	1	0.09	0.14	0.09	0.01	0.01	1	0.13	0.15	0.19	0.01	0.01
喉	C32	2	0.19	0.28	0.18	0.01	0.03	1	0.13	0.15	0.06	0.00	0.00
气管、支气管、肺	C33–C34	375	34.92	53.29	34.98	1.10	3.68	160	21.42	24.77	12.96	0.51	1.38
其他的胸腔器官	C37–C38	5	0.47	0.71	0.53	0.03	0.09	8	1.07	1.24	0.56	0.02	0.06
骨	C40–C41	9	0.84	1.28	0.77	0.04	0.06	7	0.94	1.08	0.66	0.03	0.03
皮肤的黑色素瘤	C43	0	0.00	0.00	0.00	0.00	0.00	0	0.00	0.00	0.00	0.00	0.00
其他的皮肤	C44	3	0.28	0.43	0.25	0.00	0.05	3	0.40	0.46	0.19	0.00	0.02
间皮瘤	C45	0	0.00	0.00	0.00	0.00	0.00	0	0.00	0.00	0.00	0.00	0.00
卡波西肉瘤	C46	0	0.00	0.00	0.00	0.00	0.00	0	0.00	0.00	0.00	0.00	0.00
周围神经、其他结缔组织、软组织	C47;C49	0	0.00	0.00	0.00	0.00	0.00	2	0.27	0.31	0.14	0.01	0.01
乳房	C50	1	0.09	0.14	0.09	0.01	0.01	55	7.36	8.51	5.36	0.41	0.60
外阴	C51	0	0.00	0.00	0.00	0.00	0.00	0	0.00	0.00	0.00	0.00	0.00
阴道	C52	0	0.00	0.00	0.00	0.00	0.00	0	0.00	0.00	0.00	0.00	0.00
子宫颈	C53	0	0.00	0.00	0.00	0.00	0.00	30	4.02	4.64	2.98	0.19	0.35
子宫体	C54	0	0.00	0.00	0.00	0.00	0.00	5	0.67	0.77	0.43	0.03	0.03
子宫，部位不明	C55	0	0.00	0.00	0.00	0.00	0.00	3	0.40	0.46	0.20	0.01	0.01
卵巢	C56	0	0.00	0.00	0.00	0.00	0.00	14	1.87	2.17	1.26	0.07	0.13
女性其他的生殖器	C57	0	0.00	0.00	0.00	0.00	0.00	0	0.00	0.00	0.00	0.00	0.00
胎盘	C58	0	0.00	0.00	0.00	0.00	0.00	0	0.00	0.00	0.00	0.00	0.00
阴茎	C60	0	0.00	0.00	0.00	0.00	0.00	0	0.00	0.00	0.00	0.00	0.00
前列腺	C61	12	1.12	1.71	0.98	0.01	0.05	0	0.00	0.00	0.00	0.00	0.00
睾丸	C62	0	0.00	0.00	0.00	0.00	0.00	0	0.00	0.00	0.00	0.00	0.00
男性其他的生殖器	C63	0	0.00	0.00	0.00	0.00	0.00	0	0.00	0.00	0.00	0.00	0.00
肾	C64	9	0.84	1.28	1.04	0.06	0.14	4	0.54	0.62	0.29	0.02	0.02
肾盂	C65	1	0.09	0.14	0.15	0.02	0.02	3	0.40	0.46	0.15	0.00	0.00
输尿管	C66	0	0.00	0.00	0.00	0.00	0.00	0	0.00	0.00	0.00	0.00	0.00
膀胱	C67	12	1.12	1.71	1.14	0.03	0.07	4	0.54	0.62	0.40	0.02	0.07
其他的泌尿器官	C68	0	0.00	0.00	0.00	0.00	0.00	0	0.00	0.00	0.00	0.00	0.00
眼	C69	0	0.00	0.00	0.00	0.00	0.00	0	0.00	0.00	0.00	0.00	0.00
脑、神经系统	C70–C72	27	2.51	3.84	2.70	0.12	0.35	36	4.82	5.57	3.12	0.12	0.33
甲状腺	C73	0	0.00	0.00	0.00	0.00	0.00	4	0.54	0.62	0.30	0.00	0.03
肾上腺	C74	0	0.00	0.00	0.00	0.00	0.00	0	0.00	0.00	0.00	0.00	0.00
其他的内分泌腺	C75	0	0.00	0.00	0.00	0.00	0.00	0	0.00	0.00	0.00	0.00	0.00
霍奇金病	C81	0	0.00	0.00	0.00	0.00	0.00	0	0.00	0.00	0.00	0.00	0.00
非霍奇金淋巴瘤	C82–C85;C96	11	1.02	1.56	1.19	0.06	0.14	7	0.94	1.08	0.78	0.05	0.11
免疫增生性疾病	C88	0	0.00	0.00	0.00	0.00	0.00	0	0.00	0.00	0.00	0.00	0.00
多发性骨髓瘤	C90	2	0.19	0.28	0.20	0.01	0.03	4	0.54	0.62	0.35	0.03	0.05
淋巴样白血病	C91	0	0.00	0.00	0.00	0.00	0.00	0	0.00	0.00	0.00	0.00	0.00
髓样白血病	C92–C94	1	0.09	0.14	0.07	0.00	0.00	6	0.80	0.93	0.82	0.05	0.08
白血病，未特指	C95	3	0.28	0.43	0.42	0.04	0.04	3	0.40	0.46	0.30	0.03	0.03
其他的或未指明部位	O&U	19	1.77	2.70	2.34	0.10	0.20	29	3.88	4.49	3.02	0.15	0.26
骨髓增殖性疾病	MPD	0	0.00	0.00	0.00	0.00	0.00	0	0.00	0.00	0.00	0.00	0.00
骨髓增生异常综合征	MDS	0	0.00	0.00	0.00	0.00	0.00	0	0.00	0.00	0.00	0.00	0.00
合计	ALL	1 074	100.00	152.61	103.98	4.16	11.27	747	100.00	115.63	61.05	2.69	6.15
C44 以外的部位	ALL but C44	1 071	99.72	152.19	103.72	4.16	11.22	744	99.60	115.16	60.86	2.69	6.14

表 6-113　2020 年河南省驻马店市城区恶性肿瘤发病主要指标

部位	ICD-10	男性						女性					
		病例数	构成 (%)	粗率 ($1/10^5$)	世标率 ($1/10^5$)	累积率 (%)		病例数	构成 (%)	粗率 ($1/10^5$)	世标率 ($1/10^5$)	累积率 (%)	
						0~64	0~74					0~64	0~74
唇	C00	1	0.12	0.33	0.18	0.00	0.03	1	0.11	0.30	0.09	0.00	0.00
舌	C01–C02	2	0.24	0.66	0.42	0.04	0.04	1	0.11	0.30	0.22	0.02	0.02
口	C03–C06	2	0.24	0.66	0.27	0.00	0.04	2	0.23	0.61	0.31	0.02	0.02
唾液腺	C07–C08	3	0.36	0.99	0.69	0.06	0.10	0	0.00	0.00	0.00	0.00	0.00
扁桃体	C09	0	0.00	0.00	0.00	0.00	0.00	0	0.00	0.00	0.00	0.00	0.00
其他的口咽	C10	1	0.12	0.33	0.19	0.02	0.02	0	0.00	0.00	0.00	0.00	0.00
鼻咽	C11	3	0.36	0.99	0.66	0.06	0.06	1	0.11	0.30	0.17	0.02	0.02
喉咽	C12–C13	2	0.24	0.66	0.38	0.04	0.04	0	0.00	0.00	0.00	0.00	0.00
咽，部位不明	C14	0	0.00	0.00	0.00	0.00	0.00	0	0.00	0.00	0.00	0.00	0.00
食管	C15	74	8.77	24.34	13.21	0.68	1.64	38	4.37	11.54	5.33	0.06	0.64
胃	C16	111	13.15	36.50	22.05	1.36	2.95	35	4.02	10.62	6.13	0.35	0.66
小肠	C17	4	0.47	1.32	0.60	0.02	0.05	3	0.34	0.91	0.62	0.06	0.06
结肠	C18	33	3.91	10.85	6.28	0.43	0.77	36	4.14	10.93	6.67	0.47	0.83
直肠	C19–C20	44	5.21	14.47	8.32	0.50	1.02	26	2.99	7.89	5.29	0.39	0.64
肛门	C21	0	0.00	0.00	0.00	0.00	0.00	1	0.11	0.30	0.16	0.00	0.04
肝脏	C22	107	12.68	35.19	21.25	1.79	2.36	36	4.14	10.93	5.93	0.33	0.76
胆囊及其他	C23–C24	16	1.90	5.26	3.20	0.19	0.38	13	1.49	3.95	2.47	0.15	0.35
胰腺	C25	17	2.01	5.59	3.47	0.23	0.38	15	1.72	4.55	2.50	0.17	0.22
鼻、鼻窦及其他	C30–C31	0	0.00	0.00	0.00	0.00	0.00	5	0.57	1.52	0.86	0.03	0.09
喉	C32	9	1.07	2.96	1.49	0.09	0.17	1	0.11	0.30	0.26	0.02	0.02
气管、支气管、肺	C33–C34	210	24.88	69.06	36.18	1.67	4.80	91	10.46	27.62	15.58	0.89	1.87
其他的胸腔器官	C37–C38	4	0.47	1.32	1.08	0.08	0.08	3	0.34	0.91	1.11	0.05	0.09
骨	C40–C41	5	0.59	1.64	1.43	0.12	0.17	2	0.23	0.61	0.29	0.00	0.03
皮肤的黑色素瘤	C43	1	0.12	0.33	0.40	0.02	0.02	1	0.11	0.30	0.26	0.02	0.02
其他的皮肤	C44	6	0.71	1.97	1.00	0.08	0.12	13	1.49	3.95	1.97	0.09	0.21
间皮瘤	C45	0	0.00	0.00	0.00	0.00	0.00	0	0.00	0.00	0.00	0.00	0.00
卡波西肉瘤	C46	0	0.00	0.00	0.00	0.00	0.00	0	0.00	0.00	0.00	0.00	0.00
周围神经、其他结缔组织、软组织	C47;C49	0	0.00	0.00	0.00	0.00	0.00	4	0.46	1.21	0.58	0.00	0.07
乳房	C50	0	0.00	0.00	0.00	0.00	0.00	185	21.26	56.16	39.60	3.50	4.09
外阴	C51	0	0.00	0.00	0.00	0.00	0.00	3	0.34	0.91	0.70	0.06	0.06
阴道	C52	0	0.00	0.00	0.00	0.00	0.00	3	0.34	0.91	0.45	0.00	0.07
子宫颈	C53	0	0.00	0.00	0.00	0.00	0.00	58	6.67	17.61	11.70	0.93	1.33
子宫体	C54	0	0.00	0.00	0.00	0.00	0.00	22	2.53	6.68	4.14	0.33	0.45
子宫，部位不明	C55	0	0.00	0.00	0.00	0.00	0.00	15	1.72	4.55	2.69	0.22	0.30
卵巢	C56	0	0.00	0.00	0.00	0.00	0.00	33	3.79	10.02	6.92	0.50	0.74
女性其他的生殖器	C57	0	0.00	0.00	0.00	0.00	0.00	3	0.34	0.91	0.52	0.04	0.04
胎盘	C58	0	0.00	0.00	0.00	0.00	0.00	2	0.23	0.61	0.49	0.04	0.04
阴茎	C60	1	0.12	0.33	0.15	0.02	0.02	0	0.00	0.00	0.00	0.00	0.00
前列腺	C61	33	3.91	10.85	5.80	0.29	0.71	0	0.00	0.00	0.00	0.00	0.00
睾丸	C62	0	0.00	0.00	0.00	0.00	0.00	0	0.00	0.00	0.00	0.00	0.00
男性其他的生殖器	C63	0	0.00	0.00	0.00	0.00	0.00	0	0.00	0.00	0.00	0.00	0.00
肾	C64	9	1.07	2.96	1.65	0.04	0.30	7	0.80	2.12	1.40	0.16	0.16
肾盂	C65	2	0.24	0.66	0.32	0.00	0.03	0	0.00	0.00	0.00	0.00	0.00
输尿管	C66	0	0.00	0.00	0.00	0.00	0.00	1	0.11	0.30	0.17	0.02	0.02
膀胱	C67	18	2.13	5.92	2.99	0.14	0.36	5	0.57	1.52	0.65	0.02	0.04
其他的泌尿器官	C68	0	0.00	0.00	0.00	0.00	0.00	1	0.11	0.30	0.31	0.04	0.04
眼	C69	0	0.00	0.00	0.00	0.00	0.00	0	0.00	0.00	0.00	0.00	0.00
脑、神经系统	C70–C72	8	0.95	2.63	2.24	0.12	0.18	14	1.61	4.25	2.91	0.18	0.31
甲状腺	C73	43	5.09	14.14	11.52	0.96	1.05	145	16.67	44.02	35.03	2.98	3.15
肾上腺	C74	1	0.12	0.33	0.28	0.02	0.02	0	0.00	0.00	0.00	0.00	0.00
其他的内分泌腺	C75	1	0.12	0.33	0.33	0.04	0.04	1	0.11	0.30	0.22	0.02	0.02
霍奇金病	C81	0	0.00	0.00	0.00	0.00	0.00	0	0.00	0.00	0.00	0.00	0.00
非霍奇金淋巴瘤	C82–C85;C96	22	2.61	7.24	5.25	0.42	0.61	8	0.92	2.43	1.75	0.17	0.17
免疫增生性疾病	C88	0	0.00	0.00	0.00	0.00	0.00	0	0.00	0.00	0.00	0.00	0.00
多发性骨髓瘤	C90	5	0.59	1.64	0.85	0.06	0.09	6	0.69	1.82	0.89	0.04	0.12
淋巴样白血病	C91	1	0.12	0.33	0.79	0.03	0.03	4	0.46	1.21	1.87	0.12	0.12
髓样白血病	C92–C94	8	0.95	2.63	1.76	0.09	0.21	5	0.57	1.52	1.81	0.10	0.13
白血病，未特指	C95	4	0.47	1.32	1.84	0.11	0.11	4	0.46	1.21	1.06	0.03	0.14
其他的或未指明部位	O&U	30	3.55	9.87	6.68	0.34	0.76	15	1.72	4.55	2.59	0.13	0.36
骨髓增殖性疾病	MPD	3	0.36	0.99	0.60	0.04	0.08	2	0.23	0.61	0.40	0.04	0.04
骨髓增生异常综合征	MDS	0	0.00	0.00	0.00	0.00	0.00	0	0.00	0.00	0.00	0.00	0.00
合计	ALL	844	100.00	277.56	165.78	10.20	19.86	870	100.00	264.11	175.06	12.76	18.58
C44 以外的部位	ALL but C44	838	99.29	275.59	164.78	10.12	19.73	857	98.51	260.16	173.09	12.67	18.37

表 6-114 2020 年河南省驻马店市城区恶性肿瘤死亡主要指标

部位	ICD-10	男性						女性					
		病例数	构成(%)	粗率($1/10^5$)	世标率($1/10^5$)	累积率(%)		病例数	构成(%)	粗率($1/10^5$)	世标率($1/10^5$)	累积率(%)	
						0~64	0~74					0~64	0~74
唇	C00	1	0.22	0.33	0.10	0.00	0.00	0	0.00	0.00	0.00	0.00	0.00
舌	C01–C02	1	0.22	0.33	0.34	0.03	0.03	2	0.76	0.61	0.31	0.02	0.02
口	C03–C06	2	0.44	0.66	0.20	0.00	0.00	0	0.00	0.00	0.00	0.00	0.00
唾液腺	C07–C08	0	0.00	0.00	0.00	0.00	0.00	1	0.38	0.30	0.31	0.04	0.04
扁桃体	C09	0	0.00	0.00	0.00	0.00	0.00	0	0.00	0.00	0.00	0.00	0.00
其他的口咽	C10	0	0.00	0.00	0.00	0.00	0.00	0	0.00	0.00	0.00	0.00	0.00
鼻咽	C11	1	0.22	0.33	0.19	0.02	0.02	0	0.00	0.00	0.00	0.00	0.00
喉咽	C12–C13	1	0.22	0.33	0.15	0.02	0.02	0	0.00	0.00	0.00	0.00	0.00
咽，部位不明	C14	1	0.22	0.33	0.15	0.02	0.02	0	0.00	0.00	0.00	0.00	0.00
食管	C15	52	11.45	17.10	8.20	0.20	0.92	23	8.78	6.98	3.36	0.09	0.35
胃	C16	51	11.23	16.77	9.15	0.46	1.06	19	7.25	5.77	3.24	0.21	0.35
小肠	C17	2	0.44	0.66	0.32	0.02	0.06	2	0.76	0.61	0.40	0.04	0.04
结肠	C18	9	1.98	2.96	1.13	0.02	0.09	9	3.44	2.73	1.56	0.10	0.16
直肠	C19–C20	10	2.20	3.29	1.71	0.08	0.22	9	3.44	2.73	1.21	0.07	0.07
肛门	C21	1	0.22	0.33	0.18	0.00	0.03	0	0.00	0.00	0.00	0.00	0.00
肝脏	C22	90	19.82	29.60	16.73	1.29	1.82	28	10.69	8.50	4.51	0.22	0.52
胆囊及其他	C23–C24	7	1.54	2.30	1.29	0.06	0.15	7	2.67	2.12	1.27	0.11	0.15
胰腺	C25	13	2.86	4.28	1.98	0.02	0.32	13	4.96	3.95	2.34	0.15	0.26
鼻、鼻窦及其他	C30–C31	0	0.00	0.00	0.00	0.00	0.00	1	0.38	0.30	0.13	0.00	0.00
喉	C32	2	0.44	0.66	0.27	0.00	0.04	0	0.00	0.00	0.00	0.00	0.00
气管、支气管、肺	C33–C34	127	27.97	41.77	20.72	0.82	2.50	59	22.52	17.91	8.82	0.42	0.84
其他的胸腔器官	C37–C38	2	0.44	0.66	0.38	0.02	0.02	1	0.38	0.30	0.31	0.04	0.04
骨	C40–C41	1	0.22	0.33	0.19	0.02	0.02	2	0.76	0.61	0.29	0.00	0.03
皮肤的黑色素瘤	C43	0	0.00	0.00	0.00	0.00	0.00	0	0.00	0.00	0.00	0.00	0.00
其他的皮肤	C44	2	0.44	0.66	0.20	0.00	0.00	1	0.38	0.30	0.22	0.02	0.02
间皮瘤	C45	1	0.22	0.33	0.24	0.02	0.02	0	0.00	0.00	0.00	0.00	0.00
卡波西肉瘤	C46	0	0.00	0.00	0.00	0.00	0.00	0	0.00	0.00	0.00	0.00	0.00
周围神经、其他结缔组织、软组织	C47;C49	0	0.00	0.00	0.00	0.00	0.00	0	0.00	0.00	0.00	0.00	0.00
乳房	C50	0	0.00	0.00	0.00	0.00	0.00	24	9.16	7.29	4.69	0.40	0.54
外阴	C51	0	0.00	0.00	0.00	0.00	0.00	3	1.15	0.91	0.53	0.03	0.03
阴道	C52	0	0.00	0.00	0.00	0.00	0.00	1	0.38	0.30	0.09	0.00	0.00
子宫颈	C53	0	0.00	0.00	0.00	0.00	0.00	10	3.82	3.04	1.97	0.13	0.33
子宫体	C54	0	0.00	0.00	0.00	0.00	0.00	3	1.15	0.91	0.43	0.02	0.04
子宫，部位不明	C55	0	0.00	0.00	0.00	0.00	0.00	1	0.38	0.30	0.16	0.00	0.04
卵巢	C56	0	0.00	0.00	0.00	0.00	0.00	13	4.96	3.95	2.09	0.23	0.27
女性其他的生殖器	C57	0	0.00	0.00	0.00	0.00	0.00	1	0.38	0.30	0.17	0.02	0.02
胎盘	C58	0	0.00	0.00	0.00	0.00	0.00	0	0.00	0.00	0.00	0.00	0.00
阴茎	C60	0	0.00	0.00	0.00	0.00	0.00	0	0.00	0.00	0.00	0.00	0.00
前列腺	C61	12	2.64	3.95	1.57	0.00	0.16	0	0.00	0.00	0.00	0.00	0.00
睾丸	C62	0	0.00	0.00	0.00	0.00	0.00	0	0.00	0.00	0.00	0.00	0.00
男性其他的生殖器	C63	0	0.00	0.00	0.00	0.00	0.00	0	0.00	0.00	0.00	0.00	0.00
肾	C64	5	1.10	1.64	1.05	0.06	0.15	2	0.76	0.61	0.26	0.02	0.02
肾盂	C65	1	0.22	0.33	0.18	0.00	0.03	0	0.00	0.00	0.00	0.00	0.00
输尿管	C66	0	0.00	0.00	0.00	0.00	0.00	1	0.38	0.30	0.16	0.00	0.04
膀胱	C67	6	1.32	1.97	0.64	0.00	0.00	3	1.15	0.91	0.28	0.00	0.00
其他的泌尿器官	C68	0	0.00	0.00	0.00	0.00	0.00	1	0.38	0.30	0.16	0.00	0.03
眼	C69	0	0.00	0.00	0.00	0.00	0.00	0	0.00	0.00	0.00	0.00	0.00
脑、神经系统	C70–C72	7	1.54	2.30	1.43	0.10	0.21	4	1.53	1.21	0.85	0.06	0.12
甲状腺	C73	0	0.00	0.00	0.00	0.00	0.00	2	0.76	0.61	0.40	0.04	0.04
肾上腺	C74	0	0.00	0.00	0.00	0.00	0.00	0	0.00	0.00	0.00	0.00	0.00
其他的内分泌腺	C75	0	0.00	0.00	0.00	0.00	0.00	0	0.00	0.00	0.00	0.00	0.00
霍奇金病	C81	0	0.00	0.00	0.00	0.00	0.00	0	0.00	0.00	0.00	0.00	0.00
非霍奇金淋巴瘤	C82–C85;C96	10	2.20	3.29	1.98	0.16	0.22	3	1.15	0.91	0.41	0.00	0.04
免疫增生性疾病	C88	0	0.00	0.00	0.00	0.00	0.00	0	0.00	0.00	0.00	0.00	0.00
多发性骨髓瘤	C90	3	0.66	0.99	0.49	0.00	0.06	4	1.53	1.21	0.51	0.00	0.07
淋巴样白血病	C91	0	0.00	0.00	0.00	0.00	0.00	1	0.38	0.30	0.73	0.03	0.03
髓样白血病	C92–C94	6	1.32	1.97	1.54	0.07	0.15	3	1.15	0.91	0.64	0.06	0.10
白血病，未特指	C95	3	0.66	0.99	0.46	0.00	0.06	2	0.76	0.61	0.32	0.00	0.07
其他的或未指明部位	O&U	22	4.85	7.24	4.47	0.28	0.38	3	1.15	0.91	0.34	0.00	0.04
骨髓增殖性疾病	MPD	1	0.22	0.33	0.10	0.00	0.00	0	0.00	0.00	0.00	0.00	0.00
骨髓增生异常综合征	MDS	1	0.22	0.33	0.33	0.04	0.04	0	0.00	0.00	0.00	0.00	0.00
合计	ALL	454	100.00	149.31	78.06	3.84	8.84	262	100.00	79.54	43.48	2.55	4.75
C44 以外的部位	ALL but C44	452	99.56	148.65	77.86	3.84	8.84	261	99.62	79.23	43.26	2.53	4.73

表 6-115　2020 年河南省西平县恶性肿瘤发病主要指标

部位	ICD-10	男性						女性					
		病例数	构成 (%)	粗率 ($1/10^5$)	世标率 ($1/10^5$)	累积率 (%)		病例数	构成 (%)	粗率 ($1/10^5$)	世标率 ($1/10^5$)	累积率 (%)	
						0~64	0~74					0~64	0~74
唇	C00	2	0.16	0.44	0.34	0.00	0.06	0	0.00	0.00	0.00	0.00	0.00
舌	C01–C02	3	0.24	0.65	0.48	0.03	0.03	2	0.18	0.46	0.33	0.02	0.05
口	C03–C06	3	0.24	0.65	0.52	0.00	0.09	3	0.27	0.69	0.43	0.01	0.06
唾液腺	C07–C08	1	0.08	0.22	0.41	0.00	0.00	4	0.36	0.92	0.67	0.03	0.08
扁桃体	C09	2	0.16	0.44	0.30	0.03	0.03	0	0.00	0.00	0.00	0.00	0.00
其他的口咽	C10	0	0.00	0.00	0.00	0.00	0.00	0	0.00	0.00	0.00	0.00	0.00
鼻咽	C11	4	0.32	0.87	0.65	0.04	0.07	2	0.18	0.46	0.27	0.02	0.02
喉咽	C12–C13	5	0.40	1.09	1.03	0.01	0.09	0	0.00	0.00	0.00	0.00	0.00
咽，部位不明	C14	0	0.00	0.00	0.00	0.00	0.00	0	0.00	0.00	0.00	0.00	0.00
食管	C15	140	11.23	30.55	26.04	0.51	2.62	71	6.37	16.42	10.72	0.19	0.89
胃	C16	149	11.95	32.52	25.96	0.62	3.04	55	4.93	12.72	8.14	0.25	0.91
小肠	C17	4	0.32	0.87	0.70	0.00	0.15	6	0.54	1.39	0.93	0.01	0.13
结肠	C18	43	3.45	9.38	7.49	0.34	1.00	39	3.50	9.02	6.14	0.21	0.78
直肠	C19–C20	41	3.29	8.95	7.02	0.34	0.69	44	3.95	10.17	6.97	0.30	1.00
肛门	C21	0	0.00	0.00	0.00	0.00	0.00	1	0.09	0.23	0.10	0.00	0.00
肝脏	C22	171	13.71	37.32	29.16	1.59	3.15	90	8.07	20.81	13.77	0.54	1.76
胆囊及其他	C23–C24	28	2.25	6.11	4.94	0.15	0.46	32	2.87	7.40	5.14	0.17	0.78
胰腺	C25	28	2.25	6.11	5.02	0.18	0.66	24	2.15	5.55	3.46	0.07	0.38
鼻、鼻窦及其他	C30–C31	3	0.24	0.65	0.51	0.04	0.08	1	0.09	0.23	0.19	0.02	0.02
喉	C32	8	0.64	1.75	1.45	0.04	0.09	2	0.18	0.46	0.34	0.02	0.04
气管、支气管、肺	C33–C34	368	29.51	80.31	66.76	1.81	6.94	177	15.87	40.92	27.81	1.07	3.23
其他的胸腔器官	C37–C38	2	0.16	0.44	0.31	0.03	0.03	3	0.27	0.69	0.43	0.01	0.06
骨	C40–C41	9	0.72	1.96	1.77	0.10	0.13	10	0.90	2.31	1.83	0.12	0.23
皮肤的黑色素瘤	C43	1	0.08	0.22	0.18	0.00	0.05	2	0.18	0.46	0.33	0.01	0.06
其他的皮肤	C44	3	0.24	0.65	0.50	0.04	0.08	9	0.81	2.08	1.39	0.05	0.12
间皮瘤	C45	0	0.00	0.00	0.00	0.00	0.00	0	0.00	0.00	0.00	0.00	0.00
卡波西肉瘤	C46	0	0.00	0.00	0.00	0.00	0.00	0	0.00	0.00	0.00	0.00	0.00
周围神经、其他结缔组织、软组织	C47;C49	4	0.32	0.87	0.83	0.04	0.07	3	0.27	0.69	0.50	0.03	0.06
乳房	C50	1	0.08	0.22	0.16	0.01	0.01	187	16.77	43.23	31.67	2.55	3.75
外阴	C51	0	0.00	0.00	0.00	0.00	0.00	2	0.18	0.46	0.34	0.00	0.07
阴道	C52	0	0.00	0.00	0.00	0.00	0.00	2	0.18	0.46	0.33	0.01	0.06
子宫颈	C53	0	0.00	0.00	0.00	0.00	0.00	92	8.25	21.27	15.31	1.11	1.80
子宫体	C54	0	0.00	0.00	0.00	0.00	0.00	31	2.78	7.17	5.12	0.39	0.63
子宫，部位不明	C55	0	0.00	0.00	0.00	0.00	0.00	10	0.90	2.31	1.61	0.11	0.22
卵巢	C56	0	0.00	0.00	0.00	0.00	0.00	29	2.60	6.70	5.09	0.31	0.55
女性其他的生殖器	C57	0	0.00	0.00	0.00	0.00	0.00	1	0.09	0.23	0.17	0.01	0.01
胎盘	C58	0	0.00	0.00	0.00	0.00	0.00	0	0.00	0.00	0.00	0.00	0.00
阴茎	C60	3	0.24	0.65	0.45	0.02	0.06	0	0.00	0.00	0.00	0.00	0.00
前列腺	C61	30	2.41	6.55	5.51	0.06	0.60	0	0.00	0.00	0.00	0.00	0.00
睾丸	C62	3	0.24	0.65	0.54	0.04	0.04	0	0.00	0.00	0.00	0.00	0.00
男性其他的生殖器	C63	0	0.00	0.00	0.00	0.00	0.00	0	0.00	0.00	0.00	0.00	0.00
肾	C64	14	1.12	3.06	2.44	0.15	0.25	7	0.63	1.62	1.60	0.07	0.11
肾盂	C65	0	0.00	0.00	0.00	0.00	0.00	0	0.00	0.00	0.00	0.00	0.00
输尿管	C66	2	0.16	0.44	0.56	0.02	0.02	1	0.09	0.23	0.17	0.00	0.03
膀胱	C67	31	2.49	6.77	5.83	0.20	0.46	7	0.63	1.62	1.06	0.02	0.07
其他的泌尿器官	C68	0	0.00	0.00	0.00	0.00	0.00	1	0.09	0.23	0.17	0.00	0.03
眼	C69	0	0.00	0.00	0.00	0.00	0.00	0	0.00	0.00	0.00	0.00	0.00
脑、神经系统	C70–C72	33	2.65	7.20	6.01	0.37	0.78	23	2.06	5.32	3.67	0.24	0.41
甲状腺	C73	30	2.41	6.55	5.08	0.41	0.49	57	5.11	13.18	9.59	0.90	0.96
肾上腺	C74	1	0.08	0.22	0.17	0.00	0.03	1	0.09	0.23	0.17	0.01	0.01
其他的内分泌腺	C75	0	0.00	0.00	0.00	0.00	0.00	0	0.00	0.00	0.00	0.00	0.00
霍奇金病	C81	1	0.08	0.22	0.15	0.01	0.01	2	0.18	0.46	0.33	0.02	0.06
非霍奇金淋巴瘤	C82–C85;C96	22	1.76	4.80	4.14	0.20	0.52	24	2.15	5.55	4.03	0.25	0.47
免疫增生性疾病	C88	0	0.00	0.00	0.00	0.00	0.00	2	0.18	0.46	0.35	0.02	0.05
多发性骨髓瘤	C90	9	0.72	1.96	1.51	0.03	0.23	14	1.26	3.24	2.29	0.15	0.33
淋巴样白血病	C91	5	0.40	1.09	1.20	0.08	0.10	6	0.54	1.39	1.96	0.11	0.11
髓样白血病	C92–C94	12	0.96	2.62	2.28	0.17	0.17	11	0.99	2.54	1.86	0.09	0.21
白血病，未特指	C95	7	0.56	1.53	1.33	0.07	0.10	9	0.81	2.08	1.55	0.09	0.15
其他的或未指明部位	O&U	16	1.28	3.49	2.57	0.16	0.29	15	1.35	3.47	2.48	0.18	0.24
骨髓增殖性疾病	MPD	3	0.24	0.65	0.47	0.05	0.05	1	0.09	0.23	0.17	0.00	0.03
骨髓增生异常综合征	MDS	2	0.16	0.44	0.37	0.03	0.03	0	0.00	0.00	0.00	0.00	0.00
合计	ALL	1 247	100.00	272.15	223.16	8.01	23.86	1 115	100.00	257.79	180.96	9.84	21.02
C44 以外的部位	ALL but C44	1 244	99.76	271.50	222.66	7.97	23.78	1 106	99.19	255.71	179.57	9.78	20.89

表 6-116 2020 年河南省西平县恶性肿瘤死亡主要指标

部位	ICD-10	男性						女性					
		病例数	构成(%)	粗率($1/10^5$)	世标率($1/10^5$)	累积率(%)		病例数	构成(%)	粗率($1/10^5$)	世标率($1/10^5$)	累积率(%)	
						0~64	0~74					0~64	0~74
唇	C00	0	0.00	0.00	0.00	0.00	0.00	0	0.00	0.00	0.00	0.00	0.00
舌	C01-C02	1	0.10	0.22	0.41	0.00	0.00	0	0.00	0.00	0.00	0.00	0.00
口	C03-C06	1	0.10	0.22	0.17	0.00	0.03	0	0.00	0.00	0.00	0.00	0.00
唾液腺	C07-C08	3	0.31	0.65	0.48	0.03	0.08	1	0.18	0.23	0.17	0.00	0.04
扁桃体	C09	0	0.00	0.00	0.00	0.00	0.00	1	0.18	0.23	0.17	0.00	0.04
其他的口咽	C10	0	0.00	0.00	0.00	0.00	0.00	1	0.18	0.23	0.17	0.00	0.04
鼻咽	C11	3	0.31	0.65	0.49	0.01	0.07	1	0.18	0.23	0.17	0.01	0.01
喉咽	C12-C13	2	0.21	0.44	0.35	0.00	0.07	0	0.00	0.00	0.00	0.00	0.00
咽，部位不明	C14	0	0.00	0.00	0.00	0.00	0.00	0	0.00	0.00	0.00	0.00	0.00
食管	C15	124	12.94	27.06	23.52	0.31	1.97	53	9.40	12.25	7.46	0.13	0.34
胃	C16	126	13.15	27.50	22.08	0.55	2.21	42	7.45	9.71	6.19	0.22	0.56
小肠	C17	4	0.42	0.87	0.69	0.02	0.15	2	0.35	0.46	0.33	0.00	0.06
结肠	C18	23	2.40	5.02	4.13	0.21	0.42	18	3.19	4.16	2.50	0.03	0.15
直肠	C19-C20	30	3.13	6.55	5.55	0.15	0.51	12	2.13	2.77	1.61	0.04	0.13
肛门	C21	1	0.10	0.22	0.18	0.00	0.05	0	0.00	0.00	0.00	0.00	0.00
肝脏	C22	154	16.08	33.61	27.06	1.18	2.86	71	12.59	16.42	10.98	0.40	1.36
胆囊及其他	C23-C24	34	3.55	7.42	6.40	0.08	0.90	36	6.38	8.32	5.53	0.21	0.72
胰腺	C25	21	2.19	4.58	3.74	0.11	0.54	24	4.26	5.55	3.56	0.10	0.38
鼻、鼻窦及其他	C30-C31	4	0.42	0.87	0.61	0.05	0.05	0	0.00	0.00	0.00	0.00	0.00
喉	C32	3	0.31	0.65	0.70	0.00	0.03	3	0.53	0.69	0.45	0.02	0.05
气管、支气管、肺	C33-C34	296	30.90	64.60	56.71	1.23	5.11	115	20.39	26.59	17.86	0.55	1.63
其他的胸腔器官	C37-C38	0	0.00	0.00	0.00	0.00	0.00	3	0.53	0.69	0.45	0.02	0.07
骨	C40-C41	5	0.52	1.09	0.87	0.03	0.07	2	0.35	0.46	0.33	0.02	0.05
皮肤的黑色素瘤	C43	2	0.21	0.44	0.30	0.00	0.05	0	0.00	0.00	0.00	0.00	0.00
其他的皮肤	C44	7	0.73	1.53	1.62	0.00	0.10	1	0.18	0.23	0.18	0.00	0.00
间皮瘤	C45	0	0.00	0.00	0.00	0.00	0.00	0	0.00	0.00	0.00	0.00	0.00
卡波西肉瘤	C46	0	0.00	0.00	0.00	0.00	0.00	0	0.00	0.00	0.00	0.00	0.00
周围神经、其他结缔组织、软组织	C47;C49	2	0.21	0.44	0.32	0.01	0.04	1	0.18	0.23	0.17	0.01	0.01
乳房	C50	0	0.00	0.00	0.00	0.00	0.00	35	6.21	8.09	5.88	0.32	0.66
外阴	C51	0	0.00	0.00	0.00	0.00	0.00	1	0.18	0.23	0.18	0.00	0.00
阴道	C52	0	0.00	0.00	0.00	0.00	0.00	0	0.00	0.00	0.00	0.00	0.00
子宫颈	C53	0	0.00	0.00	0.00	0.00	0.00	39	6.91	9.02	6.24	0.37	0.73
子宫体	C54	0	0.00	0.00	0.00	0.00	0.00	5	0.89	1.16	0.65	0.02	0.05
子宫，部位不明	C55	0	0.00	0.00	0.00	0.00	0.00	3	0.53	0.69	0.37	0.02	0.02
卵巢	C56	0	0.00	0.00	0.00	0.00	0.00	9	1.60	2.08	1.51	0.14	0.17
女性其他的生殖器	C57	0	0.00	0.00	0.00	0.00	0.00	1	0.18	0.23	0.17	0.00	0.03
胎盘	C58	0	0.00	0.00	0.00	0.00	0.00	0	0.00	0.00	0.00	0.00	0.00
阴茎	C60	3	0.31	0.65	0.51	0.02	0.11	0	0.00	0.00	0.00	0.00	0.00
前列腺	C61	16	1.67	3.49	3.77	0.00	0.23	0	0.00	0.00	0.00	0.00	0.00
睾丸	C62	0	0.00	0.00	0.00	0.00	0.00	0	0.00	0.00	0.00	0.00	0.00
男性其他的生殖器	C63	0	0.00	0.00	0.00	0.00	0.00	0	0.00	0.00	0.00	0.00	0.00
肾	C64	5	0.52	1.09	0.96	0.03	0.11	3	0.53	0.69	0.46	0.02	0.02
肾盂	C65	0	0.00	0.00	0.00	0.00	0.00	0	0.00	0.00	0.00	0.00	0.00
输尿管	C66	0	0.00	0.00	0.00	0.00	0.00	1	0.18	0.23	0.16	0.02	0.02
膀胱	C67	16	1.67	3.49	3.56	0.02	0.21	3	0.53	0.69	0.30	0.00	0.00
其他的泌尿器官	C68	1	0.10	0.22	0.41	0.00	0.00	0	0.00	0.00	0.00	0.00	0.00
眼	C69	0	0.00	0.00	0.00	0.00	0.00	0	0.00	0.00	0.00	0.00	0.00
脑、神经系统	C70-C72	18	1.88	3.93	3.32	0.12	0.46	12	2.13	2.77	1.98	0.08	0.28
甲状腺	C73	2	0.21	0.44	0.28	0.02	0.02	3	0.53	0.69	0.44	0.00	0.03
肾上腺	C74	1	0.10	0.22	0.41	0.00	0.00	0	0.00	0.00	0.00	0.00	0.00
其他的内分泌腺	C75	0	0.00	0.00	0.00	0.00	0.00	0	0.00	0.00	0.00	0.00	0.00
霍奇金病	C81	0	0.00	0.00	0.00	0.00	0.00	0	0.00	0.00	0.00	0.00	0.00
非霍奇金淋巴瘤	C82-C85;C96	17	1.77	3.71	3.68	0.02	0.25	13	2.30	3.01	1.98	0.07	0.23
免疫增生性疾病	C88	0	0.00	0.00	0.00	0.00	0.00	0	0.00	0.00	0.00	0.00	0.00
多发性骨髓瘤	C90	10	1.04	2.18	1.66	0.06	0.25	13	2.30	3.01	2.09	0.12	0.33
淋巴样白血病	C91	2	0.21	0.44	0.29	0.00	0.03	2	0.35	0.46	0.37	0.05	0.05
髓样白血病	C92-C94	9	0.94	1.96	1.78	0.12	0.12	11	1.95	2.54	2.34	0.09	0.22
白血病，未特指	C95	3	0.31	0.65	0.48	0.03	0.05	12	2.13	2.77	2.15	0.10	0.18
其他的或未指明部位	O&U	7	0.73	1.53	1.14	0.00	0.16	9	1.60	2.08	1.46	0.07	0.12
骨髓增殖性疾病	MPD	0	0.00	0.00	0.00	0.00	0.00	0	0.00	0.00	0.00	0.00	0.00
骨髓增生异常综合征	MDS	2	0.21	0.44	0.33	0.02	0.04	2	0.35	0.46	0.20	0.00	0.00
合计	ALL	958	100.00	209.08	178.96	4.42	17.34	564	100.00	130.40	87.21	3.26	8.76
C44 以外的部位	ALL but C44	951	99.27	207.55	177.34	4.42	17.24	563	99.82	130.17	87.03	3.26	8.76

表 6-117　2020 年河南省濮阳市华龙区恶性肿瘤发病主要指标

部位	ICD-10	男性						女性					
		病例数	构成 (%)	粗率 ($1/10^5$)	世标率 ($1/10^5$)	累积率 (%)		病例数	构成 (%)	粗率 ($1/10^5$)	世标率 ($1/10^5$)	累积率 (%)	
						0～64	0～74					0～64	0～74
唇	C00	0	0.00	0.00	0.00	0.00	0.00	0	0.00	0.00	0.00	0.00	0.00
舌	C01–C02	2	0.33	0.87	0.80	0.07	0.07	1	0.13	0.44	0.30	0.00	0.05
口	C03–C06	0	0.00	0.00	0.00	0.00	0.00	2	0.27	0.88	0.69	0.00	0.15
唾液腺	C07–C08	3	0.49	1.30	0.93	0.08	0.08	0	0.00	0.00	0.00	0.00	0.00
扁桃体	C09	1	0.16	0.43	0.35	0.03	0.03	0	0.00	0.00	0.00	0.00	0.00
其他的口咽	C10	1	0.16	0.43	0.27	0.02	0.02	0	0.00	0.00	0.00	0.00	0.00
鼻咽	C11	4	0.66	1.73	1.35	0.13	0.13	3	0.40	1.32	1.00	0.07	0.12
喉咽	C12–C13	4	0.66	1.73	1.64	0.07	0.25	1	0.13	0.44	0.26	0.02	0.02
咽，部位不明	C14	0	0.00	0.00	0.00	0.00	0.00	0	0.00	0.00	0.00	0.00	0.00
食管	C15	45	7.41	19.52	18.43	0.43	2.48	24	3.21	10.56	7.65	0.20	0.94
胃	C16	65	10.71	28.19	25.42	1.08	3.57	37	4.95	16.28	12.74	0.41	1.64
小肠	C17	1	0.16	0.43	0.35	0.00	0.06	5	0.67	2.20	1.79	0.03	0.37
结肠	C18	37	6.10	16.05	14.78	0.46	1.91	31	4.14	13.64	10.06	0.47	1.21
直肠	C19–C20	38	6.26	16.48	15.25	0.86	2.08	26	3.48	11.44	8.93	0.31	1.09
肛门	C21	0	0.00	0.00	0.00	0.00	0.00	1	0.13	0.44	0.35	0.04	0.04
肝脏	C22	61	10.05	26.46	22.07	1.24	2.67	22	2.94	9.68	7.24	0.19	1.08
胆囊及其他	C23–C24	6	0.99	2.60	2.78	0.14	0.32	7	0.94	3.08	2.12	0.08	0.18
胰腺	C25	15	2.47	6.51	5.00	0.15	0.76	9	1.20	3.96	3.07	0.14	0.43
鼻、鼻窦及其他	C30–C31	1	0.16	0.43	0.30	0.00	0.00	0	0.00	0.00	0.00	0.00	0.00
喉	C32	6	0.99	2.60	2.43	0.24	0.36	0	0.00	0.00	0.00	0.00	0.00
气管、支气管、肺	C33–C34	166	27.35	72.00	59.01	2.26	8.44	103	13.77	45.33	35.60	1.73	4.30
其他的胸腔器官	C37–C38	4	0.66	1.73	1.46	0.15	0.15	1	0.13	0.44	0.26	0.02	0.02
骨	C40–C41	2	0.33	0.87	0.98	0.06	0.06	1	0.13	0.44	0.35	0.04	0.04
皮肤的黑色素瘤	C43	1	0.16	0.43	0.05	0.00	0.00	0	0.00	0.00	0.00	0.00	0.00
其他的皮肤	C44	1	0.16	0.43	0.30	0.00	0.00	5	0.67	2.20	1.66	0.07	0.26
间皮瘤	C45	0	0.00	0.00	0.00	0.00	0.00	0	0.00	0.00	0.00	0.00	0.00
卡波西肉瘤	C46	0	0.00	0.00	0.00	0.00	0.00	0	0.00	0.00	0.00	0.00	0.00
周围神经、其他结缔组织、软组织	C47;C49	1	0.16	0.43	0.39	0.05	0.05	3	0.40	1.32	0.86	0.04	0.09
乳房	C50	0	0.00	0.00	0.00	0.00	0.00	172	22.99	75.70	58.10	4.85	6.13
外阴	C51	0	0.00	0.00	0.00	0.00	0.00	3	0.40	1.32	1.44	0.07	0.07
阴道	C52	0	0.00	0.00	0.00	0.00	0.00	0	0.00	0.00	0.00	0.00	0.00
子宫颈	C53	0	0.00	0.00	0.00	0.00	0.00	56	7.49	24.65	18.90	1.44	1.99
子宫体	C54	0	0.00	0.00	0.00	0.00	0.00	27	3.61	11.88	9.39	0.61	1.11
子宫，部位不明	C55	0	0.00	0.00	0.00	0.00	0.00	2	0.27	0.88	0.76	0.08	0.08
卵巢	C56	0	0.00	0.00	0.00	0.00	0.00	29	3.88	12.76	10.49	0.78	1.12
女性其他的生殖器	C57	0	0.00	0.00	0.00	0.00	0.00	1	0.13	0.44	0.24	0.00	0.00
胎盘	C58	0	0.00	0.00	0.00	0.00	0.00	0	0.00	0.00	0.00	0.00	0.00
阴茎	C60	4	0.66	1.73	1.72	0.08	0.32	0	0.00	0.00	0.00	0.00	0.00
前列腺	C61	22	3.62	9.54	9.14	0.05	1.26	0	0.00	0.00	0.00	0.00	0.00
睾丸	C62	0	0.00	0.00	0.00	0.00	0.00	0	0.00	0.00	0.00	0.00	0.00
男性其他的生殖器	C63	0	0.00	0.00	0.00	0.00	0.00	0	0.00	0.00	0.00	0.00	0.00
肾	C64	12	1.98	5.20	4.47	0.26	0.55	8	1.07	3.52	2.71	0.19	0.34
肾盂	C65	0	0.00	0.00	0.00	0.00	0.00	0	0.00	0.00	0.00	0.00	0.00
输尿管	C66	1	0.16	0.43	0.49	0.00	0.12	1	0.13	0.44	0.39	0.00	0.10
膀胱	C67	18	2.97	7.81	6.16	0.31	0.92	4	0.53	1.76	1.23	0.09	0.14
其他的泌尿器官	C68	0	0.00	0.00	0.00	0.00	0.00	0	0.00	0.00	0.00	0.00	0.00
眼	C69	1	0.16	0.43	0.49	0.00	0.12	0	0.00	0.00	0.00	0.00	0.00
脑、神经系统	C70–C72	8	1.32	3.47	3.28	0.20	0.44	12	1.60	5.28	4.17	0.20	0.49
甲状腺	C73	34	5.60	14.75	11.63	0.89	1.19	123	16.44	54.13	43.74	3.68	4.46
肾上腺	C74	3	0.49	1.30	1.03	0.05	0.11	2	0.27	0.88	0.64	0.05	0.05
其他的内分泌腺	C75	0	0.00	0.00	0.00	0.00	0.00	0	0.00	0.00	0.00	0.00	0.00
霍奇金病	C81	0	0.00	0.00	0.00	0.00	0.00	0	0.00	0.00	0.00	0.00	0.00
非霍奇金淋巴瘤	C82–C85;C96	14	2.31	6.07	4.61	0.17	0.78	5	0.67	2.20	1.87	0.07	0.36
免疫增生性疾病	C88	0	0.00	0.00	0.00	0.00	0.00	0	0.00	0.00	0.00	0.00	0.00
多发性骨髓瘤	C90	5	0.82	2.17	2.10	0.10	0.40	3	0.40	1.32	0.93	0.00	0.10
淋巴样白血病	C91	1	0.16	0.43	0.39	0.05	0.05	1	0.13	0.44	0.32	0.03	0.03
髓样白血病	C92–C94	4	0.66	1.73	1.64	0.05	0.30	4	0.53	1.76	1.74	0.14	0.14
白血病，未特指	C95	2	0.33	0.87	0.43	0.03	0.03	1	0.13	0.44	0.54	0.03	0.03
其他的或未指明部位	O&U	10	1.65	4.34	3.10	0.12	0.48	10	1.34	4.40	3.59	0.20	0.44
骨髓增殖性疾病	MPD	3	0.49	1.30	1.21	0.09	0.09	2	0.27	0.88	0.76	0.07	0.07
骨髓增生异常综合征	MDS	0	0.00	0.00	0.00	0.00	0.00	0	0.00	0.00	0.00	0.00	0.00
合计	ALL	607	100.00	263.27	226.23	9.97	30.67	748	100.00	329.20	256.86	16.45	29.28
C44 以外的部位	ALL but C44	606	99.84	262.84	225.94	9.97	30.67	743	99.33	327.00	255.21	16.38	29.02

表 6-118　2020 年河南省濮阳市华龙区恶性肿瘤死亡主要指标

部位	ICD-10	男性						女性					
		病例数	构成 (%)	粗率 ($1/10^5$)	世标率 ($1/10^5$)	累积率 (%)		病例数	构成 (%)	粗率 ($1/10^5$)	世标率 ($1/10^5$)	累积率 (%)	
						0~64	0~74					0~64	0~74
唇	C00	0	0.00	0.00	0.00	0.00	0.00	0	0.00	0.00	0.00	0.00	0.00
舌	C01–C02	1	0.20	0.43	0.39	0.05	0.05	2	0.61	0.88	0.54	0.00	0.05
口	C03–C06	1	0.20	0.43	0.49	0.00	0.12	1	0.30	0.44	0.30	0.00	0.05
唾液腺	C07–C08	0	0.00	0.00	0.00	0.00	0.00	0	0.00	0.00	0.00	0.00	0.00
扁桃体	C09	0	0.00	0.00	0.00	0.00	0.00	0	0.00	0.00	0.00	0.00	0.00
其他的口咽	C10	0	0.00	0.00	0.00	0.00	0.00	0	0.00	0.00	0.00	0.00	0.00
鼻咽	C11	0	0.00	0.00	0.00	0.00	0.00	2	0.61	0.88	0.69	0.00	0.15
喉咽	C12–C13	1	0.20	0.43	0.45	0.05	0.05	0	0.00	0.00	0.00	0.00	0.00
咽，部位不明	C14	0	0.00	0.00	0.00	0.00	0.00	0	0.00	0.00	0.00	0.00	0.00
食管	C15	44	8.70	19.08	15.34	0.52	2.09	22	6.67	9.68	6.48	0.12	0.52
胃	C16	58	11.46	25.16	20.87	0.37	2.87	26	7.88	11.44	8.39	0.20	0.93
小肠	C17	3	0.59	1.30	1.14	0.00	0.18	3	0.91	1.32	0.90	0.00	0.05
结肠	C18	17	3.36	7.37	5.62	0.15	0.87	14	4.24	6.16	4.49	0.11	0.36
直肠	C19–C20	22	4.35	9.54	7.58	0.31	0.97	14	4.24	6.16	4.85	0.24	0.63
肛门	C21	0	0.00	0.00	0.00	0.00	0.00	1	0.30	0.44	0.35	0.04	0.04
肝脏	C22	59	11.66	25.59	21.04	1.00	2.38	35	10.61	15.40	11.32	0.38	1.46
胆囊及其他	C23–C24	5	0.99	2.17	2.54	0.00	0.43	5	1.52	2.20	1.69	0.00	0.19
胰腺	C25	21	4.15	9.11	6.64	0.35	0.83	12	3.64	5.28	4.39	0.10	0.73
鼻、鼻窦及其他	C30–C31	0	0.00	0.00	0.00	0.00	0.00	1	0.30	0.44	0.39	0.00	0.10
喉	C32	3	0.59	1.30	1.18	0.05	0.17	0	0.00	0.00	0.00	0.00	0.00
气管、支气管、肺	C33–C34	198	39.13	85.88	69.86	1.74	9.30	91	27.58	40.05	30.55	1.15	3.56
其他的胸腔器官	C37–C38	4	0.79	1.73	1.53	0.13	0.13	0	0.00	0.00	0.00	0.00	0.00
骨	C40–C41	0	0.00	0.00	0.00	0.00	0.00	1	0.30	0.44	0.37	0.00	0.00
皮肤的黑色素瘤	C43	0	0.00	0.00	0.00	0.00	0.00	0	0.00	0.00	0.00	0.00	0.00
其他的皮肤	C44	1	0.20	0.43	0.72	0.00	0.00	1	0.30	0.44	0.39	0.00	0.10
间皮瘤	C45	0	0.00	0.00	0.00	0.00	0.00	0	0.00	0.00	0.00	0.00	0.00
卡波西肉瘤	C46	0	0.00	0.00	0.00	0.00	0.00	0	0.00	0.00	0.00	0.00	0.00
周围神经、其他结缔组织、软组织	C47;C49	0	0.00	0.00	0.00	0.00	0.00	2	0.61	0.88	0.56	0.04	0.04
乳房	C50	0	0.00	0.00	0.00	0.00	0.00	35	10.61	15.40	11.67	0.70	1.44
外阴	C51	0	0.00	0.00	0.00	0.00	0.00	2	0.61	0.88	0.72	0.04	0.04
阴道	C52	0	0.00	0.00	0.00	0.00	0.00	0	0.00	0.00	0.00	0.00	0.00
子宫颈	C53	0	0.00	0.00	0.00	0.00	0.00	19	5.76	8.36	6.83	0.49	0.73
子宫体	C54	0	0.00	0.00	0.00	0.00	0.00	6	1.82	2.64	1.76	0.10	0.15
子宫，部位不明	C55	0	0.00	0.00	0.00	0.00	0.00	0	0.00	0.00	0.00	0.00	0.00
卵巢	C56	0	0.00	0.00	0.00	0.00	0.00	6	1.82	2.64	2.21	0.12	0.31
女性其他的生殖器	C57	0	0.00	0.00	0.00	0.00	0.00	1	0.30	0.44	0.26	0.02	0.02
胎盘	C58	0	0.00	0.00	0.00	0.00	0.00	0	0.00	0.00	0.00	0.00	0.00
阴茎	C60	0	0.00	0.00	0.00	0.00	0.00	0	0.00	0.00	0.00	0.00	0.00
前列腺	C61	17	3.36	7.37	5.41	0.05	0.53	0	0.00	0.00	0.00	0.00	0.00
睾丸	C62	0	0.00	0.00	0.00	0.00	0.00	0	0.00	0.00	0.00	0.00	0.00
男性其他的生殖器	C63	0	0.00	0.00	0.00	0.00	0.00	0	0.00	0.00	0.00	0.00	0.00
肾	C64	3	0.59	1.30	1.37	0.05	0.29	1	0.30	0.44	0.30	0.00	0.00
肾盂	C65	1	0.20	0.43	0.49	0.00	0.12	0	0.00	0.00	0.00	0.00	0.00
输尿管	C66	2	0.40	0.87	0.79	0.00	0.12	0	0.00	0.00	0.00	0.00	0.00
膀胱	C67	11	2.17	4.77	4.08	0.14	0.39	4	1.21	1.76	1.09	0.00	0.00
其他的泌尿器官	C68	0	0.00	0.00	0.00	0.00	0.00	0	0.00	0.00	0.00	0.00	0.00
眼	C69	1	0.20	0.43	0.72	0.00	0.00	0	0.00	0.00	0.00	0.00	0.00
脑、神经系统	C70–C72	13	2.57	5.64	5.03	0.22	0.71	9	2.73	3.96	3.14	0.09	0.38
甲状腺	C73	1	0.20	0.43	0.35	0.00	0.06	4	1.21	1.76	1.36	0.00	0.15
肾上腺	C74	1	0.20	0.43	0.39	0.05	0.05	0	0.00	0.00	0.00	0.00	0.00
其他的内分泌腺	C75	0	0.00	0.00	0.00	0.00	0.00	0	0.00	0.00	0.00	0.00	0.00
霍奇金病	C81	0	0.00	0.00	0.00	0.00	0.00	0	0.00	0.00	0.00	0.00	0.00
非霍奇金淋巴瘤	C82–C85;C96	6	1.19	2.60	1.28	0.00	0.18	2	0.61	0.88	0.73	0.04	0.14
免疫增生性疾病	C88	0	0.00	0.00	0.00	0.00	0.00	0	0.00	0.00	0.00	0.00	0.00
多发性骨髓瘤	C90	1	0.20	0.43	0.45	0.05	0.05	0	0.00	0.00	0.00	0.00	0.00
淋巴样白血病	C91	0	0.00	0.00	0.00	0.00	0.00	0	0.00	0.00	0.00	0.00	0.00
髓样白血病	C92–C94	3	0.59	1.30	0.84	0.00	0.12	2	0.61	0.88	0.84	0.03	0.03
白血病，未特指	C95	2	0.40	0.87	0.43	0.05	0.05	0	0.00	0.00	0.00	0.00	0.00
其他的或未指明部位	O&U	5	0.99	2.17	1.83	0.02	0.15	6	1.82	2.64	1.98	0.04	0.19
骨髓增殖性疾病	MPD	1	0.20	0.43	0.30	0.00	0.00	0	0.00	0.00	0.00	0.00	0.00
骨髓增生异常综合征	MDS	0	0.00	0.00	0.00	0.00	0.00	0	0.00	0.00	0.00	0.00	0.00
合计	ALL	506	100.00	219.46	179.13	5.33	23.24	330	100.00	145.23	109.54	4.06	12.55
C44 以外的部位	ALL but C44	505	99.80	219.03	178.41	5.33	23.24	329	99.70	144.79	109.15	4.06	12.45

表 6-119　2020 年河南省三门峡市湖滨区恶性肿瘤发病主要指标

部位	ICD-10	男性						女性					
		病例数	构成 (%)	粗率 (1/10^5)	世标率 (1/10^5)	累积率 (%) 0~64	累积率 (%) 0~74	病例数	构成 (%)	粗率 (1/10^5)	世标率 (1/10^5)	累积率 (%) 0~64	累积率 (%) 0~74
唇	C00	0	0.00	0.00	0.00	0.00	0.00	0	0.00	0.00	0.00	0.00	0.00
舌	C01–C02	1	0.21	0.70	0.60	0.07	0.07	0	0.00	0.00	0.00	0.00	0.00
口	C03–C06	1	0.21	0.70	0.60	0.07	0.07	0	0.00	0.00	0.00	0.00	0.00
唾液腺	C07–C08	0	0.00	0.00	0.00	0.00	0.00	2	0.41	1.37	1.28	0.05	0.16
扁桃体	C09	1	0.21	0.70	0.60	0.07	0.07	0	0.00	0.00	0.00	0.00	0.00
其他的口咽	C10	0	0.00	0.00	0.00	0.00	0.00	0	0.00	0.00	0.00	0.00	0.00
鼻咽	C11	1	0.21	0.70	0.47	0.04	0.04	0	0.00	0.00	0.00	0.00	0.00
喉咽	C12–C13	0	0.00	0.00	0.00	0.00	0.00	1	0.21	0.69	0.29	0.00	0.00
咽，部位不明	C14	0	0.00	0.00	0.00	0.00	0.00	0	0.00	0.00	0.00	0.00	0.00
食管	C15	29	6.20	20.37	12.71	0.58	1.19	11	2.28	7.55	4.24	0.30	0.30
胃	C16	61	13.03	42.84	30.13	1.31	3.85	16	3.31	10.99	5.63	0.09	0.36
小肠	C17	3	0.64	2.11	1.36	0.08	0.22	0	0.00	0.00	0.00	0.00	0.00
结肠	C18	27	5.77	18.96	12.47	0.33	1.30	23	4.76	15.79	9.88	0.47	1.22
直肠	C19–C20	15	3.21	10.53	6.93	0.63	0.81	15	3.11	10.30	6.82	0.45	0.80
肛门	C21	0	0.00	0.00	0.00	0.00	0.00	1	0.21	0.69	0.37	0.04	0.04
肝脏	C22	36	7.69	25.28	17.02	1.29	1.90	13	2.69	8.93	4.84	0.23	0.34
胆囊及其他	C23–C24	14	2.99	9.83	6.58	0.22	0.77	14	2.90	9.61	5.59	0.12	0.58
胰腺	C25	12	2.56	8.43	6.08	0.53	0.62	9	1.86	6.18	3.49	0.11	0.33
鼻、鼻窦及其他	C30–C31	1	0.21	0.70	0.54	0.00	0.09	1	0.21	0.69	0.37	0.05	0.05
喉	C32	5	1.07	3.51	2.53	0.15	0.24	0	0.00	0.00	0.00	0.00	0.00
气管、支气管、肺	C33–C34	123	26.28	86.38	59.48	2.73	7.39	67	13.87	46.01	27.56	1.36	3.29
其他的胸腔器官	C37–C38	2	0.43	1.40	1.14	0.07	0.16	1	0.21	0.69	0.37	0.05	0.05
骨	C40–C41	1	0.21	0.70	0.54	0.00	0.09	2	0.41	1.37	0.88	0.07	0.07
皮肤的黑色素瘤	C43	1	0.21	0.70	0.41	0.03	0.03	5	1.04	3.43	2.13	0.08	0.27
其他的皮肤	C44	6	1.28	4.21	2.86	0.04	0.13	9	1.86	6.18	4.06	0.18	0.45
间皮瘤	C45	1	0.21	0.70	0.38	0.05	0.05	0	0.00	0.00	0.00	0.00	0.00
卡波西肉瘤	C46	0	0.00	0.00	0.00	0.00	0.00	0	0.00	0.00	0.00	0.00	0.00
周围神经、其他结缔组织、软组织	C47;C49	2	0.43	1.40	1.49	0.06	0.06	2	0.41	1.37	2.39	0.12	0.12
乳房	C50	1	0.21	0.70	0.54	0.00	0.09	97	20.08	66.61	40.61	2.84	4.77
外阴	C51	0	0.00	0.00	0.00	0.00	0.00	2	0.41	1.37	1.02	0.11	0.11
阴道	C52	0	0.00	0.00	0.00	0.00	0.00	0	0.00	0.00	0.00	0.00	0.00
子宫颈	C53	0	0.00	0.00	0.00	0.00	0.00	32	6.63	21.98	13.34	0.95	1.56
子宫体	C54	0	0.00	0.00	0.00	0.00	0.00	16	3.31	10.99	6.44	0.53	0.61
子宫，部位不明	C55	0	0.00	0.00	0.00	0.00	0.00	2	0.41	1.37	0.95	0.12	0.12
卵巢	C56	0	0.00	0.00	0.00	0.00	0.00	15	3.11	10.30	7.00	0.51	0.85
女性其他的生殖器	C57	0	0.00	0.00	0.00	0.00	0.00	0	0.00	0.00	0.00	0.00	0.00
胎盘	C58	0	0.00	0.00	0.00	0.00	0.00	0	0.00	0.00	0.00	0.00	0.00
阴茎	C60	4	0.85	2.81	2.20	0.04	0.42	0	0.00	0.00	0.00	0.00	0.00
前列腺	C61	23	4.91	16.15	10.73	0.08	1.12	0	0.00	0.00	0.00	0.00	0.00
睾丸	C62	0	0.00	0.00	0.00	0.00	0.00	0	0.00	0.00	0.00	0.00	0.00
男性其他的生殖器	C63	1	0.21	0.70	0.37	0.04	0.04	0	0.00	0.00	0.00	0.00	0.00
肾	C64	8	1.71	5.62	3.51	0.25	0.43	8	1.66	5.49	3.06	0.12	0.28
肾盂	C65	0	0.00	0.00	0.00	0.00	0.00	0	0.00	0.00	0.00	0.00	0.00
输尿管	C66	2	0.43	1.40	0.71	0.04	0.04	2	0.41	1.37	0.96	0.04	0.12
膀胱	C67	10	2.14	7.02	4.60	0.11	0.58	4	0.83	2.75	1.24	0.05	0.05
其他的泌尿器官	C68	0	0.00	0.00	0.00	0.00	0.00	0	0.00	0.00	0.00	0.00	0.00
眼	C69	0	0.00	0.00	0.00	0.00	0.00	0	0.00	0.00	0.00	0.00	0.00
脑、神经系统	C70–C72	11	2.35	7.73	5.01	0.28	0.51	11	2.28	7.55	5.50	0.23	0.50
甲状腺	C73	25	5.34	17.56	12.35	0.98	1.16	79	16.36	54.25	36.22	3.45	3.72
肾上腺	C74	0	0.00	0.00	0.00	0.00	0.00	1	0.21	0.69	0.29	0.00	0.00
其他的内分泌腺	C75	0	0.00	0.00	0.00	0.00	0.00	0	0.00	0.00	0.00	0.00	0.00
霍奇金病	C81	1	0.21	0.70	0.37	0.04	0.04	0	0.00	0.00	0.00	0.00	0.00
非霍奇金淋巴瘤	C82–C85;C96	11	2.35	7.73	5.34	0.36	0.78	5	1.04	3.43	2.26	0.11	0.19
免疫增生性疾病	C88	0	0.00	0.00	0.00	0.00	0.00	0	0.00	0.00	0.00	0.00	0.00
多发性骨髓瘤	C90	9	1.92	6.32	4.04	0.17	0.53	3	0.62	2.06	1.29	0.11	0.11
淋巴样白血病	C91	3	0.64	2.11	1.94	0.05	0.28	1	0.21	0.69	0.42	0.03	0.03
髓样白血病	C92–C94	6	1.28	4.21	2.43	0.17	0.17	5	1.04	3.43	2.34	0.15	0.38
白血病，未特指	C95	4	0.85	2.81	1.64	0.08	0.08	1	0.21	0.69	0.37	0.05	0.05
其他的或未指明部位	O&U	6	1.28	4.21	3.21	0.31	0.45	7	1.45	4.81	2.48	0.17	0.17
骨髓增殖性疾病	MPD	0	0.00	0.00	0.00	0.00	0.00	0	0.00	0.00	0.00	0.00	0.00
骨髓增生异常综合征	MDS	0	0.00	0.00	0.00	0.00	0.00	0	0.00	0.00	0.00	0.00	0.00
合计	ALL	468	100.00	328.67	223.86	11.36	25.87	483	100.00	331.69	205.95	13.31	22.03
C44 以外的部位	ALL but C44	462	98.72	324.46	221.00	11.32	25.74	474	98.14	325.51	201.89	13.13	21.58

表 6-120 2020 年河南省三门峡市湖滨区恶性肿瘤死亡主要指标

部位	ICD-10	男性						女性					
		病例数	构成(%)	粗率(1/10^5)	世标率(1/10^5)	累积率(%) 0~64	累积率(%) 0~74	病例数	构成(%)	粗率(1/10^5)	世标率(1/10^5)	累积率(%) 0~64	累积率(%) 0~74
唇	C00	0	0.00	0.00	0.00	0.00	0.00	0	0.00	0.00	0.00	0.00	0.00
舌	C01–C02	0	0.00	0.00	0.00	0.00	0.00	0	0.00	0.00	0.00	0.00	0.00
口	C03–C06	0	0.00	0.00	0.00	0.00	0.00	1	0.45	0.69	0.42	0.00	0.00
唾液腺	C07–C08	0	0.00	0.00	0.00	0.00	0.00	0	0.00	0.00	0.00	0.00	0.00
扁桃体	C09	0	0.00	0.00	0.00	0.00	0.00	0	0.00	0.00	0.00	0.00	0.00
其他的口咽	C10	1	0.33	0.70	0.34	0.00	0.00	0	0.00	0.00	0.00	0.00	0.00
鼻咽	C11	1	0.33	0.70	0.40	0.00	0.00	0	0.00	0.00	0.00	0.00	0.00
喉咽	C12–C13	1	0.33	0.70	0.60	0.07	0.07	0	0.00	0.00	0.00	0.00	0.00
咽，部位不明	C14	0	0.00	0.00	0.00	0.00	0.00	0	0.00	0.00	0.00	0.00	0.00
食管	C15	19	6.25	13.34	8.30	0.35	0.73	14	6.28	9.61	5.43	0.15	0.30
胃	C16	41	13.49	28.79	20.10	0.51	2.33	15	6.73	10.30	5.50	0.23	0.23
小肠	C17	2	0.66	1.40	1.14	0.07	0.16	1	0.45	0.69	0.42	0.00	0.00
结肠	C18	13	4.28	9.13	6.12	0.15	0.33	10	4.48	6.87	4.04	0.11	0.38
直肠	C19–C20	10	3.29	7.02	4.64	0.28	0.60	5	2.24	3.43	1.90	0.03	0.11
肛门	C21	0	0.00	0.00	0.00	0.00	0.00	0	0.00	0.00	0.00	0.00	0.00
肝脏	C22	25	8.22	17.56	12.73	0.54	1.61	17	7.62	11.67	6.11	0.05	0.46
胆囊及其他	C23–C24	6	1.97	4.21	3.05	0.12	0.50	12	5.38	8.24	4.90	0.07	0.57
胰腺	C25	9	2.96	6.32	4.73	0.26	0.58	9	4.04	6.18	3.34	0.03	0.26
鼻、鼻窦及其他	C30–C31	1	0.33	0.70	0.38	0.05	0.05	0	0.00	0.00	0.00	0.00	0.00
喉	C32	6	1.97	4.21	2.88	0.03	0.41	1	0.45	0.69	0.58	0.07	0.07
气管、支气管、肺	C33–C34	103	33.88	72.34	49.22	1.76	5.02	41	18.39	28.16	16.97	0.57	1.61
其他的胸腔器官	C37–C38	1	0.33	0.70	0.40	0.00	0.00	2	0.90	1.37	0.71	0.00	0.00
骨	C40–C41	1	0.33	0.70	0.57	0.00	0.14	1	0.45	0.69	0.44	0.04	0.04
皮肤的黑色素瘤	C43	0	0.00	0.00	0.00	0.00	0.00	1	0.45	0.69	0.44	0.04	0.04
其他的皮肤	C44	4	1.32	2.81	2.06	0.07	0.16	5	2.24	3.43	2.15	0.11	0.11
间皮瘤	C45	0	0.00	0.00	0.00	0.00	0.00	0	0.00	0.00	0.00	0.00	0.00
卡波西肉瘤	C46	0	0.00	0.00	0.00	0.00	0.00	0	0.00	0.00	0.00	0.00	0.00
周围神经、其他结缔组织、软组织	C47;C49	2	0.66	1.40	1.18	0.07	0.07	2	0.90	1.37	0.84	0.08	0.08
乳房	C50	0	0.00	0.00	0.00	0.00	0.00	21	9.42	14.42	10.21	0.90	1.24
外阴	C51	0	0.00	0.00	0.00	0.00	0.00	2	0.90	1.37	0.78	0.05	0.05
阴道	C52	0	0.00	0.00	0.00	0.00	0.00	1	0.45	0.69	0.42	0.00	0.00
子宫颈	C53	0	0.00	0.00	0.00	0.00	0.00	17	7.62	11.67	7.09	0.34	0.87
子宫体	C54	0	0.00	0.00	0.00	0.00	0.00	2	0.90	1.37	0.89	0.00	0.08
子宫，部位不明	C55	0	0.00	0.00	0.00	0.00	0.00	2	0.90	1.37	0.66	0.05	0.05
卵巢	C56	0	0.00	0.00	0.00	0.00	0.00	13	5.83	8.93	5.01	0.21	0.56
女性其他的生殖器	C57	0	0.00	0.00	0.00	0.00	0.00	0	0.00	0.00	0.00	0.00	0.00
胎盘	C58	0	0.00	0.00	0.00	0.00	0.00	0	0.00	0.00	0.00	0.00	0.00
阴茎	C60	1	0.33	0.70	0.34	0.00	0.00	0	0.00	0.00	0.00	0.00	0.00
前列腺	C61	20	6.58	14.05	9.38	0.00	0.37	0	0.00	0.00	0.00	0.00	0.00
睾丸	C62	0	0.00	0.00	0.00	0.00	0.00	0	0.00	0.00	0.00	0.00	0.00
男性其他的生殖器	C63	0	0.00	0.00	0.00	0.00	0.00	0	0.00	0.00	0.00	0.00	0.00
肾	C64	4	1.32	2.81	1.62	0.08	0.17	5	2.24	3.43	1.83	0.11	0.11
肾盂	C65	0	0.00	0.00	0.00	0.00	0.00	0	0.00	0.00	0.00	0.00	0.00
输尿管	C66	2	0.66	1.40	0.92	0.00	0.00	0	0.00	0.00	0.00	0.00	0.00
膀胱	C67	3	0.99	2.11	1.36	0.00	0.14	1	0.45	0.69	0.29	0.00	0.00
其他的泌尿器官	C68	0	0.00	0.00	0.00	0.00	0.00	0	0.00	0.00	0.00	0.00	0.00
眼	C69	0	0.00	0.00	0.00	0.00	0.00	0	0.00	0.00	0.00	0.00	0.00
脑、神经系统	C70–C72	9	2.96	6.32	4.77	0.27	0.50	5	2.24	3.43	3.42	0.14	0.25
甲状腺	C73	1	0.33	0.70	0.38	0.05	0.05	4	1.79	2.75	1.68	0.07	0.19
肾上腺	C74	0	0.00	0.00	0.00	0.00	0.00	1	0.45	0.69	0.29	0.00	0.00
其他的内分泌腺	C75	0	0.00	0.00	0.00	0.00	0.00	0	0.00	0.00	0.00	0.00	0.00
霍奇金病	C81	0	0.00	0.00	0.00	0.00	0.00	0	0.00	0.00	0.00	0.00	0.00
非霍奇金淋巴瘤	C82–C85;C96	4	1.32	2.81	2.32	0.07	0.36	4	1.79	2.75	1.67	0.07	0.15
免疫增生性疾病	C88	0	0.00	0.00	0.00	0.00	0.00	0	0.00	0.00	0.00	0.00	0.00
多发性骨髓瘤	C90	2	0.66	1.40	0.95	0.03	0.12	2	0.90	1.37	0.59	0.00	0.00
淋巴样白血病	C91	2	0.66	1.40	1.11	0.00	0.23	0	0.00	0.00	0.00	0.00	0.00
髓样白血病	C92–C94	5	1.64	3.51	2.27	0.22	0.22	0	0.00	0.00	0.00	0.00	0.00
白血病，未特指	C95	3	0.99	2.11	1.29	0.04	0.04	2	0.90	1.37	0.73	0.08	0.08
其他的或未指明部位	O&U	2	0.66	1.40	0.97	0.00	0.14	3	1.35	2.06	1.01	0.00	0.00
骨髓增殖性疾病	MPD	0	0.00	0.00	0.00	0.00	0.00	0	0.00	0.00	0.00	0.00	0.00
骨髓增生异常综合征	MDS	0	0.00	0.00	0.00	0.00	0.00	1	0.45	0.69	0.42	0.00	0.00
合计	ALL	304	100.00	213.50	146.52	5.12	15.13	223	100.00	153.14	91.18	3.60	7.90
C44 以外的部位	ALL but C44	300	98.68	210.69	144.46	5.04	14.97	218	97.76	149.71	89.03	3.49	7.79

表 6-121　2020 年河南省南阳市卧龙区恶性肿瘤发病主要指标

部位	ICD-10	男性						女性					
		病例数	构成 (%)	粗率 (1/10^5)	世标率 (1/10^5)	累积率 (%)		病例数	构成 (%)	粗率 (1/10^5)	世标率 (1/10^5)	累积率 (%)	
						0~64	0~74					0~64	0~74
唇	C00	1	0.07	0.21	0.21	0.03	0.03	1	0.08	0.22	0.20	0.03	0.03
舌	C01–C02	2	0.14	0.42	0.38	0.02	0.02	2	0.17	0.43	0.36	0.04	0.04
口	C03–C06	5	0.36	1.05	1.12	0.07	0.13	10	0.85	2.15	1.87	0.06	0.11
唾液腺	C07–C08	1	0.07	0.21	0.20	0.02	0.02	3	0.25	0.65	0.66	0.03	0.09
扁桃体	C09	1	0.07	0.21	0.24	0.00	0.06	1	0.08	0.22	0.20	0.03	0.03
其他的口咽	C10	3	0.22	0.63	0.67	0.00	0.05	0	0.00	0.00	0.00	0.00	0.00
鼻咽	C11	6	0.43	1.25	1.21	0.15	0.15	1	0.08	0.22	0.29	0.00	0.05
喉咽	C12–C13	4	0.29	0.84	0.82	0.04	0.04	0	0.00	0.00	0.00	0.00	0.00
咽，部位不明	C14	2	0.14	0.42	0.55	0.00	0.11	1	0.08	0.22	0.14	0.01	0.01
食管	C15	154	11.09	32.20	34.51	1.33	4.37	69	5.86	14.84	14.50	0.27	1.64
胃	C16	213	15.33	44.53	48.32	1.65	6.63	73	6.20	15.70	14.40	0.48	1.76
小肠	C17	9	0.65	1.88	2.06	0.06	0.28	8	0.68	1.72	1.84	0.03	0.23
结肠	C18	50	3.60	10.45	11.34	0.44	1.35	36	3.06	7.74	7.14	0.27	0.84
直肠	C19–C20	55	3.96	11.50	11.38	0.61	1.36	37	3.14	7.96	7.90	0.32	1.04
肛门	C21	0	0.00	0.00	0.00	0.00	0.00	2	0.17	0.43	0.39	0.00	0.00
肝脏	C22	150	10.80	31.36	30.62	1.68	3.80	48	4.07	10.33	10.21	0.41	1.33
胆囊及其他	C23–C24	18	1.30	3.76	3.83	0.17	0.45	8	0.68	1.72	1.49	0.02	0.13
胰腺	C25	17	1.22	3.55	3.74	0.19	0.46	17	1.44	3.66	3.32	0.06	0.32
鼻、鼻窦及其他	C30–C31	4	0.29	0.84	0.87	0.05	0.10	2	0.17	0.43	0.28	0.01	0.01
喉	C32	14	1.01	2.93	3.42	0.13	0.51	5	0.42	1.08	0.91	0.07	0.07
气管、支气管、肺	C33–C34	256	18.43	53.53	56.59	2.30	7.24	122	10.36	26.25	25.04	1.02	3.12
其他的胸腔器官	C37–C38	5	0.36	1.05	0.94	0.06	0.12	1	0.08	0.22	0.15	0.02	0.02
骨	C40–C41	5	0.36	1.05	1.34	0.03	0.14	6	0.51	1.29	1.61	0.07	0.17
皮肤的黑色素瘤	C43	1	0.07	0.21	0.17	0.02	0.02	8	0.68	1.72	1.79	0.00	0.26
其他的皮肤	C44	10	0.72	2.09	2.16	0.05	0.27	6	0.51	1.29	1.05	0.02	0.13
间皮瘤	C45	2	0.14	0.42	0.49	0.00	0.05	0	0.00	0.00	0.00	0.00	0.00
卡波西肉瘤	C46	0	0.00	0.00	0.00	0.00	0.00	0	0.00	0.00	0.00	0.00	0.00
周围神经、其他结缔组织、软组织	C47;C49	1	0.07	0.21	0.31	0.00	0.05	6	0.51	1.29	1.10	0.11	0.11
乳房	C50	4	0.29	0.84	0.69	0.05	0.05	210	17.83	45.18	38.45	2.81	4.43
外阴	C51	0	0.00	0.00	0.00	0.00	0.00	1	0.08	0.22	0.22	0.00	0.06
阴道	C52	0	0.00	0.00	0.00	0.00	0.00	0	0.00	0.00	0.00	0.00	0.00
子宫颈	C53	0	0.00	0.00	0.00	0.00	0.00	62	5.26	13.34	11.08	0.89	1.31
子宫体	C54	0	0.00	0.00	0.00	0.00	0.00	64	5.43	13.77	11.56	0.89	1.29
子宫，部位不明	C55	0	0.00	0.00	0.00	0.00	0.00	9	0.76	1.94	1.95	0.07	0.27
卵巢	C56	0	0.00	0.00	0.00	0.00	0.00	33	2.80	7.10	5.90	0.44	0.64
女性其他的生殖器	C57	0	0.00	0.00	0.00	0.00	0.00	2	0.17	0.43	0.38	0.04	0.04
胎盘	C58	0	0.00	0.00	0.00	0.00	0.00	0	0.00	0.00	0.00	0.00	0.00
阴茎	C60	3	0.22	0.63	0.86	0.00	0.16	0	0.00	0.00	0.00	0.00	0.00
前列腺	C61	31	2.23	6.48	7.11	0.15	0.82	0	0.00	0.00	0.00	0.00	0.00
睾丸	C62	2	0.14	0.42	0.43	0.03	0.03	0	0.00	0.00	0.00	0.00	0.00
男性其他的生殖器	C63	1	0.07	0.21	0.17	0.02	0.02	0	0.00	0.00	0.00	0.00	0.00
肾	C64	22	1.58	4.60	4.78	0.23	0.62	11	0.93	2.37	2.38	0.16	0.26
肾盂	C65	1	0.07	0.21	0.21	0.03	0.03	2	0.17	0.43	0.42	0.03	0.08
输尿管	C66	1	0.07	0.21	0.18	0.00	0.00	2	0.17	0.43	0.46	0.00	0.05
膀胱	C67	45	3.24	9.41	9.76	0.36	1.08	14	1.19	3.01	2.75	0.09	0.35
其他的泌尿器官	C68	1	0.07	0.21	0.31	0.00	0.05	0	0.00	0.00	0.00	0.00	0.00
眼	C69	2	0.14	0.42	0.55	0.02	0.02	0	0.00	0.00	0.00	0.00	0.00
脑、神经系统	C70–C72	39	2.81	8.15	7.89	0.54	0.77	30	2.55	6.45	5.95	0.31	0.78
甲状腺	C73	33	2.38	6.90	6.34	0.53	0.58	105	8.91	22.59	18.08	1.49	1.79
肾上腺	C74	0	0.00	0.00	0.00	0.00	0.00	0	0.00	0.00	0.00	0.00	0.00
其他的内分泌腺	C75	0	0.00	0.00	0.00	0.00	0.00	1	0.08	0.22	0.14	0.01	0.01
霍奇金病	C81	4	0.29	0.84	0.67	0.06	0.06	2	0.17	0.43	0.40	0.02	0.07
非霍奇金淋巴瘤	C82–C85;C96	31	2.23	6.48	6.89	0.26	0.87	22	1.87	4.73	4.58	0.21	0.52
免疫增生性疾病	C88	0	0.00	0.00	0.00	0.00	0.00	0	0.00	0.00	0.00	0.00	0.00
多发性骨髓瘤	C90	7	0.50	1.46	1.82	0.04	0.25	4	0.34	0.86	0.65	0.06	0.06
淋巴样白血病	C91	2	0.14	0.42	0.38	0.02	0.02	2	0.17	0.43	0.54	0.03	0.03
髓样白血病	C92–C94	4	0.29	0.84	0.97	0.05	0.10	3	0.25	0.65	0.79	0.03	0.08
白血病，未特指	C95	3	0.22	0.63	0.74	0.03	0.09	6	0.51	1.29	1.05	0.08	0.14
其他的或未指明部位	O&U	160	11.52	33.45	35.44	1.28	4.46	118	10.02	25.39	24.43	1.11	2.84
骨髓增殖性疾病	MPD	4	0.29	0.84	1.10	0.03	0.09	2	0.17	0.43	0.58	0.00	0.10
骨髓增生异常综合征	MDS	0	0.00	0.00	0.00	0.00	0.00	0	0.00	0.00	0.00	0.00	0.00
合计	ALL	1 389	100.00	290.42	304.79	12.80	37.99	1 178	100.00	253.43	229.62	12.14	26.74
C44 以外的部位	ALL but C44	1 379	99.28	288.33	302.63	12.76	37.72	1 172	99.49	252.13	228.57	12.12	26.61

表 6-122 2020 年河南省南阳市卧龙区恶性肿瘤死亡主要指标

部位	ICD-10	男性						女性					
		病例数	构成 (%)	粗率 ($1/10^5$)	世标率 ($1/10^5$)	累积率 (%)		病例数	构成 (%)	粗率 ($1/10^5$)	世标率 ($1/10^5$)	累积率 (%)	
						0~64	0~74					0~64	0~74
唇	C00	1	0.10	0.21	0.17	0.02	0.02	1	0.17	0.22	0.20	0.03	0.03
舌	C01–C02	2	0.20	0.42	0.35	0.02	0.02	1	0.17	0.22	0.15	0.02	0.02
口	C03–C06	2	0.20	0.42	0.46	0.03	0.09	3	0.51	0.65	0.55	0.04	0.04
唾液腺	C07–C08	3	0.30	0.63	0.76	0.02	0.07	1	0.17	0.22	0.15	0.02	0.02
扁桃体	C09	0	0.00	0.00	0.00	0.00	0.00	1	0.17	0.22	0.20	0.03	0.03
其他的口咽	C10	1	0.10	0.21	0.18	0.00	0.00	1	0.17	0.22	0.26	0.01	0.01
鼻咽	C11	3	0.30	0.63	0.71	0.03	0.08	1	0.17	0.22	0.29	0.00	0.05
喉咽	C12–C13	4	0.40	0.84	0.96	0.02	0.14	0	0.00	0.00	0.00	0.00	0.00
咽，部位不明	C14	0	0.00	0.00	0.00	0.00	0.00	1	0.17	0.22	0.14	0.00	0.00
食管	C15	135	13.58	28.23	31.45	0.62	4.03	73	12.37	15.70	14.71	0.32	1.50
胃	C16	184	18.51	38.47	42.10	1.06	5.43	83	14.07	17.86	17.22	0.36	1.74
小肠	C17	5	0.50	1.05	1.15	0.02	0.12	4	0.68	0.86	0.69	0.03	0.09
结肠	C18	26	2.62	5.44	5.57	0.20	0.63	23	3.90	4.95	4.35	0.14	0.36
直肠	C19–C20	26	2.62	5.44	5.82	0.12	0.65	22	3.73	4.73	4.60	0.18	0.33
肛门	C21	0	0.00	0.00	0.00	0.00	0.00	2	0.34	0.43	0.39	0.00	0.00
肝脏	C22	129	12.98	26.97	26.73	1.37	3.18	54	9.15	11.62	11.59	0.39	1.47
胆囊及其他	C23–C24	9	0.91	1.88	1.91	0.05	0.22	8	1.36	1.72	1.66	0.04	0.15
胰腺	C25	17	1.71	3.55	3.96	0.09	0.41	18	3.05	3.87	3.16	0.08	0.19
鼻、鼻窦及其他	C30–C31	1	0.10	0.21	0.18	0.00	0.00	0	0.00	0.00	0.00	0.00	0.00
喉	C32	6	0.60	1.25	1.34	0.00	0.17	1	0.17	0.22	0.25	0.00	0.00
气管、支气管、肺	C33–C34	214	21.53	44.74	48.71	1.39	5.84	99	16.78	21.30	20.07	0.57	2.06
其他的胸腔器官	C37–C38	3	0.30	0.63	0.68	0.02	0.07	0	0.00	0.00	0.00	0.00	0.00
骨	C40–C41	10	1.01	2.09	2.30	0.09	0.26	2	0.34	0.43	0.31	0.01	0.01
皮肤的黑色素瘤	C43	1	0.10	0.21	0.24	0.00	0.06	2	0.34	0.43	0.38	0.02	0.07
其他的皮肤	C44	5	0.50	1.05	0.93	0.01	0.07	4	0.68	0.86	0.81	0.03	0.08
间皮瘤	C45	1	0.10	0.21	0.24	0.00	0.06	0	0.00	0.00	0.00	0.00	0.00
卡波西肉瘤	C46	0	0.00	0.00	0.00	0.00	0.00	0	0.00	0.00	0.00	0.00	0.00
周围神经、其他结缔组织、软组织	C47;C49	0	0.00	0.00	0.00	0.00	0.00	0	0.00	0.00	0.00	0.00	0.00
乳房	C50	1	0.10	0.21	0.15	0.01	0.01	52	8.81	11.19	10.29	0.41	1.39
外阴	C51	0	0.00	0.00	0.00	0.00	0.00	0	0.00	0.00	0.00	0.00	0.00
阴道	C52	0	0.00	0.00	0.00	0.00	0.00	0	0.00	0.00	0.00	0.00	0.00
子宫颈	C53	0	0.00	0.00	0.00	0.00	0.00	24	4.07	5.16	4.56	0.19	0.45
子宫体	C54	0	0.00	0.00	0.00	0.00	0.00	11	1.86	2.37	2.06	0.10	0.20
子宫，部位不明	C55	0	0.00	0.00	0.00	0.00	0.00	3	0.51	0.65	0.49	0.04	0.04
卵巢	C56	0	0.00	0.00	0.00	0.00	0.00	7	1.19	1.51	1.31	0.08	0.14
女性其他的生殖器	C57	0	0.00	0.00	0.00	0.00	0.00	0	0.00	0.00	0.00	0.00	0.00
胎盘	C58	0	0.00	0.00	0.00	0.00	0.00	0	0.00	0.00	0.00	0.00	0.00
阴茎	C60	0	0.00	0.00	0.00	0.00	0.00	0	0.00	0.00	0.00	0.00	0.00
前列腺	C61	29	2.92	6.06	6.55	0.09	0.55	0	0.00	0.00	0.00	0.00	0.00
睾丸	C62	0	0.00	0.00	0.00	0.00	0.00	0	0.00	0.00	0.00	0.00	0.00
男性其他的生殖器	C63	0	0.00	0.00	0.00	0.00	0.00	0	0.00	0.00	0.00	0.00	0.00
肾	C64	9	0.91	1.88	2.09	0.04	0.20	1	0.17	0.22	0.17	0.01	0.01
肾盂	C65	1	0.10	0.21	0.17	0.02	0.02	1	0.17	0.22	0.22	0.00	0.06
输尿管	C66	1	0.10	0.21	0.18	0.00	0.00	0	0.00	0.00	0.00	0.00	0.00
膀胱	C67	11	1.11	2.30	2.66	0.03	0.23	2	0.34	0.43	0.49	0.00	0.00
其他的泌尿器官	C68	1	0.10	0.21	0.18	0.00	0.00	0	0.00	0.00	0.00	0.00	0.00
眼	C69	1	0.10	0.21	0.21	0.01	0.01	0	0.00	0.00	0.00	0.00	0.00
脑、神经系统	C70–C72	23	2.31	4.81	5.43	0.18	0.75	17	2.88	3.66	3.36	0.14	0.41
甲状腺	C73	1	0.10	0.21	0.15	0.01	0.01	6	1.02	1.29	1.17	0.04	0.14
肾上腺	C74	1	0.10	0.21	0.31	0.00	0.05	1	0.17	0.22	0.17	0.00	0.00
其他的内分泌腺	C75	1	0.10	0.21	0.31	0.00	0.05	0	0.00	0.00	0.00	0.00	0.00
霍奇金病	C81	2	0.20	0.42	0.29	0.02	0.02	2	0.34	0.43	0.39	0.01	0.07
非霍奇金淋巴瘤	C82–C85;C96	11	1.11	2.30	2.65	0.05	0.32	11	1.86	2.37	2.36	0.04	0.31
免疫增生性疾病	C88	0	0.00	0.00	0.00	0.00	0.00	0	0.00	0.00	0.00	0.00	0.00
多发性骨髓瘤	C90	5	0.50	1.05	1.18	0.01	0.25	0	0.00	0.00	0.00	0.00	0.00
淋巴样白血病	C91	3	0.30	0.63	0.62	0.01	0.01	1	0.17	0.22	0.28	0.02	0.02
髓样白血病	C92–C94	1	0.10	0.21	0.15	0.01	0.01	0	0.00	0.00	0.00	0.00	0.00
白血病，未特指	C95	3	0.30	0.63	0.67	0.05	0.05	5	0.85	1.08	0.80	0.04	0.09
其他的或未指明部位	O&U	96	9.66	20.07	21.38	0.84	2.60	41	6.95	8.82	8.11	0.27	0.73
骨髓增殖性疾病	MPD	3	0.30	0.63	0.61	0.00	0.06	0	0.00	0.00	0.00	0.00	0.00
骨髓增生异常综合征	MDS	2	0.20	0.42	0.53	0.00	0.06	0	0.00	0.00	0.00	0.00	0.00
合计	ALL	994	100.00	207.83	223.39	6.57	26.90	590	100.00	126.93	118.36	3.74	12.31
C44 以外的部位	ALL but C44	989	99.50	206.78	222.45	6.55	26.83	586	99.32	126.07	117.55	3.71	12.23

表 6-123 2020 年河南省信阳市浉河区恶性肿瘤发病主要指标

部位	ICD-10	男性						女性					
		病例数	构成(%)	粗率(1/10⁵)	世标率(1/10⁵)	累积率(%) 0~64	累积率(%) 0~74	病例数	构成(%)	粗率(1/10⁵)	世标率(1/10⁵)	累积率(%) 0~64	累积率(%) 0~74
唇	C00	3	0.40	0.88	0.53	0.02	0.02	0	0.00	0.00	0.00	0.00	0.00
舌	C01–C02	3	0.40	0.88	0.70	0.07	0.07	2	0.28	0.62	0.50	0.04	0.04
口	C03–C06	1	0.13	0.29	0.21	0.00	0.05	2	0.28	0.62	0.33	0.00	0.04
唾液腺	C07–C08	3	0.40	0.88	0.57	0.03	0.09	0	0.00	0.00	0.00	0.00	0.00
扁桃体	C09	0	0.00	0.00	0.00	0.00	0.00	0	0.00	0.00	0.00	0.00	0.00
其他的口咽	C10	0	0.00	0.00	0.00	0.00	0.00	1	0.14	0.31	0.16	0.00	0.00
鼻咽	C11	10	1.34	2.95	1.74	0.13	0.19	4	0.56	1.24	0.95	0.05	0.14
喉咽	C12–C13	2	0.27	0.59	0.35	0.04	0.04	0	0.00	0.00	0.00	0.00	0.00
咽，部位不明	C14	0	0.00	0.00	0.00	0.00	0.00	0	0.00	0.00	0.00	0.00	0.00
食管	C15	36	4.84	10.61	6.61	0.33	0.91	15	2.09	4.65	2.50	0.02	0.23
胃	C16	104	13.98	30.66	19.71	0.74	2.14	40	5.59	12.40	7.42	0.40	0.84
小肠	C17	3	0.40	0.88	0.57	0.00	0.08	0	0.00	0.00	0.00	0.00	0.00
结肠	C18	48	6.45	14.15	9.15	0.42	1.21	44	6.15	13.64	8.34	0.44	0.82
直肠	C19–C20	50	6.72	14.74	9.62	0.30	1.00	39	5.45	12.09	7.39	0.26	0.87
肛门	C21	0	0.00	0.00	0.00	0.00	0.00	1	0.14	0.31	0.17	0.00	0.04
肝脏	C22	103	13.84	30.37	19.27	0.88	2.13	42	5.87	13.02	7.94	0.32	0.93
胆囊及其他	C23–C24	5	0.67	1.47	0.84	0.02	0.08	9	1.26	2.79	1.74	0.05	0.24
胰腺	C25	22	2.96	6.49	3.96	0.23	0.51	24	3.35	7.44	4.22	0.17	0.41
鼻、鼻窦及其他	C30–C31	2	0.27	0.59	0.32	0.01	0.04	2	0.28	0.62	0.42	0.02	0.06
喉	C32	11	1.48	3.24	2.15	0.05	0.37	0	0.00	0.00	0.00	0.00	0.00
气管、支气管、肺	C33–C34	214	28.76	63.10	40.32	1.84	4.75	111	15.50	34.41	20.98	0.97	2.42
其他的胸腔器官	C37–C38	4	0.54	1.18	0.96	0.09	0.09	4	0.56	1.24	0.79	0.05	0.05
骨	C40–C41	10	1.34	2.95	2.27	0.10	0.26	10	1.40	3.10	2.70	0.18	0.26
皮肤的黑色素瘤	C43	2	0.27	0.59	0.31	0.00	0.03	1	0.14	0.31	0.17	0.00	0.04
其他的皮肤	C44	8	1.08	2.36	1.48	0.11	0.17	8	1.12	2.48	1.31	0.03	0.07
间皮瘤	C45	0	0.00	0.00	0.00	0.00	0.00	0	0.00	0.00	0.00	0.00	0.00
卡波西肉瘤	C46	0	0.00	0.00	0.00	0.00	0.00	0	0.00	0.00	0.00	0.00	0.00
周围神经、其他结缔组织、软组织	C47;C49	1	0.13	0.29	0.17	0.02	0.02	1	0.14	0.31	0.19	0.02	0.02
乳房	C50	1	0.13	0.29	0.30	0.00	0.00	163	22.77	50.53	34.17	2.51	3.65
外阴	C51	0	0.00	0.00	0.00	0.00	0.00	0	0.00	0.00	0.00	0.00	0.00
阴道	C52	0	0.00	0.00	0.00	0.00	0.00	0	0.00	0.00	0.00	0.00	0.00
子宫颈	C53	0	0.00	0.00	0.00	0.00	0.00	44	6.15	13.64	9.13	0.66	0.98
子宫体	C54	0	0.00	0.00	0.00	0.00	0.00	26	3.63	8.06	5.47	0.40	0.64
子宫，部位不明	C55	0	0.00	0.00	0.00	0.00	0.00	2	0.28	0.62	0.42	0.02	0.06
卵巢	C56	0	0.00	0.00	0.00	0.00	0.00	23	3.21	7.13	4.64	0.26	0.54
女性其他的生殖器	C57	0	0.00	0.00	0.00	0.00	0.00	0	0.00	0.00	0.00	0.00	0.00
胎盘	C58	0	0.00	0.00	0.00	0.00	0.00	0	0.00	0.00	0.00	0.00	0.00
阴茎	C60	1	0.13	0.29	0.21	0.00	0.05	0	0.00	0.00	0.00	0.00	0.00
前列腺	C61	11	1.48	3.24	2.17	0.08	0.21	0	0.00	0.00	0.00	0.00	0.00
睾丸	C62	1	0.13	0.29	0.30	0.00	0.00	0	0.00	0.00	0.00	0.00	0.00
男性其他的生殖器	C63	0	0.00	0.00	0.00	0.00	0.00	0	0.00	0.00	0.00	0.00	0.00
肾	C64	3	0.40	0.88	0.49	0.04	0.07	5	0.70	1.55	0.92	0.04	0.08
肾盂	C65	2	0.27	0.59	0.35	0.01	0.04	0	0.00	0.00	0.00	0.00	0.00
输尿管	C66	0	0.00	0.00	0.00	0.00	0.00	1	0.14	0.31	0.17	0.00	0.04
膀胱	C67	23	3.09	6.78	4.39	0.15	0.35	4	0.56	1.24	0.67	0.00	0.04
其他的泌尿器官	C68	0	0.00	0.00	0.00	0.00	0.00	1	0.14	0.31	0.19	0.02	0.02
眼	C69	0	0.00	0.00	0.00	0.00	0.00	0	0.00	0.00	0.00	0.00	0.00
脑、神经系统	C70–C72	18	2.42	5.31	3.78	0.28	0.37	10	1.40	3.10	1.82	0.06	0.23
甲状腺	C73	12	1.61	3.54	2.67	0.18	0.32	43	6.01	13.33	9.25	0.78	1.01
肾上腺	C74	1	0.13	0.29	0.18	0.01	0.01	2	0.28	0.62	0.42	0.02	0.06
其他的内分泌腺	C75	0	0.00	0.00	0.00	0.00	0.00	1	0.14	0.31	0.21	0.03	0.03
霍奇金病	C81	2	0.27	0.59	0.51	0.05	0.05	2	0.28	0.62	0.45	0.00	0.08
非霍奇金淋巴瘤	C82–C85;C96	9	1.21	2.65	1.59	0.09	0.12	9	1.26	2.79	1.81	0.12	0.16
免疫增生性疾病	C88	0	0.00	0.00	0.00	0.00	0.00	0	0.00	0.00	0.00	0.00	0.00
多发性骨髓瘤	C90	4	0.54	1.18	0.85	0.06	0.06	1	0.14	0.31	0.16	0.02	0.02
淋巴样白血病	C91	1	0.13	0.29	0.14	0.01	0.01	0	0.00	0.00	0.00	0.00	0.00
髓样白血病	C92–C94	0	0.00	0.00	0.00	0.00	0.00	3	0.42	0.93	1.05	0.03	0.06
白血病，未特指	C95	6	0.81	1.77	1.30	0.05	0.05	10	1.40	3.10	1.70	0.04	0.12
其他的或未指明部位	O&U	4	0.54	1.18	0.74	0.02	0.13	6	0.84	1.86	1.28	0.09	0.09
骨髓增殖性疾病	MPD	0	0.00	0.00	0.00	0.00	0.00	0	0.00	0.00	0.00	0.00	0.00
骨髓增生异常综合征	MDS	0	0.00	0.00	0.00	0.00	0.00	0	0.00	0.00	0.00	0.00	0.00
合计	ALL	744	100.00	219.36	141.79	6.48	16.10	716	100.00	221.95	142.17	8.17	15.45
C44 以外的部位	ALL but C44	736	98.92	217.01	140.31	6.37	15.94	708	98.88	219.47	140.86	8.13	15.38

表 6-124 2020 年河南省信阳市浉河区恶性肿瘤死亡主要指标

部位	ICD-10	男性						女性					
		病例数	构成 (%)	粗率 (1/10^5)	世标率 (1/10^5)	累积率 (%) 0~64	累积率 (%) 0~74	病例数	构成 (%)	粗率 (1/10^5)	世标率 (1/10^5)	累积率 (%) 0~64	累积率 (%) 0~74
唇	C00	1	0.18	0.29	0.14	0.00	0.00	0	0.00	0.00	0.00	0.00	0.00
舌	C01-C02	0	0.00	0.00	0.00	0.00	0.00	1	0.28	0.31	0.12	0.00	0.00
口	C03-C06	2	0.35	0.59	0.31	0.01	0.01	1	0.28	0.31	0.16	0.00	0.00
唾液腺	C07-C08	1	0.18	0.29	0.21	0.00	0.05	0	0.00	0.00	0.00	0.00	0.00
扁桃体	C09	0	0.00	0.00	0.00	0.00	0.00	0	0.00	0.00	0.00	0.00	0.00
其他的口咽	C10	0	0.00	0.00	0.00	0.00	0.00	0	0.00	0.00	0.00	0.00	0.00
鼻咽	C11	8	1.41	2.36	1.48	0.08	0.19	3	0.85	0.93	0.79	0.03	0.10
喉咽	C12-C13	1	0.18	0.29	0.18	0.00	0.03	0	0.00	0.00	0.00	0.00	0.00
咽，部位不明	C14	0	0.00	0.00	0.00	0.00	0.00	0	0.00	0.00	0.00	0.00	0.00
食管	C15	38	6.68	11.20	7.56	0.22	1.06	15	4.27	4.65	2.45	0.08	0.16
胃	C16	86	15.11	25.36	16.28	0.43	1.98	44	12.54	13.64	8.09	0.29	1.03
小肠	C17	2	0.35	0.59	0.38	0.03	0.05	1	0.28	0.31	0.23	0.00	0.04
结肠	C18	24	4.22	7.08	4.67	0.09	0.45	16	4.56	4.96	2.80	0.06	0.22
直肠	C19-C20	21	3.69	6.19	3.85	0.14	0.23	16	4.56	4.96	3.05	0.09	0.38
肛门	C21	0	0.00	0.00	0.00	0.00	0.00	2	0.57	0.62	0.39	0.00	0.00
肝脏	C22	108	18.98	31.84	19.93	1.09	2.24	46	13.11	14.26	8.64	0.37	1.03
胆囊及其他	C23-C24	1	0.18	0.29	0.18	0.00	0.03	4	1.14	1.24	0.89	0.05	0.09
胰腺	C25	23	4.04	6.78	4.05	0.19	0.50	20	5.70	6.20	3.61	0.09	0.50
鼻、鼻窦及其他	C30-C31	2	0.35	0.59	0.31	0.01	0.01	0	0.00	0.00	0.00	0.00	0.00
喉	C32	4	0.70	1.18	0.90	0.00	0.11	2	0.57	0.62	0.42	0.02	0.06
气管、支气管、肺	C33-C34	157	27.59	46.29	29.62	1.38	3.32	70	19.94	21.70	12.52	0.43	1.44
其他的胸腔器官	C37-C38	3	0.53	0.88	0.65	0.04	0.04	0	0.00	0.00	0.00	0.00	0.00
骨	C40-C41	2	0.35	0.59	0.47	0.01	0.01	4	1.14	1.24	0.70	0.02	0.02
皮肤的黑色素瘤	C43	0	0.00	0.00	0.00	0.00	0.00	0	0.00	0.00	0.00	0.00	0.00
其他的皮肤	C44	3	0.53	0.88	0.69	0.00	0.08	2	0.57	0.62	0.33	0.00	0.04
间皮瘤	C45	0	0.00	0.00	0.00	0.00	0.00	0	0.00	0.00	0.00	0.00	0.00
卡波西肉瘤	C46	0	0.00	0.00	0.00	0.00	0.00	0	0.00	0.00	0.00	0.00	0.00
周围神经、其他结缔组织、软组织	C47;C49	1	0.18	0.29	0.18	0.00	0.03	0	0.00	0.00	0.00	0.00	0.00
乳房	C50	2	0.35	0.59	0.38	0.04	0.04	27	7.69	8.37	5.05	0.23	0.51
外阴	C51	0	0.00	0.00	0.00	0.00	0.00	0	0.00	0.00	0.00	0.00	0.00
阴道	C52	0	0.00	0.00	0.00	0.00	0.00	0	0.00	0.00	0.00	0.00	0.00
子宫颈	C53	0	0.00	0.00	0.00	0.00	0.00	21	5.98	6.51	4.02	0.24	0.44
子宫体	C54	0	0.00	0.00	0.00	0.00	0.00	6	1.71	1.86	1.15	0.02	0.19
子宫，部位不明	C55	0	0.00	0.00	0.00	0.00	0.00	2	0.57	0.62	0.38	0.05	0.05
卵巢	C56	0	0.00	0.00	0.00	0.00	0.00	12	3.42	3.72	2.12	0.13	0.25
女性其他的生殖器	C57	0	0.00	0.00	0.00	0.00	0.00	0	0.00	0.00	0.00	0.00	0.00
胎盘	C58	0	0.00	0.00	0.00	0.00	0.00	0	0.00	0.00	0.00	0.00	0.00
阴茎	C60	0	0.00	0.00	0.00	0.00	0.00	0	0.00	0.00	0.00	0.00	0.00
前列腺	C61	11	1.93	3.24	2.36	0.04	0.26	0	0.00	0.00	0.00	0.00	0.00
睾丸	C62	0	0.00	0.00	0.00	0.00	0.00	0	0.00	0.00	0.00	0.00	0.00
男性其他的生殖器	C63	0	0.00	0.00	0.00	0.00	0.00	0	0.00	0.00	0.00	0.00	0.00
肾	C64	4	0.70	1.18	0.73	0.06	0.11	1	0.28	0.31	0.12	0.00	0.00
肾盂	C65	2	0.35	0.59	0.51	0.02	0.08	0	0.00	0.00	0.00	0.00	0.00
输尿管	C66	0	0.00	0.00	0.00	0.00	0.00	0	0.00	0.00	0.00	0.00	0.00
膀胱	C67	11	1.93	3.24	2.48	0.02	0.02	0	0.00	0.00	0.00	0.00	0.00
其他的泌尿器官	C68	0	0.00	0.00	0.00	0.00	0.00	1	0.28	0.31	0.12	0.00	0.00
眼	C69	0	0.00	0.00	0.00	0.00	0.00	0	0.00	0.00	0.00	0.00	0.00
脑、神经系统	C70-C72	19	3.34	5.60	3.54	0.21	0.45	11	3.13	3.41	2.40	0.13	0.25
甲状腺	C73	2	0.35	0.59	0.38	0.03	0.03	1	0.28	0.31	0.20	0.00	0.00
肾上腺	C74	1	0.18	0.29	0.18	0.01	0.01	0	0.00	0.00	0.00	0.00	0.00
其他的内分泌腺	C75	0	0.00	0.00	0.00	0.00	0.00	0	0.00	0.00	0.00	0.00	0.00
霍奇金病	C81	0	0.00	0.00	0.00	0.00	0.00	1	0.28	0.31	0.17	0.00	0.04
非霍奇金淋巴瘤	C82-C85;C96	6	1.05	1.77	1.04	0.07	0.10	6	1.71	1.86	1.20	0.02	0.13
免疫增生性疾病	C88	0	0.00	0.00	0.00	0.00	0.00	0	0.00	0.00	0.00	0.00	0.00
多发性骨髓瘤	C90	0	0.00	0.00	0.00	0.00	0.00	1	0.28	0.31	0.16	0.02	0.02
淋巴样白血病	C91	3	0.53	0.88	0.56	0.04	0.09	1	0.28	0.31	0.17	0.00	0.04
髓样白血病	C92-C94	0	0.00	0.00	0.00	0.00	0.00	2	0.57	0.62	0.83	0.04	0.04
白血病，未特指	C95	4	0.70	1.18	0.92	0.07	0.12	5	1.42	1.55	0.89	0.04	0.09
其他的或未指明部位	O&U	15	2.64	4.42	2.81	0.15	0.24	6	1.71	1.86	1.02	0.05	0.14
骨髓增殖性疾病	MPD	0	0.00	0.00	0.00	0.00	0.00	0	0.00	0.00	0.00	0.00	0.00
骨髓增生异常综合征	MDS	1	0.18	0.29	0.14	0.00	0.00	0	0.00	0.00	0.00	0.00	0.00
合计	ALL	569	100.00	167.77	108.04	4.49	12.00	351	100.00	108.80	65.20	2.49	7.30
C44 以外的部位	ALL but C44	566	99.47	166.88	107.35	4.49	11.92	349	99.43	108.18	64.86	2.49	7.26

表 6-125　2020 年河南省济源市恶性肿瘤发病主要指标

部位	ICD-10	男性						女性					
		病例数	构成 (%)	粗率 (1/10^5)	世标率 (1/10^5)	累积率 (%) 0~64	累积率 (%) 0~74	病例数	构成 (%)	粗率 (1/10^5)	世标率 (1/10^5)	累积率 (%) 0~64	累积率 (%) 0~74
唇	C00	0	0.00	0.00	0.00	0.00	0.00	1	0.10	0.28	0.32	0.00	0.00
舌	C01–C02	2	0.19	0.53	0.60	0.07	0.07	3	0.30	0.85	0.91	0.10	0.10
口	C03–C06	2	0.19	0.53	0.55	0.04	0.04	1	0.10	0.28	0.26	0.00	0.06
唾液腺	C07–C08	4	0.37	1.06	1.15	0.10	0.15	2	0.20	0.56	0.56	0.04	0.10
扁桃体	C09	0	0.00	0.00	0.00	0.00	0.00	0	0.00	0.00	0.00	0.00	0.00
其他的口咽	C10	2	0.19	0.53	0.55	0.00	0.14	2	0.20	0.56	0.55	0.04	0.04
鼻咽	C11	5	0.47	1.33	1.41	0.08	0.17	0	0.00	0.00	0.00	0.00	0.00
喉咽	C12–C13	0	0.00	0.00	0.00	0.00	0.00	2	0.20	0.56	0.53	0.06	0.06
咽，部位不明	C14	1	0.09	0.27	0.28	0.04	0.04	1	0.10	0.28	0.30	0.00	0.05
食管	C15	110	10.24	29.20	33.12	0.94	3.99	64	6.38	18.06	17.32	0.63	2.08
胃	C16	313	29.14	83.09	89.78	3.63	12.27	103	10.27	29.06	28.98	1.22	3.70
小肠	C17	4	0.37	1.06	1.14	0.14	0.14	4	0.40	1.13	1.05	0.04	0.15
结肠	C18	31	2.89	8.23	8.75	0.33	1.17	34	3.39	9.59	8.97	0.51	0.98
直肠	C19–C20	33	3.07	8.76	8.77	0.34	1.16	30	2.99	8.47	8.29	0.48	1.12
肛门	C21	0	0.00	0.00	0.00	0.00	0.00	0	0.00	0.00	0.00	0.00	0.00
肝脏	C22	102	9.50	27.08	28.60	1.67	3.59	59	5.88	16.65	16.37	0.64	2.04
胆囊及其他	C23–C24	10	0.93	2.65	3.11	0.10	0.38	22	2.19	6.21	5.89	0.16	0.56
胰腺	C25	11	1.02	2.92	2.94	0.13	0.45	16	1.60	4.51	4.37	0.24	0.40
鼻、鼻窦及其他	C30–C31	4	0.37	1.06	0.99	0.05	0.05	0	0.00	0.00	0.00	0.00	0.00
喉	C32	2	0.19	0.53	0.58	0.00	0.10	0	0.00	0.00	0.00	0.00	0.00
气管、支气管、肺	C33–C34	174	16.20	46.19	51.35	2.41	6.50	79	7.88	22.29	21.97	1.29	2.59
其他的胸腔器官	C37–C38	3	0.28	0.80	0.82	0.03	0.14	0	0.00	0.00	0.00	0.00	0.00
骨	C40–C41	13	1.21	3.45	3.46	0.20	0.41	6	0.60	1.69	2.04	0.13	0.19
皮肤的黑色素瘤	C43	4	0.37	1.06	1.12	0.09	0.14	1	0.10	0.28	0.26	0.00	0.06
其他的皮肤	C44	3	0.28	0.80	0.83	0.00	0.12	2	0.20	0.56	0.64	0.00	0.00
间皮瘤	C45	0	0.00	0.00	0.00	0.00	0.00	0	0.00	0.00	0.00	0.00	0.00
卡波西肉瘤	C46	0	0.00	0.00	0.00	0.00	0.00	0	0.00	0.00	0.00	0.00	0.00
周围神经、其他结缔组织、软组织	C47;C49	4	0.37	1.06	1.04	0.10	0.10	2	0.20	0.56	0.44	0.04	0.04
乳房	C50	2	0.19	0.53	0.52	0.04	0.04	160	15.95	45.15	42.55	3.55	4.67
外阴	C51	0	0.00	0.00	0.00	0.00	0.00	3	0.30	0.85	0.73	0.03	0.09
阴道	C52	0	0.00	0.00	0.00	0.00	0.00	0	0.00	0.00	0.00	0.00	0.00
子宫颈	C53	0	0.00	0.00	0.00	0.00	0.00	165	16.45	46.56	44.29	3.92	4.90
子宫体	C54	0	0.00	0.00	0.00	0.00	0.00	32	3.19	9.03	9.31	0.88	1.05
子宫，部位不明	C55	0	0.00	0.00	0.00	0.00	0.00	10	1.00	2.82	2.96	0.24	0.39
卵巢	C56	0	0.00	0.00	0.00	0.00	0.00	31	3.09	8.75	7.71	0.58	0.79
女性其他的生殖器	C57	0	0.00	0.00	0.00	0.00	0.00	3	0.30	0.85	0.82	0.08	0.08
胎盘	C58	0	0.00	0.00	0.00	0.00	0.00	0	0.00	0.00	0.00	0.00	0.00
阴茎	C60	2	0.19	0.53	0.52	0.03	0.03	0	0.00	0.00	0.00	0.00	0.00
前列腺	C61	30	2.79	7.96	8.78	0.04	0.86	0	0.00	0.00	0.00	0.00	0.00
睾丸	C62	0	0.00	0.00	0.00	0.00	0.00	0	0.00	0.00	0.00	0.00	0.00
男性其他的生殖器	C63	0	0.00	0.00	0.00	0.00	0.00	0	0.00	0.00	0.00	0.00	0.00
肾	C64	20	1.86	5.31	5.41	0.25	0.83	12	1.20	3.39	3.15	0.15	0.38
肾盂	C65	2	0.19	0.53	0.47	0.05	0.05	0	0.00	0.00	0.00	0.00	0.00
输尿管	C66	0	0.00	0.00	0.00	0.00	0.00	0	0.00	0.00	0.00	0.00	0.00
膀胱	C67	39	3.63	10.35	12.19	0.27	1.64	4	0.40	1.13	1.09	0.04	0.16
其他的泌尿器官	C68	0	0.00	0.00	0.00	0.00	0.00	0	0.00	0.00	0.00	0.00	0.00
眼	C69	0	0.00	0.00	0.00	0.00	0.00	3	0.30	0.85	1.26	0.10	0.10
脑、神经系统	C70–C72	35	3.26	9.29	9.90	0.68	1.10	17	1.69	4.80	4.99	0.38	0.63
甲状腺	C73	47	4.38	12.48	11.68	0.88	1.22	98	9.77	27.65	26.19	2.27	2.97
肾上腺	C74	5	0.47	1.33	1.27	0.03	0.17	1	0.10	0.28	0.30	0.00	0.05
其他的内分泌腺	C75	1	0.09	0.27	0.18	0.02	0.02	0	0.00	0.00	0.00	0.00	0.00
霍奇金病	C81	0	0.00	0.00	0.00	0.00	0.00	0	0.00	0.00	0.00	0.00	0.00
非霍奇金淋巴瘤	C82–C85;C96	8	0.74	2.12	2.20	0.08	0.27	4	0.40	1.13	1.17	0.06	0.11
免疫增生性疾病	C88	1	0.09	0.27	0.23	0.01	0.01	0	0.00	0.00	0.00	0.00	0.00
多发性骨髓瘤	C90	2	0.19	0.53	0.56	0.04	0.10	2	0.20	0.56	0.56	0.02	0.02
淋巴样白血病	C91	3	0.28	0.80	1.06	0.04	0.09	3	0.30	0.85	1.00	0.06	0.06
髓样白血病	C92–C94	6	0.56	1.59	1.97	0.06	0.22	1	0.10	0.28	0.34	0.04	0.04
白血病，未特指	C95	8	0.74	2.12	2.35	0.08	0.22	2	0.20	0.56	0.60	0.02	0.07
其他的或未指明部位	O&U	24	2.23	6.37	6.96	0.33	0.90	18	1.79	5.08	5.42	0.32	0.73
骨髓增殖性疾病	MPD	2	0.19	0.53	0.48	0.03	0.03	0	0.00	0.00	0.00	0.00	0.00
骨髓增生异常综合征	MDS	0	0.00	0.00	0.00	0.00	0.00	0	0.00	0.00	0.00	0.00	0.00
合计	ALL	1 074	100.00	285.09	307.66	13.41	39.12	1 003	100.00	283.01	274.47	18.34	31.60
C44 以外的部位	ALL but C44	1 071	99.72	284.29	306.83	13.41	39.00	1 001	99.80	282.45	273.83	18.34	31.60

表 6-126 2020 年河南省济源市恶性肿瘤死亡主要指标

部位	ICD-10	男性						女性					
		病例数	构成(%)	粗率($1/10^5$)	世标率($1/10^5$)	累积率(%)		病例数	构成(%)	粗率($1/10^5$)	世标率($1/10^5$)	累积率(%)	
						0~64	0~74					0~64	0~74
唇	C00	1	0.13	0.27	0.63	0.00	0.00	0	0.00	0.00	0.00	0.00	0.00
舌	C01–C02	0	0.00	0.00	0.00	0.00	0.00	1	0.21	0.28	0.16	0.01	0.01
口	C03–C06	2	0.26	0.53	0.54	0.00	0.07	1	0.21	0.28	0.18	0.00	0.00
唾液腺	C07–C08	1	0.13	0.27	0.29	0.00	0.05	1	0.21	0.28	0.26	0.00	0.06
扁桃体	C09	1	0.13	0.27	0.27	0.00	0.07	0	0.00	0.00	0.00	0.00	0.00
其他的口咽	C10	1	0.13	0.27	0.29	0.00	0.05	0	0.00	0.00	0.00	0.00	0.00
鼻咽	C11	2	0.26	0.53	0.56	0.04	0.10	1	0.21	0.28	0.26	0.00	0.06
喉咽	C12–C13	1	0.13	0.27	0.29	0.00	0.05	0	0.00	0.00	0.00	0.00	0.00
咽，部位不明	C14	1	0.13	0.27	0.28	0.04	0.04	0	0.00	0.00	0.00	0.00	0.00
食管	C15	99	12.87	26.28	31.22	0.75	2.74	57	11.90	16.08	14.41	0.25	1.37
胃	C16	237	30.82	62.91	74.04	2.07	7.99	100	20.88	28.22	26.77	0.55	2.47
小肠	C17	1	0.13	0.27	0.26	0.03	0.03	0	0.00	0.00	0.00	0.00	0.00
结肠	C18	21	2.73	5.57	6.77	0.15	0.65	21	4.38	5.93	5.55	0.23	0.38
直肠	C19–C20	18	2.34	4.78	4.81	0.09	0.57	10	2.09	2.82	2.55	0.16	0.21
肛门	C21	0	0.00	0.00	0.00	0.00	0.00	0	0.00	0.00	0.00	0.00	0.00
肝脏	C22	96	12.48	25.48	27.70	1.58	3.31	54	11.27	15.24	15.57	0.51	1.95
胆囊及其他	C23–C24	11	1.43	2.92	3.32	0.06	0.43	14	2.92	3.95	3.90	0.09	0.34
胰腺	C25	13	1.69	3.45	3.84	0.11	0.41	17	3.55	4.80	4.53	0.15	0.44
鼻、鼻窦及其他	C30–C31	1	0.13	0.27	0.29	0.00	0.05	0	0.00	0.00	0.00	0.00	0.00
喉	C32	2	0.26	0.53	0.60	0.04	0.09	1	0.21	0.28	0.28	0.03	0.03
气管、支气管、肺	C33–C34	136	17.69	36.10	41.48	1.20	4.74	67	13.99	18.91	17.49	0.52	2.01
其他的胸腔器官	C37–C38	3	0.39	0.80	0.89	0.04	0.14	0	0.00	0.00	0.00	0.00	0.00
骨	C40–C41	3	0.39	0.80	1.21	0.00	0.10	3	0.63	0.85	0.68	0.02	0.07
皮肤的黑色素瘤	C43	0	0.00	0.00	0.00	0.00	0.00	0	0.00	0.00	0.00	0.00	0.00
其他的皮肤	C44	2	0.26	0.53	0.50	0.00	0.00	2	0.42	0.56	0.54	0.04	0.04
间皮瘤	C45	0	0.00	0.00	0.00	0.00	0.00	0	0.00	0.00	0.00	0.00	0.00
卡波西肉瘤	C46	0	0.00	0.00	0.00	0.00	0.00	0	0.00	0.00	0.00	0.00	0.00
周围神经、其他结缔组织、软组织	C47;C49	0	0.00	0.00	0.00	0.00	0.00	2	0.42	0.56	0.55	0.00	0.11
乳房	C50	0	0.00	0.00	0.00	0.00	0.00	23	4.80	6.49	6.31	0.37	0.75
外阴	C51	0	0.00	0.00	0.00	0.00	0.00	1	0.21	0.28	0.30	0.00	0.05
阴道	C52	0	0.00	0.00	0.00	0.00	0.00	1	0.21	0.28	0.32	0.00	0.00
子宫颈	C53	0	0.00	0.00	0.00	0.00	0.00	19	3.97	5.36	5.01	0.21	0.73
子宫体	C54	0	0.00	0.00	0.00	0.00	0.00	10	2.09	2.82	2.64	0.08	0.26
子宫，部位不明	C55	0	0.00	0.00	0.00	0.00	0.00	2	0.42	0.56	0.62	0.04	0.04
卵巢	C56	0	0.00	0.00	0.00	0.00	0.00	14	2.92	3.95	3.76	0.22	0.51
女性其他的生殖器	C57	0	0.00	0.00	0.00	0.00	0.00	0	0.00	0.00	0.00	0.00	0.00
胎盘	C58	0	0.00	0.00	0.00	0.00	0.00	0	0.00	0.00	0.00	0.00	0.00
阴茎	C60	0	0.00	0.00	0.00	0.00	0.00	0	0.00	0.00	0.00	0.00	0.00
前列腺	C61	17	2.21	4.51	6.32	0.00	0.21	0	0.00	0.00	0.00	0.00	0.00
睾丸	C62	1	0.13	0.27	0.54	0.02	0.02	0	0.00	0.00	0.00	0.00	0.00
男性其他的生殖器	C63	0	0.00	0.00	0.00	0.00	0.00	0	0.00	0.00	0.00	0.00	0.00
肾	C64	9	1.17	2.39	2.73	0.05	0.32	7	1.46	1.98	1.93	0.04	0.29
肾盂	C65	0	0.00	0.00	0.00	0.00	0.00	0	0.00	0.00	0.00	0.00	0.00
输尿管	C66	0	0.00	0.00	0.00	0.00	0.00	1	0.21	0.28	0.26	0.00	0.06
膀胱	C67	13	1.69	3.45	4.60	0.06	0.34	3	0.63	0.85	0.88	0.02	0.02
其他的泌尿器官	C68	0	0.00	0.00	0.00	0.00	0.00	0	0.00	0.00	0.00	0.00	0.00
眼	C69	0	0.00	0.00	0.00	0.00	0.00	0	0.00	0.00	0.00	0.00	0.00
脑、神经系统	C70–C72	33	4.29	8.76	9.35	0.51	1.23	10	2.09	2.82	2.74	0.10	0.31
甲状腺	C73	2	0.26	0.53	0.56	0.00	0.12	3	0.63	0.85	0.80	0.04	0.04
肾上腺	C74	2	0.26	0.53	0.55	0.04	0.04	1	0.21	0.28	0.25	0.02	0.02
其他的内分泌腺	C75	0	0.00	0.00	0.00	0.00	0.00	0	0.00	0.00	0.00	0.00	0.00
霍奇金病	C81	0	0.00	0.00	0.00	0.00	0.00	0	0.00	0.00	0.00	0.00	0.00
非霍奇金淋巴瘤	C82–C85;C96	8	1.04	2.12	2.17	0.09	0.28	7	1.46	1.98	1.89	0.04	0.28
免疫增生性疾病	C88	0	0.00	0.00	0.00	0.00	0.00	0	0.00	0.00	0.00	0.00	0.00
多发性骨髓瘤	C90	2	0.26	0.53	0.56	0.04	0.10	2	0.42	0.56	0.56	0.02	0.07
淋巴样白血病	C91	2	0.26	0.53	0.51	0.05	0.05	0	0.00	0.00	0.00	0.00	0.00
髓样白血病	C92–C94	1	0.13	0.27	0.29	0.00	0.05	0	0.00	0.00	0.00	0.00	0.00
白血病，未特指	C95	8	1.04	2.12	1.88	0.10	0.17	5	1.04	1.41	1.30	0.07	0.12
其他的或未指明部位	O&U	16	2.08	4.25	4.39	0.16	0.59	18	3.76	5.08	4.66	0.19	0.54
骨髓增殖性疾病	MPD	0	0.00	0.00	0.00	0.00	0.00	0	0.00	0.00	0.00	0.00	0.00
骨髓增生异常综合征	MDS	2	0.26	0.53	0.60	0.04	0.09	0	0.00	0.00	0.00	0.00	0.00
合计	ALL	769	100.00	204.13	235.16	7.36	25.27	479	100.00	135.16	127.90	4.03	13.66
C44 以外的部位	ALL but C44	767	99.74	203.60	234.66	7.36	25.27	477	99.58	134.59	127.37	3.99	13.62